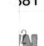

DATE DUE

SOCIAL DEVELOPMENT

Social Development
Relationships in Infancy, Childhood, and Adolescence

edited by
Marion K. Underwood
Lisa H. Rosen

THE GUILFORD PRESS
New York   London

Library of Congress Cataloging-in-Publication Data

Social development : relationships in infancy, childhood, and adolescence / edited by Marion K.
Underwood, Lisa H. Rosen.
    p. cm.
  Includes bibliographical references and index.
  ISBN 978-1-60918-233-5 (hbk. : alk. paper)
  1. Social interaction in children.   2. Social interaction in adolescence.   3. Interpersonal
relations in children.   4. Interpersonal relations in adolescence.   5. Child psychology.
6. Adolescent psychology.   I. Underwood, Marion K.   II. Rosen, Lisa H.
  BF723.S62S577 2011
  155.4′18—dc22
                                                                                2011013095

65.00

*A hundred years from now it will not matter what my bank
account was, the sort of house I lived in, or the kind of car
I drove . . . but the world may be different
because I was important in the life of a child.*
—Forest E. Whitcraft

*In memory of Duane and Linda Buhrmester,
devoted parents to Michael and Ryan
and longtime teachers of social development*

*Duane frequently taught doctoral seminars in social development
and challenged and inspired generations of students as a leading
peer relations researcher. Linda loved and cared for dozens of
infants and toddlers as a longtime home-based child care provider.
Duane and Linda fostered the development of many lives.
They are gone too soon but never forgotten.*

About the Editors

Marion K. Underwood, PhD, is an Ashbel Smith Professor of Psychological Sciences in the School of Behavioral and Brain Sciences at the University of Texas at Dallas. Dr. Underwood's research, which has been supported by the National Institutes of Health since 1995, examines anger, aggression, and gender, with special attention to the development of social aggression. Her work has been published in numerous scientific journals, and she is the author of the book *Social Aggression among Girls* (Guilford Press, 2003). She received the 2001 Chancellor's Council Outstanding Teacher of the Year Award from the University of Texas at Dallas, was granted a K02 Mid-Career Independent Scientist Award from the National Institute of Mental Health, and is a Fellow of the Association for Psychological Science.

Lisa H. Rosen, PhD, is Clinical Assistant Professor in the School of Behavioral and Brain Sciences at the University of Texas at Dallas, and works with the University's Center for Children and Families. Dr. Rosen's research examines risk factors for and consequences of peer victimization, and her work has been published in numerous scientific journals. She received the William C. Howell Award for Excellence in Undergraduate Research and Scholarship from Rice University, and was granted an Early Career Travel Award by the Society for Research in Child Development.

Contributors

Rebecca S. Bigler, PhD, Department of Psychology, University of Texas at Austin, Austin, Texas

Kristen L. Bub, EdD, Department of Human Development and Family Studies, Auburn University, Auburn, Alabama

Duane Buhrmester, PhD (deceased), School of Behavioral and Brain Sciences, The University of Texas at Dallas, Richardson, Texas

William M. Bukowski, PhD, Department of Psychology and Centre for Research in Human Development, Concordia University, Montreal, Quebec, Canada

Susan D. Calkins, PhD, Department of Human Development and Family Studies and Department of Psychology, University of North Carolina at Greensboro, Greensboro, North Carolina

Leslie J. Carver, PhD, Department of Psychology and Human Development Program, University of California, San Diego, La Jolla, California

Jennifer Connolly, PhD, Department of Psychology, York University, Toronto, Ontario, Canada

Alice J. Davidson, PhD, Department of Psychology, Rollins College, Winter Park, Florida

Jeremy A. Frimer, MA, Department of Psychology, University of British Columbia, Vancouver, British Columbia, Canada

Scott D. Gest, PhD, Department of Human Development and Family Studies, The Pennsylvania State University, University Park, Pennsylvania

Miranda Goodman, MA, Department of Psychology, University of California, Davis, Davis, California

Ashley M. Groh, MA, Department of Psychology, University of Illinois at Urbana–Champaign, Champaign, Illinois

Joan E. Grusec, PhD, Department of Psychology, University of Toronto, Toronto, Ontario, Canada

Nancy E. Hill, PhD, Graduate School of Education, Harvard University, Cambridge, Massachusetts

George W. Holden, PhD, Department of Psychology, Southern Methodist University, Dallas, Texas

Campbell Leaper, PhD, Department of Psychology, University of California, Santa Cruz, Santa Cruz, California

Jennifer S. Mackler, MA, Department of Psychology, University of North Carolina at Greensboro, Greensboro, North Carolina

Caroline McIsaac, PhD, Department of Psychology, York University, Toronto, Ontario, Canada

Sonya Negriff, PhD, School of Social Work, University of Southern California, Los Angeles, California

Margaret Tresch Owen, PhD, School of Behavioral and Brain Sciences, The University of Texas at Dallas, Richardson, Texas

Meagan M. Patterson, PhD, Department of Psychology and Research in Education, University of Kansas, Lawrence, Kansas

Glenn I. Roisman, PhD, Department of Psychology, University of Illinois at Urbana–Champaign, Champaign, Illinois

Lisa H. Rosen, PhD, School of Behavioral and Brain Sciences, The University of Texas at Dallas, Richardson, Texas

Amanda Sherman, MA, Department of Psychology, University of Toronto, Toronto, Ontario, Canada

Ross A. Thompson, PhD, Department of Psychology, University of California, Davis, Davis, California

Penelope K. Trickett, PhD, School of Social Work and Department of Psychology, University of Southern California, Los Angeles, California

Lisa Tully, MA, Department of Psychology, University of California, San Diego, La Jolla, California

Marion K. Underwood, PhD, School of Behavioral and Brain Sciences, The University of Texas at Dallas, Richardson, Texas

Brigitte Vittrup, PhD, Department of Family Sciences, Texas Woman's University, Denton, Texas

Lawrence J. Walker, PhD, Department of Psychology, University of British Columbia, Vancouver, British Columbia, Canada

Thomas S. Weisner, PhD, Department of Psychiatry, NPI–Semel Institute for Neuroscience and Center for Culture and Health, University of California, Los Angeles, Los Angeles, California

Dawn P. Witherspoon, PhD, Department of Psychology, The Pennsylvania State University, University Park, Pennsylvania

Preface

Resilience does not come from rare and special qualities, but from the everyday magic of ordinary, normative resources in the minds, brains, and bodies of children, in their families and in their relationships, and in their communities.

—Masten (2001, p. 235)

Children around the world thrive—and sometimes survive formidable adversity—in large part due to the "ordinary magic" of human relationships. The development of adaptive relationships is an amazing and never-ending story. Newborns come into the world with skills that enable them to be social partners from the beginning of life. Young children strive to form and are continuously influenced by nurturing relationships; the first is with parents, then come the bonds they develop with child care providers and teachers, the high glee and sometimes intense conflict of their relationships with siblings and early playmates, and later the companionship and solace provided by close friends and romantic partners. Children's developing relationships are forged by a set of complex, dynamic interactions between individual characteristics of the child and features of the social environment, including families, communities, schools, and the culture at large. In this book, leading scholars illuminate the development of the ordinary magic of social relationships.

This edited volume provides what we hope is a compelling and engaging intellectual guide to the field of social development from infancy through adolescence. This volume is designed for scholars—in particular, doctoral students and high-level undergraduates but also anyone desiring a thoughtful orientation to this expansive area. Each chapter is written by senior experts in the specific research area, who were asked to present the material as they would want to teach it to their favorite graduate seminars. When appropriate, chapters follow a developmental organization, providing some overview but also focusing on the most fascinating issues in each area. They highlight the creative methods used by developmental scientists to study relationships and conclude with forward-looking discussions of the most important areas for future research. The expert scholars have also provided a short list of suggested readings in each area, and the length of chapters has been strictly limited to allow chapters to be assigned in conjunction with these or other primary source readings.

This volume begins with a section on "Setting the Stage" to provide some historical context for the field of social development and to consider early building blocks of relationships. Chapter 1, by Ross A. Thompson and Miranda Goodman, provides an overview of the architecture of developmental science by highlighting the primary theories that have guided this field from its earliest origins: psychoanalytic, behavioral and cognitive social learning, cognitive-developmental, sociocultural, ethological/evolutionary, and dynamic systems approaches. Remaining mindful of these theoretical origins will help all scholars to cope with the wealth of new research findings emerging daily and to forge new theoretical models. Chapter 2, by Leslie J. Carver and Lisa Tully, provides a compelling, accessible account of the biological foundations of the developing emotional bonds between infants and caregivers. Carver and Tully discuss methods for studying the relations between brain and behavior and suggest important future directions in the emerging, exciting field of developmental social neuroscience. In Chapter 3, Susan D. Calkins and Jennifer S. Mackler discuss theories of and methods for studying temperament and self-regulation. Calkins and Mackler highlight the importance of studying these emotion-relevant processes and provide evidence that temperament predicts social competence through the development of self-regulation abilities.

The next section of the book focuses on "Self and Relationships." Chapter 4, by Lisa H. Rosen and Meagan M. Patterson, provides an overview of developmental trends in how individuals view the self. This chapter starts by discussing the first glimmerings of self-recognition in infancy and ends with a description of the complex process of identity formation that begins in adolescence. In Chapter 5, Glenn I. Roisman and Ashley M. Groh highlight the importance of early experiences with caregivers. Roisman and Groh describe individual differences in quality of attachment and discuss how these differences influence later interpersonal relationships with peers and romantic partners. Chapter 6, by George W. Holden, Brigitte Vittrup, and Lisa H. Rosen, discusses parenting and discipline as means by which parents attempt to bring children forward into the future. This chapter also marshals the existing scholarly evidence on the controversy surrounding physical discipline. In Chapter 7, William M. Bukowski, Duane Buhrmester, and Marion K. Underwood underscore the belief that peer relations matter as a source of happiness and conflict in early childhood, as opportunities for social learning and experiences, and as a unique world of potential social equality. This chapter also reminds us that friends and peers influence each other for better and for worse. Jennifer Connolly and Caroline McIsaac, in Chapter 8, provide a compelling account of how romantic relationships emerge from mixed-gender friendship groups and develop over the course of adolescence and young adulthood. The chapter also highlights the fact that romantic relationships are an emerging developmental asset and that we might be wise to focus on positive romantic development.

The third section of the volume focuses specifically on "Social Behaviors." Chapter 9, by Marion K. Underwood, provides an overview of the development of physical and social aggression in preschool, middle childhood, and adolescence. The chapter addresses origins and outcomes of individual differences and concludes with a discussion of the most effective intervention programs for preventing and reducing aggression. In Chapter 10, Lawrence J. Walker and Jeremy A. Frimer highlight the science of moral development and provide cogent, engaging descriptions of the major approaches that have guided this field, characterized as stages, schemas, orientations, domains, emotions, intuition, and personality. Walker and Frimer grapple with the fundamental challenge of how descriptive developmental science can illuminate morality's inner experience in the service of helping us all to live morally good lives.

Chapter 11, by Joan E. Grusec and Amanda Sherman, provides a scholarly and engaging account of the development of prosocial behavior, how children learn to show care and consideration for others. This chapter explains how evolutionary principles, genetic predispositions, and social experiences interact to result in children doing good and reaching out to help others in need.

The fourth section of this volume tackles the daunting challenge of examining "Contexts for Social Development." Chapter 12, by Campbell Leaper and Rebecca S. Bigler, highlights how gender shapes all aspects of human development and summarizes how gender-related thinking and gender-typed behavior are shaped by cognitive and environmental influences, including parents, language, peers, and media. Leaper and Bigler urge us to challenge the status quo and to remember that we are studying gender in a world in which men have more power and status than women. In Chapter 13, Nancy E. Hill and Dawn P. Witherspoon discuss how race, ethnicity, and socioeconomic status combine to influence social development. Given the increasing diversity in the United States, it is important to examine how ethnicity and social class affect children's experiences of prejudice, discrimination, and segregation. Margaret Tresch Owen and Kristen L. Bub present research in Chapter 14 on how child care and schools influence social development through the fascinating lens of the relationships formed between parents and child care providers and parents and teachers. Using an ecological systems approach, this chapter makes clear that the child–caregiver and teacher–student relationships are critical determinants for success in these settings and are shaped by characteristics each relationship partner brings. Chapter 15, by Thomas S. Weisner, provides a broad and sweeping view of how culture shapes social development, with fascinating examples from West Africa to Japan integrated with research on families from Europe and North America. Through these interesting illustrations, Weisner describes the many ways in which the beliefs and practices of the culture into which a child is born can influence his or her development.

The final and fifth section of this volume explores "Risk and Resilience." Chapter 16, by Penelope K. Trickett and Sonya Negriff, provides an impressive, detailed analysis of the effects of child maltreatment on attachment relationships in infancy and early childhood, on peer relationships and friendships, on romantic relationships and dating violence, and on parenting. This chapter makes clear how more sound research designs have led and will continue to lead to a more precise understanding of how children suffer from child maltreatment so that we can intervene more effectively. Finally, in Chapter 17, Scott D. Gest and Alice J. Davidson offer a valuable overview of how research on risk and resilience has evolved from identifying correlates to illuminating developmental processes to prevention science. This thoughtful chapter includes detailed discussion of model prevention programs; the effectiveness of these programs inspires great hope and suggests that the ordinary magic of relationships can be fostered even when conditions are not ideal.

We thank the outstanding scholars who contributed chapters to this volume; reading their work has broadened and deepened our own knowledge and refreshed our fascination with the never-ending story of human development. We hope this volume will inspire the next generation of scholars in social development and remind us all of the importance of investing in the life of a child and in the ordinary magic of social relationships.

MARION K. UNDERWOOD
LISA H. ROSEN

REFERENCE

Masten, A. (2001). Ordinary magic: Resilience processes in development. *American Psychologist, 56,* 227–238.

Contents

PART I. SETTING THE STAGE

1. The Architecture of Social Developmental Science: 3
Theoretical and Historical Perspectives
Ross A. Thompson and Miranda Goodman

2. Biological Correlates of Social Development   29
Leslie J. Carver and Lisa Tully

3. Temperament, Emotion Regulation, and Social Development   44
Susan D. Calkins and Jennifer S. Mackler

PART II. SELF AND RELATIONSHIPS

4. The Self and Identity   73
Lisa H. Rosen and Meagan M. Patterson

5. Attachment Theory and Research in Developmental Psychology: 101
An Overview and Appreciative Critique
Glenn I. Roisman and Ashley M. Groh

6. Families, Parenting, and Discipline   127
George W. Holden, Brigitte Vittrup, and Lisa H. Rosen

7. Peer Relations as a Developmental Context   153
William M. Bukowski, Duane Buhrmester, and Marion K. Underwood

8. Romantic Relationships in Adolescence   180
Jennifer Connolly and Caroline McIsaac

PART III. SOCIAL BEHAVIORS

9. Aggression 207
Marion K. Underwood

10. The Science of Moral Development 235
Lawrence J. Walker and Jeremy A. Frimer

11. Prosocial Behavior 263
Joan E. Grusec and Amanda Sherman

PART IV. CONTEXTS FOR SOCIAL DEVELOPMENT

12. Gender 289
Campbell Leaper and Rebecca S. Bigler

13. Race, Ethnicity, and Social Class 316
Nancy E. Hill and Dawn P. Witherspoon

14. Child Care and Schools 347
Margaret Tresch Owen and Kristen L. Bub

15. Culture 372
Thomas S. Weisner

PART V. RISK AND RESILIENCE

16. Child Maltreatment and Social Relationships 403
Penelope K. Trickett and Sonya Negriff

17. A Developmental Perspective on Risk, Resilience, and Prevention 427
Scott D. Gest and Alice J. Davidson

Author Index 455

Subject Index 470

Part I

Setting the Stage

1

The Architecture of Social Developmental Science

Theoretical and Historical Perspectives

Ross A. Thompson
Miranda Goodman

How should we understand child development? This question is posed not only by developmental researchers but also by parents, practitioners, and policymakers who are concerned with enhancing children's healthy growth. The initial answers are usually intuitive. We understand child development with reference to our own experiences of growing up and how we were raised. We do so in terms of the beliefs derived from culture, religion, and other systems of values, especially their guidance concerning the moral, intellectual, social, emotional, and other qualities characteristic of optimal growth. We also understand child development through what we learn from the media, from other authorities (such as in medicine), and, of course, from our interactions with children themselves.

Developmental science is influenced by all of these sources of knowledge, but it is also guided by formal theories of human development. Theories provide a broad conceptual framework that directs understanding and inquiry into developmental processes. Developmental theories are informed and refined by research findings, and they are also affected by the values, social needs, and prevailing beliefs of the times in which theorists work. This is especially true of the study of social development. Inquiry into social, emotional, and personality development is guided by theoretical views of the qualities and influences that are important to healthy growth. How significant, for example, is warm and nurturant care in the early years? How much do early experiences determine the course of personality development? What are the most important influences on moral growth? Cultural beliefs and research findings about these and other developmental influences have changed significantly over time. As a result, contemporary theories that influence developmental science are a reflection of research knowledge and cultural currents (especially in the Western world) and a continuing catalyst to their evolution. Historical and theoretical perspectives on the developing person are mutually influential.

One reason for attending to the theoretical and historical architecture of social developmental science, therefore, is to better understand the origins of current scientific understandings of child development. Contemporary students accept as self-evident certain conclusions about the nature of social development (such as the importance of warm, nurturant parental care) that were not so obvious to previous generations of developmental theorists. Advances in research knowledge are one reason, and another is change in theoretical assumptions and orientations that cause researchers to ask different questions, to interpret their findings differently, and to become interested in different developmental processes than was previously true. We certainly know *more* about social development than did previous generations of developmental scientists, but we also know *differently* than they did, with different questions, interests, and values that accompany theoretical and cultural changes.

This chapter opens, therefore, with a broad historical overview of changing views of the child and of human development. This historical survey puts in context several theoretical perspectives on social development that have emerged during the past century and previews the discussion of these theoretical views that follows. Six theories are profiled: (1) psychoanalytic, (2) behavioral and cognitive social learning, (3) cognitive developmental, (4) sociocultural, (5) ethological/evolutionary, and (6) dynamic systems approaches—not because they are the only theoretical perspectives that inform contemporary social development research but because they are the most influential. In a concluding section, the relevance of these theoretical and historical perspectives for future study of social development is considered.

HISTORICAL VIEWS OF THE DEVELOPING CHILD

History is an atypical source of data for developmental study, but it is a rich and valuable one. From historical sources, developmental scientists can characterize the remarkably variable social conditions in which children have grown up and their influences on social and personality growth. They can denote the connections between cultural values and how children's needs and characteristics were interpreted, the qualities that were fostered as children matured, and the perceived responsibilities of parents. Like cultural studies of human development, therefore, historical sources situate contemporary perspectives within a broader context. The overview that follows is too brief to accomplish more than highlighting major historical influences over time and hopefully provoking the reader's interest in learning more (for further historical background, consult Aries, 1962; deMause, 1974; Stone, 1977; also Collins, 2002, and Maccoby, 2006, for discussions of historical changes in social developmental science, and Parke, Ornstein, Reiser, & Zahn-Waxler, 1994, for biographical profiles of many of the developmentalists discussed here).

Early Views of Development

Throughout human history, parents and community members have been firsthand witnesses to the developmental process as they watch newborns grow into adults. It is remarkable, therefore, that a developmental perspective to the life course is a relatively recent historical emergence. Throughout much of recorded history, childhood was distinctive only because children were not yet adults. Infants and young children remained in the care of their mothers and other women until they could begin to contribute to domestic or economic labor, at which time (at about age 6 or 7) they joined the wider world of adults. Infant mortality was very high, a fact that may have undermined parents' emotional investment in young offspring who might be lost to disease or accident. Later, the influence of the Christian church conferred its own interpretive lens on childhood, portraying children as born into a state of sin with parents responsible for countering children's natural dispositions through discipline and work (Aries, 1962). Life was difficult, and although childish immaturity could be humorous at times, it was often seen as demanding and annoying, as in Shakespeare's characterization of the infant "mewling and puking in the nurse's arms" in *As You Like It* (1600/2000). Most people in traditional societies did not have the sense of human progress that we today glean from history, and in similar fashion they did not perceive human development as a progressive achievement.

With changes in Western culture, these attitudes toward childhood softened. The humanistic rationalism of the Renaissance permitted a greater appreciation of the characteristics of children for their own sake (religious art of this time began to portray the Christ child as a child, rather than a miniature adult), and children were treated more benignly and indulgently. Subsequent advances in Western philosophy paved the way for modern conceptions of the developing child. From Locke in 1690 came the idea that early experiences are important for shaping the future course of the child, who is born a "blank slate" without any innate predispositions. Child-rearing practices and education are each fundamental, according to Locke, to determining the characteristics of the adult-to-be (Locke, 1924). From Rousseau a half-century later came the idea of childhood innocence and natural goodness. Writing in *Emile* in 1792, Rousseau (1969) anticipated modern views that development will unfold naturally and best without interference, that children are not passive but will take from environmental influences what is suitable to their stage of development, and that children's natural tendencies are good and positive.

The impact of these views could be seen in a new societal interest in children and their development. As the Industrial Revolution brought large numbers of workers into the factories and mines of western Europe, laboring long hours under oppressive conditions, the novels of social reformers such as Charles Dickens (*Oliver Twist; A Christmas Carol*) and Victor Hugo (*Les Misérables*) galvanized public concern that eventually led to laws governing child labor and the movement toward compulsory public education in the 19th century (see DeMause, 1974). Children became set apart for the first time because of their unique needs and vulnerabilities.

Scientific Study of Development

A strong interest of those concerned with childhood in these eras was social–emotional growth: the child's moral dispositions, capacities for self-control, and emotions, as well as education, were the focus. The dawn of the 20th century saw the beginnings of the scientific study of child development and, perhaps unsurprisingly, similar concerns were apparent. Charles Darwin's (1877) "baby biography" of his son, nicknamed Doddy, was one of several efforts of the time to meticulously record firsthand accounts of early behavior and its causes, and in Darwin's account Doddy's emergent emotions were a primary focus. These observations were incorporated into Darwin's (1872/1955) seminal volume, *The Expression of the Emotions in Man and Animals*, published earlier in that decade, and foreshadowed Piaget's similar use of systematic observations of his own offspring. G. Stanley Hall (e.g., 1904) used questionnaires to gather information about children's characteristics, including their feelings, self-control of emotions and intentions, individual differences in moral behavior, and a range of other attributes. In doing so, he helped to inaugurate the child study movement of the turn of the century and also drew new attention to the "storm and stress" of adolescence. He founded the research journal that later was renamed *Journal of Genetic Psychology* and advanced the view that human development recapitulates aspects of the evolution of the species. These early scientific inquiries into child development share in common the influence of Darwinian theory on culture and science, especially the view that human behavior can be understood in terms of its origins, whether phylogenetically or ontogenetically. It is the inaugural theoretical influence on social developmental science.

Behaviorism

As the influence of Darwinian theory illustrates, theoretical understanding of social development is often appropriated from other areas of scientific study. This was also true of the emergence of behaviorism in psychology in the United States early in the 20th century. John Watson's (1913) "behaviorist manifesto" drew on the classical conditioning studies of Ivan Pavlov to argue that conditioned learning is alone sufficient to explain human behavior, including social dispositions, emotional reactions, and love. The implications of this view for child development were elucidated in Watson's (1928) *Psychological Care of Infant and Child*, which was a national best-seller. Children should be treated objectively and systematically, with parents thoughtfully aware of how their reactions are shaping the behavior of their offspring and judiciously avoiding behavior (such as indulgence and sentimentality) that might inadvertently encourage dependency or undermine self-control in their children.

Watson's environmentalism contrasted strongly with the maturationism underlying the normative–descriptive developmental studies of contemporaries such as Hall, Arnold Gesell (e.g., 1928) and others of the time and heightened the nature–nurture tension that has become a classic issue in developmental thinking. Compare, for example, Watson's claim that fears derive from conditioned learning in infancy with the maturational view that fears (such as stranger anxiety) emerge according to an innate timetable, with the implication that the former can be changed, the latter accommodated. The rapid growth of interest in understanding child development in the context of clashing theoretical views made this an exciting period for scholars, parents, and practitioners. Gesell's normative developmental standards provided them with benchmarks against which a child's developmental progress could be compared, and Watson's views about the influence of conditioning in child development met a responsive audience in parents of that era who were interested in using the tools of scientific experts to raise children who were independent and self-reliant and for whom, Watson argued, "mother love is a dangerous instrument" (Watson, 1928, p. 87). Several decades later, learning approaches to child development were resurgent with Skinner's (e.g., 1948, 1953, 1971) applications of operant conditioning to understanding behavior and development—especially as they were popularized through his provocative, widely read books (*Walden Two; Beyond Freedom and Dignity*)—and Bandura's cognitive social learning theory (Bandura, 1977; Bandura & Walters, 1963).

Freud and Psychoanalytic Thinking

Across the Atlantic, psychological thinking in Europe was being shaped by the ideas of psychoanalytic scholars. Freud's personality theory was as much a product of the Victorian-era Viennese society in which he lived as Watson's behaviorism was a function of American can-do practicality, but each approach shared a developmental emphasis on the role of parents and the influence of early experience. However, the psychoanalytic focus on the centrality of emotional experience, unconscious influences on psychological growth, and the interaction of innate psychological needs with parental demands and support offered a unique approach to understanding social development that was shaped both by the influence of Darwin's ideas on Freud's thinking and by the repressive sexuality of the Victorian era.

Psychoanalytic ideas influenced developmental theory through several avenues. First, the World War II-era immigration to the United States and Britain of many leading psychoanalytic scholars from Germany and occupied countries (including Freud himself) broadened the influence of psychoanalytic thinking and its applications to developmental psychology. As postwar America later turned attention again to matters of child rearing and children's emotional well-being, psychoanalytic ideas offered insights that maturational and learning approaches did not. Second, contributing to this influence were several groups of researchers in the United States—most notably, Miller and Dollard (1941), Sears, Maccoby, and Levin (1957), and Sears, Rau, and Alpert (1965)—who sought to recast classic psychoanalytic ideas about behavior and development in terms more appropriate to the empirical analysis of learning theory. The Freudian concept of identification with the parent, for example, was studied in terms of child imitative behavior, permitting more systematic research than would have been possible if researchers had tried to operationalize directly the internal emotional qualities of identification. Finally, in the years that followed Freud's publications, several neoanalytic scholars, such as Erik Erikson (1963), Rene Spitz (1965), and Margaret Mahler (Mahler, Pine, & Bergman, 1975), offered influential developmental approaches (such as Erikson's idea of the "identity crisis") that many scholars in the United States found more congenial than orthodox Freudian theory.

The Rise of Theory

By the middle of the 20th century, therefore, developmental research had become theory-driven. Social developmental scientists had, in particular, a handful of provocative, well-developed theoretical frameworks within which to consider and study the importance of parent–child relationships, the role of peers in social growth, the development of emotional self-regulation, and many other processes. Psychologists appreciated, moreover, that developmental research was necessary to testing key propositions of major psychological theories, especially concerning the early origins of enduring competencies, personality characteristics, and social dispositions. As a consequence, several major longitudinal studies were inaugurated in the late 1920s to systematically assess a variety of developmental processes and influences from infancy through adulthood. These studies included the Oakland Growth Study and the Berkeley Guidance Study (Clausen, 1993) and the Fels Longitudinal Study (Kagan & Moss, 1962), each inaugurated when participants were infants and continuing through their adulthood. Not surprisingly, each study showed that predicting adult social and personality characteristics is complex, not deriving straightforwardly from early patterns of child

rearing but instead encompassing early temperamental dispositions, the child's interpretation of experience, and the varieties of unique events occurring throughout the
life course (Elder, 1974).

Piaget

Throughout this period, another European view was emerging in the theory and
research of Jean Piaget. It was not until the 1960s, however, that Piaget's ideas became
well known in the United States owing, in part, to a national concern with children's
cognitive achievement deriving from the scientific competition between the United
States and the Soviet Union. Piaget's constructivist theory identified sequences and
processes of cognitive development that became highly influential in developmental
science and education and influenced classroom practices of the time. Moreover, as
the first uniquely developmental theory, it influenced other fields of psychological
inquiry. Piaget's cognitive-developmental theory contributed to developmental psychologists' rediscovery of the child (and infant) who is active in the process of creating
psychological understanding rather than the passive recipient of socialization influences. Piaget's theory was thus important to the study of social development, not only
because Piaget (1932) extended his ideas to moral judgment and peer relationships but
also because his ideas influenced others who studied the development of social understanding through the prism of his structuralist account. Kohlberg's (1969) theory of
moral judgment, for example, explicitly incorporated the theoretical assumptions of
Piaget's cognitive-developmental model (see also Walker & Frimer, Chapter 10, this
volume), as did Selman's (1980) theory of the development of social perspective taking
and a wide range of other approaches to the development of social cognition in the
1970s and 1980s. In many respects, contemporary research on developing theory of
mind bears the enduring legacy of Piaget's thinking and its implications for the growth
of social understanding.

New Theories

During the past several decades, the vigor of developmental science has contributed
to the emergence of several new theoretical perspectives on social development that
are discussed later. Although it is yet unclear whether these approaches—sociocultural theory, ethological/evolutionary approaches, and dynamic systems theory—will
achieve the scope of applications of classic learning, psychoanalytic, and cognitive-
developmental theories, they each provide social developmental scientists with valuable conceptual tools.

Social developmental science at the beginning of the 21st century is thus at a
conceptually exciting but paradoxical crossroads. There is a wealth of theoretical perspectives to provoke and guide inquiry into social, emotional, and personality growth,
many of these conceptual perspectives drawn from other fields of study and few
unique to the study of social development. These theories have emerged in the context
of historically evolving conceptions of the child, changing cultural values and beliefs
influencing theorists' views of development, and the growth of research understanding. But the field of social development is changing rapidly and, in particular, the value
of these theoretical perspectives may be increasingly questioned in the future by the
growing influence of biological approaches to social development that appear to be
atheoretical in orientation. Work in behavioral and molecular genetics, developmental

neuroscience, and developmental biology appears to be primarily data-driven; after all, interpreting a functional magnetic resonance image (fMRI) or genotyping a DNA sample seems to be minimally influenced by the theoretical views of the researcher (Miller, 2002). Such a conclusion leads to the question: What use are theories to social developmental science? Do they continue to be valuable?

THEORETICAL VIEWS OF THE DEVELOPING CHILD

One way to answer these questions above is to look at the historical development of the field. Social developmental science has grown in sophistication and depth in response to the emergence of new conceptual perspectives that have raised new questions, provoked new interpretations, and directed inquiry to new aspects of social, emotional, and personality development. Indeed, it could be argued that the growth of the field is more attributable to the development of theory than to the expansion of the research literature insofar as theory has historically played a pivotal role in changing the direction of research. Thus the proliferation of psychoanalytic ideas in American psychology in the postwar era led to new attention to the importance of maternal nurturance to early emotional health, the growth of attachment theory, and a rejection of the "danger" of mother love from the behaviorist tradition. Similarly, the "cognitive revolution" inspired by the discovery of Piaget's theory in the 1960s by American researchers led to a new appreciation of the child's construction of understanding by cognitive developmentalists and a new awareness of the construction of social understanding by social developmentalists and paved the way for the emergence of sociocultural approaches in later years. In many ways, therefore, the field is advanced by theoretical developments as much as by empirical advances.

In addition, theory and its influence are often hidden in the unspoken assumptions of the researcher. When a developmental scientist attributes a child's aggressive behavior to the example of a violent parent, a learning view is underlying this interpretation rather than a sociocultural or constructivist perspective. When attachment theorists describe a child's response to a story-completion probe as reflecting nonconscious mental models of relationships, it reflects a uniquely psychoanalytic influence. Thus the apparently atheoretical, data-driven interpretation of research findings by contemporary developmental scientists often reflects implicit theoretical commitments. In this regard, the materialism underlying contemporary developmental neuroscience or molecular genetics research—that is, the view that complex social, emotional, and cognitive processes can be ultimately understood as the activation of relevant brain areas and gene transcription guiding protein synthesis—is itself a theoretical view.

Theories are important, therefore, for guiding developmental research, directing attention to important new areas of study, providing foundational assumptions about developmental processes, and generating scholarly interest in new areas. Despite their importance, however, developmental scientists are rarely unitheoretical. In other words, they tend to be eclectic in their use of theories to explain and illuminate research findings. This tendency derives, in part, from an appreciation of the strengths and weaknesses of different theoretical views and no clear consensus that one theory best explains the variety of developmental processes that scientists seek to understand. Most of the time, this theoretical eclecticism enables developmentalists to create multilayered, robust explanations for developmental processes. Attachment research is one example of this eclectic approach, because attachment theory incorporates elements of multiple theoretical views, including psychoanalytic, ethological/evolutionary, and cognitive developmental (some would also add sociocultural theory to this list). In the survey of theoretical viewpoints that follows, we illustrate this by drawing on the ideas of attachment research on several occasions to illustrate how it has included ideas from multiple approaches (see Miller, 2002, for an expanded analysis of each of these and other developmental theories).

Psychoanalytic Theory

Psychoanalytic theory, developed by Viennese neurologist Sigmund Freud in the early decades of the 20th century, is in many ways the foundation for *all* theories of social development. Freud first posed questions that developmental scientists are still trying to answer concerning, for example, the influence of early experiences and relationships, the nature of developmental stages, the effects of nonconscious representations, the connection between maturational needs and the responsiveness of the social environment, and the role of conflict in psychological growth. Moreover, his developmental theory has influenced subsequent efforts to understand developmental processes that he first studied, including moral development, parent–child relationships, self-regulation, and gender identity (see, e.g., Freud, 1935/1960, 1924/1964).

These contributions are notable for the fact that Freud's theories derived entirely from his work with adults, not with children. Indeed, Freud was perhaps best known for the treatment of adult psychiatric patients—a legacy that would seem quite independent of theories of social development, if not for the fact that Freud's adult patients consistently reported experiences of early childhood trauma during the course of their treatment. From these therapeutic encounters came the idea that early experiences have a profound and enduring influence on later development, and Freud was among the first theorists not only to articulate this view but also to attempt to uncover the specific mechanisms that link past experiences to present social and personality functioning. Although his work remained strictly retrospective, gleaning inferences about typical child development from adults experiencing atypical pathologies, Freud set the stage for modern views of human development.

The Structure of Personality

Freud's focus on the formative influence of early experiences emphasized the first 5 years of life, when the structures of personality (id, ego, superego) first emerge and personality development is guided through the initial stages of psychosexual growth. Freud believed that these stages are a universal maturational sequence but that they also contribute to the emergence of individual differences in personality based on the success with which the child resolves the challenges represented by each of these stages. In each of the four stages (oral, anal, phallic, genital), a different area of the child's body is a primary source of pleasure or gratification, and conflict emerges between the child's desire for gratification and the constraints that society (which early in life consists primarily of the child's caregivers) places on that desire. In the oral stage during infancy, for example, the child derives pleasure through the mouth, particularly during feeding interactions with the caregiver. Individual differences in development at this stage primarily emerge in how outside influences support or frustrate the need for oral gratification, such as in feeding interactions that are abrupt or create anxiety or cases in which the baby is offered food when he or she is upset. Early social experiences of this kind can color adult personality structure (e.g., foreshadowing the development of an adult who clings to close relational partners) by shaping modes of internal functioning that have implications for social relatedness. Each of the subsequent three stages brings with it similar implications for adult functioning.

As these psychosexual stages suggest, central to Freud's developmental theory was the belief that, from birth onward, children have strong emotional needs and desires. Indeed, Freud conceptualized infants as being *all* strong emotion and desire because they have yet to develop the personality structures that grant them the ability to delay gratification or control instinctual drives. The reason, according to Freud's structural theory, is that infants are equipped only with an *id*, the most primitive personality structure guided by the pleasure principle (to avoid discomfort by any means possible). Unfortunately for the infant, not all desires can be immediately satisfied, and some (such as tasting an object that could pose a choking hazard) may even be prohibited. Although initially the regulation of impulses comes from external sources (particularly parents, who can either acquiesce or prohibit), with increasing age, regulation occurs internally, as a second personality structure emerges out of the id. The *ego*, which functions according to the reality principle (trying to appease the desires of the id while still adhering to the demands and limitations of the real world), provides the child with a developing capacity for self-regulation when faced with an inappropriate impulse. It does so not only through well-known defensive processes (e.g., repression) but also through other ego functions, such as affect regulation, reality testing, judgment, and impulse control.

The development of the third personality structure, the *superego*, is arguably the most strongly influenced by the social context in which the child lives. The superego is the internalization of the rules and expectations of society that may require children to ignore their own desires in favor of adhering to societal standards. The superego is composed of the conscience (derived from parents' prohibitions) and the ego ideal (consisting of aspirational standards of conduct). Both facets of the superego develop from the preschooler's identification with the same-sex parent, a process that occurs somewhat differently for boys and girls in Freud's theory. Identification has other implications for social development, including the growth of gender identity.

The Influence of Psychoanalytic Theory

Many specific claims of Freud's developmental theory have not withstood critical examination or research inquiry, and at worst this theory has been viewed as being unscientific, obsolete, or even misogynistic (Emde, 1992). But even a casual reading of this brief summary should also underscore how significantly Freudian ideas have influenced contemporary thinking about social development, even to the extent of these ideas having become so incorporated into other formulations that they are no longer recognized as Freudian. The importance of the parent–child relationship early in life; the centrality of emotion to early psychological experience; the influence of conflict on psychological growth (anticipating similar ideas in the theories of Piaget and Kohlberg); the growth of self-regulatory capacities in early childhood; and the development of moral values and gender identity through identification with the same-sex parent—these are all formulations with currency to contemporary thinking about social and personality development. Psychoanalytic thinking has also been very influential for the study of developmental psychopathology, particularly in the views that normal and atypical development share many common characteristics, that individuals are shaped by the success with which they confront age-salient developmental challenges, that developmental growth is influenced by the interaction of internal needs with the responsiveness of the social world, and that risk and protective factors are important to developmental adaptation (Cicchetti & Cohen, 1995).

Neo-Freudian Theory

Freud's legacy to social developmental science also includes the neo-Freudian developmental theorists he inspired, including Erik Erikson (1963), Rene Spitz (1965), Anna Freud (Freud's daughter; 1965), and Margaret Mahler (Mahler et al., 1975). Most notable for his contributions to social development is Erik Erikson, who developed his own stagelike theory of psychosocial development. Erikson departed from Freud in his belief that development is lifelong, and instead of focusing on the significance of sexuality, Erikson instead emphasized the social influences on individual growth. But he shared with Freud a conviction about the enduring legacy of early experiences, and his ideas about how the establishment of basic trust in early care would shape developing capacities to trust in later relationships became a foundational view of contemporary attachment theory. Erikson is also the source of other ideas that are current to social developmental science, including the establishment of identity in adolescence, the importance of personal generativity in middle adulthood, and how later life requires perspective on the choices and decisions of the life course.

Attachment Theory

Attachment theory is rooted in psychoanalytic ideas (see Bowlby, 1969, 1972). This is unsurprising given that the founder of attachment theory, John Bowlby, was a British psychoanalyst. From this background emerged Bowlby's view that the quality of an infant's earliest relationships can have lifelong significance and that early attachments influence later personality development, social relationships, and, in some cases, even psychopathology. Although Bowlby raised strong objections to the emphasis on unconscious processes of classic psychoanalytic theory, attachment theory has helped to provide a way to explore how conscious and nonconscious mental representations of relationships, which Bowlby termed "internal working models," are shaped by relational experience and guide social and personality growth (see Roisman & Groh, Chapter 5, this volume, for a more extensive discussion of attachment theory).

Attachment theory has not only benefited from psychoanalytic ideas but has also made significant contributions to the growth of psychoanalytic thinking by reframing classic Freudian ideas in terms more congenial to contemporary developmental science and encouraging their empirical testing. One of the best known research initiatives deriving from attachment theory is the Minnesota Study of Risk and Adaptation, a longitudinal study that began in the 1970s and continues to this day (Sroufe, Egeland, Carlson, & Collins, 2005). The researchers credit Freud with many of their central hypotheses, including "the idea that early experience has special significance, that the emotional life of infants is of great importance, and that early primary relationships are central in the shaping of personality" (Sroufe et al., 2005, p. 34). The Minnesota researchers began their study by recruiting pregnant women from at-risk populations and then studied them and their offspring from infancy through adulthood and even into the next generation, as the original children from the study started families of their own. This intensive longitudinal study assessed participants across a wide range of social, emotional, and personality measures, making it possible to test some of the basic formulations of Freud's psychoanalytic developmental theory. They found that the legacy of early parent–infant attachments could be observed initially in how children created and maintained new relationships with other partners and that the long-term effects of early attachment could sometimes still be seen much later in life, even as they were modified by subsequent experiences and relationships. The Minnesota Study is a unique contribution to social developmental science, but it is also representative of the large number of studies from within and outside attachment theory that have been inspired by some of the provocative ideas first formulated within psychoanalytic theory.

Behavioral and Cognitive Social Learning Theories

Behavioral Theory

The legacy of psychoanalytic theory can be found not only among developmentalists interested in expanding on Freud's ideas but also in the theories that emerged in direct opposition to the psychoanalytic viewpoint. Behavioral theory is an example. Both Watson (1913) and Skinner (e.g., 1948, 1953, 1971) explicitly eschewed consideration of unconscious motives in favor of a focus on observable behavior and testable laws of learning. From this different perspective, behavioral theory provided social developmental science with extremely powerful models of learning with which to understand behavioral development throughout the life course. Cognitive social learning theory, in turn, addressed some of the shortcomings of the behavioral analysis through its attention to the cognitive processes mediating learning in children.

Watson articulated the behavioral perspective in 1913 that psychology should abandon its interest in unconscious (and, by his logic, thereby unknowable) processes in favor of studying observable behavior and the influences of learning. Instructed by Pavlov's (1927) studies, Watson was so convinced of the power of classical conditioning to shape human behavior and development that he offered this well-known claim concerning the malleability of children's growth:

> Give me a dozen healthy infants, well-formed, and my own specified world to bring them up in and I'll guarantee to take any one at random and train him to become any type of specialist I might select—doctor, lawyer, artist, merchant-chief, and, yes, even beggar-man and thief—regardless of his talents, penchants, tendencies, abilities, vocation, and race of his ancestors. (Watson, 1924, p. 104)

Even at the time of this writing Watson was aware that this boast was unrealistic, but it underscores his conviction of the importance of early learning experiences as being of paramount importance in shaping the kinds of persons that children become. Watson rejected the psychoanalytic claim of the significance of early maternal nurturance to psychological adjustment, reasoning instead that early emotions could and should be conditioned by parents to help the child develop adequate self-regulation. Although he was incorrect about the danger of sensitive care, Watson's studies of emotional conditioning showed how emotions and other behavioral reactions can readily be conditioned, sometimes by the inadvertent creation of learned associations among salient environmental events. The significance of classical conditioning in understanding learned emotional reactions (such as fear, love, and anxiety), particularly to social partners, remains part of Watson's legacy and contributes to his contemporary influence.

Later, in the 1950s, B. F. Skinner developed his own version of radical behaviorism that focused on the role of reinforcement and punishment in the operant conditioning of behavior. Like Watson, Skinner was not a developmental scientist, but he believed that these laws of learning were applicable to explaining the growth of behavior through deliberate and unintended learning experiences. Whether a young child responds to frustration with crying, problem solving, or help seeking, for example, is likely to be affected by how prior responses to frustrating experiences have been reinforced in the past by caregivers. Parents were therefore encouraged to perceive their influence as one of appropriately reinforcing good behavior while judiciously punishing bad conduct in a manner of socialization that was unidirectional (Maccoby, 2006). Although developmental scientists later recognized how much infants and children reciprocally reinforce the behavior of their caregivers (Bell, 1968), Skinner's arguments nevertheless underscore how much the explicit and informal social reinforcements of everyday family interaction shape social and personality development.

The ideas of Watson and Skinner and their followers, as valuable as they remain, nevertheless failed to constitute a comprehensive developmental theory for several reasons. First, straightforward conditioning processes were overextended to create tortured and, ultimately, inadequate explanations for complex developmental achievements, such as language (Chomsky, 1959). It became apparent that the nature of learning and development in children was different, in important ways, from that of pigeons and rats. Second, many rich and interesting developmental achievements in social and personality growth, such as conscience development, attachment, and sex typing, became highly simplified and sterile when reduced to a conditioning analysis and failed to encompass the diverse developmental outcomes associated with these achievements. Explaining mother–infant attachment in terms of the association of mother with primary reinforcers such as food, for example, failed to explain many important features of attachment formation (Harlow, 1958). Third, and most important, developmental scientists began to appreciate the significant cognitive mediators of learning in children and adults. Understanding the influence of learning in humans requires understanding the mental processes associated with it.

Cognitive Social Learning Theory

Cognitive social learning theory emerged in response to some of these problems with traditional behavioral analysis. A major tenet of social learning theory is that children learn by imitating the behavior of others (observational learning) in conjunction with reinforcement for behavioral imitation (Bandura, 1977; Bandura & Walters, 1963). Observational learning provides a much more flexible network of learning influences with which to understand the growth of social behavior and personality characteristics in children. Learning can also occur through symbolic means, such as children's observations of others through television and storytelling. Even more important are the cognitive processes identified by Bandura (1986) that mediate observations of behavior and their enactment by the observer. These include the child's interpretation of what is observed, cognitive representations of that behavior, the consistency of observed behavior with preexisting schemas and beliefs, self-efficacy, and other conceptual incentives for acting in a manner similar to what was observed. All of these cognitive constituents of social learning change significantly with psychological growth, suggesting that learning processes occur in developmentally evolving ways. Finally, cognitive social learning theory moves beyond the unidirectional socialization model of traditional behavioral analysis to argue for the reciprocal determinism of behavior that derives from an interaction between the psychological and cognitive characteristics of the child, the child's behavior, and the environment. Environmental influences are important, as traditional behavioral analysis argues, but so also are the ways in which the child affects the environment, which, in turn, subsequently influence the child's behavior and internal characteristics.

Taken together, the conceptual tools of traditional behavioral analysis and cognitive social learning theory provide important ways of comprehending children's social development and also have important applications to understanding and treating behavioral problems. One illustration of these applications is the work of the Oregon Social Learning Center (OSLC), which was begun by Gerald Patterson (1982) in the 1960s and continues to this day. The OSLC was created to assist troubled families, and Patterson found that traditional clinical methods were ineffective in treating children with aggressive behavioral problems. He discovered that rather than working directly and exclusively with the children, the most effective treatments targeted how parents were inadvertently reinforcing their children's aggressive behavior. Parents often did so through negative reinforcement, such as by backing off from reasonable behavioral expectations when the child was aggressively resistant and thus inadvertently reinforcing the child's defiance. Instead, Patterson concluded, parents needed to be trained to provide appropriate consequences for child behavior, consistently sanctioning bad conduct as well as ensuring consistent rewards for good conduct. More recent work has also focused on the cognitions underlying parent–child interactions, including parents' hostile attribution biases that cause them to interpret child conduct as deliberately resistant and thus to respond in a coercive rather than a competent manner (Snyder, Cramer, Afrank, & Patterson, 2005). The continuing work of the OSLC illustrates the applications of modern cognitive social learning theory to the analysis of family problems that incorporates cognitive and behavioral methods and an understanding of the reciprocal processes that are involved in social development.

Despite these valuable contributions, learning approaches offer a limited understanding of behavioral development because, in part, none of the leading learning theorists was developmental in orientation. Bandura's attention to the cognitive mediators of learning in children was important but also highlighted the further need to understand developmental changes in the cognitive constructions of experience that influence how children respond to everyday events. Fortunately, during the period in which cognitive social learning theory was prominent, another theorist in Europe was building a comprehensive theory of cognitive development that would significantly alter how developmental scientists think of the developing child and of that child's social development.

Cognitive-Developmental Theory

That theorist was Jean Piaget. Piaget (e.g., 1952, 1970) came to the study of children's cognitive development through philosophy and an interest in how knowledge was created. In describing himself as a "genetic epistemologist," Piaget assumed the challenge of understanding developmental changes in the process of knowing and the organization of knowledge. Such an approach put the developing mind—rather than emotions or behavior—squarely at the heart of developmental analysis and led to a theory with significant implications for the study of cognitive development, education, and social development.

Although Piaget's stage theory is the best known aspect of his developmental formulation, other aspects of Piaget's theory have had a greater and more enduring impact on developmental psychology (Flavell, 1963). Perhaps the most important of these is constructivism, the idea that children actively construct knowledge through their interactions with objects and events. Essential to this view is the portrayal of the child as an active reasoner rather than a passive recipient of stimulation or reinforcement and the idea that the child's current structures of reasoning mediate between environmental events and the knowledge that is derived from them. Children at different stages of cognitive development, Piaget argued, are likely to apply different understanding to a common experience, such as when a preschooler and a grade-schooler are each asked to select a delectable snack for Mommy or to think about what Grandma was like when she was a child. In his emphasis on how current reasoning structures mediate between experience and knowledge, Piaget contributed to developmental psychology the view that knowledge is never a copy of reality but is rather constructed (and reconstructed) from the interaction of experience and reasoning. In his emphasis on the child's activity as a core component of knowledge acquisition, furthermore, Piaget contributed to developmental thinking that the child's engagement in events is more provocative of conceptual growth than is what is done or told to the child (a view also adopted by sociocultural theorists). These ideas have profound implications for the construction of social understanding and knowledge about people.

In this theory, Piaget was fundamentally concerned with the mental structures of reasoning and how they change with development. A conflict model is central to Piaget's portrayal of cognitive development. In this portrayal, children often assimilate new events and experiences to preexisting structures of reasoning, tailoring their interpretation of those experiences to conform to prior knowledge and expectations. Seeing mother in tears as she greets her parents after a long time away, for example, a preschooler might naturally conclude that mother is sad about their arrival. Assimilation induces cognitive growth as new experiences broaden preexisting cognitive structures. But some experiences are not easily assimilated to prior understanding. The preschooler may notice that mother is also smiling through her tears as she says how glad she is to see her parents again. Comprehending this requires a further cognitive step of changing—or accommodating—preexisting structures of reasoning to this new experience. The preschooler may derive a new realization that people (especially adults) sometimes look different than they really feel or that people may experience different emotions at the same time. This is where conceptual growth also arises, and without the disequilibrium generated by discordant experiences of cognitive conflict, new or modified cognitive structures do not develop.

In this manner—through the dual processes of assimilation and accommodation—infants and children proceed through the four stages of cognitive development in Piaget's stage theory. The first stage, *sensorimotor,* lasting during the first 2 years, is an initial prerepresentational stage of cognition in which thinking is based on sensory experience and motor activity. During this period, the newborn's reflex activity evolves into the toddler's sophisticated capacities for learning about the properties of objects and associations among them, and behavior becomes increasingly strategic in acquiring new understanding. The second stage, *preoperational,* lasting roughly from ages 2 to 6, is marked by the child's capacity to use mental symbols (including language) in thinking and reasoning. Even so, Piaget's depiction of this stage focuses also on the limitations in the preschooler's thinking—such as egocentrism, a reliance on intuition and perceptual features of events, and reasoning that is inflexible and irreversible—that can yield misleading judgments, including those with implications for social understanding. By the time the child reaches the third stage of *concrete operations*, lasting from ages 6 to 11, these deficiencies are remedied by the emergence of logical reasoning structures that enable school-age children to approach situations more objectively, systematically, and rationally. It is no accident, therefore, that this is the period in which children typically enter formal education. The fourth stage, *formal operations*, completes the process of cognitive development in Piaget's stage theory by correcting the remaining limitation in the school-age child's thinking, that of concrete reasoning. Children in early adolescence can, for example, interpret the proverb "the squeaky wheel gets the grease" with reference to its lesson for human relations rather than for bicycle maintenance and can exhibit their capacities for abstract, hypothetical reasoning also in their thinking about love, justice, the meaning of life, and other abstract notions.

These stages are described here because their implications for social, moral, and emotional understanding were readily understood by Piaget and other developmentalists. Piaget (1932) himself wrote about the implications of children's cognitive growth for the development of moral judgment, distinguishing the rigid, authority-oriented heteronomous morality of the preoperational child from the more flexible, cooperatively autonomous morality of the concrete-operational child. Kohlberg (1969) also drew on Piaget's ideas for his own theory of the development of moral judgment. Kohlberg explained the differences in reasoning, for example, between the preconventional morality of the preschooler and the conventional morality of the school-age child in terms of the egocentric, consequentialist orientation of the younger child. Likewise, conventional morality is different from the postconventional morality of the older child because of the latter's reliance on abstract ethical values. Kohlberg's theory of the development of moral judgment is much more than a derivative of Piagetian theory, of course, but his work helped to alert students of social development to the implications of Piaget's cognitive theory for their own research.

The 1970s and 1980s witnessed burgeoning research into social cognitive development based on cognitive-developmental theory and especially on the limits of preschoolers' egocentrism for social understanding (see, e.g., Miller & Aloise, 1989). These efforts included applications of Piagetian ideas to the development of role taking and social communication (Flavell, 1968), social perspective taking (Selman, 1980), self-awareness and self-understanding (Harter, 2001), prosocial reasoning (Mussen & Eisenberg-Berg, 1977), gender identity (Kohlberg, 1966), and many other areas. Bowlby's (1969) attachment theory enlisted Piaget's stages to explain the growth of attachment formation in the early years. For many years, the field of social cognition was defined by the application of Piagetian insights to the study of social understanding.

Piaget's theory has had other implications for the study of social development. Most contemporary developmental researchers have a constructivist orientation based on Piaget's work because they recognize that the child's active interpretation of experience is essential to the influence of events on behavior and understanding. Understanding the effects of divorce on children critically depends, for example, on developmental changes in children's interpretive construction of that experience (see Wallerstein & Kelly, 1996). Moreover, because cognitive growth arises, in part, from the disequilibrium evoked by the conflict between preexisting knowledge structures and experience, Piaget recognized that social experiences could be potent sources of cognitive conflict when children are confronted with another's ideas that cannot readily be assimilated into the child's prior beliefs. However, by contrast with the predominant focus of his contemporaries on parental socialization, Piaget viewed peer relationships as more influential instigators of cognitive change because peers are on a more equal conceptual footing in relation to each other. Peer relationships are crucial, for example, to children's progress toward more flexible, cooperative forms of moral judgment, in which children have experience in shared rule making and its application to their play activity. A similar view was subsequently adopted by Kohlberg in his arguments concerning the importance of socio-moral conflict as a catalyst to growth in moral judgment through interactions with peers.

Cognitive-developmental theory thus remains a very influential approach to understanding cognitive growth and social development, even though its influence has waned in recent decades with the emergence of alternative approaches to understanding cognitive development. One reason for its diminishing influence is Piaget's stage theory. Current students of cognitive development have concluded that conceptual growth is not necessarily stage-like in its emergence and that Piaget also underestimated the cognitive skills of infants and young children in his theory. Concerning the latter: In his insistence on using exacting assessments, Piaget sometimes presented young children with tasks (such as those requiring verbal justifications) that may have masked their true abilities. Using simpler methods, cognitive developmentalists today recognize that very young children are more conceptually and representationally sophisticated than Piaget had estimated and that preschoolers are not egocentric in the manner in which Piaget characterized them (Flavell, Miller, & Miller, 2001). This has important implications for research on social cognitive development that is based on Piaget's ideas. Egocentric thinking is not, for example, the significant limitation on social understanding that it was earlier thought to be. To illustrate, new research on early conscience development suggests that preschoolers have a much more humanistic, relational moral orientation than was earlier believed and that it incorporates their rapidly developing understanding of others' feelings and desires (Thompson, 2009). This new view of the growth of conscience contrasts markedly with Kohlberg's portrayal of preconventional morality based on Piagetian egocentrism and suggests that contemporary students of moral and social cognitive development may have to reexamine some of their conclusions in light of newer discoveries about early cognitive growth in this post-Piagetian era (see Walker & Frimer, Chapter 10, this volume).

Sociocultural Theory

The prevailing metaphor of the child from cognitive-developmental theory is as a scientist who is actively experimenting on the world to derive new insights about it. Sociocultural theorists also embrace a view of the child's active reasoning about the world, but they also believe that cognitive development derives from a collaboration between the child and others who are more experienced and knowledgeable. Sociocultural theorists seek to explain conceptual development as an interaction between the remarkably inquisitive mind of the child (without viewing the child in isolation) and the remarkable sensitivity of adults in structuring developing understanding (without viewing the child as the passive recipient of instruction). Such a view has important implications for students of social and personality development.

Sociocultural theory originated in a much different cultural context than did other theories discussed thus far—in the theoretical work of Lev Vygotsky (1962, 1978). Early after the dawn of the Soviet republic, Vygotsky began in the 1920s and

1930s to construct a cultural–historical theory of psychological development based on Marxist ideas about the relation between the individual and the collective. Cognitive development is the outcome, in his view, of the child's ongoing interactions with other people in social settings and using cultural tools that guide developing thinking and reasoning. Vygotskian theory thus emphasizes the socially constituted creation of knowledge and the cultural relativity of intellectual skills, underscoring that modes of learning (individual, collaborative, technological) and their outcomes will vary depending on the social context in which the child lives. Whereas the sociocultural features of Vygotsky's theory are readily understood by developmental theorists, the roots of Vygotskian ideas in the historical materialism of Marxism—the view that modes of work and the tools of labor are a foundation for a culture's ideology—is a more radical formulation for a developmental theory.

A central concept of Vygotskian theory reflects these ideas: the "zone of proximal development." It describes the difference between the child's current developmental achievements as they are independently exhibited and the higher level of capability that can be demonstrated only with the guidance of a more experienced partner. In a sense, the "zone" reflects a domain of potential development-in-the-making, and the important feature of this concept is that interaction with a mentor not only enables the child to function more competently but is also a catalyst for psychological growth. An example of this process is how sharing recollections about events in the recent past with an adult not only enables young children to remember these events better but also contributes to the growth of mnemonic ability (Ornstein, Haden, & Hedrick, 2004). Why does this occur? One reason is that in sensitive social collaboration, a mentor scaffolds the task in a manner that draws on the child's current capabilities while providing support and guidance for the expansion of those skills so the child can accomplish more. In shared reminiscing, for example, a sensitive adult prompts memory for events in their temporal sequence, helping the child remember each event in relation to what preceded it, offering memory prompts when needed ("And then we went to Burger ... ?" to which the child responds "King!"), adding elaborative detail, drawing logical connections between sequential events, and in so doing modeling effective memory reconstruction skills. This kind of scaffolding is common to interaction between parents and young children and has been termed "guided participation" by Rogoff (1990), a neo-Vygotskian theorist.

What kinds of skills are learned in this manner? By contrast with the focus of most developmental theorists on universal cognitive accomplishments, sociocultural theorists underscore the cultural relativity of the cognitive skills that children acquire. Children in different cultures worldwide learn similar and different skills, which may include reading, managing farm animals, mathematics, understanding seasonal weather patterns, refined visual discrimination (such as in farming or hunting), social discriminations, and many other abilities. The cultural tools relevant to these skills are equally variable and may include a computer, an abacus, a loom, a sling, a pencil or a brush for writing, or knowledge of how to consult a village elder. To contemporary sociocultural theorists, these reflect the cultural construction of knowledge. To Vygotsky, they also reflect the historical reconstruction of development, such as when illiterate peasants in Russian society began developing skills in concept formation, logical reasoning, and problem solving relevant to their new participation in Soviet economic life.

Language is a preeminent cultural tool that guides the growth of understanding because it is both a cultural construction (with different language systems incorporating cultural meanings, beliefs, and assumptions) and a means of the social transmission of knowledge that eventually becomes internalized by the child into how he or she thinks. In addition, language is a means of self-regulation, as young children initially talk to themselves (what Vygotsky called "private speech"), sometimes using the words they have been provided to guide their thinking and actions, and progressively internalize this speech so it becomes an internal, nonverbal behavior regulator ("inner speech"). As 3-year-olds talk to themselves during their activities ("Now I color red ... " while painting at an easel), Vygotsky believed that this overt self-talk eventually goes underground to constitute the child's internal monologue. This developmental progression from the intermental (between-minds) to the intramental (within-mind) through language illustrates how deeply mental growth is a function of social activity and of the cultural context within which it occurs. Rogoff (1990) adds to this concept the recognition that the child's active mind can transform others' guidance as it is appropriated; for instance, a preschooler listens to a parent's careful explanation of dinosaurs and later explains to a peer how the cowboys rode on dinosaurs to round up the cattle.

The ideas of Vygotsky and subsequent theorists such as Rogoff (1990) and Cole (1996) have contributed to contemporary sociocultural theory, which has influenced the study of social and personality development in several ways. First, it has inspired cultural studies of social growth that have revealed how significantly the societal context shapes children's conceptions of themselves and other people (see Weisner, Chapter 15, this volume). This begins early in the different patterns of parent–infant interaction that orient the developing sense of self and modes of relating to other people (Keller, 2007) and continues as children begin to be included in activities of the adult world.

Second, and equally important, sociocultural theory has also influenced how we conceptualize and study social development. Concepts such as guided participation, in which the sensitive scaffolding of a caregiver's prompts interacts with the child's inquisitive mind, offer a way of thinking about the development of social skills and understanding in a manner that significantly extends the formulations of traditional cognitive social learning and cognitive-developmental theories. Considerable research, for example, has examined the influence of parent–child conversation not only on reminiscing but also on developing emotion understanding, conscience, self-understanding, and other aspects of social development, showing how the content and quality of parental discourse scaffolds developing psychological understanding in young children who are in the process of comprehending mental events (see Thompson, 2006; Thompson, Laible, & Ontai, 2003). Taken together, sociocultural theoretical concepts of guided participation or children as "apprentices in thinking" that reflect social scaffolding of emergent abilities have been highly influential in research on social development. Although the contributions of sociocultural theory are often complementary to other developmental theories—with Rogoff's (1990) provocative integration of Vygotskian and Piagetian formulations an example—they provide essential conceptual tools.

Ethological and Evolutionary Theories

In the views of Vygotsky and his followers, the developing child is inseparable from the cultural context. Ethological/evolutionary theories also situate the child within a broader context: species evolution. These approaches are complementary in their contextual orientation, but they are very different in their primary emphasis on universal or local (e.g., cultural) processes. In viewing child development within the context of the adaptational requirements of natural selection, ethological and evolutionary theories portray many aspects of social development as biologically deeply rooted within humans.

Ethology is the branch of the biological sciences dedicated to the study of animal behavior. Ethological theory is drawn from evolutionary biology and the view that the behavior we observe in animals evolved due to the advantages it offers for species survival and reproductive success in their particular ecological niche. Consequently, ethologists are especially focused on observing animals in their natural environments in order to understand what influences shape biologically adaptive behavior. It is useful to note that the ethological perspective gained traction in American psychology in the second half of the 20th century due, in part, to a growing recognition that there were limits to the application of straightforward learning analyses to animal behavior (Grusec & Lytton, 1988). For example, attempts to train pigs to put wooden discs into a piggy bank were thwarted by the pigs' natural instinct to drop the coins to the ground and root around with them. This forced researchers to acknowledge that even in animals far less complex than humans, conditioning principles were not fully adequate in behavioral analysis.

The work of Konrad Lorenz (1957, 1966), an Austrian zoologist who studied precocial birds (i.e., birds who are relatively mature at hatching and can therefore leave the nest quickly), illustrates the ethological focus on biologically adaptive behavior in the natural environment. Working with geese, Lorenz was interested in the behavioral processes that keep young birds close to their mothers—and thus relatively safe from harm—despite their ability to wander away. Lorenz discovered that, soon after hatching, goslings "imprinted" on a moving object near the nest, revealed in their following this object and preferring it to others. In nearly all instances (except experimental interventions), of course, the moving object is the mother bird, and thus imprinting contributes to the survival of the young by ensuring that it stays close to the mother for protection and nurturance. Lorenz determined that imprinting happened during a very specific period of time (i.e., a critical period) after hatching and that it was irreversible once formed. Although human infants are incapable of rapid mobility after birth, infants are also more likely to survive if they also have behavioral processes for remaining close to nurturant caregivers. Determining what these adaptive behaviors are for human infants was the focus of Bowlby's (1969) attachment theory, discussed shortly.

An ethological respect for the functions of behavior in its natural setting has been incorporated into developmental research on many topics. To many students of social development, careful observations of parent–infant interaction, peer play behavior, classroom activity, and other aspects of social interaction in natural settings are an essential complement to laboratory studies because they enable researchers to observe how social behavior functions in the everyday contexts in which it occurs. Ethological theory has also encouraged social developmentalists to denote parallels in the behavior of human children and the young of other animal species (e.g., play) when they are responding to similar adaptive challenges.

It is easy to see how ethological research derived from Darwinian theory. Contemporary evolutionary psychology is also derived from Darwinian theory and consists of an explicit effort to understand how psychological functioning derives from natural selection (Buss, 2009a). At the core of evolutionary psychology is the belief that many psychological behaviors and characteristics have evolved in response to recurrent problems in the human environment of evolutionary adaptedness. Evolutionary psychologists have applied these principles to understanding many human behaviors across virtually all disciplines of psychology, including fears and phobias, kinship patterns, individual differences in personality, aggression, and family relationships (Buss, 2009b).

The ideas of evolutionary analysis have also been applied to child development in the field of evolutionary developmental psychology (Ellis & Bjorklund, 2005). Many biological adaptations have evolved that enable infants and children to survive to maturity. For example, some developmentalists believe that male and female children first begin practicing the sex-differentiated skills that are carried forward into adulthood, with boys more likely to play in ways related to establishing dominance or conflict resolution and girls more likely to play in cooperative ways (Bjorklund & Yunger, 2001). These skills are thought to derive from the evolved behavioral patterns of males and females related to sexual competition or parental investment. Although an evolutionary account is not the only way of understanding the origins of sex differences in play, of course, it can potentially contribute to a better understanding of why these and other behaviors develop and endure.

Attachment theory is based in the ideas of psychoanalytic theory, as earlier noted, but it is also founded on ethological and evolutionary theories. Bowlby (1969) hypothesized that the close bond between infant and parent is not just psychologically significant for the baby but also critical for the infant's survival. Because human infants are born incapable of caring for themselves and are defenseless against predators, they require the nurturance and protection of the adults, just as precocial birds do. Attachment behaviors such as crying, reaching, and clinging to an adult evolved, Bowlby believed, to keep caregivers close—particularly during stress or danger—and also provided the child an opportunity to learn survival skills from the parent. The development of an emotional attachment between baby and parent contributes crucially, in this view, to the motivation for parents and infants to remain in proximity. In this way, according to Bowlby, attachment promotes the long-term survival of the child.

In developing these views, Bowlby was influenced by the thinking of Darwin (as well as of Freud) and Lorenz's ethological studies of imprinting. He was also influenced by Harlow's studies with infant rhesus monkeys. Harlow found that when baby monkeys were separated from their mothers and placed with one of two wire surrogates, they preferred the surrogate that was soft and warm (full of "contact comfort," according to Harlow) over a wire surrogate that was their sole source of food (Harlow, 1958). Bowlby concurred with Harlow's conclusion that these findings were inconsistent with conditioning explanations of infant–parent attachment that emphasize affection for the mother as a derivative of her provision of food and pointed to an independent motivational system governing attachment relationships. Bowlby found that motivational system in the biologically adaptive requirements of the human species related to the nurturance and protection of the young.

Attachment theory illustrates how evolutionary thinking can illuminate central questions for sociopersonality development when thoughtfully integrated into a broader theoretical formulation. Careful applications of evolutionary theory require comparative ethological analysis of other species with similar adaptational requirements, as well as cultural–historical analyses, to evaluate the contextual variability in behavior that is presumed to have a biological foundation. This kind of careful work is far different from the casual theorizing that yields post hoc evolutionary "explanations" for complex behavior in humans. Likewise, developmental researchers have learned that generalizing to humans from ethological studies of other animal species is far more complex than simply identifying homologous behaviors in each. For example, critical periods may be far less common in humans than are more flexible sensitive periods because of the more complex determinants of human functioning (Bornstein, 1989). When these cautions are taken into consideration, however, ethological and evolutionary theory can offer unique and valuable contributions to the study of social development.

Dynamic Systems Theory

Dynamic systems theory is described as a "minitheory" by Miller (2002, p. 432) but also as an "influential and promising" one. As the newest of the theories described in this chapter, the potential of dynamic systems theory in elucidating issues of social development remains to be fully realized, but there is little doubt that it offers a creative and provocative perspective.

Dynamic systems thinking in developmental psychology derives from a collection of theories in the natural sciences (including mathematics, physics, meteorology, and biology) that are fundamentally concerned with the self-organization of complex systems. A dynamic systems theorist asks how new forms of psychological organization emerge out of simpler components. This is, in a sense, a question common to developmental theories (consider, e.g., Piaget's description of the reorganization of mental structures with each new stage of cognitive development), but dynamic systems theorists approach this challenge with a formal analysis, inclusiveness, and scope of application that is unique among developmental theories. They begin with the conviction that understanding development requires considering the continuous, interdependent interaction among the multiple components of a developing system as they function on all levels, from the molecular to the cultural. This general systems view is complemented by the belief that developmental analysis encompasses many time scales, from changes that occur over milliseconds to those requiring years (see Lewis, 2000; Thelen & Smith, 2006). In a sense, the complexity of understanding child development is likened to predicting the weather. The challenge in each case is in understanding how an extraordinarily complex system becomes organized in a dynamic manner involving multiple influences over many levels of complexity across immediate and long periods of time.

The central concept in a dynamic systems perspective is *self-organization*: the spontaneous emergence and stabilization of order through recursive interactions among antecedent, simpler elements without a predetermined blueprint. How does this occur? In the language of dynamic systems theorists, systemic phase transitions (or reorganizations) can result from changes in elements of the context or within the organism to result in a new "preferred state." This new stabilization may or may not endure, although each new reorganization of the system is constrained by the previous pattern and, in general, preferred states tend to become increasingly stable over time. Critical elements of the system, known as control parameters, may determine the new organization that emerges and also the disorganization of the system when control parameters pass critical thresholds. This dynamic reorganization of the system can occur repeatedly in periods of a few seconds, minutes, or years in developmental analysis.

Although this brief overview does not do justice to the richness of dynamic systems theory, it is sufficient to illustrate what many developmentalists find attractive about the theory. First, dynamic systems theory adopts a holistic, inclusive analysis: Rather than breaking complex systems into their component parts, as most theories do, it adopts a comprehensive systems view instead. Second, the theory is domain-general: It is not primarily concerned with cognitive, emotional, or behavioral development, but can potentially be used to study any feature of development and any developing system. Third, the boundaries between the child and context—so carefully delineated in other developmental formulations—disappear with the incorporation of the child and the context into a single complex system. Fourth, the preferred states that emerge from system reorganizations may or may not resemble those of another complex system; there is room in this theory for both consistent and unique developmental outcomes. This is important to developmental analysis owing to how frequently children's responses in research studies differ from expectations; within this view, variability in behavior owing to contextual influences, performance factors, motivation, fatigue, and other influences are part of the same self-organizing system. Finally (perhaps most important), dynamic systems theory seeks to address directly the conceptual challenge for all developmental theorists: How do new forms of psychological organization emerge from old ones?

The heuristic power of this theory is undeniable. Moreover, dynamic systems ideas have usefully been enlisted to explain early motor development, in which the transition from the neonatal stepping reflex to voluntary stepping and walking is viewed as being governed less by maturational changes than by a complex self-organizing system of kinesthetics, muscle strength, and the gravitational dynamics of early locomotion (Thelen, 1989). Dynamic systems approaches have also been applied to the study of language development (Smith, 1995), communication (Fogel & Thelen, 1987), mother–infant interaction (Lewis, Lamey, & Douglas, 1999), and emotional development (see contributors to Lewis & Granic, 2000). One of the challenges in the application of dynamic systems thinking is that it is far easier to identify how dynamic systems ideas can provide thought-provoking interpretations of well-known research findings than it is to generate testable hypotheses involving novel applications of the theory to new empirical initiatives. It is, of course, the testability of a theory that is important to developmental science, and this is one of the future challenges for work in this area.

PERSPECTIVE AND FUTURE DIRECTIONS

The theories discussed in this chapter certainly do not exhaust the range of theoretical views relevant to social development. Social information-processing theory (Crick & Dodge, 1994), ecological systems theory (Bronfenbrenner, 1979; Bronfenbrenner & Morris, 2006), socioemotional selectivity theory (Carstensen, 2006), and the range of neo-analytic developmental theories identified earlier, among others, further attest to the vitality of theory relevant to the field of social development. Those selected for discussion in this chapter are the most influential in the field and the most developmentally oriented in their analysis, but the value of theory for the field is reflected in the continued generation of new perspectives.

The historical, cultural, and scientific context of contemporary social development theory is, of course, different from that of the past. Concerning science, contemporary theorists face a far more exciting, vast—and daunting—range of research findings to explain and incorporate into a conceptual framework, with advances in research technology contributing complexity, as well as insight, to research data. Growing scholarly enthusiasm for biological approaches to understanding social development from developmental neurobiology, developmental biology, and molecular genetics encourages contemporary developmental theorists to comprehend the influence of biological processes in ways that previous developmental theorists tended to neglect. This is especially important in light of the scientific obsolescence of the classic nature–nurture debate that in the past has impeded rather than advanced developmental understanding. In addition, the increasing specialization and narrowness of knowledge within research fields in developmental psychology means that future theories of social development are more likely to be domain-specific (e.g., concerning peer relationships or adult emotional growth) than domain-general. Indeed, it is common to hear developmental psychologists conclude that the era of grand psychological theories is over and that the field will never again be dominated by the influence of comprehensive approaches such as behavioral or Piagetian theory as it once was. Whether or not this is true, other fields of scientific study with narrowly specialized fields continue to be guided by broad theoretical perspectives, and it remains to be seen whether this will also be true of the future of social developmental science.

The historical and cultural context of social development research has also changed considerably since the dawn of the child study movement in the United States a century ago. Developmental theory has been a contributor to evolving cultural values concerning children that have expanded national attention to their nurturance and education. A public that has become convinced by developmental studies of the importance of the early years (motivated by popular awareness of research on brain development and a national concern with increasing school readiness), the significance of parental nurturance, and the marvel of the "scientist in the crib" is a receptive audience for new understanding of social and emotional development.

But there are also important challenges ahead for social developmental science. One is providing understanding of the connections between traditionally disconnected developmental domains—cognition, emotion, personality, language, sociability—that are more deeply integrated than science and public awareness often recognize. Another is conceptualizing the unique risks and vulnerabilities of social development in the early years—which has been the focus of much scientific attention—compared with other periods of the life course. A third is connecting expanding understanding of social and emotional development with the practical implications of intervention, particularly for at-risk populations of children for whom socioemotional challenges are paramount to their developmental outcomes.

These are formidable challenges. Developmental theories provide a map for navigating these and other new issues concerning social development in a cultural context of public receptivity to new understanding. It is an exciting time for social developmental science.

SUGGESTED READINGS

Collins, A. (2002). Historical perspectives on contemporary research in social development. In P. K. Smith & C. H. Hart (Eds.), *Blackwell handbook of childhood social development* (pp. 3–23). Malden, MA: Blackwell.

Grusec, J. E., & Lytton, H. (1988). *Social development: History, theory and research.* New York: Springer-Verlag.

Maccoby, E. E. (2006). Historical overview of socialization theory and research. In J. E. Grusec & P. D. Hastings (Eds.), *Handbook of socialization* (pp. 13–41). New York: Guilford Press.

Miller, P. H. (2002). *Theories of developmental psychology* (4th ed.). New York: Worth.

Parke, R. D., Ornstein, P. A., Reiser, J. J., & Zahn-Waxler, C. (Eds.). (1994). *A century of developmental psychology*. Washington, DC: American Psychological Association.

REFERENCES

Aries, P. (1962). *Centuries of childhood*. New York: Random House.

Bandura, A. (1977). *Social learning theory*. Morristown, NJ: General Learning Press.

Bandura, A. (1986). *Social foundations of thought and action*. Englewood Cliffs, NJ: Prentice-Hall.

Bandura, A., & Walters, R. H. (1963). *Social learning and personality development*. New York: Holt, Rinehart & Winston.

Bell, R. Q. (1968). A reinterpretation of the direction of effects in studies of socialization. *Psychological Review, 75*, 81–95.

Bjorklund, D. F., & Yunger, J. (2001). Evolutionary developmental psychology: A useful framework for evaluating the evolution of parenting. *Parenting: Science and Practice, 1*, 63–66.

Bornstein, M. H. (1989). Sensitive periods in development: Structural characteristics and causal interpretations. *Psychological Bulletin, 105*, 179–197.

Bowlby, J. (1969). *Attachment and loss: Vol. 1. Attachment*. New York: Basic Books.

Bowlby, J. (1972). *Attachment and loss: Vol. 2. Separation: Anxiety and anger*. New York: Basic Books.

Bronfenbrenner, U. (1979). *The ecology of human development*. Cambridge, MA: Harvard University Press.

Bronfenbrenner, U., & Morris, P. A. (2006). The bioecological model of human development. In R. M. Lerner & W. Damon (Eds.), *Handbook of child psychology: Vol. 1. Theoretical models of human development* (6th ed., pp. 793–828). Hoboken, NJ: Wiley.

Buss, D. M. (2009a). The great struggles of life: Darwin and the emergence of evolutionary psychology. *American Psychologist, 64*, 140–148.

Buss, D. M. (2009b). How can evolutionary psychology successfully explain personality and individual differences? *Perspectives on Psychological Science, 4*, 359–366.

Carstensen, L. (2006). The influence of a sense of time on human development. *Science, 312*, 1913–1915.

Chomsky, N. (1959). A review of *Verbal behavior,* by B. F. Skinner. *Language, 35*, 26–58.

Cicchetti, D., & Cohen, D. J. (1995). Perspectives on developmental psychopathology. In D. Cicchetti & D. J. Cohen (Eds.), *Developmental psychopathology: Vol. 1. Theory and methods* (pp. 3–20). New York: Wiley.

Clausen, J. A. (1993). *American lives*. New York: Free Press.

Cole, M. (1996). *Cultural psychology*. Cambridge, MA: Harvard University Press.

Collins, A. (2002). Historical perspectives on contemporary research in social development. In P. K. Smith & C. H. Hart (Eds.), *Blackwell handbook of childhood social development* (pp. 3–23). Malden, MA: Blackwell.

Crick, N. R., & Dodge, K. A. (1994). A review and reformulation of social information-processing mechanisms in children's social adjustment. *Psychological Bulletin, 115*, 74–101.

Darwin, C. (1877). A biographical sketch of an infant. *Mind, 2*, 285–294.

Darwin, C. (1955). *The expression of the emotions in man and animals*. Oxford, UK: Philosophical Library. (Original work published 1872)

deMause, L. (Ed.) (1974). *The history of childhood*. New York: Harper & Row.

Elder, G. (1974). *Children of the Great Depression*. Boulder, CO: Westview.

Ellis, B. J., & Bjorklund, D. F. (Eds.). (2005). *Origins of the social mind*. New York: Guilford Press.

Emde, R. (1992). Individual meaning and increasing complexity: Contributions of Sigmund Freud and René Spitz to developmental psychology. *Developmental Psychology, 28*, 347–359.

Erikson, E. (1963). *Childhood and society*. New York: Norton.

Flavell, J. (1963). *The developmental psychology of Jean Piaget*. Princeton, NJ: Van Nostrand.

Flavell, J. H. (1968). *The development of role-taking and communication skills in children*. Oxford, UK: Wiley.

Flavell, J. H., Miller, P. H., & Miller, S. A. (2001). *Cognitive development* (4th ed.). Englewood Cliffs, NJ: Prentice-Hall.

Fogel, A., & Thelen, E. (1987). Development of early expressive and communicative action: Reinterpreting the evidence from a dynamic systems perspective. *Developmental Psychology, 23*, 747–761.

Freud, A. (1965). *The writings of Anna Freud: Vol. 6. Normality and pathology in childhood: Assessments of development*. New York: International Universities Press.

Freud, S. (1960). *A general introduction to psychoanalysis*. New York: Washington Square Press. (Original work published 1935)

Freud, S. (1964). An outline of psychoanalysis. In J. Strachey (Ed. & Trans.), *The standard edition of the complete psychological works of Sigmund Freud, Vol. 19*. London: Hogarth Press. (Originally work published 1924)

Gesell, A. (1928). *Infancy and human growth*. New York: Macmillan.

Grusec, J. E., & Lytton, H. (1988). *Social development*. New York: Springer-Verlag.

Hall, G. S. (1904). *Adolescence*. New York: Appleton-Century-Crofts.

Harlow, H. F. (1958). The nature of love. *American Psychologist, 13*, 673–685.

Harter, S. (2001). *The construction of the self*. New York: Guilford Press.

Kagan, J., & Moss, H. A. (1962). *Birth to maturity*. New York: Wiley.

Keller, H. (2007). *Cultures of infancy*. Mahwah, NJ: Erlbaum.

Kohlberg, L. (1966). A cognitive-developmental analysis of children's sex-role concepts and attitudes. In E. E. Maccoby (Ed.), *The development of sex differences* (pp. 82–133). Stanford, CA: Stanford University Press.

Kohlberg, L. (1969). Stage and sequence: The cognitive-developmental approach to socialization. In D. A. Goslin (Ed.), *Handbook of socialization theory and research* (pp. 347–480). Chicago: Rand McNally.

Lewis, M. D. (2000). The promise of dynamic systems approaches for an integrated account of human development. *Child Development, 71*, 36–43.

Lewis, M. D., & Granic, I. (Eds.) (2000). *Emotion, development, and self-organization*. New York: Cambridge University Press.

Lewis, M. D., Lamey, A. V., & Douglas, L. (1999). A new dynamic systems method for the analysis of early socioemotional development. *Developmental Science, 2*, 457–475.

Locke, J. (1924). *An essay concerning human understanding*. Oxford: Clarendon. (Original work published 1690)

Lorenz, K. (1957). Companionship in bird life: Fellow members of social behavior. In C. H. Schiller (Ed.), *Instinctive behavior* (pp. 120–152). New York: International Universities Press.

Lorenz, K. Z. (1966). *On aggression*. San Diego, CA: Harcourt Brace Jovanovich.

Maccoby, E. E. (2006). Historical overview of socialization theory and research. In J. E. Grusec & P. D. Hastings (Eds.), *Handbook of socialization* (pp. 13–41). New York: Guilford Press.

Mahler, M., Pine, F., & Bergman, A. (1975). *The psychological birth of the human infant*. New York: Basic Books.

Miller, N. E., & Dollard, J. (1941). *Social learning and imitation*. New York: McGraw-Hill.

Miller, P. H. (2002). *Theories of developmental psychology* (4th ed.). New York: Worth.

Miller, P. H., & Aloise, P. A. (1989). Young children's understanding of the psychological causes of behavior: A review. *Child Development, 60*, 257–285.

Mussen, P., & Eisenberg-Berg, N. (1977). *Roots of caring, sharing, and helping: The development of prosocial behavior in children*. Oxford, UK: Freeman.

Ornstein, P. A., Haden, C. A., & Hedrick, A. M. (2004). Learning to remember: Social-communicative exchanges and the development of children's memory skills. *Developmental Review, 24*, 374–395.

Parke, R. D., Ornstein, P. A., Reiser, J. J., & Zahn-Waxler, C. (Eds.). (1994). *A century of developmental psychology*. Washington, DC: American Psychological Association.

Patterson, G. R. (1982). *Coercive family processes*. Eugene, OR: Castalia.

Pavlov, I. (1927). *Conditioned reflexes: An investigation of the physiological activity of the cerebral cortex.* Oxford, UK: Oxford University Press.

Piaget, J. (1932). *The moral judgment of the child.* London: Routledge & Kegan Paul.

Piaget, J. (1952). *The origins of intelligence in children.* New York: International Universities Press. (Original work published 1936)

Piaget, J. (1970). Piaget's theory. In P. H. Mussen (Ed.), *Carmichael's manual of child psychology* (Vol. 1, pp. 703–732). New York: Wiley.

Rogoff, B. (1990). *Apprenticeship in thinking.* New York: Oxford University Press.

Rousseau, J. J. (1969). *Emile.* New York; Dutton. (Original work published 1792)

Sears, R. R., Maccoby, E. E., & Levin, H. (1957). *Patterns of child rearing.* Evanston, IL: Row Peterson.

Sears, R. R., Rau, L., & Alpert, R. (1965). *Identification and child rearing.* Stanford, CA: Stanford University Press.

Selman, R. L. (1980). *The growth of interpersonal understanding.* Orlando, FL: Academic.

Shakespeare, W. (2004). *As you like it.* New York: Simon & Schuster. (Original work published 1600)

Skinner, B. F. (1948). *Walden two.* Indianapolis, IN: Hackett.

Skinner, B. F. (1953). *Science and human behavior.* New York: Macmillan.

Skinner, B. F. (1971). *Beyond freedom and dignity.* New York: Knopf.

Smith, L. B. (1995). Self-organizing processes in learning to learn new words: Development is not induction. In C. A. Nelson (Ed.), *Minnesota Symposia in Child Psychology: Vol. 28. New perspectives on learning and development* (pp. 1–32). Mahwah, NJ: Erlbaum.

Snyder, J., Cramer, A., Afrank, J., & Patterson, G. R. (2005). The contributions of ineffective discipline and parental hostile attributions of child misbehavior to the development of conduct problems at home and school. *Developmental Psychology, 41,* 30–41.

Spitz, R. (1965). *The first year of life.* Oxford, UK: International Universities Press.

Sroufe, L. A., Egeland, B., Carlson, E. A., & Collins, W. A. (2005). *The development of the person: The Minnesota Study of Risk and Adaptation from Birth to Adulthood.* New York: Guilford Press.

Stone, L. (1977). *The family, sex and marriage in England, 1500–1800.* New York: Harper & Row.

Thelen, E. (1989). Self-organization in developmental processes: Can systems approaches work? In M. R. Gunnar & E. Thelen (Eds.), *Minnesota Symposia on Child Psychology: Vol. 22. Systems and development* (pp. 77–118). Hillsdale, NJ: Erlbaum.

Thelen, E., & Smith, L. B. (2006). Dynamic systems theories. In R. M. Lerner & W. Damon (Eds.), *Handbook of child psychology: Vol. 1. Theoretical models of human development* (6th ed., pp. 258–312). Hoboken, NJ: Wiley.

Thompson, R. A. (2006). The development of the person: Social understanding, relationships, self, conscience. In W. Damon & R. M. Lerner (Series Eds.) & N. Eisenberg (Vol. Ed.), *Handbook of child psychology: Vol. 3. Social, emotional, and personality development* (pp. 24–98). New York: Wiley.

Thompson, R. A. (2009). Early foundations: Conscience and the development of moral character. In D. Narvaez & D. Lapsley (Eds.), *Personality, identity, and character: Explorations in moral psychology* (pp. 159–184) New York: Cambridge University Press.

Thompson, R. A., Laible, D. J., & Ontai, L. L. (2003). Early understanding of emotion, morality, and the self: Developing a working model. In R.V. Kail (Ed.), *Advances in child development and behavior* (Vol. 31, pp. 137–171). San Diego: Academic.

Vygotsky, L. (1962). *Thought and language.* Cambridge, MA: MIT Press. (Original work published 1934)

Vygotsky, L. (1978). *Mind in society.* Cambridge, MA: Harvard University Press. (Original work published 1930)

Wallerstein, J. S., & Kelly, J. B. (1996). *Surviving the breakup.* New York: Basic Books.

Watson, J. (1913). Psychology as the behaviorist views it. *Psychological Review, 20,* 158–177.

Watson, J. B. (1924). *Behaviorism.* New York: Norton.

Watson, J. B. (1928). *Psychological care of infant and child.* New York: Norton.

2

Biological Correlates of Social Development

Leslie J. Carver
Lisa Tully

From the earliest days of development, infants engage with their caregivers to establish what may be the most important relationship of their lives. Despite the importance of this relationship, we know relatively little about events at the heart of its development. What are the biological events that lead to the emotional linking between two people? We know surprisingly little about what happens during the construction of relationships from a biological perspective, especially in humans. However, we have an increasingly large literature on the biology of parent–infant bonds in animals (especially about what happens to mothers) to form some ideas about the biological basis for relationships in humans.

This chapter has two main purposes. First, we digress briefly to discuss methods used to study the brain and behavior in humans, with an emphasis on how difficult these methods are to apply to the question of social relationships. Second, we describe the biological factors that are thought to lead to the development of the bond between infant and mother. We focus on this relationship because it is one of the most well-understood human relationships and because some of the same mechanisms seem to be at play in later romantic relationships, which we briefly touch on. The biology of important relationships between infancy and adulthood, primarily those between children and their peers, is largely unstudied. Finally, we describe briefly the interplay between social relationships and the biological basis of specific social behaviors. We propose future research that might elucidate some of the many questions that arise from considering this issue.

Although there is a large and growing literature on the neural correlates of cognition, attention, and perception in development, developmental social neuroscience has been much slower to emerge. This has been in large part due to the constraints that exist in the kinds of methodologies that can be applied to early brain–behavior relations. Many of the methods that have provided important information about brain–behavior relations in adults are difficult to use in children, and even those that are usable with children and infants are highly constrained. For example, in functional neuroimaging studies, blood flow is measured as participants watch stimuli and perform cognitive tasks. Because of the relatively long time course of blood flow in the brain, participants need to remain very still during these tasks. In electrophysiology studies, electrodes are placed on the scalp of the participant, and electrical activity produced by the brain is measured. In event-related potential (ERP) studies, brain responses are time locked to the presentation of discrete stimuli. Because the signals generated by these stimuli are small and there is a great deal of background electro-encephalographic (EEG) activity, the signal-to-noise ratio in such studies is small. In order to acquire an interpretable signal in this context, stimuli need to be displayed very briefly and repeated many times.

Constraints such as these make it difficult to explore social phenomena, which, by their nature, are fluid events that develop over time. Nevertheless, progress has been made, primarily by combining behavioral measures with brain and biological measures. For example, Striano and colleagues (Striano, Reid, & Hoehl, 2006; Striano & Stahl, 2005) have used clever manipulations of joint attention, along with ERP measures, to show how the developing brain allocates attention differently when in a shared-attention context than when in a context in which an observer is seen looking at an object but without sharing attention with the infant being tested. This and other recent creative methodological developments have led to the emergence of a developmental social neuroscience, in which the developmental antecedents of social behavior and social cognition have begun to be explored.

One area that remains of interest, and in which there are relatively few data, is on the influence of relationships on how these brain systems develop. In order to begin to address these issues, we start with the area in which the most is probably known, albeit due to studies of animals. This is the bidirectional influence of neurochemicals and hormones in close, intimate relationships. We focus here on the relationship between a mother and her newborn infant, although note that many of the same mechanisms appear to be at work in later adolescent and adult romantic relationships (e.g. Gordon et al., 2008).

BIOLOGICAL ASPECTS OF SOCIAL DEVELOPMENT

The fundamental units of communication in the brain are neurotransmitters. Neurotransmitters are neurochemicals that are released at the junction between two synapses, typically in response to depolarization of the presynaptic neuron. After release from the presynaptic axon terminal, neurotransmitters are taken up by receptors located on the postsynaptic cell. Excess amounts of neurotransmitters left in the gap between neurons are returned to the presynaptic terminal through reuptake mechanisms. In this section, we summarize what is known about three major neurochemicals that are likely to be involved in social interactions, their functions and contributions to the early development of the attachment relationship, and how they develop.

Serotonin

The Function of Serotonin

Serotonin (5-HT) is an inhibitory neurotransmitter in the central nervous system and can be measured in the blood, cerebrospinal fluid (CSF), through positron emission tomography (PET) scans, and by genetic testing. Central levels of serotonin can be measured in CSF (5-HIAA). Serotonin has a variety of functions, including regulating mood, aggression, and anger. Measures of serotonin levels in rhesus macaques indicate that early maternal interaction has lasting effects on the levels of serotonin (Ichise et al., 2006; Maestripieri, Hoffman, Anderson, Carter, & Higley, 2009), and genotype studies in humans point to the differential susceptibility to the influence of maternal interaction (Barry, Kochanska, & Philibert, 2008; Spangler, Johann, Ronai, & Zimmermann, 2009).

Serotonin and Attachment

One way to measure serotonin without drawing blood is with PET scans, which allow the accurate quantitative imaging of serotonin transporter (SERT) binding. Maternal deprivation in the first 6 months of a rhesus monkey's life can affect the development of the serotonergic system by decreasing SERT binding potential in various critical regions of the brain (Ichise et al., 2006).

The effects of maternal deprivation can also be seen in CSF 5-HIAA concentrations as early as 14 days of life (Shannon et al., 2005). Infant monkeys who were hand-raised in nurseries had significantly lower CSF 5-HIAA concentrations over the first 5 months of life than infants who were reared by their mothers since birth. For both groups, CSF 5-HIAA concentrations declined over time, whereas individual differences remained stable.

Total maternal deprivation is not necessary for this difference to occur. Rhesus macaque infants who experienced high rates of maternal rejection in the first 6 months of life also have lower CSF 5-HIAA concentrations than infants who experienced low rates of rejection (Maestripieri et al., 2009; Maestripieri, McCormack, Lindell, Higley, & Sanchez, 2006). The effect was found both for infants raised by their biological mothers and for those who were cross-fostered (e.g., raised by an unrelated female since birth), suggesting that experience might be driving the association, rather than pure genetic inheritance (Maestripieri et al., 2006). Although it is possible that infants with low CSF 5-HIAA concentrations behave in a way that might cause an adult to be more rejecting, this is probably not the case, because rhesus macaque mothers who are rejecting are generally rejecting to *all* infants in their care across time and are not selectively rejecting (Maestripieri, Lindell, Ayala, Gold, & Higley, 2005). Infants who experienced high rates of maternal rejection displayed more anxiety in the second year of life than those who experienced low rates of rejection, suggesting that the atypical serotonin levels might also be expressed in abnormal social behavior.

Those cross-fostered female infants then went on to have children of their own when they were 4–5 years of age. The rates of rejection displayed by the adult cross-fostered females over the first 3 months of motherhood were positively associated with the rates of rejection they experienced from their foster mothers (Maestripieri, Lindell, & Higley, 2007). In addition, most of the cross-fostered females with lower CSF 5-HIAA in the second year of life exhibited higher rates of rejection of their own infants. This suggests that the biological impact of the early caregiving environment can have effects across generations.

Another study found the opposite result, with abusive mothers evincing significantly higher CSF 5-HIAA concentrations than nonabusive mothers (Maestripieri et al., 2005). The CSF 5-HIAA levels were also positively correlated with maternal rejection of the infant. This study measured CSF 5-HIAA levels in adulthood, whereas the previous study measured childhood levels, so it is possible that the relation between early experience and serotonin activity changes over the course of development. Levels of serotonin diminish at different rates over time for maltreated and nonmaltreated rhesus macaques (Shannon et al., 2005).

In addition, maternal separation has been found to have a differential effect on young rhesus monkeys based on their baseline levels of withdrawal behavior 2 weeks before separation (Erickson et al., 2005). At 6–7 months of age, the infants were separated from their mothers for the first time. Highly withdrawn infants had significantly higher 5-HIAA levels during separation than infants who displayed moderate or low withdrawal behavior. This study did not measure maternal behavior, so it is not known whether the quality of the maternal interaction influenced the intensity of the withdrawal behavior or the level of 5-HIAA concentrations. It is also possible that there was an interaction of genetic predisposition on the impact of the environmental stressor, but this possibility has not yet been measured directly in rhesus macaques.

Genetic correlations between serotonin and social behavior have been evaluated in human infants. The 5-HTTLPR gene codes for serotonin transcription efficiency, transporter levels, and serotonin uptake. The short allele (s) has been associated with diminished serotonin capacity compared with the long allele (l), thus conferring risk for a number of emotional and behavioral disorders (Barry et al., 2008).

The evidence for an association between attachment style and 5-HTTLPR genotype is mixed. When data from infants homozygous for the short allele (ss) were combined with those from infants carrying heterozygous alleles (sl), an association was found (Barry et al., 2008). However, in a second study, the sl and ll groups' data were combined, and there was no relation between genotype and attachment security. Instead, relations between genotype and infant fearfulness were mediated by caregiver behavior (Pauli-Pott, Friedl, Hinney, & Hebebrand, 2009). Because the former study also found that all infants who were classified as disorganized or unclassifiable carried at least one short allele (ss/sl), it seems likely that it is the presence of a single (s) allele that confers risk for the development of insecure attachment. It is possible that the latter study's method of combining the infants with ll and sl genotypes washed out any possible effects.

However, attachment is most likely not determined by genotype alone. The environmental variable that has received the most attention for its influence on attachment security is maternal sensitivity. A meta-analysis revealed that the relationship between attachment security and maternal sensitivity was moderately strong, indicating that although maternal sensitivity is important, it is not the sole determinant of attachment style (De Wolff & van IJzendoorn, 1997).

The combination of environmental risk (i.e., maternal sensitivity) and genetic risk (i.e., short 5-HTTLPR allele) increases the likelihood of developing an insecure attachment (Barry et al., 2008; Spangler et al., 2009). For infants with mothers who are low in responsiveness, risk for developing disorganized attachment increased with the number of short alleles (Spangler et al., 2009). There was no association between genotype and attachment disorganization for the infants who experienced high maternal sensitivity. In another study, infants with at least one short allele (*ss/sl*) were more likely to be securely attached at age 15 months if their mothers had been highly responsive at 7 months of age than infants whose mothers were relatively unresponsive (Barry et al., 2008). The attachment security of children who were homozygous for long alleles (*ll*) was not influenced by the degree of maternal sensitivity experienced at 7 months of age. Both studies found that mother's responsiveness was not related to child genotype, which suggests that genotype was not driving the infants to behave in a manner that caused their mothers to be more or less sensitive.

Summary

Maternal interactions can permanently alter the levels of serotonin in rhesus monkey infants, with maternal deprivation and abuse leading to lower levels of serotonin. Genetic predispositions cause human infants to be differentially susceptible to the effects of maternal sensitivity. Infants carrying at least one short allele of the 5-HTTLPR gene are at greater risk of developing an insecure attachment if they also have mothers who do not respond in a sensitive manner.

Oxytocin

The Function of Oxytocin

Oxytocin (OT) is a neuropeptide that can be measured peripherally in the blood (plasma OT) and centrally in the cerebrospinal fluid (CSF OT). Human studies mostly use the less invasive peripheral measures, and it is not known how these measures relate to central OT levels (Campbell, 2008). It is well documented that oxytocin contributes to the onset of maternal care behavior and adult pair bonding (Feldman, Weller, Zagoory-Sharon, & Levine, 2007; Tops, Van Peer, Korf, Wijers, & Tucker, 2007). In human mothers, OT decreases anxiety and stress and enhances feelings of bonding with their infants (see Campbell, 2008, for review). It also works to lessen the stress response as it decreases the release of stress hormones (see Heinrichs, von Dawans, & Domes, 2009; Lee, Macbeth, Pagani, & Young, 2009, for review).

Oxytocin and Maternal Behavior

Unlike serotonin, plasma oxytocin is not related to maternal rejection in rhesus monkeys (Maestripieri et al., 2009). It is, however, related to maternal warmth, which includes nursing, cradling, and grooming the infant. These behaviors could influence the attachment of the infant to the mother, but there are no data on whether or not this influences the levels of OT found in the infant.

Plasma OT levels during pregnancy are also positively related to postpartum maternal warmth in humans, as well as to maternal cognitive representations of attachment and bonding to the infant (Feldman et al., 2007). Levels of plasma OT were found to be consistent across pregnancy and the postpartum period, and they predicted postpartum maternal behavior. Again, there are no data on how this reflects on the levels of OT found in infants.

It seems possible that OT levels influence mothers to act in a manner that behaviorally increases the likelihood of developing secure attachment in infants. However, we know very little about the developmental influences of oxytocin in infants. Because

OT and OT receptors (OTR) are modulated by estrogen, it is possible that OT functions in different ways across the life cycle. Most of the infant research has been conducted on rodents, but a few studies have been conducted with primates.

Oxytocin and Attachment

In rats, early experience can change the levels of OTR binding, as well as influence subsequent maternal care behavior in adulthood (Champagne & Meaney, 2007). There appears to be some plasticity in that multiple environmental influences can have a unique impact on the levels of OTR binding in rats. If the rearing environment is normal, early maternal care will influence the levels of OTR binding, with low maternal care leading to lower levels of OTR binding. The effects of early maternal care are minimized if the infant then experiences an environment that is outside the normal experience (either enriched or impoverished). The pups in this study had only 1 week of maternal care, so we do not know much about a possible critical period to this plasticity. The levels of OTR binding were also expressed behaviorally in the levels of licking and grooming behavior these rats displayed to their own infants.

Similar correlations are seen in primates. Rhesus monkeys who were raised in isolation for the first 45–60 days of life and then placed with peers exhibited decreased CSF OT levels compared with monkeys who had been raised by their mothers for the first year of life (Winslow, Noble, Lyons, Sterk, & Insel, 2003). These differences were consistent from 18 to 36 months of age. The monkeys raised in isolation also exhibited less affiliative social behavior and more solitary and repetitive behavior compared with the mother-reared monkeys. Plasma OT levels did not correlate with CSF OT levels or with infant behavior.

Although OT has not been measured in human infants, it has been measured in older children and adults. In one study, OT levels were measured in children after interactions with their mothers and an unfamiliar woman. All children in this study were currently experiencing typical home environments, but some children had experienced severe deprivation while being raised in impoverished orphanages early in development and were currently living in adoptive homes. OT levels were lower in the children who had a history of institutionalization than in the comparison sample (Wismer Fries, Ziegler, Kurian, Jacoris, & Pollak, 2005). In addition, baseline levels of another neuropeptide important for social interaction, vasopressin, were lower for the postinstitutionalized sample. This finding suggests that early experience has an important impact on how the brain responds to social interactions. In adults, higher plasma OT levels in college students were related to self-reporting of greater bonding with parents and lower levels of psychological distress (Gordon et al., 2008). Higher plasma OT levels in women are associated with a greater tendency to share emotional experiences with friends (Tops et al., 2007).

OT is also involved in the early stages of face processing, a crucial skill for developing social bonds and attachments. When OT is administered intranasally to males, their recognition accuracy for faces improves, whereas there is no effect for nonsocial stimuli (Rimmele, Hediger, Heinrichs, & Klaver, 2009). OT may also improve memory for happy faces in particular (Guastella, Mitchell, & Mathews, 2008). It is possible that OT helped participants focus on positive social information, information that is used in the creation of social bonds. In both studies, OT did not affect people's perception of the stimuli, but rather only their feelings of familiarity with the stimuli. Information on whether or not OT functions in the same way in infancy is currently missing. Because face recognition in infancy is one of the building blocks for forming attachment, the role of OT is critical for our understanding of how attachment develops in infancy.

Summary

Early rearing conditions have lasting effects on central OT levels in primates and peripheral OT levels in rodents, as well as on social behavior in both species. Research indicates that OT levels are associated with social bonding in adults, but currently there are no data on the developmental function of OT in human infants. Because OT is responsive to estrogen, it does not seem safe to simply assume that OT functions in the same way in infancy as it does in adulthood.

Not only does OT increase social bonding, but it also works as an anxiolytic. In this way, OT functioning is tied to cortisol functioning in that it dampens cortisol's response to stress. Measuring cortisol may be one way of measuring the brain's sensitivity to OT. It is possible that early experience can alter the brain's sensitivity to OT as seen through cortisol levels. Compared with control subjects, college-age men who had experienced prolonged or permanent separation from one parent before the age of 13 exhibited smaller decreases in cortisol after receiving OT intranasally relative to receiving a placebo (Meinlschmidt & Heim, 2007). This result indicates that men with early parental separation were not benefiting from the additional OT as much as men who did not experience an early separation and, in turn, did not experience a decrease in cortisol. In this way, differences in cortisol levels may reflect dysfunction in other systems.

Cortisol

The Function of Cortisol

Cortisol is a hormone commonly referred to as the "stress hormone." Although responsible for a variety of functions, it is best known for regulating the body's response to stressors. Cortisol is released in higher levels during stress and aids in the onset of the physiological changes associated with the activation of the sympathetic nervous system. There are developmental changes in normative basal levels of cortisol and its circadian patterns through the day. In contrast to adults, who have a single peak in basal cortisol levels during the day, newborn infants have two peaks (Francis et al., 1987). By 3 months of age, infants show a morning peak in cortisol levels, similarly to adults, and a dip in the evening (Price, Close, & Fielding, 1983). An important component of the cortisol system is a well-understood circuit involving the adrenal gland, the pituitary, and the hypothalamus, among other brain areas. This system responds to stressful events and is regulated through feedback loops in the brain (see de Kloet, Fitzsimons, Datson, Meijer, & Vreugdenhil, 2009). Cortisol levels can be measured in saliva, blood, and urine. Currently, little is known about the consequences of differences in measurement.

Cortisol and Social Relationships

Supportive social relationships and OT are thought to modulate the release of cortisol. College-age men had lower cortisol levels following a speech stressor when their best friends were present compared with men who did not have the support of a friend (Heinrichs, Baumgartner, Kirschbaum, & Ehlert, 2003). Although OT did not have as large an effect on cortisol levels, OT and social support both increased feelings of calmness and decreased feelings of anxiety during the stressor.

Individual differences in cortisol levels may affect an individual's ability to benefit from the buffering effects of social relationships. And as the data on men who experienced early parental separation indicate, it is possible that different experiences in life alter this ability (Meinlschmidt & Heim, 2007).

Cortisol and Attachment

Lower plasma cortisol levels in women during pregnancy were predictive of greater levels of mothers' attention, such as gaze, affect, touch, and vocalization, directed toward their babies (Feldman et al., 2007). Once again, these maternal behaviors may increase the likelihood of a secure attachment in their infants; however, we do not know whether maternal cortisol levels influence infant cortisol levels.

In rhesus macaques, maternal interaction has lasting effects on an infant's cortisol response to stress. When presented with a stressor, mother-reared monkeys exhibited a reduced cortisol response when in the presence of a familiar peer (Winslow et al., 2003). This response was not seen in monkeys that had been raised in a nursery with human caretakers attending to their physical needs. Mother-reared monkeys also exhibited an increase in social contact and a reduction in abnormal repetitive behavior. Thus these nursery-reared monkeys were not able to benefit from social support in the same way as mother-reared monkeys. From these data, it is not possible to determine whether being deprived of maternal interaction prevented the cortisol system from developing properly or prevented the monkey from learning how to behave in a way that reaps the benefits of social support. It would be beneficial to know whether a nursery-reared monkey could subsequently be taught how to interact in a socially positive manner and whether that would have any effects on cortisol levels. It is interesting to note that the basal plasma cortisol levels did not differ between nursery-reared monkeys and monkeys who were raised by their mothers for the first year of life (Winslow et al., 2003). This seems to indicate that maternal interaction has effects only on an infant's response to a stressor and not on everyday stress levels. However, the mother-raised monkeys had experienced a 4-week separation from their mothers before cortisol levels were measured, during which time basal cortisol levels may have changed.

There is a small literature on connections between social relationships and cortisol activity in humans. Although most studies involve the extremes of caregiving environments, there is evidence that the cortisol system is dysregulated in children who have experienced maltreatment (Hart, Gunnar, & Cicchetti, 1995), neglect (Wismer Fries, Shirtcliff, & Pollak, 2008), or harsh parenting (Bugental, Martorell, & Barraza, 2003).

The quality of the maternal interaction may also shape the stress response. Young rhesus monkey infants who were more protected by their mothers had higher plasma cortisol levels (Maestripieri et al., 2009). The infants were trapped and placed into a squeeze cage overnight before cortisol levels were measured the following day. It is possible that these infants experienced the trapping procedure as more stressful because they were accustomed to having the security of their mothers.

In the same vein, it is possible that there is a similar correlation in humans. Preliminary evidence suggests that human maternal insensitivity during diaper changing coincides with increased salivary cortisol levels in infants (Morelius, Nelson, & Gustafsson, 2006). Although this association was not addressed statistically and age effects seemed to be present, it is an interesting model that deserves further consideration in light of the evidence from rhesus monkeys.

Attachment security has been directly associated with cortisol levels. Disorganized attachment, in particular, is related to higher levels of cortisol following the stress-inducing Strange Situation procedure in both at-risk and low-risk toddlers (Hertsgaard, Gunnar, Erickson, & Nachmias, 1995; Spangler & Grossmann, 1993). Insecurely attached toddlers exhibited an increase in cortisol, whereas securely attached toddlers experienced a decrease following the Strange Situation procedure. As with the monkeys, the initial cortisol levels of these toddlers did not differ based on attachment style (Spangler & Grossmann, 1993). Once again, cortisol levels seem to be influenced by either knowing how to use social support or having social support available in the face of stress. Behavioral differences were not seen between the attachment groups, perhaps in part because cortisol is a slowly acting system.

When low-risk toddlers were left at day care for the first time, those who were securely attached showed less increase in cortisol levels than those who were insecurely attached (Ahnert, Gunnar, Lamb, & Barthel, 2004). So once again, the insecurely attached toddlers had an increased cortisol response to a stressor compared with the securely attached toddlers. Because behavioral measures of social interaction were not taken, there is no evidence to suggest whether the relationship is a result of being better able to use the social support of peers, of the comforting effects of an increased expectation that the mother will return, or purely of the functioning of the cortisol system.

Other factors have also been found to moderate the relationship between attachment style and cortisol levels. When infants were separated into a high-fearful group and a low- to average-fearful group based on parent report, cortisol levels in response to a well-baby immunization shot at 15 months and the Strange Situation at 18 months differed by attachment style only if the infant was also in the high-fearful group (Gunnar, Brodersen, Machmian, Buss, & Rigatuso, 1996). For low- to average-fearful children, attachment style was not associated with cortisol levels. It is important to note that fearfulness was not associated with attachment style. Compared with insecurely attached toddlers, securely attached toddlers had mothers who were more sensitive and responsive to them during their 2- and 6-month well-baby shots. Securely attached toddlers also had significantly lower basal cortisol levels at 2–6 months of age than insecurely attached toddlers. However, cortisol response to inoculations and crying behavior did not predict later attachment security. This pattern is different from that seen in rhesus monkeys, which may be due to the different ages at which cortisol measures were taken, as well as the type of measure (central vs. peripheral).

It is possible that maternal behavior influences a child's ability to cope with stress. One study separated children into high- and low-inhibition groups based on parent reports of the children's response to new situations. Insecure children with higher inhibition had higher cortisol levels than secure children with higher inhibition after experiencing a highly stimulating and/or stressful event (Nachmias, Gunnar, Mangelsdorf, & Parritz, 1996). Mothers who encouraged their infants to approach the novel stimuli more and gave more comfort had toddlers with higher post-session cortisol. This may shed some light on the mechanism by which maternal interaction contributes to later attachment security. Although the results may appear counterintuitive, the authors suggest that by being too intrusive, mothers may be interfering with an inhibited child's natural coping mechanism and thereby causing greater stress. It is possible that forcing an inhibited child to explore a highly stimulating situation too quickly will produce an amount of stress that is beyond what maternal comfort can counteract. It is also possible that this form of parenting could be considered insensitive given the child's individual temperament.

Fearfulness and inhibition seem to be related personality factors. It would be beneficial to explore whether or not these factors are associated with the serotonin genotype. Variations in serotonin-related genotype have also been differentially associated with risk of insecure attachment. Research on the developmental implications of this genotype for personality development might provide important insight into gene–environment interaction in the development of mother–infant relationships.

Summary

Social support buffers adult humans from the effects of stressors, and, in the same way, a highly responsive mother can lessen the impact of stressors for her child. What is unclear is whether or not cortisol functioning is actively shaping a child's ability to form a social bond or merely reflecting the outcome of another system. This last line of research, measuring maternal responsiveness, child attachment, and cortisol, should be combined with measures of OT and serotonin to get a more complete picture of how biology is involved in the development of attachment relationships in infancy.

INFLUENCE OF SOCIAL RELATIONSHIPS ON BRAIN DEVELOPMENT

Other research has focused on the effects of various kinds of social experience on the developing brain. Early studies used PET to measure glucose utilization in institutionalized children (Chugani, Phelps, & Mazziotta, 1987). In general, these studies have found that glucose utilization and brain size are smaller in children who experienced severe deprivation in institutions. However, early studies did not always measure correlates of social behavior, so it is not entirely clear what effects this reduction in brain size and blood flow had on social behavior. More recent research has shown that the volume of the superior posterior cerebellar lobes is smaller in children who experienced severe neglect and that the size of this brain area is related to cognitive functioning (Bauer, Hanson, Pierson, Davidson, & Pollak, 2009).

One area in which relations between social interactions and brain development have been reasonably well described is response to faces and facial expressions of emotions. In one study, brain responses to facial expressions of emotions were measured in Romanian children who were currently placed in poor-quality orphanages, children who had been in orphanages but were randomly assigned to a foster care program, and control children living with their families of origin (Moulson, Fox, Zeanah, & Nelson, 2009). Although the ability to differentiate emotional expressions was not affected, overall brain responses were lowest in children who remained in the orphanage, but responses were intermediate in the foster care group. This result suggested that an improvement in social environment led to an overall improvement in brain function.

Another series of studies has been conducted with children who have suffered severe abuse and neglect. In these children, behavioral evidence suggests increased sensitivity to emotional signals (Pollak, Cicchetti, Hornung, & Reed, 2000; Pollak & Sinha, 2002). In one study (Shackman, Shackman, & Pollak, 2007), children who had been severely abused saw pictures of emotional faces, some posed by their mothers (who were confirmed to be the abusers in all cases) and some posed by a stranger. At the same time, children heard their mothers' voices and a stranger's voice uttering phrases in the same emotions. On some trials the emotion displayed on faces and that heard spoken were consistent with each other, and on other trials they were incongruent. Children were instructed to attend to faces in one study and to voices in another and to press a button when they detected a specific emotion in whichever modality they were instructed to attend to. Children who had been abused showed increased amplitude in an ERP component that is associated with attention in response to their mothers' faces posing angry emotions. There were no differences in responses to stranger's voices posing anger and no differences in responses to happy and sad voices. When instructed to attend to the voices, children who had been abused showed an increase in attentional response to anger, although this response was not specific to their mothers, as it was for faces. And, even when the angry emotion was not relevant to the task (e.g., the target was happy or sad), children who had been abused showed increased attentional ERP responses. This finding, along with behavioral evidence from the same lab, suggests that attentional systems in the brain are changed by negative social experiences.

There is relatively little information about effects of more typical social experiences on brain and biological development. In one series of studies, we (Swingler, Carver, & Sweet, 2010; Swingler, Sweet, & Carver, 2007) have sought to relate infants' brain responses to their mothers' faces and a stranger's face to their behavior on separation from their mothers. We tested very young infants (6 months old). They were separated from their caregivers for a short period of time, and we examined their behavior in response to the separation and on reunion with the caregivers. In this sample of children experiencing a typical range of caregiving environments, we found that proximity-seeking behaviors in 6-month-olds were predictive of brain responses, especially to the mothers' faces (Swingler et al., 2007), and, in a subsequent analysis (Swingler et al., 2010), that distress on separation was the primary driver of this relation in these very young infants. It remains to be seen whether these relations between brain responses to faces and social behavior are due to the relationship between the infant and his or her caregiver or whether they are the effect of temperamental factors the infant brings to the relationship. One possibility is that our separation procedure activated the attachment system in these infants and thus that the brain activity patterns we observed were the result of physiological responses driven by the activation of this behavioral system. In future research, this procedure might be a useful index of the kinds of physiological responses that drive infants to form relationships with caregivers. These data hint that the caregiving environment is related to important social functions, although of course it is not possible to tell what causal mechanisms are at work here.

FUTURE DIRECTIONS

Thus far, we have described some of the research on the bidirectional relations between biological and social development. Although the preceding review shows that there has been some progress in identifying the biological correlates of social development, primarily in animals, there is a small literature on the effects of social interaction on brain development, and there are still many steps that need to be taken.

Although we are learning a great deal from animal models about the physiological and neural correlates and consequences of relationships, there is much that we still do not know. Many of the studies of neurochemicals and their roles in social behavior have been limited to nonhuman species. Future research on how these mechanisms function in humans would provide important information toward understanding the biology of social development. In addition, advances in genetics research can inform us about how genes and environment can interact to produce relationships and their consequent effects on social behavior.

Of primary importance is the need to bring these new developments together with theories about the development of social behavior and social cognition. For example, we (Carver & Cornew, 2009) have described a putative brain system that is thought to develop in support of social cognition. In brief, this system involves cortical areas known to be involved in social information processing (Anderson et al., 2004; Ochsner et al., 2004) and emotion detection (Adolphs, Baron-Cohen, & Tranel, 2002; Adolphs et al., 2005) and develops as a more primitive system of obligatory attention feeds into a higher volitional attention system after repeated experiences (Rueda, Posner, & Rothbart, 2005). However, in our previous discussion of this putative social cognitive system, the factor that remained unaddressed was the role of relationships in the development of the system. Relationships are integral to the model we proposed: The experiences that drive the putative transitions between obligatory attention to social, shared volitional attention involve interactions with another person, and, in infancy, that person is most likely the primary caregiver.

The nature of the relationship between the infant and the caregiver and, indeed, the very fact of that relationship are essential components in the development of social cognition. As children develop, other relationships begin to take center stage. Although peer relationships are extraordinarily important for children, almost nothing is known about the role of brain and biological factors in how children form them. In addition, in the same way that maternal relationships shape biological systems in infancy, peer relationships likely have some effect on social brain systems and their physiology. Future theory on how the brain system that underlies multiple aspects of social behavior develops should carefully consider the role of social relationships.

SUGGESTED READINGS

Barry R. A., Kochanska G., & Philibert R. A. (2008). G x E interaction in the organization of attachment: Mothers' responsiveness as a moderator of children's genotypes. *Journal of Child Psychology and Psychiatry, 49*, 1313–1320.

Carver, L. J., & Vaccaro, B. G. (2007). Twelve-month-old infants allocate increased neural resources to stimuli associated with negative parental expressions, *Developmental Psychology, 43*, 54–69.

Maestripieri, D., Hoffman, C. L., Anderson, G. M., Carter, C. S., & Higley, J. D. (2009). Mother–infant interactions in free-ranging rhesus macaques: Relationships between physiological and behavioral variables. *Physiology and Behavior, 96*, 613–619.

Striano, T., Reid, V. M., & Hoehl, S. (2006). Neural mechanisms of joint attention in infancy. *European Journal of Neuroscience, 23*, 2819–2823.

Swingler, M. M., Sweet, M., & Carver, L. J. (2007). Relation between mother–child interactions and the neural correlates of face perception in 6-month-old infants. *Infancy, 11*, 63–86.

Winslow, J. T., Noble, P. L., Lyons, C. K., Sterk, S. M., & Insel, T. R. (2003). Rearing effects on cerebrospinal fluid oxytocin concentration and social buffering in rhesus monkeys. *Neuropsychopharmacology, 28*, 910–918.

REFERENCES

Adolphs, R., Baron-Cohen, S., & Tranel, D. (2002). Impaired recognition of social emotions following amygdala damage. *Journal of Cognitive Neuroscience, 14*(8), 1264–1274.

Adolphs, R., Gosselin, F., Buchanan, T. W., Tranel, D., Schyns, P., & Damasio, A. R. (2005). A mechanism for impaired fear recognition after amygdala damage. *Nature, 433*, 68–72.

Ahnert, L., Gunnar, M. R., Lamb, M. E., & Barthel, M. (2004). Transition to child care: Associations with infant–mother attachment, infant negative emotion, and cortisol elevations. *Child Development, 75*, 639–650.

Anderson, M. C., Ochsner, K. N., Kuhl, B., Cooper, J., Robertson, E., Gabrieli, S. W., et al. (2004). Neural systems underlying the suppression of unwanted memories. *Science, 303*, 232–235.

Barry, R. A., Kochanska, G., & Philibert, R. A. (2008). G × E interaction in the organization of attachment: Mothers' responsiveness as a moderator of children's genotypes. *Journal of Child Psychology and Psychiatry, 49*, 1313–1320.

Bauer, P. M., Hanson, J. L., Pierson, R. K., Davidson, R. J., & Pollak, S. D. (2009). Cerebellar volume and cognitive functioning in children who experienced early deprivation. *Biological Psychiatry, 66*, 1100–1106.

Bugental, D. B., Martorell, G. A., & Barraza, V. (2003). The hormonal costs of subtle forms of infant maltreatment. *Hormones and Behavior, 43*, 237–244.

Campbell, A. (2008). Attachment, aggression and affiliation: The role of oxytocin in female social behavior. *Biological Psychology, 77*, 1–10.

Carver, L. J., & Cornew, L. (2009). Development of social information gathering in infancy: A model of neural substrates and developmental mechanisms. In M. de Haan & M. Gunnar (Eds.), *Handbook of developmental social neuroscience* (pp. 122–141). New York: Guilford Press.

Champagne, F. A., & Meaney, M. J. (2007). Transgenerational effects of social environment on variations in maternal care and behavioral response to novelty. *Behavioral Neuroscience, 121*, 1353–1363.

Chugani, H. T., Phelps, M. E., & Mazziotta, J. C. (1987). Positron emission tomography study of human brain functional development. *Annals of Neurology, 22*, 487–497.

de Kloet, E. R., Fitzsimons, C. P., Datson, N. A., Meijer, O. C., & Vreugdenhil, E. (2009). Glucocorticoid signaling and stress-related limbic susceptibility pathway: About receptors, transcription machinery and microRNA. *Brain Research, 1293*, 129–141.

De Wolff, M., & van IJzendoorn, M. H. (1997). Sensitivity and attachment: A meta-analysis on parental antecedents of infant attachment. *Child Development, 68*, 571–591.

Erickson, K., Gabry, K. E., Schulkin, J., Gold, P., Lindell, S., Higley, J. D., et al. (2005). Social withdrawal behaviors in nonhuman primates and changes in neuroendocrine and monoamine concentrations during a separation paradigm. *Developmental Psychobiology, 46*, 331–339.

Feldman, R., Weller, A., Zagoory-Sharon, O., & Levine, A. (2007). Evidence for a neuroendocrinological foundation of human affiliation: Plasma oxytocin levels across pregnancy and the postpartum period predict mother–infant bonding. *Psychological Science, 18*, 965–970.

Francis, S. J., Walker, R. F., Riad-Fahmy, D., Hughes, D., Murphy, J. F., & Gray, O. P. (1987). Assessment of adrenocortical activity in term newborn infants using salivary cortisol determinants. *Journal of Pediatrics, 111*, 129–133.

Gordon, I., Zagoory-Sharon, O., Schneiderman, I., Leckman, J. F., Weller, A., et al. (2008). Oxytocin and cortisol in romantically unattached young adults: Associations with bonding and psychological distress. *Psychophysiology, 45*, 349–352.

Guastella, A. J., Mitchell, P. B., & Mathews, F. (2008). Oxytocin enhances the encoding of positive social memories in humans. *Biological Psychiatry, 64*, 256–258.

Gunnar, M. R., Brodersen, L., Machmian, M., Buss, K., & Rigatuso, J. (1996). Stress reactivity and attachment security. *Developmental Psychobiology, 29*, 191–204.

Hart, J., Gunnar, M., & Cicchetti, D. (1995). Salivary cortisol in maltreated children: Evidence of relations between neuroendocrine activity and social competence. *Development and Psychopathology, 7*, 11–26.

Heinrichs, M., Baumgartner, T., Kirschbaum, C., & Ehlert, U. (2003). Social support and oxytocin interact to suppress cortisol and subjective responses to psychosocial stress. *Biological Psychiatry, 54,* 1389–1398.

Heinrichs, M., von Dawans, B., & Domes, G. (2009). Oxytocin, vasopressin, and human social behavior. *Frontiers in Neuroendocrinology, 30,* 548–557.

Hertsgaard, L., Gunnar, M., Erickson, M. F., & Nachmias, M. (1995). Adrenocortical responses to the Strange Situation in infants with disorganized/disoriented attachment relationships. *Child Development, 66,* 1100–1106.

Ichise, M., Vines, D. C., Gura, T., Anderson, G. M., Suomi, S. J., Higley, J. D., et al. (2006). Effects of early life stress on [^{11}C]DASB positron emission tomography imaging of serotonin transporters in adolescent peer- and mother-reared rhesus monkeys. *Journal of Neuroscience, 26,* 4638–4643.

Lee, H., Macbeth, A. H., Pagani, J. H., & Young, W. S. (2009). Oxytocin: The great facilitator of life. *Progress in Neurobiology, 88,* 127–151.

Maestripieri, D., Hoffman, C. L., Anderson, G. M., Carter, C. S., & Higley, J. D. (2009). Mother–infant interactions in free-ranging rhesus macaques: Relationships between physiological and behavioral variables. *Physiology and Behavior, 96,* 613–619.

Maestripieri, D., Lindell, S. G., Ayala, A., Gold, P. W., & Higley, J. D. (2005). Neurobiological characteristics of rhesus macaque abusive mothers and their relation to social and maternal behavior. *Neuroscience and Biobehavioral Reviews, 29,* 51–57.

Maestripieri, D., Lindell, S. G., & Higley, J. D. (2007). Intergenerational transmission of maternal behavior in rhesus macaques and its underlying mechanisms. *Developmental Psychobiology, 49,* 165–171.

Maestripieri, D., McCormack, K., Lindell, S. G., Higley, J. D., & Sanchez, M. M. (2006). Influence of parenting style on the offspring's behaviour and CSF monoamine metabolite levels in crossfostered and noncrossfostered female rhesus macaques. *Behavioural Brain Research, 175,* 90–95.

Meinlschmidt, G., & Heim, C. (2007). Sensitivity to intranasal oxytocin in adult men with early parental separation. *Biological Psychiatry, 61,* 1109–1111.

Morelius, E., Nelson, N., & Gustafsson, P. A. (2006). Salivary cortisol response in mother–infant dyads at high psychosocial risk. *Child: Care, Health and Development, 33,* 128–136.

Moulson, M. C., Fox, N. A., Zeanah, C. H., & Nelson, C. A. (2009). Early adverse experiences and the neurobiology of facial emotion processing. *Developmental Psychology, 45,* 17–30.

Nachmias, M., Gunnar, M., Mangelsdorf, S., & Parritz, R. H. (1996). Behavioral inhibition and stress reactivity: The moderating role of attachment security. *Child Development, 67,* 508–522.

Ochsner, K. N., Knierim, K., Ludlow, D. H., Hanelin, J., Ramachandran, T., Glover, G., et al. (2004). Reflecting upon feelings: An fMRI study of neural systems supporting the attribution of emotion to self and other. *Journal of Cognitive Neuroscience, 16,* 1746–1772.

Pauli-Pott, U., Friedl, S., Hinney, A., & Hebebrand, J. (2009). Serotonin transporter gene polymorphism (5-HTTLPR), environmental conditions, and developing negative emotionality and fear in early childhood. *Journal of Neural Transmission, 116,* 503–512.

Pollak, S. D., Cicchetti, D., Hornung, K., & Reed, A. (2000). Recognizing emotion in faces: Developmental effects of child abuse and neglect. *Developmental Psychology, 36,* 679–688.

Pollak, S. D., & Sinha, P. (2002). Effects of early experience on children's recognition of facial displays of emotion. *Developmental Psychology, 38,* 784–791.

Price, D. A., Close, G. C., & Fielding, B. A. (1983). Age of appearance of circadian rhythm in salivary cortisol values in infancy. *Archives of Disease in Childhood, 58,* 454–456.

Rimmele, U., Hediger, K., Heinrichs, M., & Klaver, P. (2009). Oxytocin makes a face in memory familiar. *Journal of Neuroscience, 29,* 38–42.

Rueda, M. R., Posner, M. I., & Rothbart, M. K. (2005). The development of executive attention: Contributions to the emergence of self-regulation. *Developmental Neuropsychology, 28,* 573–594.

Shackman, J. E., Shackman, A. J., & Pollak, S. D. (2007). Physical abuse amplifies attention to threat and increases anxiety in children. *Emotion, 7,* 838–852.

Shannon, C., Schwandt, M. L., Champoux, M., Shoaf, S. E., Suomi, S. J., Linnoila, M., et al. (2005).

Maternal absence and stability of individual differences in CSF 5-HIAA concentrations in rhesus monkey infants. *American Journal of Psychiatry, 162,* 1658–1664.

Spangler, G., & Grossmann, K. E. (1993). Biobehavioral organization in securely and insecurely attached infants. *Child Development, 64,* 1439–1450.

Spangler, G., Johann, M., Ronai, Z., & Zimmermann, P. (2009). Genetic and environmental influence on attachment disorganization. *Journal of Child Psychology and Psychiatry, 50,* 952–961.

Striano, T., Reid, V. M., & Hoehl, S. (2006). Neural mechanisms of joint attention in infancy. *European Journal of Neuroscience, 23,* 2819–2823.

Striano, T., & Stahl, D. (2005). Sensitivity to triadic attention in early infancy. *Developmental Science, 8,* 333–343.

Swingler, M. M., Sweet, M., & Carver, L. J. (2007). Relation between mother–child interactions and the neural correlates of face perception in 6-month-old infants. *Infancy, 11,* 63–86.

Swingler, M. M., Sweet, M. A., & Carver, L. J. (2010). Brain–behavior correlations: Relationships between mother–stranger face processing and infants' behavioral responses to a separation from mother. *Developmental Psychology, 46,* 669–680.

Tops, M., Van Peer, J. M., Korf, J., Wijers, A. A., & Tucker, D. M. (2007). Anxiety, cortisol, and attachment predict plasma oxytocin. *Psychophysiology, 44,* 444–449.

Winslow, J. T., Noble, P. L., Lyons, C. K., Sterk, S. M., & Insel, T. R. (2003). Rearing effects on cerebrospinal fluid oxytocin concentration and social buffering in rhesus monkeys. *Neuropsychopharmacology, 28,* 910–918.

Wismer Fries, A. B., Shirtcliff, E. A., & Pollak, S. D. (2008). Neuroendocrine dysregulation following early social deprivation in children. *Developmental Psychobiology, 50,* 588–599.

Wismer Fries, A. B., Ziegler, T. E., Kurian, J. R., Jacoris, S., & Pollak, S. D. (2005). Early experience in humans is associated with changes in neuropeptides critical for regulating social behavior. *Proceedings of the National Academy of Science, 102,* 17237–17240.

3

Temperament, Emotion Regulation, and Social Development

Susan D. Calkins
Jennifer S. Mackler

Social competence has long been considered a hallmark of adaptive functioning in early childhood. At its core, social competence refers to how one forms and maintains relationships with others (Burt, Obradovic, Long, & Masten, 2008). A number of components of social competence have been studied, but in this chapter, we use the term to refer to social skills and peer relationships, including friendships and indicators of peer liking. Failures of social competence resulting in peer rejection (Miller-Johnson, Coie, Maumary-Gremaud, Bierman, & Conduct Problems Research Group, 2002) or withdrawal from the peer group (Hanish & Guerra, 2002; Hodges, Boivin, Vitaro, & Bukowski, 1999) are associated with numerous negative outcomes. Although early work on the predictors of social skills and peer relationships focused on how children were *thinking* about social partners (e.g., processing social cues and generating responses to specific peer behaviors; Dodge, Pettit, McClaskey, & Brown, 1986), most recent work has focused on the *emotion-relevant behaviors* that children exhibit in the peer environment and that may predict how they respond to the behavior of others (Denham et al., 2003; Eisenberg, Fabes, Guthrie, & Reiser, 2000; Graziano, Keane, & Calkins, 2007). Emotion-related behaviors may include children's own tendencies to react to the positive and negative behavior of others (i.e., their temperament) and how well they manage those reactions (i.e. their emotion regulation ability; Calkins & Hill, 2007).

In this chapter, we focus on the role of these two specific emotion-related processes—temperament and emotion regulation—as predictors of child functioning and social competence. We present evidence suggesting that the way in which early temperament influences later outcomes, including social competence, is through the emotion regulation skills and strategies that young children develop. We review this evidence with an emphasis on early childhood, as this is the age period in which most research has been conducted. We review the history and theory behind work in the areas of temperament and emotion regulation, examine how temperament affects the development of emotion regulation, and focus on how emotion processes are linked across development to particular indices of adjustment and social competence. Finally, we provide suggestions for future research that might help to fill gaps in our knowledge about how emotion regulation and social competence are linked.

TEMPERAMENT

The construct of temperament has been the focus of considerable developmental and clinical psychology research because it has the potential to capture the contribution of the child to early developmental processes. Temperament refers to individual characteristics that are assumed to have a biological or genetic basis, that determine the individual's affective, attentional, and motoric responding cross-situationally, and that play a role in subsequent social interactions and social functioning. Early temperament research focused on establishing taxonomies of temperament dimensions, addressing measurement issues, and examining stability of temperament across time. More recent longitudinal research has focused on the extent to which temperament affects adjustment and the development of psychopathology. In this section, we describe theoretical approaches to the construct of temperament, with a focus on Rothbart's influential theory. We also discuss the development and measurement of the construct and highlight the important role of biological processes in understanding the behavioral aspects of temperament.

Temperament Theory

The construct of temperament is typically viewed as the basic organization of personality that is observable as early as infancy. Temperament becomes elaborated over the course of development as the individual's skills, abilities, cognitions, and motivations become more sophisticated (Rothbart & Bates, 1998; Shiner & Caspi, 2003). Temperament thus refers primarily to early differences in emotional and behavioral characteristics that are relatively stable traits with genetic and biological components (DiLalla & Jones, 2000; Goldsmith, Lemery, Aksan, & Buss, 2000).

Current theorizing about infant and child temperament and its role in emotional functioning and social adjustment has its roots in the work of Thomas and Chess (Thomas, Birch, Chess, Hertzig, & Korn, 1964; Thomas & Chess, 1977; Thomas, Chess, & Birch, 1970). Thomas and Chess conducted a longitudinal study of children's behavioral styles, later termed *temperament*, in an effort to understand how children's personalities emerged and interacted with their environments. On the basis of interviews with parents about children's reactions to a variety of stimuli and situations, Thomas and Chess described nine different behavioral dimensions that clustered into three types, labeled *easy*, *difficult*, and *slow-to-warm-up* temperaments. Children displaying these different profiles exhibited characteristic patterns of responding across a variety of situations. Importantly, though, Thomas and Chess viewed the critical predictor of this adaptation to be the "goodness of fit" between a child's temperament and the environment. With their work, Thomas and Chess introduced the idea that children bring with them to their development, and to their interactions with others, their own style that plays a role in subsequent behavioral adaptation.

Thomas and Chess's work stimulated a number of researchers interested in early socioemotional development to explore the notion that inborn characteristics of the child contributed substantively to later behavior and to try to develop measurement strategies to capture these characteristics. Subsequent theories of temperament have varied in the numbers of temperament dimensions proposed, the emphasis on emotion versus behavior, and the extent to which the environment influences these initial tendencies (Fox, Henderson, & Marshall, 2001; Goldsmith et al., 1987; Rothbart & Bates, 1998).

For example, Seifer and colleagues (Seifer & Sameroff, 1986; Seifer, Schiller, Sameroff, Resnick, & Riordan, 1996) have extended Thomas and Chess's theory to incorporate the notion that the goodness-of-fit between parent and child is influenced by a number of factors, including infant behavior, parent expectations and parenting practices, and the context in which these interactions occur. Alternatively, Goldsmith and Campos focused on the expression of specific emotions in specific contexts (Goldsmith & Campos, 1990), with less attention to the potential interactional nature of temperament. Kagan (1994; Kagan & Snidman, 1991) focused his temperament theory on two extreme types of children—inhibited and uninhibited—that, he argued, represented distinct biobehavioral profiles leading to patterns of approach versus withdrawal tendencies across childhood. Inhibited children are sensitive to novelty and withdraw from stimulation, whereas uninhibited children are more outgoing and tend to be eager to approach new stimuli.

Rothbart and colleagues (Derryberry & Rothbart, 1997; Rothbart, 1981; Rothbart & Bates, 1998) have articulated one of the most influential theories of early temperament and one that has generated a great deal of research on infant development over the past 10 years (Buss & Goldsmith, 1998; Stifter & Braungart, 1995; Calkins & Fox, 1992; Calkins, Dedmon, Gill, Lomax, & Johnson, 2002). This theory defines temperament along two broad dimensions of reactivity and self-regulation, which then subsume six subscales that place a greater emphasis on basic emotion, attention, and motor processes.

With respect to the reactive dimension of temperament, Rothbart notes that the initial responses of an infant may be characterized by his or her physiological and behavioral reactions to sensory stimuli of different qualities and intensities. This reactivity is believed to be present and observable at birth and reflects a relatively stable characteristic of the infant (Rothbart, Derryberry, & Hershey, 2000). Moreover, infants will differ initially in their level of reactivity to stimuli that elicit negative affect (e.g., Calkins, Fox & Marshall, 1996). These initial affective responses, which are characterized by vocal and facial indices of negativity, are presumed to reflect generalized distress. Thus this initial negative reactivity has neither the complexity nor the range of later emotional responses. Rather, it is a rudimentary form of the more sophisticated and differentiated emotions that will in later infancy be labeled as fear, anger, and sadness. These emotions undergo further differentiation with cognitive development and the emergence of self-awareness during early childhood (Bronson, 2000).

The second dimension proposed by Rothbart, self-regulation, has been described largely in terms of attentional and motoric control mechanisms that emerge across early development. For example, the development of attention and its use in the control of emotional reactivity begins to emerge in the first year of life and continues through-out the preschool and school years (Posner & Rothbart, 2000; Rothbart, 1989; Roth-bart & Bates, 1998). Individual differences in the ability to voluntarily sustain focus or shift attention are paramount to the self-control of attention. In particular, attentional orienting skills have been identified as a critical component of the regulatory process, as orienting has the direct effect of amplifying at a neural level the stimuli toward which attention is directed, thus changing the affective experience of the individual (Rothbart, Posner, & Rosicky, 1994). Thus orienting skills assist in the management of both negative and positive emotions and, consequently, in the development of adap-tive control of emotion and behavior. Qualitative shifts in attention skills across the first 12 months of life may be integral to the qualitative shifts in emotional regulation that are observed during this period. However, there are clear individual differences in the ability to utilize attention to successfully control emotion. For example, Roth-bart (1981, 1986) found increases in positive affect and decreases in distress from 3 to 6 months during episodes of focused attention, suggesting that control of attention is tied to affective experience. Moreover, negative affectivity is believed to interfere with the child's ability to deploy attention to explore and learn about the environment (Rothbart, et al., 1994; Ruff & Rothbart, 1996). Clearly, attention must be considered a central process that links temperamental reactivity to later adjustment very early in development.

In sum, although a number of different approaches to conceptualizing and study-ing early temperament have been proposed, Rothbart's theory of temperament has the potential to elucidate processes related to adjustment and social competence. Rothbart views the very young infant as a highly reactive organism whose behavior becomes, with development, increasingly controlled by regulatory processes. Research and the-ory on the relations between temperament and social adjustment, reviewed later, have largely focused on the negative and reactive dimensions of temperament (such as anger and fear). However, it is the emergence and recruitment of regulatory processes that may ultimately determine the young child's degree of success at mastering developmen-tal achievements such as social skills (Calkins, 2009).

Development of Temperament

Dimensions of temperament have been assessed across development, including certain temperament traits that have been detected before birth. For example, fetal activity level at 36 prenatal weeks has been found to predict later temperament traits. In a study conducted by DiPietro, Hodgson, Costigan, and Johnson (1996), more active fetuses were found to be more unadaptable, difficult, and unpredictable at 3 and 6 months of age. Infants develop the ability to modulate levels of arousal such that at around 2–3 months they engage in self-soothing behaviors (e.g., thumb sucking). From 3 to 9 months infants begin to change their behaviors to respond to the envi-ronment through activities such as reaching and grasping (Kopp, 1982). During this time, other temperamental traits, such as distress and avoidance, emerge (Rothbart, 2007). Although these traits are thought to be relatively stable, temperament may appear to change in childhood as a consequence of both developmental processes and interactions with caregivers. So, for example, specific parenting behaviors, such as warm and sensitive caregiving, may heighten temperamental traits such as positive affectivity and approach and minimize temperamental tendencies to be fussy, fear-ful, or angry. Thus, as parents teach behaviors to control emotion, the appearance of early traits such as distress or negative affectivity may be altered (Putnam & Stifter, 2008).

There is also evidence that early temperament traits are moderately stable into adolescence, although the research on this developmental time period has shifted to focus on emerging personality traits rather than rudimentary traits such as those seen in infancy and early childhood (Ganiban, Saudino, Ulbricht, Neiderhiser, & Reiss, 2008). For example, in a sample of children followed from 4 months to 15 years, those identified as highly reactive were found to exhibit behaviors such as facial tension or infrequent smiling throughout childhood and early adolescence (Kagan, Snidman, Kahn, & Towsley, 2007). The expression of these traits may still be influenced by the environment; however, from middle childhood to early adolescence a transactional relationship still exists between child temperament and caregiver influences. During this time, parents may use strategies such as emotion coaching to help children manage their temperament-driven emotional reactivity. And certain temperament traits, such as anger reactivity, might influence parenting practices and the parent–adolescent relationship (Katainen, Raikkonen, & Keltikangas-Jarvinen, 1998; Lengua, 2006). The development of temperament over time, although initially driven by biological processes, continues to be influenced by the environment, which may yield changes in the expression of temperament traits from childhood to adolescence.

Measurement of Temperament

Efforts to assess the endogenous behavioral traits that are described in temperament theory and that may influence subsequent personality development and childhood adjustment have generated a variety of methodologies. These approaches include both laboratory and questionnaire techniques. Thomas and Chess construed temperament in terms of behavioral style, which is thought to be stable over time. This style is reflected in the similarity of children's responses to situations commonly confronted during the course of early development and readily observable to parents. Thus Thomas and Chess's approach relied largely on parent reports of children's temperament. Other temperament theorists have proposed particular dimensions of temperament that reflect, in general, the child's emotionality, activity level, and attention (Buss & Plomin, 1984; Rothbart, 1981; Thomas & Chess, 1977). Most of these approaches are similar in that the measurement of these traits is achieved through the completion of a questionnaire that requires mothers to rate the frequency of particular infant behaviors observed during the previous week.

The measurement of specific temperament dimensions using questionnaire techniques has led to a great deal of research concerning the stability of temperament, its convergent validity with observations of behavior, and its role in developing social relationships. Direct observations of temperament in the home or laboratory have been used as one means of validating maternal assessments via questionnaire. The Laboratory Temperament Assessment Battery (LAB-TAB; Goldsmith & Rothbart, 1993), developed in the tradition of Rothbart's model of temperament, utilizes a standard set of tasks that may be used to assess temperament in the laboratory and that are scored along a number of dimensions, yielding measurements of such temperament dimensions as fear, positive affectivity, and frustration. A number of recent studies have utilized such batteries to assess temperament and its relation to social development and adjustment (Buss & Goldsmith, 1998; Calkins & Dedmon, 2000). For example, we (Calkins & Dedmon, 2000) utilized the LAB-TAB battery with 2-year-old children to elicit reactions ranging from fear to empathy and recorded heart rate reactivity during these tasks. These reactions were then used to determine factors that underlie early adjustment difficulties. However, it is important to note that the primary emphasis in many studies is on the emotional reactivity component of the child's response to a particular task or situation, including the latency, intensity, and duration of distress, with less explicit emphasis on the potential regulatory component of the child's response. In addition, observational methods are vulnerable to distortion, as well, because the period of observation is short and the range of behaviors observed may be constricted. Matheny and others (Calkins et al., 2002; Matheny, Riese, & Wilson, 1985; Rothbart & Bates, 1998) have argued in favor of multimethod assessments that include both laboratory and maternal assessments. Such multimethod approaches validate maternal assessment and provide a measure of temperament that takes into account behaviors that are observed over the course of several days or weeks.

Psychobiological Assessments of Temperament

In addition to finding reliable and valid measurement instruments with which to assess the behavioral component of temperament, it is useful for temperament theorists to try to account for the biological or physiological component of the construct, as well. That is, if, as temperament theorists propose, temperamental types or characteristics reflect the behavioral manifestation of some underlying biological process, it would be helpful to observe convergent validity of behavior and biology. Three primary types of measures have been used to study relations between physiology and emotional responsivity to a variety of elicitors: measures of heart rate, brain electrical activity, and adrenocortical activity. Excellent reviews of the use of these three measures in both the adult and child literature have been conducted (Henderson & Fox, 2007; Porges, 1991; Stansbury & Gunnar, 1994). Briefly, we describe these measures and representative findings from the temperament literature.

Measures of Heart Rate

Numerous studies have examined individual differences in heart rate and heart rate variability among different groups of infants and children (cf., Calkins et al., 2002). Fox and Gelles (2006) found that infants differing on level of heart rate variability also differed in degree of facial expressivity. Kagan, Reznick, and Snidman (1987) found that behaviorally inhibited children display faster and less variable heart rates compared with behaviorally extroverted children. This variability is thought to reflect differences in the degree of sympathetic activation between the two groups. Other studies have examined individual differences in vagal tone, or heart rate variability that occurs at the frequency of breathing (respiratory sinus arrhythmia, RSA), which is thought to reflect parasympathetic activity, and its relation to emotional reactivity in infancy (Calkins et al., 2002; Porges, Doussard-Roosevelt, Portales, & Greenspan, 1996; Stifter, Fox, & Porges, 1989; Stifter & Fox, 1990). In a series of studies, Porges and his colleagues have demonstrated that vagal tone is related to both emotional reactivity and regulation (Porter, Porges, & Marshall, 1988; Stifter et al., 1989). Infants with high vagal tone tend to be more reactive emotionally, and, as Porges speculates, this responsivity may be predictive of better regulatory ability. Further, developmental changes in vagal tone may be a contributor to normative changes in emotion expression observed during infancy (Porges, 1991).

Recent work has examined a measure of cardiac activity that may be more directly related to the kinds of self-regulatory behaviors children begin to display in toddlerhood and early childhood. This measure is vagal regulation of the heart as indexed by a decrease (suppression) in RSA during situations in which coping or emotional and behavioral regulation is required. Vagal regulation in the form of suppression of RSA during demanding tasks may reflect physiological processes that allow the child to shift focus from internal homeostatic demands to demands that require the generation of coping strategies to control affective or behavioral arousal. Thus suppression of RSA is thought to be a physiological strategy that permits sustained attention and behaviors indicative of active coping that are mediated by the parasympathetic nervous system (Porges, 1991, 1996; Wilson & Gottman, 1996).

Brain Electrical Activity

A second physiological measure that has recently been utilized in the study of infant temperament is the electroencephalogram (EEG). EEG is low level electrical activity recorded off the scalp. Researchers interested in the pattern of activation between the right and left hemispheres have computed ratio scores of the difference in power or energy between the two hemispheres. These ratio or difference scores present relative differences in power and a score that reflects the degree to which one hemisphere or region in a hemisphere exhibits greater activation than a homologous region. In applying these methods to the study of infant emotion, Fox and Davidson (Davidson & Fox, 1982, 1989; Fox & Davidson, 1988) examined whether differences in hemispheric asymmetry are markers for individual differences in emotionality or temperament in infancy. In their study of infants' reactions to maternal separation, they found that infants who displayed less left-sided activation in the frontal region during a baseline condition were more likely to cry in response to brief separation (Fox & Davidson, 1987). Fox and Davidson (1991) argued that infants who show a characteristic right-sided frontal activation may have a lower threshold for experiencing negative emotion. More recently, this work has been extended to examine differences among behaviorally inhibited and uninhibited children. Data from several longitudinal cohorts of infants and children suggest that infants selected for temperamental characteristics predictive of inhibition are more likely to exhibit greater relative right frontal activation (Calkins et al., 1996) and that children who continue to show inhibited and shy behavior in childhood also display a similar frontal asymmetry (Fox, Schmidt, Calkins, Rubin, & Coplan, 1996).

Adrenocortical Activity

A third physiological measure that has recently been applied to the study of temperament is adrenocortical activity as measured in plasma and salivary cortisol. Cortisol is the primary hormone of the adrenocortical system whose production varies fairly rhythmically during the course of the 24-hour day–night cycle. In addition, however, cortisol levels change in response to both physiological and psychological elicitors (see Carver & Tully, Chapter 2, this volume). In using cortisol as a measure of emotional reactivity, then, the aim is to compare changes in cortisol levels from basal to stressor conditions, with consideration to the activity of the system relative to its daily cycle (Gunnar & Davis, 2003; Stansbury & Gunnar, 1994). Measurement of adrenocortical activity in infants is further complicated by the developmental changes occurring in the pattern of daily cortisol activity during the first year of life. Nevertheless, recent improvements in the radioimmune assays used to analyze salivary cortisol make this method of obtaining psychophysiological data from very young infants quite feasible.

Summary of Temperament Theory and Methods

In sum, many theories of temperament focus largely on the dimensions of emotionality, particularly emotional reactivity, which is thought to be biologically based and relatively stable across time. Measurement of temperament, whether by observation or through maternal report, has focused largely on the emotional reactivity component of temperament. Psychobiological work has examined relations between particular physiological systems and both reactivity and the regulation of emotion.

The important question of *how* temperament might affect subsequent adjustment and the development of behavior problems in childhood is receiving increasing attention (Rothbart & Bates, 1998; Shiner & Caspi, 2003). Studies that have reported modest direct effects of temperament have motivated theorists and researchers to search for *causal mechanisms* between temperament and social competence and social functioning (Hinshaw, 2002). Multiple models of such mechanisms have been proposed, including, most frequently, those that focus on the moderational role of the caregiving environment (see Bates & McFadyen-Ketchum, 2000, for a review of these studies). However, less work has focused on the processes that might mediate the relation between such temperament dimensions as distress or negativity, caregiving contexts, and different behavioral outcomes. One hypothesis that follows directly from Rothbart's theory is that *temperament exerts its effects on child behavior via the developing self-regulatory system, and in particular, through its effect on emerging emotion regulation skills.* Next, we explore how the processes that reflect temperament, particularly the processes related to regulation, are related to later development, including indicators of child adjustment and social competence.

EMOTION REGULATION

Defining Emotion Regulation

Numerous definitions have been offered for the construct of emotion regulation from within both the child and adult emotion literatures (Gross & Thompson, 2007). Our definition reflects recent theoretical and empirical work in both developmental (Cole, Martin, & Dennis, 2004; Fox & Calkins, 2003) and clinical (Keenan, 2000) psychology that highlights the fundamental role played by emotion processes in both child development and child functioning (Eisenberg et al., 2000) and, importantly, that is anchored in the measurement of such processes *during* emotionally evocative situations (Calkins & Hill, 2007). Consistent with many of our colleagues (Gross & Thompson 2007; Eisenberg, Hofer, & Vaughan, 2007), we view emotion regulation processes as those behaviors, skills, and strategies, whether conscious or unconscious, automatic or effortful, that serve to modulate, inhibit, and enhance emotional experiences and expressions (Calkins & Hill, 2007).

We also view the dimension of emotional reactivity as part of the emotion regulation process, although we, like some of our colleagues (Gross & Thompson, 2007), see a value in examining this element of the process as distinct from the efforts to manage it, what we refer to as the control dimension (Fox & Calkins, 2003). The emotion regulation process is clearly a dynamic one in which reactive and control dimensions alter one another across time. Moreover, in our view, the reactive dimension, as opposed to the control dimension, is present and functional early in neonatal life, as it is strongly influenced by genetic and biological factors (Fox & Calkins, 2003) and is reflective of the child's innate temperament.

Development of Emotion Regulation

Although some children appear to be quite proficient in the use of basic emotion regulation skills at a relatively early age, it is clear that dramatic growth occurs in the acquisition and display of emotion regulation skills and abilities early in development. The process may be described broadly as one in which the relatively passive and reactive neonate becomes a child capable of self-initiated behaviors that serve an emotion regulatory function. The infant moves from near complete reliance on caregivers for regulation (e.g., via physical soothing provided when the infant is held) to independent emotion regulation (e.g., choosing to find another toy to play with, rather than having a tantrum, when the desired toy is taken by a companion), although the variability in such regulation across children, in terms of both style and efficacy, is considerable (Buss & Goldsmith, 1998; Calkins, 2009). As the infant makes this transition to greater independence, the caregiver's use of specific strategies and behaviors within dyadic interactions becomes integrated into the infant's repertoire of emotion regulation skills across both biological and behavioral levels of functioning (Calkins & Dedmon, 2000; Calkins & Hill, 2007). The child may then draw on this repertoire in a variety of contexts, in both conscious, effortful ways (e.g., walking away from a confrontation with a peer) and in nonconscious, automatic ways (e.g., reducing vagal regulation of the heart to facilitate behavior coping; Calkins, Graziano, Berdan, Keane, & Degnan, 2008).

From infancy to toddlerhood, emotional development consists of differentiating emotional expressions and developing language to describe these emotions (Zeman, Cassano, Perry-Parrish, & Stegall, 2006). Verbal abilities begin to develop in infancy, and as children move into the preschool period, verbal abilities significantly contribute to their ability to regulate and deal with emotional content. As such, the development of language is considered a "major milestone" in the development of emotion regulation (Campos, Frankel, & Camras, 2004, p. 387). With the development of language, and through interactions with family and caregivers, children continue to develop increasingly complex regulation strategies. The family is thought to influence emotion regulation through parenting practices related to emotional understanding and regulation strategies, through the emotional climate of the family, and through the child's direct observation of emotional processes (Morris, Silk, Steinberg, Myers, & Robinson, 2007). Through this process, children become aware of culture-specific display rules for emotions and their own emotional responses so that they can utilize their own regulatory processes to elicit appropriate reactions from the environment (Fox & Calkins, 2003). Regulation strategies become more flexible over time to meet contextual demands, allowing children to inhibit or activate behavior accordingly through context-appropriate arousal, planning, and accurate processing of social information in the environment (Eisenberg et al., 2007; Thompson, Lewis, & Calkins, 2008). As children continue to develop regulatory abilities via modeling, language acquisition, and social interactions, regulation increases while reactivity decreases, though these trajectories are affected by early levels of physiological regulation, at least to some degree (Blandon, Calkins, Keane, & O'Brien, 2008).

The practice of these newly emerging skills during the preschool period leads to greater automaticity so that, by the time the child is ready to enter the arena of formal schooling, greater effort may be directed toward more demanding academic and social challenges. Importantly, these expanding interactional contexts will place demands on the child to integrate emotional and cognitive skills in the service of achieving diverse academic and social goals. School-age children are capable of more active and planned regulation strategies, including increasing abilities to distract themselves and to reevaluate frustrating and disappointing situations in a more positive manner (Kalpidou, Power, Cherry, & Gottfried, 2004; Stansbury & Sigman, 2000). However, young children's strategies for controlling their reactivity to challenging events are not always successful, and early emerging patterns of problematic behavior begin to become entrenched, affecting children's social and academic success (Burt et al., 2008)

Late childhood into adolescence is a time of transition, both biologically and environmentally. Recent evidence from developmental neuroscience suggests that the regions of the brain associated with the emotion regulation process include the prefrontal cortex, anterior cingulate cortex, and the amygdala, which continue to mature through childhood and into adolescence (Beauregard, Levesque, & Paquette, 2004). During this time there is also a shift in children's developmental contexts, with a shift in emphasis to the peer group and peer influences (Steinberg, 2005). As such, these transitions are influenced by and also affect the individual's emotional experience. Changes within the brain, in hormone levels, and in physical growth are the biological mechanisms of adolescent development, but there is a reciprocal effect between the social world and the environment that adolescents reside in and these physical changes. The environmental systems organize themselves around the emerging biological changes, and how these systems adapt to these biological changes affects long-term outcomes (Granic, Dishion, & Hollenstein, 2003). During early adolescence, arousal is heightened due to the onset of puberty before the full maturation of regulation and the systems of risk-and-reward detection, and this offset provides links to observed sensation seeking, reckless behaviors, and increased risk for emotional problems (Steinberg, 2004). Further, the increase and instability in hormone levels during adolescence may be implicated in the more labile and negative emotional experiences during this time (Rosenblum & Lewis, 2003). However, it is also during this time that adolescents develop the ability to distinguish between both long- and short-term means of regulation given that they can better identify long-term consequences of their behaviors (Moilanen, 2007).

Although there is considerable growth in emotion regulation from late childhood into adolescence, research suggests that there is also stability in individual differences in emotion regulation (e.g., Raffaelli, Crockett, & Shen, 2005). During this time, caregiver influences continue to affect children's emotion regulation abilities. For example, adolescents whose mothers dampen or invalidate displays of positive affect engage in dysregulated strategies that are related to depressive symptomatology, and those adolescents are, in turn, likely to also engage in negative behaviors with their mothers (Yap, Allen, & Ladouceur, 2008). This research suggests that regulatory processes, although grounded in early biological processes, are subject to environmental influences throughout development.

Measurement of Emotion Regulation

The broad construct of emotion regulation has been studied in many ways across early development (Cole et al., 2004), including through the use of parent reports, psychophysiological measures, and direct observation. Our approach entails the examination of the child's use of specific strategies in emotionally demanding contexts and the effects of these strategies on emotion experience and expression (Calkins & Dedmon, 2000). We have borrowed extensively from the LAB-TAB protocol (Goldsmith, Reilly, Lemery, Longley, & Prescott, 1995) to elicit emotion in the laboratory and then measured the child's response to the situation once the emotion was observed. We also measure the physiological response of the child to the emotional challenge, assuming that behavioral strategies to deal with emotional arousal are at least in part dependent on biological efforts to control arousal (Calkins, 1997). So, for example, we have observed that specific emotion regulation strategies such as self-comforting, help seeking, and self-distraction may assist the young child in managing early temperament-driven frustration and fear responses and that such reactions are observable in laboratory assessments using standard assessment batteries (Calkins & Dedmon, 2000). We have also found that a physiological change is observed under such conditions (Calkins & Keane, 2004) and that such behavioral and physiological strategies may also be observed in real-world situations in which the control of negative emotions may be necessary, such as with peers or in school (Calkins, Gill, Johnson, & Smith, 1999; Graziano, Keane, & Calkins, 2007).

Another approach to the measurement of emotion regulation relies on parent report or, with older children, self-report. For example, the Emotion Regulation Checklist (ERC; Shields & Cicchetti, 1997) requires parents to report on their child's negativity/lability and emotion regulation—that is, the child's tendency to be negative and the ability to modulate that negativity, respectively. The Adolescent Self-Regulatory Inventory (Moilanen, 2007) is a measure that taps multiple dimensions of regulation, as well as the outcomes of particular regulation strategies. Like temperament questionnaires, these measures are subject to the biases of the reporter and are best used as a complement to direct observations.

Temperament and the Development of Emotion Regulation

There are several possible ways that temperament may affect the display and development of emotion regulation and, consequently, the development of social skills or problematic behavior (Calkins, 1994, 2004). One hypothesis is that temperament directly constrains the development of specific regulatory behaviors that are integral to behavioral control and social functioning (Calkins & Johnson, 1998). A second hypothesis is that temperament is moderated by specific kinds of caregiving behaviors or environments that then alter the trajectories of self-regulation. A third hypothesis is that temperament might be mediated by other basic regulatory processes, such as attention or physiology (Harman, Rothbart, & Posner, 1997; Calkins & Dedmon, 2000; Shipman, Schneider, & Brown, 2004), that then affect the development of emotional regulation in context.

Much research has focused on how early infant temperament influences subsequent emotion regulation. Characteristics of the infant that are most often explored in the study of emotional self-regulation are temperamental dimensions such as proneness to distress (Calkins & Fox, 1992; Mangelsdorf, Gunnar, Kestenbaum, Lang, &

Andreas, 1990; Seifer et al., 1996). Hypothetically, one might imagine an infant who is highly negatively reactive to novel stimuli. Such an infant might cry easily, intensely, and for a long duration when exposed to new people, objects, or environments. Given the level of behavioral disorganization that might accompany such a response, this child might be unable to display, and therefore practice, the skills that typically lead to a reduction in the experience and expression of negative affect. Under repeated exposures to novelty, the opportunities for the acquisition of early regulatory behaviors become limited. As the child develops, the likelihood of having a rich behavioral repertoire of strategies to draw on also becomes limited. In this way, temperamental reactivity to novelty may function to minimize concurrent strategy use, as well as the practice and development of more sophisticated skills that build on early primitive strategies and that are critical to adaptive functioning across a range of more challenging contexts.

A small number of studies examining the role of temperament in displays of emotional regulation support this hypothesis. For example, in a recent series of studies, we and others have suggested that frustration reactivity, elicited in response to physical restraint or denial, may constrain both the use and the development of appropriate regulatory behaviors (Calkins, 1994; Calkins & Fox, 1992; Fox & Calkins, 1993; Stifter & Fox, 1990). In one study, Rothbart and colleagues (Rothbart, Posner, & Boylan, 1990) observed that at least one specific emotion regulation behavior, attentional control, is related to decreases in negative emotionality in infancy. Buss and Goldsmith (1998) further observed that a number of different regulatory behaviors that infants display when in frustrating or constraining situations appear to reduce negative affect.

In our work, we have demonstrated that there is a relationship between level of reactivity to frustration, both behaviorally and physiologically, and emotional and physiological regulation. For example, the magnitude of baseline resting heart rate variability, or vagal tone, which is often used as a marker of temperament, predicted the magnitude of physiological regulation in response to frustration during infancy, toddlerhood, and preschool (Calkins, 1997; Calkins et al., 2002; Calkins, Smith, Gill, & Johnson, 1998). We have also demonstrated that there are relations between regulatory behaviors and the tendency to be distressed in response to frustrating situations during toddlerhood (Calkins & Johnson, 1998). And we found that a group of infants characterized by low frustration tolerance differed from less frustrated infants in terms of physiological regulation, emotion regulation strategies, attention, and activity level (Calkins et al., 2002). Similarly, a group of toddlers characterized by disruptive behavior displayed fewer emotion regulation behaviors and poorer physiological regulation (Calkins & Dedmon, 2000). The implications of these behavioral and physiological profiles for longer term emotional regulation are unclear. However, the notion that certain behaviors serve to minimize frustration reactivity has clear support, as has the hypothesis that greater levels of frustration are linked both to less regulation and to the use of less adaptive types of regulation.

A second issue with respect to the direct effect of temperament is its effect on developing regulatory ability over time. Braungart-Rieker and Stifter (1996) demonstrated that frustration reactivity at 5 months of age was related to the use of fewer emotion regulation behaviors at 10 months of age. What is unclear, though, is whether some types of emotion regulation behaviors are more likely to be associated with heightened frustration over time than others. A small number of studies conducted with children of various ages suggest that it might be possible to identify profiles of infants at higher risk for regulatory difficulties. For example, Aksan and colleagues (1999) report that a preschool temperament type characterized by uncontrolled expressive behavior was predicted by infant distress in response to limitations. Thus there seems to be evidence that the dimension of frustration, as it is displayed in infancy at least, is linked both concurrently and predictively to the use of less adaptive emotion regulation skills.

A second way that temperament might affect emotional regulation is in its moderation by some environmental influence, such as parenting behavior (Calkins, 1994). Such a hypothesis implies that temperament affects emotional regulation when it is displayed in the context of a specific type of parenting. So, for example, an infant who has a tendency to be easily frustrated might have difficulties developing appropriate emotion regulation skills only when the infant's caregiver does not provide sensitive and responsive care. Such an infant might be forced to rely on immature or ineffective self-regulation skills because the caregiver is not providing the appropriate and, indeed, necessary emotional support that will allow the child to become a skilled practitioner of emotion regulation even in the absence of the caregiver.

There is considerable evidence that caregiving behavior is directly related to both proximal and distal measures of emotion regulation, as well as to both behavioral and biological measures of such behavior (Calkins et al., 1998; Diener, Mangelsdorf, McHale, & Frosch, 2002; Nachmias, Gunnar, Mangelsdorf, Parritz, & Buss, 1996). Empirical investigations of the hypothesis that temperament is moderated by caregiving interactions with respect to proximal measures of emotion regulation are quite uncommon. Gilliom, Shaw, Beck, Schonberg, and Lukon (2002), however, conducted a study that examined maternal factors as a moderating factor in preschoolers' use of specific anger control strategies during a waiting paradigm. Specific strategies involving the control of attention were found to predict the anger reaction of the children in this situation; however, maternal negative control was found to moderate this temperament effect. Children who displayed a difficult temperament and whose mothers used more negative control developed different, potentially less effective, strategies for regulating anger when they were of school age (Gilliom et al., 2002).

A third way that temperament may affect the development of emotional regulation is through processes or mechanisms that mediate this relation. As defined by Baron and Kenny (1986), a mediator is a variable that serves as the mechanism through which a predictor affects an outcome. Because mediational analyses allow one to specify possible mechanisms or processes that explain how one variable affects another, they are quite useful in understanding developmental processes. Although few studies have specified the goal of understanding the mechanism through which temperament affects regulation, it is possible to extrapolate, at least on a theoretical level, some of these processes given the existing literature. For example, one hypothesized central process in the emergence of emotion regulation is the control of attention (Kopp, 2002). A number of investigators have reported that specific attention-regulating behaviors have a direct influence on the experience and expression of both positive and negative affective states (Calkins et al., 2002; Rothbart et al., 1994; Stifter & Moyer, 1991). Clearly, attention must be a central process that links temperamental reactivity to early emotional regulation.

Another process that may also link temperament to emotion regulation in early development may be physiological in nature. For example, Fox (1994) has noted that the frontal lobes of the brain are differentially specialized for approach versus avoidance and that these tendencies influence the behaviors that children engage in when emotionally and behaviorally aroused. He further notes that maturation of the frontal cortex provides a mechanism for the more sophisticated and planned regulatory behaviors of older children versus infants. Porges (1996) also describes an important role for biological maturation, specifically maturation of the parasympathetic nervous system that plays a key role in regulation of state, motor activity, and emotion. Moreover, Porges notes that individual differences in nervous system functioning might mediate the expression and regulation of emotion (Porges, Doussard-Roosevelt, & Maita, 1994). The degree to which the individual experiences physiological arousal as reflected in heart rate variability may affect the successful generation of emotional coping skills because of the capacity to regulate physiological arousal. So, for example, childhood psychological problems that have been linked to temperamental reactivity may, in fact, be due to the failure of these children to acquire adaptive regulatory skills to cope with their physiological reactivity to novelty and uncertainty (Calkins, 1994, 2009).

In sum, within the framework outlined here, temperament is hypothesized to affect children's social competence and psychological functioning via its influence on developing emotional regulation. Relations between specific dimensions of self and emotional regulation and specific childhood outcomes are now the focus of much developmental and clinical psychology research, with somewhat greater emphasis on the emotion–psychopathology associations. By and large, this research has focused on early and middle childhood, perhaps in recognition of the fact that once these patterns are set, they are unlikely to change. In the next section, we review research that supports these links in childhood.

Effects of Emotion Regulation on Child Functioning and Social Competence

It should not be surprising that emotion regulation skills predict children's adjustment and social competence. Emotion regulation processes begin to develop very early in life in the context of children's earliest social relationships: those with the primary caregivers (Diener et al., 2002; Thompson & Lagattuta, 2006; Zeman et al., 2006). One important assumption of much of the research on the acquisition of emotional self-regulation is that parental caregiving practices may support or undermine such development and thus contribute to observed individual differences among young children's emotional skills displayed in the peer and school environments (Morris et al., 2007; Thompson, 1994). In fact, Sroufe (1996) has argued that emotional development is inextricably linked with social development, with the course of emotional development described as the transition from dyadic regulation of affect with caregivers to self-regulation of affect in other contexts. He argues that the ability to self-regulate arousal levels is embedded in affective interactions between the infant and caregiver. These interactions provide infants with the experience of arousal escalation and reduction as a function of caregiver interventions, distress reactions that are relieved through caregiver actions, and positive interactions with the caregiver (Sroufe, 1996). Such experiences contribute to the working model of affect-related expectations that will transfer from the immediate caregiving environment to the larger social world of peers and others. As such, early emotion regulation processes have implications for a range of childhood behaviors in both social and nonsocial domains (Blair, Denham, Kochanoff, & Whipple, 2004; Calkins, 1994; Calkins et al., 1998; Cicchetti, Ganiban, & Barnett, 1991). Here, we review evidence linking emotion regulation to psychological, social, and school adjustment.

Considerable research on emotion regulation demonstrates that successful regulation of affect influences children's psychological functioning and social skills, including aggressive behavior and peer rejection. Some of the most influential work in this area has been conducted by Nancy Eisenberg and her colleagues (Eisenberg, 2001; Eisenberg, Spinrad, & Morris, 2002; Murphy, Shepard, Eisenberg, & Fabes, 2004). In their early work, Eisenberg, Fabes, and colleagues reported in several studies that individuals who were highly emotional in response to anger-inducing events and low in regulation were likely to be aggressive with others (Eisenberg, Fabes, Bernzweig, & Karbon, 1993; Fabes & Eisenberg, 1992). More recent work demonstrates that the relations between emotion regulation and peer acceptance are mediated by social skills (Maszk, Eisenberg, & Guthrie, 1999). Similarly, other research has found that preschoolers who were high on negative emotionality and who used predominantly passive coping strategies (avoiding and denying emotions) were at risk for acting-out behavior problems (Blair et al., 2004). Finally, children high in social competence report engaging in more effective coping strategies when faced with peer rejection (Reijntjes, Stegge, & Terwogt, 2006). These data suggest that there are complex relations among emotion regulation, problem behaviors, social processes, and peer acceptance. One challenge to this work has been sorting out the pathways through which these different processes may exert their effects (Blandon, Calkins, Grimm, Keane, & O'Brien, 2010).

Given that children enter the peer milieu of preschool or school with some skills and tendencies already present, it is especially useful to examine emotion regulation very early in development to see what role it may play in emerging social behaviors (Blandon et al., 2010). In our own research we have studied children with early-onset acting-out behavior problems. We have followed these children over time and found that poor emotion regulation skills predict the severity and trajectory of ongoing behavior problems (Degnan, Calkins, Keane, & Hill-Soderlund, 2008) and compromise early peer interactions (Calkins, Gill, & Williford, 1999; Keane & Calkins, 2004). However, we also found that the impact of early behavior problems on children's subsequent functioning varies as a function of the kind of caregiving experience children receive. For children who were at low risk of developing persistent externalizing behavior problems, those who evidenced better emotion regulation at 2 years of age and who had mothers who were warm and responsive were more liked by their classmates in kindergarten. In contrast, children with equally well-developed emotion regulation strategies but who had mothers who were not warm and responsive were less well liked by their classmates in kindergarten (Blandon et al., 2008). These results lend further evidence that the emotional climate of mother–child interactions is important for children to successfully use their emotion regulation strategies in social situations involving peers.

Although there has been less focus on peers and the development of emotion regulation, it is clear that by the time children enter school, peers also help with the development of these important self-regulatory skills. Peers serve as sources of emotional support during times of stress (Hartup, 1996) but also provide feedback about the appropriateness of emotional displays. Anger expression, bossiness, aggression, and impulsivity are all negatively related to peer status (Eisenberg et al., 1993; Keane & Calkins, 2004); rejected children are also more effusive in their display of emotion (e.g., happiness) to positive events (Hubbard, 2001). Taken together, these studies suggest that both positive and negative high-intensity emotional behavior play a role in determining concurrent peer status. The peer group may also attempt to socialize children's emotion regulation through specific negative treatment, such as peer victimization or exclusion (Salisch, 2001).

Most research has examined the relations between behavioral indicators of emotion regulation and child outcomes; however, a small number of studies have focused on the biological indicators of emotion regulation. Although relatively few studies have examined the role of vagal regulation in social development, the initial evidence suggests a positive relation. Despite a small sample, Porges and colleagues (Porges, Doussard-Roosevelt, Portales, & Greenspan, 1996) demonstrated that infants with vagal regulation difficulties during a social-attention task at 9 months of age had significantly more behavioral problems at 3 years of age. We also found that 2-year-old children with symptoms of externalizing problems displayed significant and consistent lower vagal regulation during challenging situations than did children with no behavior problems (Calkins & Dedmon, 2000). Vagal regulation has also been associated with children's behavioral regulation strategies during affect-eliciting situations and has been identified as a protective factor against externalizing problems associated with parental conflict (Calkins, 1997; El-Sheikh, 2001; El-Sheikh, Harger, & Whitson, 2001). Three studies have assessed the relation between vagal regulation and children's positive social behavior. Cole, Zahn-Waxler, Fox, Usher, and Welsh (1996) found no significant difference between the vagal regulation of expressive and inexpressive groups. The study was limited, however, by the use of only one brief mood-induction story to obtain a vagal regulation measure. In contrast, Stifter and Corey (2001) found that infants with greater vagal regulation during a cognitive challenge task were rated by the experimenters as more social. Graziano et al. (2007) found that higher RSA was related to more positive peer relationships. Thus there is partial support for the hypothesis that children who are better at regulating vagal tone have a greater capacity for social functioning.

A few studies have examined the relations between emotion regulation and other indicators of childhood adjustment. For example, in terms of early school success, Shields and colleagues (2001) found that preschoolers with good emotion regulation skills at the beginning of the school year were reported by their teachers to have better school functioning (acquired early academic skills, adapted to routines, complied with rules, formed positive relationships) at the end of the year. Blair (2002) proposes that inefficient emotion regulation inhibits the use of higher order cognitive regulation. In support of this proposal, Trentacosta and Izard (2007) found that, after controlling for verbal ability, children who were reported by their teachers to be able to successfully regulate their emotions in kindergarten attended more to academic tasks and subsequently had higher academic achievement in the first grade. They also found that emotion knowledge in kindergarten was directly and positively associated with academic skills in the first grade.

In sum, emotion regulation skills that allow the child to manage both physiological and behavioral indicators of emotional arousal are implicated in a range of outcomes. Emotion regulation appears to play a significant role in preparing children to be ready for school, as defined by both social and academic indicators, and is implicated in psychological adjustment. And, although there is less research examining this issue, it appears that good emotion regulation skills contribute to adaptive functioning throughout childhood and adolescence (Morris et al., 2007; Raffaelli, Crockett, & Shen, 2005).

DIRECTIONS FOR FUTURE RESEARCH

Despite considerable progress in our understanding that emotion is influential in children's adjustment generally and social competence specifically, many unanswered questions remain about *how* this occurs. This knowledge gap exists, in part, because of a number of conceptual and empirical challenges to the study of temperament, emotion, and emotional regulation. In this section, we focus on issues that we consider paramount to furthering our understanding of how emotion processes, child adjustment, and social competence are linked. We focus on emotion regulation as the central mechanism that links these domains and the challenges this conceptualization poses for empirical work.

Emotion Regulation Is a Dynamic Process

Most researchers agree that the process of reacting to an emotional stimulus (which may be more temperament-driven) is distinct from efforts to regulate that response, and most measurement strategies reflect this view. However, the distinction becomes artificial unless one acknowledges that the two processes are often difficult to disentangle and that they interact dynamically across time. Static measurement of either is bound to obscure individual differences in such things as initial level of reactivity, success or failure of particular strategies over time, and whether reactivity constrains regulation or vice versa. In fact, few studies have attempted either to measure cross-time patterns of both processes (Buss & Goldsmith, 1998) or to discern patterns of time-linked responding across children.

The dynamic nature of emotion responding leads to the possibility that there are several different dimensions of this responding that may be relevant to specific indices of adjustment and social functioning. So it is possible that the relevant aspect of emotion regulation that we should be interested in when trying to understand particular psychological disorders or social skills will vary depending on the particular features of the domain or skill. Reactivity to provocation, for example, is likely to be very important in understanding peer acceptance and rejection, but it may be less important if one is interested in how children develop anxiety disorders. Greater specificity concerning dimensions of emotion and emotion regulation is needed if we are to describe more process-oriented models of development.

Emotion Regulation Is a Multilevel Process

Implicit, and sometimes explicit, in the research on emotion regulation is the acknowledgement that emotion regulation is never a purely emotional process. Emotion regulation draws on fundamental neurological, physiological, cognitive, and behavioral processes. We believe that emotion regulation and other behavioral and cognitive control processes are linked in fundamental ways to more basic biological and attentional processes and have consequences for later-developing and more sophisticated social and cognitive skills. And we, like some of our colleagues (Blair & Razza, 2007; Eisenberg et al., 2007; Rothbart & Sheese, 2007), embed these processes within the larger construct of self-regulation.

One way to conceptualize emotion regulation is to consider it as one component of the larger self-regulatory system, which we describe as a system of adaptive control that may be observed at the level of physiological, attentional, emotional, behavioral, cognitive, and interpersonal or social processes (Calkins & Fox, 2002; Calkins & Marcovitch, 2010). Control at these various levels emerges, at least in primitive form, across the prenatal, infancy, toddler, and early childhood periods of development. Fundamental to this developmental process is the maturation of different neural systems and processes that provide a functional mechanism for the behavioral integration we ultimately observe as children mature (Lewis & Todd, 2007). Importantly, though, the mastery of earlier regulatory tasks becomes an important component of later competencies, and, by extension, the level of mastery of these early skills may constrain the development of later skills. Thus understanding the development of specific control processes, such as emotion regulation or executive functions, becomes integral to understanding the emergence of other childhood skills and adaptive functioning across developmental domains (Calkins & Fox, 2002).

Emotion Regulation Is a Dyadic Process

From a contextual standpoint, the mechanism(s) responsible for growth in emotion regulation processes that support adaptive skills, as opposed to maladaptive behavioral patterns, are to be found in the interactions between very early child characteristics and the contexts in which development is occurring: social relationships. In infancy, there is an almost exclusive reliance on parents for the regulation of emotion. Over time, interactions with parents in emotion-laden contexts teach children that particular strategies may be more useful for the reduction of emotional arousal than other strategies (Sroufe, 1996). Once children move into the school environment, teachers and peers take on the role of partners in the emotion regulation process by providing input, feedback, and modeling in contexts that may place multiple demands on the child.

The implications for this perspective are that assessment tools that allow us to capture the dyadic nature of emotion regulation may be more informative than tasks that yield information about the individual in isolation. Given that symptoms of many psychological disorders include aspects of social relationships and relationship functioning, some emphasis on these relations may yield information about the dimensions of emotion regulation that are integral to successful functioning. In addition, as the expression of temperament and regulation changes into late childhood and early adolescence, social interactions likely change as well. Although we have highlighted how dysregulation affects numerous domains of adjustment, including social competence, there is little focus on how these factors may affect other critical factors, such as friend selection. Certain temperament traits may influence the selection of social agents. For example, do inhibited children seek out similarly inhibited children, and what are the consequences for social development in these relationships? Similarly, more research is necessary to clarify the role of socialization agents beyond the caregiver in the acquisition of regulatory strategies. As noted in our review, peers and siblings are thought to play an important role in the development of emotion regulation, but there is little research on these effects (Thompson & Meyer, 2007). Specifically considering peer influences, if temperament traits enhance friend selection and friends influence regulation, then the consequences of a maladaptive peer group may have broad-reaching implications for emotional development.

Emotion Regulation Is Developmentally Defined

Although some children appear to be quite proficient in the use of basic emotion regulation skills at a relatively early age, it is clear that across early development dramatic growth occurs in the acquisition and display of emotion regulation skills and abilities. The practice of these newly emerging skills leads to greater automaticity, so that by the time the child is ready to enter the arena of formal schooling, greater effort may be directed toward more demanding academic and social challenges. Moreover, because of its dependence on the maturation of prefrontal–limbic connections, the development of the broader domain of self-regulatory skills is relatively protracted (Beauregard et al., 2004), from the emergence of basic and automatic regulation of biological processes in early childhood to the more self-conscious and intentional regulation of behavior and cognition emerging in middle childhood and adolescence that require and are supported by biological processes (Ochsner & Gross, 2004).

The implication of a developmental framework for conceptualizing emotion regulation is that any empirical investigation of the phenomena requires an appreciation of what emotion regulation is, or consists of, at any particular point in development. That is, it is important to appreciate that early in development, fundamental biological and attentional processes are likely to be the best index of emotion regulation, whereas among older children emotion awareness and appraisal may be more important to the emotion regulation process. Understanding where a child is functioning developmentally leads to measurement of the most relevant emotion regulation processes, which may lead to greater appreciation of the specific skills and deficits that lead to adjustment versus maladjustment.

Emotion Processes Are Amenable to Intervention

Finally, much of the research on temperament, emotion regulation, and social development has been correlational in nature. Thus more experimental research is needed, as is research that examines potential intervention and prevention efforts to enhance regulation and social competence. For example, Izard and colleagues (2008) recently tested the effectiveness of an intervention that focuses exclusively on the development of emotion regulation. The Emotion-Based Prevention Program (EBP) teaches emotion knowledge and regulation of the most common and basic emotions (happiness, sadness, fear, anger, interest and contempt). Children are encouraged to use language to express and respond to their emotions, thereby facilitating control of emotions. Tests of specific interventions that are effective in altering basic control processes are needed to demonstrate the causal role of these processes in children's functioning.

ACKNOWLEDGMENT

The writing of this chapter was supported in part by a National Institute of Health Research Scientist Career Development Award (K02) to Susan D. Calkins (MH 74077).

SUGGESTED READINGS

Blandon, A. Y., Calkins, S. D., Grimm, K., Keane, S. P., & O'Brien, M. (2010). Testing a developmental cascade model of emotional and social competence and peer acceptance. *Development and Psychopathology, 22,* 737–748.

Eisenberg, N., Fabes, R. A., Guthrie, I. K., & Reiser, M. (2000). Dispositional emotionality and regulation: Their role in predicting quality of social functioning. *Journal of Personality and Social Psychology, 78,* 136–157.

Eisenberg, N., Hofer, C., & Vaughan, J. (2007). Effortful control and its socioemotional consequences. In J. J. Gross (Ed.), *Handbook of emotion regulation* (pp. 287–306). New York: Guilford Press.

Moilanen, K. L. (2007). The Adolescent Self-Regulatory Inventory: The development and validation of a questionnaire of short-term and long-term self-regulation. *Journal of Youth and Adolescence, 36,* 835–848.

Rothbart, M. K. (2004). Temperament and the pursuit of an integrated developmental psychology. *Merrill–Palmer Quarterly, 50,* 492–505.

Rothbart, M. K. (2007). Temperament, development, and personality. *Current Directions in Psychological Science, 16,* 207–212.

Rothbart, M. K., Ahadi, S. A., Hershey, K. L., & Fisher, P. (2001). Investigation of temperament at three to seven years: The Children's Behavior Questionnaire. *Child Development, 72,* 1394–1408.

Steinberg, L. (2005). Cognitive and affective development in adolescence. *Trends in Cognitive Sciences, 9,* 69–74.

REFERENCES

Aksan, N., Goldsmith, H. H., Smider, N., Essex, M., Clark, R., Klein, M., et al. (1999). Derivation and prediction of temperamental types among preschoolers. *Developmental Psychology, 35,* 958–971.

Baron, R. M., & Kenny, D. A. (1986). The moderator–mediator variable distinction in social psychological research: Conceptual, strategic, and statistical considerations. *Journal of Personality and Social Psychology, 51,* 1173–1182.

Bates, J. E., & McFadyen-Ketchum, S. (2000). Temperament and parent–child relations as interacting factors in children's behavioral adjustment. In V. J. Molfese & D. L. Molfese (Eds.), *Temperament and personality development across the lifespan* (pp. 141–176). Mahwah, NJ: Erlbaum.

Beauregard, M., Levesque, J., & Paquette, V. (2004). Neural basis of conscious and voluntary self-regulation of emotion. In M. Beauregard (Ed.), *Consciousness, emotional self-regulation and the brain* (pp. 163–194). Amsterdam: Benjamins.

Blair, C. (2002). School readiness: Integrating cognition and emotion in a neurobiological conceptualization of children's functioning at school entry. *American Psychologist, 57,* 111–127.

Blair, C., & Razza, R. P. (2007). Relating effortful control, executive function, and false belief understanding to emerging math and literacy ability in kindergarten. *Child Development,* 78(2), 647–663.

Blair, K. A., Denham, S. A., Kochanoff, A., & Whipple, B. (2004). Playing it cool: Temperament, emotion regulation, and social behavior in preschoolers. *Journal of School Psychology, 42,* 419–443.

Blandon, A. Y., Calkins, S. D., Grimm, K. J., Keane, S. P., & O'Brien, M. (2010). Testing a developmental cascade model of emotional and social competence and early peer acceptance. *Development and Psychopathology, 22,* 737–748.

Blandon, A. Y., Calkins, S. D., Keane, S. P., & O'Brien, M. (2008) Individual differences in trajectories of emotion regulation processes: The effects of maternal depressive symptomatology and children's physiological regulation. *Developmental Psychology, 44,* 1110–1123.

Braungart-Rieker, J. M., & Stifter, C. A. (1996). Infants' responses to frustrating situations: Continuity and change in reactivity and regulation. *Child Development, 67,* 1767–1779.

Bronson, M. B. (2000). *Self-regulation in early childhood: Nature and nurture.* New York: Guilford Press.

Burt, K. B., Obradovic, J., Long, J. D., & Masten, A. S. (2008). The interplay of social competence and psychopathology over 20 years: Testing transactional and cascade models. *Child Development, 79,* 359–374.

Buss, A. H., & Goldsmith, H. H. (1998). Fear and anger regulation in infancy: Effects on the temporal dynamics of affective expression. *Child Development, 69,* 359–374.

Buss, A. H., & Plomin, R. (1984). *Temperament: Early developing personality traits.* Hillsdale, NJ:
Erlbaum.

Calkins, S. D. (1994). Origins and outcomes of individual differences in emotion regulation. *Monographs of the Society for Research in Child Development, 59,* 53–72.

Calkins, S. D. (1997). Cardiac vagal tone indices of temperamental reactivity and behavioral regulation in young children. *Developmental Psychology, 31,* 125–135.

Calkins, S. D. (2004). Temperament and emotional regulation: Multiple models of early development. In M. Beauregard (Ed.), *Consciousness, emotional self-regulation and the brain* (pp.
35–59). Amsterdam: Benjamins.

Calkins, S. D. (2009). Regulatory competence and early disruptive behavior problems: The role of
physiological regulation. In S. Olson & A. Sameroff (Eds.), *Regulatory processes in the development of behavior problems: Biological, behavioral, and social–ecological interactions* (pp.
86–115). New York: Cambridge University Press.

Calkins, S. D., & Dedmon, S. E. (2000). Physiological and behavioral regulation in two-year-old
children with aggressive/destructive behavior problems. *Journal of Abnormal Child Psychology, 28*(2), 103–118.

Calkins, S. D., Dedmon, S., Gill, K., Lomax, L., & Johnson, L. (2002). Frustration in infancy:
Implications for emotion regulation, physiological processes, and temperament. *Infancy, 3,*
175–198.

Calkins, S. D., & Fox, N. A. (1992). The relations among infant temperament, security of attachment, and behavioral inhibition at 24 months. *Child Development, 63,* 1456–1472.

Calkins, S. D., & Fox, N. A. (2002). Self-regulatory processes in early personality development: A
multilevel approach to the study of childhood social withdrawal and aggression. *Development
and Psychopathology, 14,* 477–498.

Calkins, S. D., Fox, N. A., & Marshall, T. R. (1996). Behavioral and psychological antecedents of
inhibition in infancy. *Child Development, 67,* 523–540.

Calkins, S. D., Gill, K., Johnson, M. C., & Smith, C. (1999). Emotional reactivity and emotion
regulation strategies as predictors of social behavior with peers during toddlerhood. *Social
Development, 8,* 310–341.

Calkins, S. D., Gill, K. A., & Williford, A. (1999). Externalizing problems in two-year-olds: Implications for patterns of social behavior and peers' responses to aggression. *Early Education and
Development, 10,* 266–288.

Calkins, S. D., Graziano, P. A., Berdan, L. E., Keane, S. P., & Degnan, K. A. (2008). Predicting
cardiac vagal regulation in early childhood from maternal–child relationship quality during
toddlerhood. *Developmental Psychobiology, 50*(8), 751–766.

Calkins, S. D., & Hill, A. (2007). Caregiver influences on emerging emotion regulation. In J. J. Gross
(Ed.), *Handbook of emotion regulation* (pp. 229–248). New York: Guilford Press.

Calkins, S. D., & Johnson, M. C. (1998). Toddler regulation of distress to frustrating events: Temperamental and maternal correlates. *Infant Behavior and Development, 21*(3), 379–395.

Calkins, S. D., & Keane, S. P. (2004). Cardiac vagal regulation across the preschool period: Stability, continuity, and implications for childhood adjustment. *Developmental Psychobiology, 45,*
101–112.

Calkins, S. D., & Marcovitch, S. (2010). Emotion regulation and executive functioning in early
development: Mechanisms of control supporting adaptive functioning. In S. D. Calkins &
M. A. Bell (Eds.), *Child development at the intersection of emotion and cognition* (pp. 37–57).
Washington, DC: APA Books.

Calkins, S. D., Smith, C. L., Gill, K. L., & Johnson, M. C. (1998). Maternal interactive style across
contexts: Relations to emotional, behavioral, and physiological regulation during toddlerhood.
Social Development, 7, 350–369.

Campos, J. J., Frankel, C. B., & Camras, L. (2004). On the nature of emotion regulation. *Child
Development, 75,* 377–394.

Cicchetti, D., Ganiban, J., & Barnett, D. (1991). Contributions from the study of high-risk populations to understanding the development of emotion regulation. In J. Garber & K. A. Dodge

(Eds.), *The development of emotion regulation and dysregulation* (pp. 15–48). New York: Cambridge University Press.

Cole, P. M., Martin, S. E., & Dennis, T. A. (2004). Emotion regulation as a scientific construct: Methodological challenges and directions for child development research. *Child Development, 75,* 317–333.

Cole, P. M., Zahn-Waxler, C., Fox, N. A., Usher, B. A., & Welsh, J. D. (1996). Individual differences in emotion regulation and behavior problems in preschool children. *Journal of Abnormal Psychology, 105,* 518–529.

Davidson, R. J., & Fox, N. A. (1982). Asymmetrical brain activity discriminates between positive versus negative affective stimuli in human infants. *Science, 218,* 1235–1237.

Davidson, R. J., & Fox, N. A. (1989). Frontal brain asymmetry predicts infants' response to maternal separation. *Journal of Abnormal Psychology, 98,* 127–131.

Degnan, K. A., Calkins, S. D., Keane, S. P., & Hill-Soderlund, A. L. (2008). Profiles of disruptive behavior across early childhood: Contributions of frustration reactivity, physiological regulation, and maternal behavior. *Child Development, 79*(5), 1357–1376.

Denham, S. A., Blair, K. A., DeMulder, E., Levitas, J., Sawyer, K., Auerbach-Major, S., et al. (2003). Preschool emotional competence: Pathway to social competence? *Child Development, 74,* 238–256.

Derryberry, D., & Rothbart, M. K. (1997). Reactive and effortful processes in the organization of temperament. *Development and Psychopathology, 9,* 633–652.

Diener, M. L., Mangelsdorf, S. C., McHale, J. L., & Frosch, C. A. (2002). Infants' behavioral strategies for emotion regulation and with fathers and mothers: Associations with emotional expression and attachment quality. *Infancy, 3,* 153–174.

DiLalla, L. F., & Jones, S. (2000). Genetic and environment influences on temperament in preschoolers. In V. J. Molfese & J. A. Card (Eds.), *Temperament and personality development across the life span* (pp. 33–55). Mahwah, NJ: Erlbaum.

DiPietro, J. A., Hodgson, D. M., Costigan, K. A., & Johnson, T. R. B. (1996). Fetal antecedents of infant temperament. *Child Development, 67,* 2568–2583.

Dodge, K. A., Pettit, G. S., McClaskey, C. L., & Brown, M. M. (1986). Social competence in children. *Monographs of the Society for Research in Child Development, 51*(2), 1–85.

Eisenberg, N. (2001). The core and correlates of affective social competence. *Social Development, 10,* 120–124.

Eisenberg, N., Fabes, R. A., Bernzweig, J., & Karbon, M. (1993). The relations of emotionality and regulation to preschoolers' social skills and sociometric status. *Child Development, 64*(5), 1418–1438.

Eisenberg, N., Fabes, R. A., Guthrie, I. K., & Reiser, M. (2000). Dispositional emotionality and regulation: Their role in predicting quality of social functioning. *Journal of Personality and Social Psychology, 78,* 136–157.

Eisenberg, N., Hofer, C., & Vaughan, J. (2007). Effortful control and its socioemotional consequences. In J. J. Gross (Ed.), *Handbook of emotion regulation* (pp. 287–306). New York: Guilford Press.

Eisenberg, N., Spinrad, T. L., & Morris, A. S. (2002). Regulation, resiliency, and quality of social functioning. *Self and Identity, 1,* 121–128.

El-Sheikh, M. (2001). Parental drinking problems and children's adjustment: Vagal regulation and emotional reactivity as pathways and moderators of risk. *Journal of Abnormal Psychology, 110,* 499–515.

El-Sheikh, M., Harger, J., & Whitson, S. M. (2001). Exposure to interparental conflict and children's adjustment and physical health: The moderating role of vagal tone. *Child Development, 72,* 1617–1636.

Fabes, R. A., & Eisenberg, N. (1992). Young children's coping with interpersonal anger. *Child Development, 63,* 116–128.

Fox, N. A. (1994). Dynamic cerebral processes underlying emotion regulation. In N. A. Fox (Ed.), The development of emotion regulation: Behavioral and biological considerations. *Monographs of the Society for Research in Child Development, 59*(2–3, Serial No. 240), 152–166.

Fox, N. A., & Calkins, S. D. (1993). Pathways to aggression and social withdrawal: Interactions among temperament, attachment and regulation. In K. Rubin & J. Asendorpf (Eds.), *Social withdrawal, shyness and inhibition in childhood* (pp. 81–100). Hillsdale, NJ: Erlbaum.

Fox, N. A., & Calkins, S. D. (2003). The development of self-control of emotion: Intrinsic and extrinsic influences. *Motivation and Emotion, 27,* 7–26.

Fox, N. A., & Davidson, R. J. (1987). Electroencephalogram asymmetry in response to the approach of a stranger and maternal separation in 10-month-old infants. *Developmental Psychology, 23,* 233–240.

Fox, N. A., & Davidson, R. J. (1988). Patterns of brain electrical activity during the expression of discrete emotions in ten-month-old infants. *Developmental Psychology, 24,* 230–236.

Fox, N. A., & Davidson, R. J. (1991). Hemispheric asymmetry and attachment behaviors: Developmental processes and individual differenes in separation protest. In J. L. Gewirtz & W. M. Kurtines (Eds.), *Intersections with attachment* (pp. 147–164). Hillsdale, NJ: Erlbaum.

Fox, N. A., & Gelles, M. (2006). Face-to-face interaction in term and preterm infants. *Infant Mental Health Journal, 5,* 192–205.

Fox, N. A., Henderson, H. A., & Marshall, P. J. (2001). The biology of temperament: An integrative approach. In C. A. Nelson & M. Luciana (Eds.), *The handbook of developmental cognitive neuroscience* (pp. 631–646). Cambridge, MA: MIT Press.

Fox, N. A., Schmidt, L. A., Calkins, S. D., Rubin, K. H., & Coplan, R. J. (1996). The role of frontal activation in the regulation and dysregulation of social behavior during the preschool years. *Development and Psychopathology, 8,* 89–102.

Ganiban, J. M., Saudino, K. J., Ulbricht, H., Neiderhiser, J. M., & Reiss, D. (2008). Stability and change in temperament during adolescence. *Journal of Personality and Social Psychology, 95,* 222–236.

Gilliom, M., Shaw, D., Beck, J., Schonberg, M., & Lukon, J. (2002). Anger regulation in disadvantaged preschool boys: Strategies, antecedents, and the development of self-control. *Developmental Psychology, 38,* 222–235.

Goldsmith, H. H., Buss, K. A., Plemin, R., Rothbart, M., Thomas, A., Chess, S., et al. (1987). Roundtable: What is temperament? Four approaches. *Child Development, 58,* 505–529.

Goldsmith, H. H., & Campos, J. J. (1990). The structure of temperamental fear and pleasure in infants: A psychometric perspective. *Child Development, 61,* 1944–1964.

Goldsmith, H. H., Lemery, K. S., Aksan, N., & Buss, K. A. (2000). Temperamental substrates of personality. In V. J. Molfese & D. L. Molfese (Eds.), *Temperament and personality development across the life span* (pp. 1–32). Mahwah, NJ: Erlbaum.

Goldsmith, H. H., Reilly, J., Lemery, K. S., Longley, S., & Prescott, A. (1995). *Preliminary manual for the Preschool Temperament Assessment Battery* (Version 1.0 Technical Report). Madison: University of Wisconsin, Department of Psychology.

Goldsmith, H. H., & Rothbart, M.K. (1993). *The Laboratory Temperament Assessment Battery (LAB-TAB).* Madison: University of Wisconsin.

Granic, I., Dishion, T. J., & Hollenstein, T. (2003). The family ecology of adolescence: A dynamic systems perspective on normative development. In G. R. Adams & M. D. Berzonsky (Eds.), *Blackwell handbook of adolescence* (pp. 60–91). Malden, MA: Blackwell.

Graziano, P. A., Keane, S. P., & Calkins, S. D. (2007). Cardiac vagal regulation and early peer status. *Child Development, 78,* 264–278.

Gross, J. J., & Thompson, R. A. (2007). Emotion regulation: Conceptual foundations. In J. J. Gross (Ed.), *Handbook of emotion regulation* (pp. 3–24). New York: Guilford Press.

Gunnar, M. R., & Davis, E. P. (2003). Stress and emotion in early childhood. In R. M. Lerner, M. A. Easterbrooks, & J. Mistry (Eds.), *Handbook of psychology: Developmental psychology* (pp. 113–134). Hoboken, NJ: Wiley.

Hanish, L. D., & Guerra, N. G. (2002). A longitudinal analysis of patterns of adjustment following peer victimization. *Development and Psychopathology,14*(1), 69–89.

Harman, C., Rothbart, M. K., & Posner, M. I. (1997). Distress and attention interactions in early infancy. *Motivation and Emotion, 21,* 27–43.

Hartup, W. W. (1996). The company they keep: Friendships and their developmental significance. *Child Development, 67*(1), 1–13.

Henderson, H. A., & Fox, N. A. (2007). Considerations in studying emotion in infants and children. In J. A. Coan & J. J. B. Allen (Eds.), *Handbook of emotion elicitation and assessment* (pp. 349–360). New York: Oxford University Press.

Hinshaw, S. P. (2002). Process, mechanism, and explanation related to externalizing behavior in developmental psychopathology. *Journal of Abnormal Child Psychology, 30,* 431–446.

Hodges, E. V. E., Boivin, M., Vitaro, F., & Bukowski, W. M. (1999). The power of friendship: Protection against an escalating cycle of peer victimization. *Developmental Psychology, 35*(1), 94–101.

Hubbard, J. A. (2001). Emotion expression processes in children's peer interaction: The role of peer rejection, aggression, and gender. *Child Development, 72*(5), 1426–1438.

Izard, C., King, K. A., Trentacosta, C. J., Morgan, J. K., Laurenceau, J., Krauthamer-Ewing, S. E., et al. (2008). Accelerating the development of emotion competence in Head Start children: Effects on adaptive and maladaptive behavior. *Development and Psychopathology, 20,* 369–397.

Kagan, J. (1994). On the nature of emotion. In N. A. Fox (Ed.). The development of emotion regulation: Behavioral and biological considerations. *Monographs of the Society for Research in Child Development, 59*(2–3, Serial No. 240), 7–24.

Kagan, J., Reznick, J. S., & Snidman, N. (1987). The physiology and psychology of behavioral inhibition in children. *Child Development, 58,* 1459–1473.

Kagan, J., & Snidman, N. (1991). Temperamental factors in human development. *American Psychologist, 46,* 856–862.

Kagan, J., Snidman, N., Kahn, V., & Towsley, S. (2007). The preservation of two infant temperaments into adolescence. *Monographs of the Society for Research in Child Development, 72,* 1–95.

Kalpidou, M. D., Power, T. G., Cherry, K. E., & Gottfried, N. W. (2004). Regulation of emotion and behavior among 3- and 5-year-olds. *Journal of General Psychology, 131,* 159–178.

Katainen, S., Raikkonen, K., & Keltikangas-Jarvinen, L. (1998). Development of temperament: Childhood temperament and the mother's childrearing attitudes as predictors of adolescent temperament in a 9-year follow-up study. *Journal of Research on Adolescence, 8,* 485–509.

Keane, S. P., & Calkins, S. D. (2004). Predicting kindergarten peer social status from toddler and preschool problem behavior. *Journal of Abnormal Child Psychology, 32,* 409–423.

Keenan, K. (2000). Emotion dysregulation as a risk factor for child psychopathology. *Clinical Psychology: Science and Practice, 7*(4), 418–434.

Kopp, C. B. (1982). Antecedents of self-regulation: A developmental perspective. *Developmental Psychology, 18,* 199–214.

Kopp, C. B. (2002). Commentary: The codevelopments of attention and emotion regulation. *Infancy, 3*(2), 199–208.

Lengua, L. J. (2006). Growth in temperament and parenting as predictors of adjustment during children's transition to adolescence. *Developmental Psychology, 42,* 819–832.

Lewis, M. D., & Todd, R. M. (2007). The self-regulating brain: Cortical–subcortical feedback and the development of intelligent action. *Cognitive Development, 22,* 406–430.

Mangelsdorf, S., Gunnar, M., Kestenbaum, R., Lang, S., & Andreas, D. (1990). Infant proneness-to-distress temperament, maternal personality, and mother–infant attachment: Associations and goodness of fit. *Child Development, 61,* 820–831.

Maszk, P., Eisenberg, N., & Guthrie, I. K. (1999). Relations of children's social status to their emotionality and regulation: A short-term longitudinal study. *Merrill–Palmer Quarterly, 45,* 468–492.

Matheny, A. P., Riese, M. L., & Wilson, R. S. (1985). Rudiments of infant temperament: Newborn to 9 months. *Developmental Psychology, 21,* 486–494.

Miller-Johnson, S., Coie, J. D., Maumary-Gremaud, A., Bierman, K., & Conduct Problems Prevention Research Group. (2002). Peer rejection and aggression and early starter models of conduct disorder. *Journal of Abnormal Child Psychology, 30*(3), 217–230.

Moilanen, K. L. (2007). The Adolescent Self-Regulatory Inventory: The development and validation of a questionnaire of short-term and long-term self-regulation. *Journal of Youth and Adolescence, 36,* 835–848.

Morris, A. S., Silk, J. S., Steinberg, L., Myers, S. S., & Robinson, L. R. (2007). The role of the family context in the development of emotion regulation. *Social Development, 16,* 361–388.

Murphy, B. C., Shepard, S. A., Eisenberg, N., & Fabes, R. A. (2004). Concurrent and across time prediction of young adolescents' social functioning: The role of emotionality and regulation. *Social Development, 13,* 56–86.

Nachmias, M., Gunnar, M., Mangelsdorf, S., Parritz, R., & Buss, K. (1996). Behavioral inhibition and stress reactivity: The moderating role of attachment security. *Child Development, 67,* 508–522.

Ochsner, K. N., & Gross, J. J. (2004). Thinking makes it so: A social cognitive neuroscience approach to emotion regulation. In R. F. Baumeister & K. D. Vohs (Eds.), *Handbook of self-regulation: Research, theory, and applications* (pp. 229–255). New York: Guilford Press.

Porges, S. W. (1991). Vagal tone: An autonomic mediator of affect. In J. A. Garber & K. A. Dodge (Eds.), *The development of affect regulation and dysregulation* (pp. 111–128). New York: Cambridge University Press.

Porges, S. W. (1996). Physiological regulation in high-risk infants: A model for assessment and potential intervention. *Development and Psychopathology, 8,* 43–58.

Porges, S. W., Doussard-Roosevelt, J., & Maita, A. K. (1994). Vagal tone and the physiological regulation of emotion. *Monographs of the Society for Research in Child Development, 59* (Nos. 2–3, Serial No. 240), 167–186.

Porges, S. W., Doussard-Roosevelt, J. A., Portales, A. L., & Greenspan, S. I. (1996). Infant regulation of the vagal "brake" predicts child behavior problems: A psychobiological model of social behavior. *Developmental Psychobiology, 29,* 697–712.

Porter, F. L., Porges, S. W., & Marshall, R. E. (1988). Newborn pain cries and vagal tone: Parallel changes in response to circumcision. *Child Development, 59,* 495–505.

Posner, M. I., & Rothbart, M. K. (2000). Developing mechanisms of self-regulation. *Development and Psychopathology, 12,* 427–441.

Putnam, S. P., & Stifter, C. A. (2008). Reactivity and regulation: The impact of Mary Rothbart on the study of temperament. *Infant and Child Development, 17,* 311–320.

Raffaelli, M., Crockett, L. J., & Shen, Y. (2005). Developmental stability and change in self-regulation from childhood to adolescence. *Journal of Genetic Psychology, 166,* 54–75.

Reijntjes, A., Stegge, H., & Terwogt, M. M. (2006). Children's coping with peer rejection: The role of depressive symptoms, social competence, and gender. *Infant and Child Development, 15,* 89–107.

Rosenblum, G. D., & Lewis, M. (2003). Emotional development in adolescence. In G. R. Adams & M. D. Berzonsky (Eds.), *Blackwell handbook of adolescence* (pp. 269–289). Malden, MA: Blackwell.

Rothbart, M. K. (1981). Measurement of temperament in infancy. *Child Development, 52,* 569–578.

Rothbart, M. K. (1986). Longitudinal observation of infant temperament. *Developmental Psychology, 22,* 356–365.

Rothbart, M. K. (1989). Temperament and development. In G. Kohnstamm, J. Bates, & M. K. Rothbart (Eds.), *Temperament in childhood* (pp. 187–248). Chichester, UK: Wiley.

Rothbart, M. K. (2007). Temperament and the pursuit of an integrated developmental psychology. In G. W. Ladd (Ed.), *Appraising the human developmental sciences: Essays in honor of Merrill–Palmer Quarterly* (pp. 83–96). Detroit, MI: Wayne State University Press.

Rothbart, M. K., & Bates, J. E. (1998). Temperament. In W. Damon (Series Ed.) & N. Eisenberg (Vol. Ed.), *Handbook of child psychology: Vol. 4. Social, emotional, and personality development* (5th ed., pp. 105–176). New York: Wiley.

Rothbart, M. K., Derryberry, D., & Hershey, K. (2000). Stability of temperament in childhood: Laboratory infant assessment to parent report at seven years. In V. Molfese & D. Molfese (Eds.), *Temperament and personality development across the lifespan* (pp. 85–119). Mahwah, NJ: Erlbaum.

Rothbart, M. K., Posner, M. I., & Boylan, A. (1990). Regulatory mechanisms in infant development. In J. Erms (Ed.), *The development of attention: Research and theory* (pp. 139–160). Amsterdam: Elsevier.

Rothbart, M. K., Posner, M. I., & Rosicky, J. (1994). Orienting in normal and pathological development. *Development and Psychopathology, 6,* 635–652.

Rothbart, M. K., & Sheese, B. E. (2007). Temperament and emotion regulation. In J. J. Gross (Ed.), *Handbook of emotion regulation* (pp. 331–350). New York: Guilford Press.

Ruff, H., & Rothbart, M. K. (1996). *Attention in early development.* New York: Oxford University Press.

Salisch, M. V. (2001). Children's emotional development: Challenges in their relationships to parents, peers, and friends. *International Journal of Behavioral Development, 25*, 310–319.

Seifer, R., & Sameroff, A. J. (1986). The concept, measurement, and interpretation of temperament in young children: A survey of research issues. *Advances in Developmental and Behavioral Pediatrics, 7*, 1–43.

Seifer, R., Schiller, M., Sameroff, A., Resnick, S., & Riordan, K. (1996). Attachment, maternal sensitivity, and infant temperament during the first year of life. *Developmental Psychology, 32*, 12–25.

Shields, A., & Cicchetti, D. (1997). Emotion regulation in school-age children: The development of a new criterion Q-sort scale. *Developmental Psychology, 33*, 906–916.

Shields, A., Dickstein, S., Seifer, R., Gusti, L., Magee, K. D., & Spritz, B. (2001). Emotional competence and early school adjustment: A study of preschoolers at risk. *Early Education and Development, 12*, 73–96.

Shiner, R., & Caspi, A. (2003). Personality differences in childhood and adolescence: Measurement, development, and consequences. *Journal of Child Psychology and Psychiatry and Allied Disciplines, 44*, 2–33.

Shipman, K., Schneider, R., & Brown, A. (2004). Emotion dysregulation and psychopathology. In M. Beauregard (Ed.), *Consciousness, emotional self-regulation and the brain* (pp. 61–85). Amsterdam: Benjamins.

Sroufe, A. L. (1996). *Emotional development: The organization of emotional life in the early years.* New York: Cambridge University Press.

Stansbury, K., & Gunnar, M. R. (1994). Adrenocortical activity and emotion regulation. In N. A. Fox (Ed.), The development of emotion regulation: Biological and behavioral considerations. *Monographs of the Society for Research in Child Development, 59*(2–3, Serial No. 240, pp. 108–134).

Stansbury, K., & Sigman, M. (2000). Responses of preschoolers in two frustrating episodes: Emergence of complex strategies for emotion regulation. *Journal of Genetic Psychology, 161*, 182–202.

Steinberg, L. (2004). Risk taking in adolescence: What changes, and why? In R. E. Dahl (Ed.), *Adolescent brain development: Vulnerabilities and opportunities* (pp. 51–58). New York: New York Academy of Sciences.

Steinberg, L. (2005). Cognitive and affective development in adolescence. *Trends in Cognitive Sciences, 9*, 69–74.

Stifter, C. A., & Braungart, J. M. (1995). The regulation of negative reactivity in infancy: Function and development. *Developmental Psychology, 31*, 448–455.

Stifter, C. A., & Corey, J. M. (2001). Vagal regulation and observed social behavior in infancy. *Social Development, 10*, 189–201.

Stifter, C. A., & Fox, N. A. (1990). Infant reactivity: Physiological correlates of newborn and 5-month temperament. *Developmental Psychology, 26*, 582–588.

Stifter, C. A., Fox, N. A., & Porges, S.W. (1989). Facial expressivity and vagal tone in five- and ten-month old infants. *Infant Behavior and Development, 12*, 127–137.

Stifter, C. A., & Moyer, D. (1991). The regulation of positive affect: Gaze aversion activity during mother–infant interaction. *Infant Behavior and Development, 14*, 111–123.

Thomas, A., Birch, H., Chess, S., Hertzig, M., & Korn, S. (1964). *Behavioral individuality in early childhood.* New York: New York University Press.

Thomas, A., & Chess, S. (1977). *Temperament and development.* New York: Brunner/Mazel.

Thomas, A., Chess, S., & Birch, H. G. (1970). The origins of personality. *Scientific American, 223*, 102–109.

Thompson, R. A. (1994). Emotion regulation: A theme in search of definition. *Monographs of the Society for Research in Child Development, 59*, 250–283.

Thompson, R. A., & Lagattuta, K. H. (2006). Feeling and understanding: Early emotional development. In K. McCartney & D. Philips (Eds.), *Blackwell handbook of early childhood development* (pp. 317–337). Malden, MA: Blackwell.

Thompson, R. A., Lewis, M. D., & Calkins, S. D. (2008). Reassessing emotion regulation. *Child Development Perspectives, 2*, 124–131.

Thompson, R. A., & Meyer, S. (2007). Socialization of emotion regulation in the family. In J.J. Gross (Ed.), *Handbook of emotion regulation* (pp. 249–268). New York: Guilford Press.

Trentacosta, C. J., & Izard, C. E. (2007). Kindergarten children's emotion competence as a predictor of their academic competence in first grade. *Emotion, 7,* 77–88.

Wilson, B., & Gottman, J. (1996). Attention: The shuttle between emotion and cognition: Risk, resiliency, and physiological bases. In E. Hetherinton & E. Blechman (Eds.), *Stress, coping and resiliency in children and families* (pp. 189–228). Mahwah, NJ: Erlbaum.

Yap, M. B. H., Allen, N. B., & Ladouceur, C. D. (2008). Maternal socialization of positive affect: The impact of invalidation on adolescent emotion regulation and depressive symptomatology. *Child Development, 79,* 1415–1431.

Zeman, J., Cassano, M., Perry-Parrish, C., & Stegall, S. (2006). Emotion regulation in children and adolescents. *Developmental and Behavioral Pediatrics, 27,* 155–168.

Part II

Self and Relationships

4

The Self and Identity

Lisa H. Rosen
Meagan M. Patterson

When four and a half months old, he repeatedly smiled at my image and his own in a mirror, and no doubt mistook them for real objects.
—DARWIN *discussing his son's response to mirror images* (1877, p. 289)

No, I don't really think about who I am, well it happens sometimes ... I think about how I am towards others. I want to be friends with everyone I meet ... I don't want to be unpleasant....
—*Adolescent describing himself* (in Adamson, Hartman, & Lyxell, 1999, p. 25)

Self-understanding develops throughout life; an infant is unable to recognize his or her reflection, but an adolescent is capable of reflecting on him- or herself along multiple dimensions and in relation to others. This chapter describes the development of self-understanding from infancy through late adolescence. We begin this chapter by describing how theorists have conceptualized the self. This chapter then describes infants' emerging sense of self, including discrimination of self from others, a growing sense of personal agency, and self-recognition. Next, we depict the development of the self-concept, or the manner in which one defines oneself. The self-concept includes perceptions of one's personal characteristics and roles (Brinthaupt & Lipka, 1985; Damon & Hart, 1988; McConnell & Strain, 2007). Then we discuss self-esteem, which refers to the extent to which one's overall evaluation of oneself is positive or negative. That is, self-esteem is the *evaluative* element of the self-concept. Self-esteem includes evaluations of competence, as well as liking of oneself or feelings about one's worthiness as a person (Brown & Marshall, 2006). The chapter concludes by detailing the manner in which adolescents reach a well-developed definition of the self by forging a unique identity. A mature sense of identity entails a strong, coherent understanding of who one is, what one values, and one's future life course (Erikson, 1980; Marcia, 2002a).

DUALITY OF SELF

Ever since the work of William James (1890), the tendency has been for researchers to differentiate between the self as subject and self as object (Harter, 2003; Leary & Tangney, 2003; Lewis & Brooks-Gunn, 1979; Ross, 1992). The self as subject, also known as the "I-self" or the existential self, refers to understanding the self in terms of its functions as knower and actor. Understanding the self as subject entails four types of self-processes: (1) a sense of personal agency, (2) a sense of distinctness, (3) a sense of self-continuity, and (4) a sense of self-awareness (Butterworth, 1992; Damon & Hart, 1988; Harter, 2003). The self as object, also known as the "Me-self" or the categorical self, refers to the self as known. Understanding the self as object includes perceptions of one's characteristics and roles and is often referred to as the self-concept (Damon & Hart, 1988; Leary & Tangney, 2003; Ross, 1992). The self as object includes perceptions of material attributes (e.g., one's physical characteristics and belongings), social attributes (e.g., social roles and relationships), and what James referred to as "spiritual" attributes (e.g., thoughts, psychological processes; Damon & Hart, 1988; Harter, 1998; James, 1890).

The self as subject develops before the self as object; "before we can know what we are like, we first need to know that we exist" (Brown, 1998, p. 91). The I-self is evident from a very early point in infancy and likely has its roots in the processes of sensory perception (Butterworth, 1990). The beginnings of self–other differentiation and a sense of personal agency may be evident within the first few months of life (Lewis & Brooks-Gunn, 1979; Rochat & Striano, 2000). Newborn infants are able to distinguish between their own cries and those of other infants (Dondi, Simion, & Caltran, 1999). A newborn is also more likely to display the rooting response in reaction to external stimulation (i.e., an experimenter touching his or her cheek) than to self-stimulation (i.e., touching his or her own cheek; Rochat & Striano, 2000). Young infants are capable of imitation, which suggests the ability to detect equivalences between one's own behavior and that of others (Meltzoff, 1990, 2007). With development, individuals come to understand the self as distinct from others, as manifested in their unique combinations of attributes, as well as subjective experiences (Damon & Hart, 1988).

Young infants also demonstrate an early sense of personal agency, or the understanding that they can influence some events in their environments. Infants come to realize that they can control objects in their environments, as well as influence people (Rochat & Striano, 2000). For example, based on expectations that they have formed, infants may attempt to elicit certain behaviors from caregivers by behaving in a certain way, such as extending both arms toward the caregiver. As the child acquires language, this sense of personal agency is echoed in sentiments of toddlers such as, "I doed it myself" (Wigfield & Karpathian, 1991, p. 233).

Knowledge of the self as object (i.e., the self-concept) follows from knowledge of the self as subject. Young children begin to describe the self in terms of concrete, observable characteristics such as physical attributes, possessions, and family roles (Brinthaupt & Lipka, 1985; Damon & Hart, 1982; Harter, 1998). With development, individuals come to describe the self in terms of abstract psychological characteristics such as attitudes, beliefs, and feelings (Damon & Hart, 1982; Harter, 1998; Ross, 1992), as is discussed in more detail later.

SELF-RECOGNITION AND THE EMERGING SELF

Self-recognition entails identification of the self in a mirror, photograph, or video recording, along with an understanding that the image is a visual representation of the self. Lewis and Brooks-Gunn (1979) have studied the development of self-recognition extensively; they believe that "self-recognition is a window on the emerging concept of self and, by necessity, implies a concept of self" (p. 222). Self-recognition is often examined using a procedure known as the mark test or the rouge test. This procedure was pioneered by Gallup (1970) and Amsterdam (1972). Gallup (1970) was examining self-recognition in chimpanzees, and Amsterdam (1972) was examining self-recognition in infants. As part of Gallup's procedure, he anesthetized the chimpanzees and put a small amount of red dye on the eyebrow and the opposite ear. When the chimpanzees awoke and were put in front of a mirror, they engaged in mark-directed behaviors (e.g., touching the marked areas on their faces, visually inspecting the marked area), providing evidence of self-recognition.

A version of this test has been applied to the study of self-recognition in infants (Lewis & Brooks-Gunn, 1979). The caregiver covertly applies a bit of rouge to the infant's nose, often under the guise of wiping dirt from the face. The infant is then given the opportunity to observe him- or herself in a mirror. In this paradigm, self-recognition is operationally defined as mark-directed behavior, because this behavior implies an understanding that an image of the self is reflected in the mirror and that the mark lies not on the mirror image but on the infant's face (Brooks-Gunn & Lewis, 1984). This procedure has since been used by many researchers to examine self-recognition in infancy and the toddler years. Some researchers have modified this procedure; for example, one research group covertly placed stickers on participants' legs as they were sitting in a high chair to demonstrate that mirror self-recognition extends to other parts of the body in addition to the face (Nielsen, Suddendorf, & Slaughter, 2006).

There is a developmental progression in infants' responses to their mirror images before they engage in mark-directed behavior (Amsterdam, 1972; Brooks-Gunn & Lewis, 1984; Lewis & Brooks-Gunn, 1979; Lewis, Brooks-Gunn, & Jaskir, 1985). Initially, infants tend to display social behavior toward their mirror images, as if looking at a playmate. Infants may smile at, vocalize toward, or touch their mirror images, as they might with another infant. Mirror-directed social behavior is most common between 5 and 18 months of age and then decreases across the second year of life. Infants react in a self-conscious fashion when viewing their mirror images at around 15 months of age. These self-conscious reactions suggest a sense of self-awareness and are reflected in behaviors characteristic of self-admiration and embarrassment (e.g., strutting, grooming, glancing in a coy fashion, blushing). Mark-directed behavior, which is indicative of self-recognition, first appears around 15 months of age and is evident in the majority of 18- to 24-month olds. An infant who notices that his or her face has been marked may try to wipe off the mark or use the mirror to scrutinize the spot on his or her nose.

The development of self-recognition is associated with the emergence of personal pronoun usage (e.g., *me, I*; Lewis & Ramsay, 2004). Infants who display mark-directed behavior in the rouge test use more personal pronouns than those who fail to display behavior indicative of self-recognition. Thus, the use of personal pronouns further suggests a rudimentary concept of self. Only a small percentage of infants demonstrate self-recognition at 15 months of age, and, likewise, the use of personal pronouns is rare at this time. The use of personal pronouns increases during the second year of life (Bates, 1990; Lewis & Ramsay, 2004). Many children also begin to use their own names around 18–20 months of age (Bates, 1990).

Although developmental trends in self-recognition have been widely documented, there are individual differences within age groups (Brooks-Gunn & Lewis, 1984). The emerging sense of self develops within the context of one's social world, and early experiences with caregivers may influence the development of self-recognition (Keller et al., 2004). Secure attachment may be associated with greater knowledge of self at 2–3 years of age; securely attached infants demonstrated greater success than insecurely attached infants on featural knowledge tasks, including the rouge/mark test and identifying the self with verbal labels (Pipp, Easterbrooks, & Harmon, 1992). Infants with secure attachments use their caregivers as a secure base from which to explore their environments, and this greater exploration may help to account for advanced self-recognition in securely attached infants (Schneider-Rosen & Cicchetti, 1984).

In addition to influencing self-recognition, caregiver behaviors can also affect the development of autobiographical memory or recollections of distinct events in one's personal past (Fivush & Nelson, 2004; Harley & Reese, 1999). Most adults and older children are unable to recall events that occurred within the first few years of their lives. This inability to retrieve events that took place prior to age 3 is referred to as infantile or childhood amnesia (Harley & Reese, 1999; Howe, 1998). The emergence of autobiographical memory follows achievement of self-recognition as assessed by the mark test. A concept of the self allows for memories to be stored in reference to the self; Howe suggests this enables encoding of experiences as ones that "happened to a 'me'" (1998, p. 479). Parents reflect on past events with their children, such as a visit to a park or a family trip. Some parents rely on an elaborative style of reminiscing— that is, they talk about these events with a greater level of detail with their children. Parents who demonstrate an elaborative style also employ open-ended questions to elicit detailed recollections from their children; for example, a mother may ask "and what'd daddy do on the boat?" (Harley & Reese, 1999, p. 1341). A maternal elaborative style of reminiscing contributes to the development of autobiographical memory (Fivush & Nelson, 2004; Harley & Reese, 1999).

SELF-CONCEPT DEVELOPMENT

Self-description follows the emergence of self-recognition. The ability to recognize oneself suggests the beginnings of the Me-self. The Me-self becomes elaborated to include descriptive information about the self (Stipek, Gralinski, & Kopp, 1990), and this self-concept changes with development. The manner in which children describe themselves first centers on concrete terms and becomes more abstract with development (Brinthaupt & Lipka, 1985; Montemayor & Eisen, 1977). Self-descriptions shift from the social exterior (e.g., physical, demographic, and behavioral attributes) to the psychological interior (e.g., attitudes, emotions); Rosenberg writes, "as the child grows older, he becomes less of a demographer, less of a behaviorist, more of a psychological clinician" (Rosenberg, 1979, p. 202). Although qualitative changes take place in children's prototypical self-descriptions with age, it is important to note that these changes do not progress in an all-or-none fashion. There is evidence that children may sometimes describe themselves in social and psychological terms beginning at a young age. Likewise, older children and adolescents continue to describe the self in physical terms (Damon & Hart, 1982, 1988). The self-concept becomes more differentiated with age, and adolescents are able to describe themselves along a greater number of dimensions than are younger children (Montemayor & Eisen, 1977). We describe the development of the self-concept in greater detail, focusing on how children answer the question "Who am I?" at different periods of development.

Early Childhood

Preschool-age children will commonly mention observable characteristics when they are asked to describe themselves (Harter, 1998, 2003). For example, a typical pre-schooler may describe him- or herself as follows:

> I'm 3 years old and I live in a big house with my mother and father, and my brother Jason, and my sister, Lisa. I have blue eyes and a kitty that is orange and a television in my own room. I know all my ABC's listen: A, B, C, D, E, F, G, H, J, L, K, O, M, P, Q, X, Z. I can run real fast. I like pizza and I have a nice teacher at preschool. I can count up to 100, want to hear me? I love my dog Skipper. I can climb to the top of the jungle gym, I'm not scared! I'm never scared! I'm always happy. I have brown hair and I go to preschool. I'm really strong. I can lift this chair, watch me! (in Harter, 1999, p. 37)

In describing themselves, young children often mention their physical attributes (e.g., blue eyes, brown hair) and possessions (e.g., kitty, television). They may also make mention of their typical behavior or actions that they can accomplish (Keller, Ford, & Meacham, 1978); these descriptions focus on specific behaviors (e.g., "I can count up to 100"; Harter, 1999).

Although young children's self-descriptions focus on observable attributes, there is some evidence to suggest that they possess a rudimentary understanding of their psychological characteristics. Eder (1990) presented young children with a forced-choice task that was less dependent on verbal abilities than were previous studies in which young children were asked to describe themselves. Children were presented with pairs of statements, one of which represented the high end point and one of which represented the low end point of a series of psychological dimensions (e.g., achievement, aggression, social closeness), and they selected the statement that they found to best describe themselves. For example, children selected one of the following statements as most self-descriptive: "It's more fun to do things with other people than by myself" or "It's more fun to do things by myself than with other people" (Eder, 1990, p. 853). Children answered in a consistent fashion, and responding was stable across time. These findings suggest an incipient understanding of the self along psychological dimensions.

Middle Childhood

Children become able to describe themselves in terms of their psychological charac-teristics with development. This is exemplified by the following description offered by an 11½-year-old girl:

> My name is A. I'm a human being. I'm a girl. I'm a truthful person. I'm not pretty. I do so-so in my studies. I'm a very good cellist. I'm a very good pianist. I'm a little bit tall for my age. I like several boys. I like several girls. I'm old-fashioned. I play tennis. I am a very good swimmer. I try to be helpful. I'm always ready to be friends with anybody. Mostly I'm good, but I lose my temper. I'm not well-liked by some girls and boys. I don't know if I'm liked by boys or not. (in Montemayor & Eisen, 1977, pp. 317–318)

During middle childhood, individuals begin to describe themselves in terms of traits, which are generalizations based on the combination of specific behaviors (Brown, 1998; Harter, 1999, 2003). In the preceding example, the child describes herself as helpful; this assessment may be based on helping her parents with the dishes, assisting her younger sibling with his homework, and volunteering to pass back papers for her teacher. During this developmental period, there is also an increasing tendency to describe the self in terms of interpersonal qualities (e.g., not well liked, ready to be friends with anyone).

In middle childhood, children increasingly engage in social comparisons, evaluating their own behavior in light of their peers' performance (Harter, 1999; Ruble, Boggiano, Feldman, & Loebl, 1980). The girl in the preceding example may have come to see herself as a good swimmer because she often swims faster than her peers and receives more positive feedback from her coach. The self-portrait of middle childhood includes more information regarding the psychological interior than that of early childhood and is also more dependent on how one relates to peers.

Adolescence

Adolescents' own beliefs, values, and moral positions are often included in their self-descriptions (Harter, 1999; Montemayor & Eisen, 1977). For example, a 17-year-old girl described herself in the following terms:

> I am a human being. I am a girl. I am an individual. I don't know who I am. I am a Pisces. I am a moody person. I am an indecisive person. I am an ambitious person. I am a very curious person. I am not an individual. I am a loner. I am an American (God help me). I am a Democrat. I am a liberal person. I am a radical. I am a conservative. I am a pseudoliberal. I am an atheist. I am not a classifiable person (i.e., I don't want to be). (in Montemayor & Eisen, 1977, p. 318)

Adolescents may describe themselves in terms of their political affiliation (e.g., Democrat) and religious views (e.g., atheist).

Adolescents are able to combine different traits to formulate more abstract descriptions of themselves. For example, an adolescent may describe him- or herself as follows: "At school, I'm pretty intelligent. I know that because I'm smart when it comes to how I do in classes, I'm curious about learning new things, and I'm also creative when it comes to solving problems" (Harter, 1999, p. 60). This description reflects the ability to integrate specific traits (i.e., smart, curious, and creative) into a higher order conceptualization of the self (i.e., intelligent).

Furthermore, adolescents come to view themselves differently depending on social context and partners (Griffin, Chassin, & Young, 1981). The self becomes progressively more differentiated with development as adolescents come to realize that they behave differently at home and school or when interacting with friends, teachers, and family members (Harter & Monsour, 1992). There are even differences in adolescents' self-descriptions in the role of son or daughter when referencing their relation to their mothers and to their fathers (Griffin et al., 1981).

The proliferation of different role-dependent selves may result in a sense of confusion over what constitutes the true self (Harter & Monsour, 1992). Adolescents behave differently in diverse contexts, and awareness of opposing self-attributes may be disconcerting. For instance, a teenager may be baffled over how she can be outgoing with her very close friends but shy in front of the entire class. During early adolescence, individuals are less likely to notice and be troubled by conflicting self-attributes because they do not yet have the cognitive ability to compare abstract self-descriptors. Even though those in middle adolescence possess the cognitive ability to compare abstract self-attributes, they are not yet able to integrate these seemingly opposing self-conceptions into an organized and consistent self-portrait. Individuals in middle adolescence are most likely to recognize and be upset by opposing self-attributes. During this developmental period, adolescents may be troubled by differences in their behavior as a function of interactional context. For example, one adolescent participant expressed such a concern noting that "I really think of myself as a happy person, and I want to be that way with everyone because I think that's my true self, but I get depressed with my family and it bugs me because that's not what I want to be like" (Harter & Monsour, 1992, p. 253). In later adolescence, individuals become able to integrate these potential inconsistencies into a coherent self-theory and thus are less likely to acknowledge and be concerned about potentially opposing attributes. As an illustration, one adolescent remarked: "Yeah, I can be both depressed and cheerful because I am a moody person" (Harter & Monsour, 1992, p. 256). This developmental progression makes clear that the self-concept of late adolescence has evolved dramatically from the concrete descriptions of early childhood.

SELF-ESTEEM

Self-esteem refers to the evaluative aspect of the self-concept and has been a topic of interest and debate throughout the history of psychology. We first provide an overview of the self-esteem literature before focusing on the developmental factors that influence self-esteem and how self-esteem changes with development.

Consequences of Self-Esteem

Self-esteem has been linked to a number of concurrent and subsequent life outcomes. Low self-esteem in childhood and adolescence is associated with various negative outcomes, including depression and other mental health issues, substance abuse, school dropout, risky sexual behavior and teenage pregnancy, lower relationship satisfaction, and criminal behavior (Barry, Grafeman, Adler, & Pickard, 2007; Crockenberg & Soby, 1989; Ethier et al., 2006; Harter, 1999; Lan & Lanthier, 2003; Reinherz et al., 1993; Roberts, Gotlib, & Kassel, 1996; Rumberger, 1995; Trzesniewski et al., 2006).

Some psychologists have questioned whether self-esteem is a useful construct (Baumeister, Campbell, Kreuger, & Vohs, 2003). These researchers argue that high self-esteem is an effect, rather than a cause, of positive life outcomes. Other researchers (Swann, Chang-Schneider, & McClarty, 2007) have argued that self-esteem is, in fact, a useful construct and does influence individuals' choices; these researchers argue that the predictive power of self-esteem is greatest when the self-view measured is closely tied to the outcome of interest (e.g., academic self-concept will predict grades better than general self-esteem).

Behavioral Correlates of Self-Esteem

In young children, who lack the ability to verbalize their global self-esteem, measurement of behavioral correlates of self-esteem is especially important. According to research with early childhood educators, young children with high self-esteem are confident and independent in their behavior and display adaptive reactions to stress (Harter, 1990).

In addition to behaviors that reflect self-esteem, individuals may engage in certain behaviors designed to preserve self-esteem. For example, individuals who do not expect to be successful or receive positive feedback in a particular domain may disidentify with that domain or state that the domain is not important to them and thus that their success or failure in that domain is not relevant to their sense of overall self-esteem (Crocker & Major, 1989; Major, Spencer, Schmader, Wolfe, & Crocker, 1998).

Promotion of Positive Self-Esteem

Recently, some researchers have argued that individuals born in the 1970s, '80s, and '90s have been influenced by parents' and teachers' attempts to promote self-esteem to such an extent that they now possess inflated self-esteem, reflecting positive self-views that are not consistent with actual accomplishments or abilities (Twenge, 2006). However, a recent evaluation of trends in self-esteem and self-enhancement indicates that these phenomena have not increased over time (Trzesniewski, Donnellan, & Robins, 2008).

Due to the importance of self-esteem and its relationship with various behavioral outcomes, a number of interventions aimed at raising individuals' self-esteem have been implemented. Intervention programs can be successful at increasing self-esteem and performance in related domains, such as academics. In order to be most effective, intervention programs should be theory-based and specifically focused on raising self-esteem (Haney & Durlak, 1998).

Self-Esteem as a Reflection of Ability

In early childhood, self-esteem levels are generally unrelated to children's actual competence (Harter, 1999). With increasing age, children's self-evaluations become more accurate (e.g., perceptions of academic ability are more closely related to school grades for older children than for younger children; Chapman & Tunmer, 1995). This increase in accuracy is due to changes in criteria used to evaluate competence, as well as cognitive development (Bouffard, Markovits, Vezeau, Boisvert, & Dumas, 1998; Stipek & Mac Iver, 1989). Among elementary school-age children, those with higher levels of cognitive development have more accurate self-perceptions than same-age peers with lower levels of cognitive development (Bouffard et al., 1998).

Developmental Influences on Self-Esteem

Heredity

Behavioral genetic research indicates that both overall self-esteem and specific elements of self-concept (e.g., perceived academic or athletic competence) are influenced by genetics. Several studies indicate that genetics and nonshared environment have greater influences on self-esteem than shared (family) environment (McGuire et al., 1999; Neiss, Sedikides, & Stevenson, 2002). For example, McGuire et al. (1999) found that identical twins' self-concepts were twice as correlated as those of fraternal twins and nontwin siblings. This relationship may be due to the influence of genes on characteristics strongly related to self-esteem, such as physical attractiveness (Harter, 2006).

Gender

Researchers have observed consistent gender differences in self-esteem. Gender differences in self-views tend to be consistent with gender stereotypes, with girls and women having higher self-esteem in areas such as reading and interpersonal relationships and boys and men having higher self-esteem in areas such as mathematics, sports, and physical appearance (Harter, 1999). Multiple explanations have been suggested for gender differences in self-evaluations, including the influence of gender stereotypes, socialization by parents and other adults, and motivational differences (see Pomerantz, Saxon, & Kenney, 2001, for review).

Attachment Style

Attachment theorists have argued that early relationships with caregivers influence children's views of themselves, their caregivers, and interpersonal relationships in general (Bowlby, 1973, 1979). These views, called *internal working models*, are carried with the individual throughout life and influence many aspects of life, including relationship quality and self-esteem. In *Attachment and Loss*, Bowlby claimed that "in the working model of the self that anyone builds a key feature is his notion of how acceptable or unacceptable he himself is in the eyes of his attachment figures" (Bowlby, 1973, p. 203).

Children who have a secure attachment to the attachment figure view the attachment figure as accepting and reliable and view themselves as worthy of acceptance and love. These positive internal working models of the self are, in turn, associated with high self-esteem (Cassidy, 1988; Mikulincer, 1995; Verschueren, Marcoen, & Schoefs, 1996). Conversely, children who have developed an insecure attachment will form working models of attachment figures as uninterested or rejecting and of the self as devalued, unlovable, or incompetent (Bretherton & Munholland, 1999). Specific mother–child attachment styles are associated with particular patterns of self-views. Securely attached children generally have positive but realistic self-views, whereas insecurely attached children more frequently have negative or idealized self-views (Cassidy, 1988).

Parenting Behaviors

Influences of parenting on children's self-esteem do not stop after infancy. Effects of parenting style or parenting behaviors on self-esteem have been found from early childhood through adolescence. Preschool-age children typically have highly positive self-views and high self-esteem, but their tendency to view the world in a rigid, all-or-none fashion can lead to universally negative self-views in the case of abuse or insecure attachment (Crittenden & Ainsworth, 1989; Toth, Cicchetti, Macfie, & Emde, 1997). In middle childhood, high self-esteem is linked to an authoritative parenting style in which parents are warm and affectionate while setting clear limits for acceptable behavior (Lamborn, Mounts, Steinberg, & Dornbusch, 1991). Children whose parents are abusive may continue to hold the undifferentiated (e.g., universally negative) self-views typical of younger children (Harter, 1999). In adolescence, views of the mother as controlling or unaffectionate, as well as views of the self as defiant, untrusting, or debilitated (i.e., high in anxiety and self-blame), are related to lower self-esteem (Ojanen & Perry, 2007). Perceived support from parents is related to high self-esteem within the context of the parent–adolescent relationship (Harter, Waters, & Whitesell, 1998).

Others' Appraisals

In addition to parents' behaviors, parents' (and others') views of the child also have a meaningful influence on self-esteem. The role of others' views in the development of self-esteem was first examined by Cooley (1902), who developed the concept of the "looking glass self," a self-concept formed by learning of others' perceptions and evaluations of oneself. Modern approaches to the influence of others' views on self-esteem have often focused on reflected appraisals (i.e., an individual's perceptions of others' perceptions and evaluations of him or her). Reflected appraisals may be consistent or inconsistent with the individual's self-appraisals and with others' actual appraisals of the individual, though self-appraisals are generally more strongly related to reflected appraisals than to others' actual appraisals (Berndt & Burgy, 1996). The influence of reflected appraisals on self-esteem may be stronger for characteristics that are heavily dependent on the perceptions of others, such as physical attractiveness (Felson, 1985).

Social Comparisons

Social comparison is the process by which individuals compare their skills, abilities, or performance to that of others. Early researchers argued that social comparison is most common when one is uncertain about one's ability and information from objective sources is insufficient to resolve the uncertainty (Festinger, 1954); later researchers have examined the role of comparisons that enhance or confirm existing self-views (Brown, 1986; Swann, Pelham, & Krull, 1989).

Children younger than 7 rarely use social comparison information to evaluate their own abilities; use of social comparison increases during the early elementary school years and may decrease in the later elementary school years (Ruble et al., 1980; Ruble & Frey, 1991). Young children are most likely to judge their performance relative to absolute standards, such as working all problems correctly. Throughout the lifespan, social comparison continues to occur, with same-age peers serving as the most frequent comparison targets (Suls & Mullen, 1982). Older children may move away from direct social comparisons and toward more subtle social comparisons as explicit comparisons come to be seen as "bragging" or otherwise socially undesirable (Pomerantz, Ruble, Frey, & Greulich, 1995).

Developmental Changes in Self-Esteem

Large cross-sectional studies indicate that, overall, self-esteem is high in childhood, drops over the course of adolescence, rises over early and middle adulthood, and drops in old age (Marsh, 1989; Robins, Trzesniewski, Tracy, Gosling, & Potter, 2002). Along with these general developmental trends, however, there is evidence that individuals' self-esteem is fairly consistent over time (Robins et al., 2002; Shapka & Keating, 2005). That is, a person with high self-esteem in childhood will likely also have high self-esteem in adolescence and adulthood.

There is substantial evidence that self-esteem becomes more differentiated with development, though some researchers have argued that differentiation primarily occurs between early childhood and early adolescence (Harter, 1999; Marsh, 1989). With development, the number of measurable domains of self-esteem increases. For example, a commonly used measure of self-esteem in middle childhood includes the domains of scholastic competence, athletic competence, physical appearance, peer acceptance, behavioral conduct, and global self-worth; the corresponding measure for adolescents adds assessments of job competence, close friendships, and romantic relationships (Harter, 1999).

Early Childhood

Young children are able to indicate their self-esteem in relevant domains, such as cognitive competence and peer acceptance (Harter & Pike, 1984). Young children are generally unable to discuss their global self-esteem, although there are behavioral indicators of global self-esteem, such as displays of confidence and adaptive reactions to failure and change, that can be reliably measured through observation (Haltiwanger, 1989; Harter, 1990; Harter & Pike, 1984).

Middle Childhood

In middle childhood, children show increasing use of social comparison information and increasing awareness of the expectations of others (such as parents and teachers); these factors contribute to a decrease in overall self-esteem and an increase in the accuracy of self-perceptions relative to early childhood (Oosterwegel & Oppenheimer, 1993; Ruble & Frey, 1991).

Adolescence

Much research in adolescence has focused on differences in levels of global self-esteem across different situations or contexts. The valence (positive or negative) of adolescents' self-descriptions, as well as their perceptions of how much they like themselves as people, often vary based on the environment or relationship context (Harter, Bresnick, Bouchey, & Whitesell, 1997; Harter et al., 1998). Self-esteem in a given interpersonal context is related to the level of support and approval the individual perceives as being provided in that relationship (Harter et al., 1998). Self-esteem in adolescence tends to be highly dependent on the adolescent's perceptions of others' views of him or her (i.e., reflected appraisals); this reliance on the views of others may lead to volatility in self-esteem (Harter, 2006; Harter & Whitesell, 2003; Rosenberg, 1986).

IDENTITY

Adolescents' self-conceptions and self-evaluations provide the framework for the identity formation process. Identity has been conceptualized as "a sense of who one is, based on who one has been and who one can realistically imagine oneself to be in the future" (Marcia, 2002a, p. 202). One's sense of identity is multifaceted (Finkenauer, Engels, Meeus, & Oosterwegel, 2002) and includes both chosen and assigned components (Grotevant, 1992). Forging an identity entails making important decisions regarding career directions, ideological positions (e.g., religious and political beliefs), and interpersonal relationships (e.g., dating and gender roles; Bennion & Adams, 1986). We first describe Erikson's and Marcia's theories of identity formation regarding these chosen aspects of identity. However, individuals are not able to make choices about some aspects of his or her identity. Membership in social groups, such as gender, race, and ethnicity, can form an important element of one's personal identity (Brewer & Gardner, 1996; Ruble et al., 2004), although the relative importance of a particular social identity can vary across individuals and contexts (Turner & Brown, 2007; Yip & Fuligni, 2002). We end our discussion of identity by discussing ethnic and gender identity.

Erikson's Psychosocial Theory

Erik Erikson posited that forging a sense of identity was the major developmental task of adolescence (Erikson, 1950, 1968, 1980). According to Erikson's psychosocial theory, individuals must successfully resolve conflicts at eight different developmental stages in order to form a healthy personality (Erikson, 1980; Marcia, 2002a). He believed that success at each stage was contingent upon successful resolution of the previous stages. Identity versus identity confusion is the fifth developmental stage in Erikson's model; successful resolution of this stage requires the formation of a mature identity, whereas unsuccessful resolution is characterized by a sense of confusion about one's role. Erikson coined the term *identity crisis* (Hopkins, 1995) to describe the conflict occurring at this stage, but he noted that this term does not necessarily imply an imminent traumatic experience but rather a developmental turning point away from childhood (Erikson, 1968; Kroger, 2003).

Marcia's Identity Statuses

James Marcia built on Erikson's theory of identity, positing that individuals employ qualitatively different styles in the identity formation process (Kroger, 2000). These different styles of negotiating identity result in four potential outcomes of the identity formation process, known as identity statuses, which are based on two dimensions: exploration and commitment (see Figure 4.1; Marcia, 1966, 1994, 2002a; Patterson, Sochting, & Marcia, 1992; Rogow, Marcia, & Slugoski, 1983). A period of exploration in identity development is characterized by active questioning and consideration of different alternatives. Commitment refers to having made firm decisions about one's goals and values and behaving accordingly (Crocetti, Rubini, & Meeus, 2008; Marcia, 1966, 1994, 2002a; Waterman, 1992).

The four different identity statuses—identity achievement, identity foreclosure, identity moratorium, and identity diffusion—can be assessed by interviews or questionnaires. The revised version of the Extended Objective Measure of Ego Identity

		Undergone Period of Exploration	
		Yes	No
Commitment	Yes	Identity Achievement	Identity Foreclosure
	No	Identity Moratorium	Identity Diffusion

FIGURE 4.1. Marcia's identity statuses.

Status is one of the commonly used questionnaires to assess the identity statuses; we cite one item representative of each status for illustrative purposes (Adams, 1998; Bennion & Adams, 1986). Those classified as in identity achievement status have made commitments to values and goals following a period of exploration. Identity-achieved individuals may endorse a statement such as, "it took me a long time to decide but now I know for sure what direction to move in for a career" (Adams, 1998). Individuals classified as in identity foreclosure status are also committed to values and goals, but they have made these commitments without exploring alternatives. Identity-foreclosed individuals often accept the values and goals of their parents or other authority figures and may endorse a statement such as "my parents decided a long time ago what I should go into for employment and I'm following through their plans" (Adams, 1998). Individuals in identity moratorium status are currently exploring different alternatives and seeking information; they have yet to make firm commitments but are working toward making these decisions. An adolescent in identity moratorium may endorse a statement such as "I'm still trying to decide how capable I am as a person and what work will be right for me" (Adams, 1998). Individuals in identity diffusion status also lack firm commitments, but unlike those in moratorium, they are not actively exploring potential values and goals. Those in identity diffusion status often do not appear concerned about their lack of commitments and may endorse statements such as "I'm not really interested in finding the right job, any job will do. I just seem to flow with what is available" (Adams, 1998).

Identity development may proceed along different trajectories. Some individuals stay in the same status; however, many individuals progress from less mature identity statuses (i.e., identity foreclosure and identity diffusion) to more mature identity statuses (i.e., identity moratorium and identity achievement). A cross-sectional study of males between the ages of 12 and 24 years found that an increasing number of individuals are classified as identity-achieved with age, and correspondingly there are a decreasing number of individuals classified at less mature statuses (i.e., identity foreclosure and identity diffusion; Meilman, 1979). Similar results were found for a cross-sectional study that included females; there was an increase in the number of individuals classified as identity-achieved across development (Archer, 1982). Marcia (2002a) speculated that the most typical developmental course is to begin in identity foreclosure and transition to identity moratorium and then to identity achievement.

By late adolescence, many individuals remain in the less mature states of identity foreclosure and identity diffusion (Archer, 1982; Meilman, 1979), suggesting that not all individuals follow the same path of identity development and that identity continues to develop across the lifespan (Arnett, 2000; Erikson, 1968; Kroger, 2003; Marcia, 2002b; Sneed, Whitbourne, & Culang, 2006; Stephen, Fraser, & Marcia, 1992). Changes in identity status may occur across adulthood, often triggered by disequilibrating events (e.g., divorce, death of a loved one, job loss, retirement; Marcia, 2002a, 2002b). Many individuals undergo an achievement–moratorium–achievement cycle following these life changes (Marcia, 2002b); however, it is also possible to transition from identity achievement to a less mature identity status (Stephen et al., 1992).

Contextual Influences on Identity Development

A number of environmental factors influence identity development, and these factors may either facilitate or hinder the formation of a mature identity (Beyers & Cok, 2008; Markstrom-Adams, 1992; Yoder, 2000). Identity development can be conceptualized as a process of person–context interactions (Beyers & Cok, 2008; Bosma & Kunnen, 2001). Adolescents' relationships with parents and peers can affect the extent to which adolescents explore and make identity decisions. Likewise, both the school environment and the larger sociohistorical context shape identity development. Although contextual factors can largely influence identity development, it is important to remember that there still are individual differences (Bosma & Kunnen, 2001).

Parents

Parents influence their adolescents' identity development by the extent to which they provide their children with emotional support and the independence to explore (Campbell, Adams, & Dobson, 1984; Grotevant & Cooper, 1985; Markstrom-Adams, 1992; Papini, 1994). Adolescents classified as in identity achievement or in identity moratorium statuses are likely to have parents who allow them the independence to explore but at the same time provide a secure base, offering their children affection and the opportunity to communicate. Identity-foreclosed adolescents often have extremely close emotional attachments to their parents; they tend to rely heavily on their parents as a source of security at the cost of exploration. Adolescents in the identity diffusion status do not appear to have strong emotional attachments to their parents and may view their parents as rejecting.

Peers

Peers may also provide a secure base for identity exploration. Adolescents learn about themselves by interacting with their peers (see Bukowski, Buhrmester, & Underwood, Chapter 7, this volume). Close friendships, in particular, can serve as a source of emotional support as adolescents discuss identity alternatives (Azmitia, 2002). Empirical evidence for the facilitative effects of friendship on identity formation comes from the study of career development in undergraduate students; strong attachments to friends predicted exploration of career options and occupational commitment (Felsman & Blustein, 1999).

School

Characteristics of the school environment influence identity development. Teachers can provide emotional support for identity exploration and encourage this process of self-discovery in their students (Pascarella & Terenzini, 2005). Some educators may promote exploration by exposing their students to a wide range of identity alternatives. They may do so through classroom activities such as open discussions of identity-related issues and hosting events such as career day (Waterman, 1989). Further, teachers may foster self-reflection through pedagogical exercises such as assigning students to write about themselves (Waterman, 1989). Courses that incorporate service learning may also promote identity development (Pascarella & Terenzini, 2005; Yates & Youniss, 1996). Community service may lead adolescents to reflect on politics and social programs and the roles they might play in these arenas.

Sociohistorical Context

Identity development occurs within the context of the adolescent's larger sociohistorical context, which is replete with factors that can facilitate or impede identity development (Baumeister & Muraven, 1996; Bosma & Kunnen, 2001; Côté & Levine, 1987; Erikson, 1968). Certain conditions usually associated with high-status individuals in industrialized nations foster identity exploration (Côté & Levine, 1987). However, there are also potential barriers, or external limitations, that constrain identity exploration and commitment. These barriers may result from factors such as geographic isolation, socioeconomic status, lack of educational opportunities, overbearing parents, and political zeitgeist. For instance, some parents may prohibit their adolescent daughters from working and expect them to commit to arranged marriages according to cultural beliefs (Yoder, 2000; see also Weisner, Chapter 15, this volume).

Political, economic, and social factors that influence identity development change with the course of history (Baumeister & Muraven, 1996). An example of how historical forces influence identity formation was provided by the economic restructuring that took place in New Zealand in the 1980s. The country transitioned from a partially socialized nation to one with a free market economy, and these changes resulted in a rising unemployment rate. Kroger (1993) examined identity status in college students before and after this changeover. There were more female identity foreclosures following the transition than there were beforehand. The distribution of identity statuses among males did not change across this period. Females were especially affected by rising unemployment because they made up a large portion of the part-time workforce, which was largely reduced. These conditions limited women's options and may have made them more likely to accept their parents' values, as these might have offered a sense of security.

Personality, Cognitive, and Behavioral Correlates

Researchers have identified certain characteristics and behaviors that are commonly associated with adolescents in the different identity statuses (Kroger, 2003). In interpreting these findings, it is important to note that this research is correlational in nature. In addition, one must keep in mind that these relationships are far from perfect, holding true for many but not all individuals in a particular identity status (Archer,

1989). Furthermore, it has been hypothesized that some attributes connected with the different identity statuses (e.g., personality dimensions) both influence and are influenced by the identity formation process (Clancy & Dollinger, 1993).

Identity Achievement

Individuals characterized as in identity achievement status tend to be low on neuroticism and high on conscientiousness and extraversion (Clancy & Dollinger, 1993). Those who are identity achieved often demonstrate the planned, rational decision making characteristic of formal operational thought and a high level of moral reasoning (Kroger, 2003; Leadbeater & Dionne, 1981; Rowe & Marcia, 1980). Identity-achieved individuals tend to persevere when faced with difficult problems, avoid procrastination, and perform well in academic settings (Cross & Allen, 1970; Marcia, 1966; Shanahan & Pychyl, 2007). They often exhibit prosocial tendencies and behaviors, such as helping others (Hardy & Kisling, 2006). Identity-achieved individuals also have relationships that are characterized by a high level of intimacy (Fitch & Adams, 1983; Hoegh & Bourgeois, 2002; Kroger, 2003; Orlofsky, Marcia, & Lesser, 1973).

Identity Foreclosure

Individuals characterized in identity foreclosure status are low on openness to experience (Clancy & Dollinger, 1993). Adolescents in identity foreclosure status demonstrate less cognitive complexity and lower levels of formal operational thought than those in identity achievement or identity moratorium status (Leadbeater & Dionne, 1981; Slugoski, Marcia, & Koopman, 1984). These individuals are likely to demonstrate high levels of conformity and endorsement of authoritarian values (Kroger, 2003; Marcia, 1966, 1967). Identity-foreclosed individuals demonstrate low levels of autonomy and high reliance on parents (Orlofsky et al., 1973).

Identity Moratorium

Individuals characterized as in identity moratorium status are high on neuroticism and low on conscientiousness (Clancy & Dollinger, 1993). Adolescents in identity moratorium often demonstrate formal operational thinking when considering identity-related issues (Leadbeater & Dionne, 1981). These individuals may have a tendency to procrastinate (Shanahan & Pychyl, 2007). Adolescents in identity moratorium also have close, intimate relationships but may have not yet committed to a partner (Fitch & Adams, 1983; Kroger, 2003).

Identity Diffusion

Individuals characterized as in identity diffusion status are high on neuroticism and low on conscientiousness and agreeableness (Clancy & Dollinger, 1993). Similarly to those in identity foreclosure status, individuals in identity diffusion status demonstrate less cognitive complexity and lower levels of formal operational thought than those in identity achievement or identity moratorium (Leadbeater & Dionne, 1981; Slugoski et al., 1984). There is a positive relationship between identity diffusion and procrastination, and those in identity diffusion may avoid dealing with identity-related issues (Leadbeater & Dionne, 1981; Shanahan & Pychyl, 2007). These individuals are also often reluctant to trust others, lack close relationships, and may be isolated (Hoegh & Bourgeois, 2002; Kroger, 2003; Orlofsky et al., 1973).

Identity and Adjustment

Successful identity development is associated with psychological well-being (Adams, Berzonsky, & Keating, 2006; Meeus, Iedema, Helsen, & Vollebergh, 1999; Waterman, 1992). The capacities for exploration and commitment that characterize the status of identity achievement may facilitate successful navigation of a changing world and are therefore associated with positive adjustment outcomes (Archer, 1989). Individuals in the identity achievement status report positive psychosocial resources, including feelings of hope and a sense of purpose, competence, and control over their environment (Adams et al., 2006). Individuals in the identity foreclosure status often demonstrate rigid thinking (Marcia, 1994, 2006). It has been suggested that those in identity foreclosure status may be anxious and fearful of exploration or disagreement with their parents (Marcia, 1994). However, some empirical findings suggest that adolescents in identity foreclosure status are similarly well adjusted to those in identity achievement status and demonstrate low levels of general anxiety (Marcia, 1967; Meeus et al., 1999). Individuals in identity moratorium status may demonstrate anxiety or confusion as a result of identity exploration (Marcia, 1967, 1994; Waterman, 1992). Identity diffusion is negatively related to reports of environmental mastery, sense of purpose and personal growth, and positive relationships (Vleioras & Bosma, 2005). Individuals in the identity diffusion status may attempt to avoid confronting problems and are most likely to report alcohol and drug use (Berzonsky, 1992a, 1992b; Jones, 1992). Given the relationship between identity development and adjustment, some researchers and clinicians have called for interventions to facilitate healthy identity formation through education and/or psychotherapy (Archer, 1989; Josselson, 1994). Particular attention has been given to the potential effectiveness of curriculum-based interventions in the schools as a means of promoting identity development (Waterman, 1989).

Ethnic Identity

Ethnic identity refers to the affiliation with and sense of oneself as a member of a racial or ethnic group, particularly for members of minority or nondominant ethnic groups. Components of ethnic identity include identification as a group member, a sense of belonging to the group, attitudes toward the ethnic group, and involvement with the ethnic group such as participation in cultural practices (Phinney, 1990; see also Hill & Witherspoon, Chapter 13, this volume and Weisner, Chapter 15, this volume).

Models of Ethnic Identity Development

Phinney (1989) proposed a three-stage model of ethnic identity development. The first stage is an unexamined ethnic identity, in which individuals are uninterested in their ethnic identity and heritage (diffusion) or have their ethnic identity largely dictated by their parents or the dominant culture (foreclosure). The second stage is a time of exploration, in which individuals actively explore the history and culture of their ethnic group and consider the meaning of these factors in relation to their individual ethnic identity (moratorium). In the third and final stage, an ethnic identity is achieved or committed to; individuals are comfortable with themselves as members of their ethnic group (achievement). Possession of an achieved ethnic identity is associated with positive psychological adjustment (Phinney, 1989). With development, perceptions of racial or ethnic discrimination may increase (Brown & Bigler, 2005), and these perceptions of discrimination may influence ethnic identity (Hughes et al., 2006).

A related body of research has examined ethnic identity in the context of acculturation, or integration of ethnic identification and identification with the dominant culture (Berry, 1980; Berry, Trimble, & Olmedo, 1986). Researchers describe four possible acculturative strategies (Berry, 1997): assimilation (integration into majority culture without maintenance of cultural identity), separation (maintenance of cultural identity and separation from majority culture), integration (participation in majority culture and maintenance of cultural identity), and marginalization (lack of identification with either culture).

Gender Identity

Gender identity, in its most basic form, describes a person's sense of self as male or female (Zucker & Bradley, 1995). The first step in this process is children's emerging awareness of themselves as male or female, typically measured by the ability to apply a gender label to the self. This ability typically emerges around age 2½ (Campbell, Shirley, & Caygill, 2002; Ruble et al., 2007). As children develop, gender identity moves beyond labeling to include perceptions of one's interests in gender-typed activities; possession of gender-typed characteristics, traits, and abilities; friendship and relationship preferences; and the overall subjective sense of oneself as gender typical or atypical (see Ruble, Martin, & Berenbaum, 2006, for a detailed discussion of gender identity within a broader gender development context).

Many models of the development of gender identity and gender-typed behavior exist (e.g., Bussey & Bandura, 1999; Liben & Bigler, 2002; Martin, Ruble, & Szkrybalo, 2002). Whereas most models have focused on the influence of gender-related cognitions (such as identity) on behavior, Liben and Bigler (2002) presented two pathways for the development of gender-related beliefs, attitudes, and behaviors: an attitudinal and a personal pathway. In the attitudinal-pathway model, gender-related beliefs (such as identity and stereotype endorsement) influence personal preferences and behavior. Conversely, in the personal-pathway model, individual characteristics and preferences influence gender-related beliefs. Also included in both models is the notion of gender schematicity—whether the individual considers gender to be an important personal construct. Both individual and situational factors can influence gender schematicity. Liben and Bigler (2002) argue that both the personal- and attitudinal-pathway processes typically occur within an individual; the model that predominates may vary due to personal, situational, or developmental factors.

Perceptions of gender typicality are an important element of gender identity for older children and adolescents. Gender typicality includes an individual's perception of him- or herself as typical or atypical for his or her gender (Egan & Perry, 2001). The emergence of self-perceived gender typicality may be related to social comparison processes (Perry, 2004). What leads an individual to feel typical or atypical is somewhat idiosyncratic. For example, one girl may feel atypical because she excels in math, whereas another girl may feel atypical due to a preference for boys as friends. (See Leaper & Bigler, Chapter 12, this volume.)

FUTURE DIRECTIONS

The study of the self and identity is rapidly progressing with the application of new methodologies to this field. Recently, advanced neuroimaging techniques have been applied to the study of the self (LeDoux & Debiec, 2003). These techniques have been used with adult participants to examine self-face and self-voice recognition (Kaplan, Aziz-Zadeh, Uddin, & Iacoboni, 2008), self–other differentiation (Heatherton et al., 2006), and self-reflection across time (D'Argembeau et al., 2008). However, it is more challenging to use neuroimaging equipment with infants and young children, and thus there are fewer psychophysiological studies with these age groups. Despite these difficulties, some researchers have begun to examine infants and children who have been referred for magnetic resonance imaging (MRI) examination to assess for possible neurological problems. In one such investigation, Lewis and Carmody (2008) studied children 15–30 months of age who were being tested for but did not demonstrate neurological problems. They created a self-representation score for each child based on behavioral assessments of mirror recognition and pretend play and maternal reports of personal pronoun usage. MRI technology was used to acquire structural images of the brain. Comparing behavioral measures with those obtained from neuroimaging revealed a relationship between self-representation and a particular region of the brain; specifically, self-representation was associated with maturation of the temporoparietal junction, independent of age. Future studies employing similar techniques will enable researchers to examine how environmental factors and brain development interact to influence self-representation, as well as many other questions related to development of the self.

Researchers are also applying theories of the self originally developed and empirically tested with adult participants to child and adolescent samples. Self-verification theory is one such theory that has recently attracted attention in the literature. After discovering that self-verification was a motivator of adult behavior, recent work has begun to address self-verification strivings in children and adolescents. According to self-verification theory, individuals want others to view them in the same manner that they view themselves and often take steps in their interactions to ensure that this is the case (Swann & Ely, 1984). Individuals may self-verify because this process provides them with a sense of psychological coherence and helps to facilitate harmonious social interactions (Swann, Stein-Seroussi, & Giesler, 1992). Children and adolescents, like adults, solicit self-verifying feedback; that is, they desire feedback congruent with their own self-views (Cassidy, Aikins, & Chernoff, 2003; Cassidy, Ziv, Mehta, & Feeney, 2003; Swann et al., 1989). Future research will likely examine self-verification in the context of childhood and adolescent relationships (e.g., peer relations, early romantic relationships, and parent–child relationships), as well as the consequences of the self-verification process. Adults prefer self-verifying partners (Swann & Pelham, 2002), and, likewise, children and adolescents with low self-esteem may continually seek out negative feedback and affiliate with those who see them in a negative light. These behaviors would create an environment in which depression is likely to emerge and be self-maintaining (Giesler, Josephs, & Swann, 1996; Joiner, 1995; Swann, 1997; Swann, Wenzlaff, Krull, & Pelham, 1992); future research is needed to examine these processes in childhood and adolescence.

In terms of the study of identity, a great number of studies have examined the four identity statuses following their introduction by Marcia in the 1960s. The majority of this extant research has been conducted with European American middle- to upper-class youths who are college-bound or attending universities (Kroger, 2000; Yoder, 2000). The limited work that has addressed differences between working and college-bound youths between the ages of 18 and 21 years has documented differences between these groups. Working youths may commit to an identity at an earlier age than those attending college (Munro & Adams, 1977). The homogeneity of participants in past identity research has led preeminent scholars in the field to express the need for the study of identity-related issues in a diverse sample of adolescents in many contexts (Kroger, 2000; Yoder, 2000). Future empirical research on identity development and its consequences for youths should include individuals from different socioeconomic classes, religious backgrounds, and ethnic groups. Many important research questions remain to be answered regarding the self and identity, and these questions can best be answered by studying diverse samples of children and adolescents.

SUGGESTED READINGS

Adams, G. R., Gullotta, T. P., & Montemayor, R. (1992). *Adolescent identity formation.* Thousand Oaks, CA: Sage.

Damon, W., & Hart, D. (1988). *Self-understanding in childhood and adolescence.* New York: Cambridge University Press.

Harter, S. (1999). *The construction of the self.* New York: Guilford Press.

Kroger, J. (2003). Identity development during adolescence. In G. R. Adams & M. D. Berzonsky (Eds.), *Blackwell handbook of adolescence* (pp. 205–226). Oxford, UK: Blackwell.

Lewis, M., & Ramsay, D. (2004). Development of self-recognition, personal pronoun use, and pretend play during the second year. *Child Development, 75,* 1821–1831.

REFERENCES

Adams, G. R. (1998). *The objective measure of ego identity status: A reference manual.* Guelph, Ontario: Author.

Adams, G. R., Berzonsky, M. D., & Keating, L. (2006). Psychosocial resources in first-year university students: The role of identity processes and social relationships. *Journal of Youth and Adolescence, 35,* 81–91.

Adamson, L., Hartman, S. G., & Lyxell, B. (1999). Adolescent identity: A qualitative approach: Self-concept, existential questions and adult contacts. *Scandinavian Journal of Psychology, 40,* 21–31.

Amsterdam, B. (1972). Mirror self-image reactions before age two. *Developmental Psychobiology, 5,* 297–305.

Archer, S. L. (1982). The lower age boundaries of identity development. *Child Development, 53,* 1551–1556.

Archer, S. L. (1989). The status of identity: Reflections on the need for intervention. *Journal of Adolescence, 12,* 345–359.

Arnett, J. J. (2000). Emerging adulthood: A theory of development from the late teens through the twenties. *American Psychologist, 55,* 469–480.

Azmitia, M. (2002). Self, self-esteem, conflicts, and best friendships in early adolescence. In T. M. Brinthaupt & R. P. Lipka (Eds.), *Understanding early adolescent self and identity: Applications and interventions* (pp. 167–192). Albany: University of New York Press.

Barry, C. T., Grafeman, S. J., Adler, K. K., & Pickard, J. D. (2007). The relations among narcissism, self-esteem, and delinquency in a sample of at-risk adolescents. *Journal of Adolescence, 30,* 933–942.

Bates, E. (1990). Language about me and you: Pronominal reference and the emerging concept of self. In D. Cicchetti & M. Beeghly (Eds.), *The self in transition: Infancy to childhood* (pp. 165–182). Chicago: University of Chicago Press.

Baumeister, R. F., Campbell, J. D., Kreuger, J. I., & Vohs, K. D. (2003). Does high self-esteem cause better performance, interpersonal success, happiness, or healthier lifestyles? *Psychological Science in the Public Interest, 4*, 1–44.

Baumeister, R. F., & Muraven, M. (1996). Identity as adaptation to social, cultural, and historical context. *Journal of Adolescence, 19*, 405–416.

Bennion, L. D., & Adams, G. R. (1986). A revision of the extended version of the Objective Measure of Ego Identity Status: An identity instrument for use with late adolescents. *Journal of Adolescent Research, 1*, 183–197.

Berndt, T. J., & Burgy, L. (1996). The social self-concept. In B. A. Bracken (Ed.), *Handbook of self-concept: Developmental, social, and clinical considerations* (pp. 171–209). Oxford, UK: Wiley.

Berry. J. W. (1980). Social and cultural change. In H. C. Triandis & R. Brislin (Eds.), *Handbook of cross-cultural psychology: Vol. 5. Social psychology* (pp. 211–279). Boston: Allyn & Bacon.

Berry, J. W. (1997). Immigration, acculturation, and adaptation. *Applied Psychology: An International Review, 46*, 5–68.

Berry, J. W., Trimble, J. E., & Olmedo, E. L. (1986). Assessment of acculturation. In W. J. Lonner & J. W. Berry (Eds.), *Cross-cultural research and methodology: Vol. 8. Field methods in cross-cultural research* (pp. 291–324). Thousand Oaks, CA: Sage.

Berzonsky, M. D. (1992a). A process perspective on identity and stress management. In G. R. Adams, T. P. Gullotta, & R. Montemayor (Eds.), *Adolescent identity formation* (pp. 193–215). Thousand Oaks, CA: Sage.

Berzonsky, M. D. (1992b). Identity style and coping strategies. *Journal of Personality, 60*, 771–788.

Beyers, W., & Cok, F. (2008). Adolescent self and identity development in context. *Journal of Adolescence, 31*, 147–150.

Bosma, H. A., & Kunnen, E. S. (2001). Determinants and mechanisms in ego identity development: A review and synthesis. *Developmental Review, 21*, 39–66.

Bouffard, T., Markovits, H., Vezeau, C., Boisvert, M., & Dumas, C. (1998). The relation between accuracy of self-perception and cognitive development. *British Journal of Educational Psychology, 68*, 321–330.

Bowlby, J. (1973). *Attachment and loss: Volume 2. Separation: Anxiety and anger.* New York: Basic Books.

Bowlby, J. (1979). *The making and breaking of affectional bonds.* London: Tavistock.

Bretherton, I., & Munholland, K. A. (1999). Internal working models in attachment relationships: A construct revisited. In J. Cassidy & P. R. Shaver (Eds.), *Handbook of attachment: Theory, research, and clinical applications* (pp. 89–111). New York: Guilford Press.

Brewer, M. B., & Gardner, W. (1996). Who is this "We"? Levels of collective identity and self representations. *Journal of Personality and Social Psychology, 71*, 83–93.

Brinthaupt, T. M., & Lipka, R. P. (1985). Developmental differences in self-concept and self-esteem among kindergarten through twelfth-grade students. *Child Study Journal, 15*, 207–221.

Brooks-Gunn, J., & Lewis, M. (1984). The development of early visual self-recognition. *Developmental Review, 4*, 215–239.

Brown, C. S., & Bigler, R. S. (2005). Children's perceptions of discrimination: A developmental model. *Child Development, 76*, 533–553.

Brown, J. D. (1986). Evaluations of self and others: Self-enhancement biases in social judgments. *Social Cognition, 4*, 353–376.

Brown, J. D. (1998). *The self.* New York: McGraw-Hill.

Brown, J. D., & Marshall, M. A. (2006). The three faces of self-esteem. In M. H. Kernis (Ed.), *Self-esteem issues and answers* (pp. 4–9). New York: Psychology Press.

Bussey, K., & Bandura, A. (1999). Social cognitive theory of gender development and differentiation. *Psychological Review, 106*, 676–713.

Butterworth, G. (1990). Self-perception in infancy. In D. Cicchetti & M. Beeghly (Eds.), *The self in transition: Infancy to childhood* (pp. 119–137). Chicago: University of Chicago Press.

Butterworth, G. (1992). Origins of self-perception in infancy. *Psychological Inquiry, 3*, 103–111.

Campbell, E., Adams, G. R., & Dobson, W. R. (1984). Familial correlates of identity formation in late adolescence: A study of the predictive utility of connectedness and individuality in family relations. *Journal of Youth and Adolescence, 13*, 509–525.

Campbell, A., Shirley, L., & Caygill, L. (2002). Sex-typed preferences in three domains: Do two-year-olds need cognitive variables? *British Journal of Psychology, 93,* 203–217.

Cassidy, J. (1988). Child–mother attachment and the self in six-year-olds. *Child Development, 59,* 121–134.

Cassidy, J., Aikins, J. W., & Chernoff, J. J. (2003). Children's peer selection: Experimental examination of the role of self-perceptions. *Developmental Psychology, 39,* 495–508.

Cassidy, J., Ziv, Y., Mehta, T. G., & Feeney, B. C. (2003). Feedback seeking in children and adolescents: Associations with self-perceptions, attachment representations, and depression. *Child Development, 74,* 612–628.

Chapman, J. W., & Tunmer, W. E. (1995). Development of young children's reading self-concepts: An examination of emerging subcomponents and their relationship with reading achievement. *Journal of Educational Psychology, 87,* 154–167.

Clancy, S. M., & Dollinger, S. J. (1993). Identity, self, and personality: I. Identity status and the five-factor model of personality. *Journal of Research on Adolescence, 3,* 227–245.

Cooley, C. H. (1902). *Human nature and the social order.* New York: Charles Scribner's Sons.

Côté, J. E., & Levine, C. (1987). A formulation of Erikson's theory of ego identity formation. *Developmental Review, 7,* 273–325.

Crittenden, P. M., & Ainsworth, M. D. S. (1989). Child maltreatment and attachment theory. In D. Cicchetti & V. Carlson (Eds.), *Child maltreatment: Theory and research on the causes and consequences of child abuse and neglect* (pp. 432–463). New York: Cambridge University Press.

Crocetti, E., Rubini, M., & Meeus, W. (2008). Capturing the dynamics of identity formation in various ethnic groups: Development and validation of a three-dimensional model. *Journal of Adolescence, 31,* 207–222.

Crockenberg, S. B., & Soby, B. A. (1989). Self-esteem and teenage pregnancy. In A. M. Mecca, N. J. Smelser, & J. Vasconcellos. *The social importance of self-esteem* (pp. 125–164). Berkeley: University of California Press.

Crocker, J., & Major, B. (1989). Social stigma and self-esteem: The self-protective properties of stigma. *Psychological Review, 96,* 608–630.

Cross, H. J., & Allen, J. G. (1970). Ego identity status, adjustment, and academic achievement. *Journal of Consulting and Clinical Psychology, 34,* 288.

Damon, W., & Hart, D. (1982). The development of self-understanding from infancy through adolescence. *Child Development, 53,* 841–864.

Damon, W., & Hart, D. (1988). *Self-understanding in childhood and adolescence.* New York: Cambridge University Press.

D'Argembeau, A., Feyers, D., Majerus, S., Collette, F., Van der Linden, M., Maquet, P., et al. (2008). Self-reflection across time: Cortical midline structures differentiate between present and past selves. *Social Cognitive and Affective Neuroscience, 3,* 244–252.

Darwin, C. (1877). A biographical sketch of an infant. *Mind, 2,* 285–294.

Dondi, M., Simion, F., & Caltran, G. (1999). Can newborns discriminate between their own cry and the cry of another newborn infant? *Developmental Psychology, 35,* 418–426.

Eder, R. A. (1990). Uncovering young children's psychological selves: Individual and developmental differences. *Child Development, 61,* 849–863.

Egan, S. K., & Perry, D. G. (2001). Gender identity: A multidimensional analysis with implications for psychosocial adjustment. *Developmental Psychology, 37,* 451–463.

Erikson, E. H. (1950). *Childhood and society.* New York : Norton.

Erikson, E. H. (1968). *Identity: Youth and crisis.* New York: Norton.

Erikson, E. H. (1980). *Identity and the life cycle.* New York: Norton.

Ethier, K. A., Kershaw, T. S., Lewis, J. B., Milan, S., Niccolai, L. M., & Ickovics, J. R. (2006). Self-esteem, emotional distress and sexual behavior among adolescent females: Interrelationships and temporal effects. *Journal of Adolescent Health, 38,* 268–274.

Felsman, D. E., & Blustein, D. L. (1999). The role of peer relatedness in late adolescent career development. *Journal of Vocational Behavior, 54,* 279–295.

Felson, R. B. (1985). Reflected appraisal and the development of self. *Social Psychology Quarterly, 48,* 71–78.

Festinger, L. (1954). A theory of social comparison processes. *Human Relations, 7,* 117–140.

Finkenauer, C., Engels, R. C. M. E., Meeus, W., & Oosterwegel, A. (2002). Self and identity in early adolescence: The pains and gains of knowing who and what you are. In T. M. Brinthaupt & R. P. Lipka (Eds.), *Understanding early adolescent self and identity: Applications and interventions* (pp. 25–56). Albany: University of New York Press.

Fitch, S. A., & Adams, G. R. (1983). Ego identity and intimacy status: Replication and extension. *Developmental Psychology, 19*, 839–845.

Fivush, R., & Nelson, K. (2004). Culture and language in the emergence of autobiographical memory. *Psychological Science, 15*, 573–577.

Gallup, G. G. (1970). Chimpanzees: Self-recognition. *Science, 167*, 86–87.

Giesler, R. B., Josephs, R. A., & Swann, W. B. (1996). Self-verification in clinical depression: The desire for negative evaluation. *Journal of Abnormal Psychology, 105*, 358–368.

Griffin, N., Chassin, L., & Young, R. D. (1981). Measurement of global self-concept versus multiple role-specific self-concepts in adolescents. *Adolescence, 16*, 49–56.

Grotevant, H. D. (1992). Assigned and chosen identity components: A process perspective on their integration. In G. R. Adams, T. P. Gullotta, & R. Montemayor (Eds.), *Adolescent identity formation* (pp. 73–90). Thousand Oaks, CA: Sage.

Grotevant, H. D., & Cooper, C. R. (1985). Patterns of interaction in family relationships and the development of identity exploration in adolescence. *Child Development, 56*, 415–428.

Haltiwanger, J. (1989, April). *Behavioral referents of presented self-esteem in young children.* Paper presented at the meeting of the Society for Research in Child Development, Kansas City, MO.

Haney, P., & Durlak, J. A. (1998). Changing self-esteem in children and adolescents: A meta-analytic review. *Journal of Clinical Child Psychology, 27*, 423–433.

Hardy, S. A., & Kisling, J. W. (2006). Identity statuses and prosocial behaviors in young adulthood: A brief report. *Identity, 6*, 363–369.

Harley, K., & Reese, E. (1999). Origins of autobiographical memory. *Developmental Psychology, 35*, 1338–1348.

Harter, S. (1990). Causes, correlates, and the functional role of global self-worth: A life-span perspective. In R. Sternberg & J. Kolligan (Eds.), *Competence considered* (pp. 67–97). New Haven, CT: Yale University Press.

Harter, S. (1998). The development of self-representations. In W. Damon (Series Ed.) & Nancy Eisenberg (Vol. Ed.), *Handbook of child psychology: Vol. 3. Social, emotional, and personality development* (5th ed.). New York: Wiley.

Harter, S. (1999). *The construction of the self.* New York: Guilford Press.

Harter, S. (2003). The development of self-representations during childhood and adolescence. In M. R. Leary & J. P. Tangney (Eds.), *Handbook of self and identity* (pp. 610–642). New York: Guilford Press.

Harter, S. (2006). The self. In W. Damon & R. M. Lerner (Series Eds.) & B. Eisenberg (Volume Ed.), *Social, emotional, and personality development: Handbook of child psychology* (6th ed., pp. 505–570). Hoboken, NJ: Wiley.

Harter, S., Bresnick, S., Bouchey, H. A., & Whitesell, N. R. (1997). The development of multiple role-related selves during adolescence. *Development and Psychopathology, 9*, 835–853.

Harter, S., & Monsour, A. (1992). Development analysis of conflict caused by opposing attributes in the adolescent self-portrait. *Developmental Psychology, 28*, 251–260.

Harter, S., & Pike, R. (1984). The pictorial scale of perceived competence and social acceptance for young children. *Child Development, 55*, 1969–1982.

Harter, S., Waters, P., & Whitesell, N. R. (1998). Relational self-worth: Differences in perceived worth as a person across interpersonal contexts among adolescents. *Child Development, 69*, 756–766.

Harter, S., & Whitesell, N. R. (2003). Beyond the debate: Why some adolescents report stable self-worth over time and situation, whereas others report changes in self-worth. *Journal of Personality, 71*, 1027–1058.

Heatherton, T. F., Wyland, C. L., Macrae, C. N., Demos, K. E., Denny, B. T., & Kelley, W. M. (2006). Medial prefrontal activity differentiates self from close others. *Social Cognitive and Affective Neuroscience, 1*, 18–25.

Hoegh, D. G., & Bourgeois, M. J. (2002). Prelude and postlude to the self: Correlates of achieved identity. *Youth and Society, 33*, 573–594.

Hopkins, J. R. (1995). Erik Homburger Erikson (1902–1994): Obituary. *American Psychologist, 50*, 796–797.

Howe, M. L. (1998). Language is never enough: Memories are more than words reveal. *Applied Cognitive Psychology, 12*, 475–481.

Hughes, D., Rodriguez, J., Smith, E., Johnson, D., Stevenson, H., & Spicer, P. (2006). Parents' ethnic–racial socialization practices: A review of research and directions for future study. *Developmental Psychology, 42*, 747–770.

James, W. (1890). *Principles of psychology*. New York: Holt.

Joiner, T. E. (1995). The price of soliciting and receiving negative feedback: Self-verification theory as a vulnerability to depression theory. *Journal of Abnormal Psychology, 104*, 364–372.

Jones, R. M. (1992). Ego identity and adolescent problem behavior. In G. R. Adams, T. P. Gullotta, & R. Montemayor (Eds.), *Adolescent identity formation* (pp. 216–233). Thousand Oaks, CA: Sage.

Josselson, R. (1994). The theory of identity development and the question of intervention: An introduction. In S. L. Archer (Ed.), *Interventions for adolescent identity development* (pp. 12–25). Thousand Oaks, CA: Sage.

Kaplan, J. T., Aziz-Zadeh, L., Uddin, L. Q., & Iacoboni, M. (2008). The self across the senses: An fMRI study of self-face and self-voice recognition. *Social Cognitive and Affective Neuroscience, 3*, 218–223.

Keller, A., Ford, L. H., & Meacham, J. A. (1978). Dimensions of self-concept in preschool children. *Developmental Psychology, 14*, 483–489.

Keller, H., Yovsi, R., Borke, J., Kärtner, J., Jensen, H., & Papaligoura, Z. (2004). Developmental consequences of early parenting experiences: Self-recognition and self-regulation in three cultural communities. *Child Development, 75*, 1745–1760.

Kroger, J. (1993). The role of historical context in the identity formation process of late adolescence. *Youth and Society, 24*, 363–376.

Kroger, J. (2000). Ego identity status research in the new millennium. *International Journal of Behavioral Development, 24*, 145–148.

Kroger, J. (2003). Identity development during adolescence. In G. R. Adams & M. D. Berzonsky (Eds.), *Blackwell handbook of adolescence* (pp. 205–226). Oxford, UK: Blackwell.

Lamborn, S. D., Mounts, N. S., Steinberg, L., & Dornbusch, S. M. (1991). Patterns of competence and adjustment among adolescents from authoritative, authoritarian, indulgent, and neglectful families. *Child Development, 62*, 1049–1065.

Lan, W., & Lanthier, R. (2003). Changes in students' academic performance and perceptions of school and self before dropping out of schools. *Journal of Education for Students Placed at Risk, 8*, 309–332.

Leadbeater, B. J., & Dionne, J. (1981). The adolescent's use of formal operational thinking in solving problems related to identity resolution. *Adolescence, 16*, 111–121.

Leary, M. R., & Tangney, J. P. (2003). The self as an organizing construct in the behavioral and social sciences. In In M. R. Leary & J. P. Tangney (Eds.), *Handbook of self and identity* (pp. 3–14). New York: Guilford Press.

LeDoux, J. E., & Debiec, J. (2003). Preface: The self: From soul to brain. *Annals of the New York Academy of Sciences, 1001*, vii–viii.

Lewis, M., & Brooks-Gunn, J. (1979). *Social cognition and the acquisition of self*. New York: Plenum Press.

Lewis, M., Brooks-Gunn, J., & Jaskir, J. (1985). Individual differences in visual self-recognition as a function of mother–infant attachment relationship. *Developmental Psychology, 21*, 1181–1187.

Lewis, M., & Carmody, D. P. (2008). Self-representation and brain development. *Developmental Psychology, 44*, 1329–1334.

Lewis, M., & Ramsay, D. (2004). Development of self-recognition, personal pronoun use, and pretend play during the second year. *Child Development, 75*, 1821–1831.

Liben, L. S., & Bigler, R. S. (2002). The developmental course of gender differentiation: Conceptualizing, measuring, and evaluating constructs and pathways. In W. F. Overton (Series Ed.), *Monographs of the Society for Research in Child Development* (Serial No. 269, Vol. 67). Boston: Wiley-Blackwell.

Major, B., Spencer, S., Schmader, T., Wolfe, C., & Crocker, J. (1998). Coping with negative stereotypes about intellectual performance. *Personality and Social Psychology Bulletin, 24*, 34–50.

Marcia, J. E. (1966). Development and validation of ego-identity status. *Journal of Personality and Social Psychology, 3*, 551–558.

Marcia, J. E. (1967). Ego identity status: Relationship to change in self-esteem, "general maladjustment," and authoritarianism. *Journal of Personality, 35*, 119–133.

Marcia, J. E. (1994). Identity and psychotherapy. In S. L. Archer (Ed.), *Interventions for adolescent identity development* (pp. 29–46). Thousand Oaks, CA: Sage.

Marcia, J. E. (2002a). Adolescence, identity, and the Bernardone family. *Identity, 2*, 199–209.

Marcia, J. E. (2002b). Identity and psychosocial development in adulthood. *Identity, 2*, 7–28.

Marcia, J. E. (2006). Ego identity and personality disorders. *Journal of Personality Disorders, 20*, 577–596.

Markstrom-Adams, C. (1992). A consideration of intervening factors in adolescent identity formation. In G. R. Adams, T. P. Gullotta, & R. Montemayor (Eds.), *Adolescent identity formation* (pp. 173–192). Thousand Oaks, CA: Sage.

Marsh, H. W. (1989). Age and sex effects in multiple dimensions of self-concept: Preadolescence to early adulthood. *Journal of Educational Psychology, 81*, 417–430.

Martin, C. L., Ruble, D. N., & Szkrybalo, J. (2002). Cognitive theories of early gender development. *Psychological Bulletin, 128*, 903–933.

McConnell, A. R., & Strain, L. M. (2007). Content and structure of the self-concept. In C. Sedikides & S. Spencer (Eds.), *The self* (pp. 51–73). New York: Psychology Press.

McGuire, S., Manke, B., Saudino, K. J., Reiss, D., Heatherington, E. M., & Plomin, R. (1999). Perceived competence and self-worth during adolescence: A longitudinal behavioral genetic study. *Child Development, 70*, 1283–1296.

Meeus, W., Iedema, J., Helsen, M., & Vollebergh, W. (1999). Patterns of adolescent identity development: Review of literature and longitudinal analysis. *Developmental Review, 19*, 419–461.

Meilman, P. (1979). Cross-sectional age changes in ego identity status during adolescence. *Developmental Psychology, 15*, 230–231.

Meltzoff, A. N. (1990). Foundations for developing a concept of self: The role of imitation in relating self to other and the value of social mirroring, social modeling, and self practice in infancy. In D. Cicchetti & M. Beeghly (Eds.), *The self in transition: Infancy to childhood* (pp. 139–164). Chicago: University of Chicago Press.

Meltzoff, A. N. (2007). "Like me": A foundation for social cognition. *Developmental Science, 10*, 126–134.

Mikulincer, M. (1995). Attachment style and the mental representation of the self. *Journal of Personality and Social Psychology, 69*, 1203–1215.

Montemayor, R., & Eisen, M. (1977). The development of self-conceptions from childhood to adolescence. *Developmental Psychology, 13*, 314–319.

Munro, G., & Adams, G. R. (1977). Ego-identity formation in college students and working youth. *Developmental Psychology, 13*, 523–524.

Neiss, M. B., Sedikides, C., & Stevenson, J. (2002). Self-esteem: A behavioural genetic perspective. *European Journal of Personality, 16*, 351–368.

Nielsen, M., Suddendorf, T., & Slaughter, V. (2006). Mirror self-recognition beyond the face. *Child Development, 77*, 176–185.

Ojanen, T., & Perry, D. G. (2007). Relational schemas and the developing self: Perceptions of mother and of self as joint predictors of early adolescents' self-esteem. *Developmental Psychology, 43*, 1474–1483.

Oosterwegel, A., & Oppenheimer, L. (1993). *The self-system: Developmental changes between and within self-concepts.* Hillsdale, NJ: Erlbaum.

Orlofsky, J. L., Marcia, J. E., & Lesser, I. M. (1973). Ego identity status and the intimacy versus isolation crisis of young adulthood. *Journal of Personality and Social Psychology, 27*, 211–219.

Papini, D. R. (1994). Family interventions. In S. L. Archer (Ed.), *Interventions for adolescent identity development* (pp. 47–61). Thousand Oaks, CA: Sage.

Pascarella, E., & Terenzini, P. (2005). *How college affects students: A third decade of research.* San Francisco, CA: Jossey-Bass.

Patterson, S. J., Sochting, I., & Marcia, J. E. (1992). The inner space and beyond: Women and identity. In G. R. Adams, T. P. Gullotta, & R. Montemayor (Eds.), *Adolescent identity formation* (pp. 9–24). Thousand Oaks, CA: Sage.

Perry, D. G. (2004, April). *Gender identity and gender relevance beliefs: Two components of a causal cognitive system underlying gender differentiation?* Paper presented at the Gender Development Conference, San Francisco, CA.

Phinney, J. (1989). Stages of ethnic identity in minority group adolescents. *Journal of Early Adolescence, 9,* 34–49.

Phinney, J. S. (1990). Ethnic identity in adolescents and adults: Review of research. *Psychological Bulletin, 108,* 499–514.

Pipp, S., Easterbrooks, M. A., & Harmon, R. J. (1992). The relation between attachment and knowledge of self and mother in one- to three-year-old infants. *Child Development, 63,* 738–750.

Pomerantz, E. M., Ruble, D. N., Frey, K. S., & Greulich, F. (1995). Meeting goals and confronting conflict: Children's changing perceptions of social comparison. *Child Development, 66,* 723–738.

Pomerantz, E. M., Saxon, J. L., & Kenney, G. W. (2001). Self-evaluation: The development of sex differences. In G. B. Moscowitz (Ed.), *Cognitive social psychology: The Princeton Symposium on the Legacy and Future of Social Cognition.* Mahwah, NJ: Erlbaum.

Reinherz, H. Z., Giaconia, R. M., Pakiz, B., Silverman, A. B., Frost, A. K., & Lefkowitz, E. S. (1993). Psychosocial risks for major depression in late adolescence: A longitudinal community study. *Journal of the American Academy of Child and Adolescent Psychiatry, 32,* 1155–1163.

Roberts, J. E., Gotlib, I. H., & Kassel, J. D. (1996). Adult attachment security and symptoms of depression: The mediating roles of dysfunctional attitudes and low self-esteem. *Journal of Personality and Social Psychology, 70,* 310–320.

Robins, R. W., Trzesniewski, K. H., Tracy, J. L., Gosling, S. D., & Potter, J. (2002). Global self-esteem across the life span. *Psychology and Aging, 17,* 423–434.

Rochat, P., & Striano, T. (2000). Perceived self in infancy. *Infant Behavior and Development, 23,* 513–530.

Rogow, A. M., Marcia, J. E., & Slugoski, B. R. (1983). The relative importance of identity status interview components. *Journal of Youth and Adolescence, 12,* 387–400.

Rosenberg, M. (1979). *Conceiving the self.* New York: Basic Books.

Rosenberg, M. (1986). Self-concept from middle childhood through adolescence. In J. Suls & A. G. Greenwald (Eds.), *Psychological perspectives on the self* (Vol. 3, pp. 107–135). Hillsdale, NJ: Erlbaum.

Ross, A. O. (1992). *The sense of self: Research and theory.* New York: Springer.

Rowe, I., & Marcia, J. E. (1980). Ego identity status, formal operations, and moral development. *Journal of Youth and Adolescence, 9,* 87–99.

Ruble, D. N., Alvarez, J., Bachman, M., Cameron, J., Fuligni, A., Garcia Coll, C., et al. (2004). The development of a sense of "we": The emergence and implications of children's collective identity. In M. Bennett & F. Sani (Eds.), *The development of the social self* (pp. 29–76). New York: Psychology Press.

Ruble, D. N., Boggiano, A. K., Feldman, N. S., & Loebl, J. H. (1980). Developmental analysis of the role of social comparison in self-evaluation. *Developmental Psychology, 16,* 105–115.

Ruble, D. N., & Frey, K. S. (1991). Changing patterns of comparative behavior as skills are acquired: A functional model of self-evaluation. In J. Suls & T. A. Wills (Eds.), *Social comparison: Contemporary theory and research* (pp. 79–113). Hillsdale, NJ: Erlbaum.

Ruble, D. N., Martin, C. L., & Berenbaum, S. A. (2006). Gender development. In W. Damon & R. M. Lerner (Series Eds.) and N. Eisenberg (Vol. Ed.), *Handbook of child psychology: Vol. 3. Social, emotional, and personality development* (pp. 505–570). Hoboken, NJ: Wiley.

Ruble, D. N., Taylor, L. J., Cyphers, L., Greulich, F. K., Lurye, L. E., & Shrout, P. E. (2007). The role of gender constancy in early gender development. *Child Development, 78,* 1121–1136.

Rumberger, R. W. (1995). Dropping out of middle school: A multilevel analysis of students and schools. *American Educational Research Journal, 32,* 583–625.

Schneider-Rosen, K., & Cicchetti, D. (1984). The relationship between affect and cognition in maltreated infants: Quality of attachment and the development of visual self-recognition. *Child Development, 55,* 648–658.

Shanahan, M. J., & Pychyl, T. A. (2007). An ego identity perspective on volitional action: Identity status, agency, and procrastination. *Personality and Individual Differences, 43,* 901–911.

Shapka, J. D., & Keating, D. P. (2005). Structure and change in self-concept during adolescence. *Canadian Journal of Behavioural Science, 37,* 83–96.

Slugoski, B. R., Marcia, J. E., & Koopman, R. F. (1984). Cognitive and social interactional characteristics of ego identity statuses in college males. *Journal of Personality and Social Psychology, 47,* 646–661.

Sneed, J. R., Whitbourne, S. K., & Culang, M. E. (2006). Trust, identity, and ego integrity: Modeling Erikson's core stages over 34 years. *Journal of Adult Development, 13,* 148–157.

Stephen, J., Fraser, E., & Marcia, J. E. (1992). Moratorium-achievement (Mama) cycles in lifespan identity development: Value orientations and reasoning system correlates. *Journal of Adolescence, 15,* 283–300.

Stipek, D. J., Gralinski, J. H., & Kopp, C. B. (1990). Self-concept development in the toddler years. *Developmental Psychology, 26,* 972–977.

Stipek, D., & Mac Iver, D. (1989). Developmental change in children's assessment of intellectual competence. *Child Development, 60,* 521–538.

Suls, J., & Mullen, B. (1982). From the cradle to the grave: Comparison and self-evaluation across the life-span. In J. Suls (Ed.), *Psychological perspectives on the self* (Vol. 1, pp. 97–125). Hillsdale, NJ: Erlbaum.

Swann, W. B. (1997). The trouble with change: Self-verification and allegiance to the self. *Psychological Science, 8,* 177–180.

Swann, W. B., & Ely, R. J. (1984). A battle of wills: Self-verification versus behavioral confirmation. *Journal of Personality and Social Psychology, 46,* 1287–1302.

Swann, W. B., & Pelham, B. (2002). Who wants out when the going gets good? Psychological investment and preference for self-verifying college roommates. *Self and Identity, 1,* 219–233.

Swann, W. B., Stein-Seroussi, A., & Giesler, R. B. (1992). Why people self-verify. *Journal of Personality and Social Psychology, 62,* 392–401.

Swann, W. B., Wenzlaff, R. M., Krull, D. S., & Pelham, B. W. (1992). Allure of negative feedback: Self-verification strivings among depressed persons. *Journal of Abnormal Psychology, 101,* 293–306.

Swann, W. B., Jr., Chang-Schneider, C., & McClarty, K. (2007). Do our self-views matter?: Self-concept and self-esteem in everyday life. *American Psychologist, 62,* 84–94.

Swann, W. B., Jr., Pelham, B. W., & Krull, D. S. (1989). Agreeable fancy or disagreeable truth? Reconciling self-enhancement and self-verification. *Journal of Personality and Social Psychology, 57,* 782–791.

Toth, S. L., Cicchetti, D., Macfie, J., & Emde, R. N. (1997). Representations of self and others in the narratives of neglected, physically abused, and sexually abused preschoolers. *Development and Psychopathology, 9,* 781–796.

Turner, K. L., & Brown, C. S. (2007). The centrality of gender and ethnic identities across individuals and contexts. *Social Development, 16,* 700–719.

Trzesniewski, K. H., Donnellan, M. B., Moffitt, T. E., Robins, R. W., Poulton, R., & Caspi, A. (2006). Low self-esteem during adolescence predicts poor health, criminal behavior, and limited economic prospects during adulthood. *Developmental Psychology, 42,* 381–390.

Trzesniewski, K. H., Donnellan, M. B., & Robins, R. W. (2008). Do today's young people really think they are so extraordinary?: An examination of secular trends in narcissism and self-enhancement. *Psychological Science, 19,* 181–188.

Twenge, J. M. (2006). *Generation Me: Why today's young Americans are more confident, assertive, entitled—and more miserable than ever before.* New York: Free Press.

Verschueren, K., Marcoen, A., & Schoefs, V. (1996). The internal working model of the self, attachment, and competence in five-year-olds. *Child Development, 67,* 2493–2511.

Vleioras, G., & Bosma, H. A. (2005). Are identity styles important for psychological well-being? *Journal of Adolescence, 28,* 397–409.

Waterman, A. S. (1989). Curricula interventions for identity change: Substantive and ethical considerations. *Journal of Adolescence, 12,* 389–400.

Waterman, A. S. (1992). Identity as an aspect of optimal psychological functioning. In G. R. Adams,

T. P. Gullotta, & R. Montemayor (Eds.), *Adolescent identity formation* (pp. 50–72). Thousand Oaks, CA: Sage.

Wigfield, A., & Karpathian, M. (1991). Who am I and what can I do? Children's self-concepts and motivation in achievement situations. *Educational Psychologist, 26,* 233–261.

Yates, M., & Youniss, J. (1996). Community service and political–moral identity in adolescents. *Journal of Research on Adolescence, 6,* 271–284.

Yip, T., & Fuligni, A. J. (2002). Daily variation in ethnic identity, ethnic behaviors, and psychological well-being among American adolescents of Chinese descent. *Child Development, 73,* 1557–1572.

Yoder, A. E. (2000). Barriers to ego identity status formation: A contextual qualification of Marcia's identity status paradigm. *Journal of Adolescence, 23,* 95–106.

Zucker, K. J., & Bradley, S. J. (1995). *Gender identity disorder and psychosexual problems in children and adolescents.* New York: Guilford Press.

5

Attachment Theory and Research in Developmental Psychology

An Overview and Appreciative Critique

Glenn I. Roisman
Ashley M. Groh

A decade into the new millennium, attachment theory—one of the last remaining "grand theories" of social development—stands as a dominant framework in our field (see, e.g., Dixon's 2002 survey, in which 1,500 doctoral-level members of the Society for Research in Child Development voted Bowlby's [1969/1982] *Attachment and Loss* and Ainsworth, Blehar, Waters, and Wall's [1978] "Patterns of Attachment" the third and fourth "most revolutionary" studies in child psychology since 1950). Why attachment research currently occupies such a central place in modern developmental science is clear: This corpus of work reflects a paradigmatic example of how research in our field can be productive in terms of advancing both basic research and applied goals via empirical and methodological rigor. Consider: in just over 50 years, attachment research has: (1) emerged from testable theoretical propositions based on clinical and naturalistic observations of humans and other primates (Bowlby 1969/1982, 1973, 1980; Harlow & Zimmerman, 1959); (2) inspired assessments of complex interpersonal phenomena that have been enhanced by crucial tests of their psychometric properties (e.g., Ainsworth et al., 1978; Fraley & Spieker, 2003; Main, Kaplan, & Cassidy, 1985); and (3) generated a large corpus of cross-sectional, longitudinal, and, more recently, experimental data on the developmental significance of these vital relationships (e.g., Cassidy & Shaver, 2008; Grossmann, Grossmann, & Waters, 2006; Sroufe, Egeland, Carlson, & Collins, 2005).

The purpose of this chapter is twofold. First and most critically, we wish to communicate to new developmental scholars: (1) the basic logic of Bowlby's theory, (2) a working knowledge of the primary methods that have been developed to test it, and (3) the status of evidence for the core proposals of the theory. Second, where applicable, we also offer an "appreciative critique" of this important area of research. One sign of a mature scientific theory is the emergence of reliable evidence that its predictions have been able to withstand empirical scrutiny, particularly in the context of theoretically "risky" tests of core propositions. Paradoxically, perhaps, the flip side of this is that, when the core of a theory has gained considerable support, a mature area of research has greater potential to be open to thoughtful critique. As such, in this chapter we have made a special effort to contrast "canonical" perspectives on the status of support for the major hypotheses of attachment theory with relevant empirical evidence. In this context, wherever possible, we privilege conclusions drawn from meta-analyses, which provide quantitative reviews of both what is known and not known in relation to what has become a very large corpus of relevant findings focused on attachment (in)security and its antecedents, correlates, and consequences (e.g., De Wolff & van IJzendoorn, 1997; Fearon, Bakermans-Kranenburg, van IJzendoorn, Lapsley, & Roisman, 2010; van IJzendoorn, 1995).

All of this said, this chapter should be regarded merely as an overview and broad introduction to this area of research for at least two reasons. First, this necessarily focused review in general emphasizes the way in which attachment theory has been engaged by *developmental* psychologists. One of the more remarkable aspects of attachment theory is that it has been used generatively across a number of disciplines within and outside of psychological science. Although we personally do not regard studies inspired by attachment theory of, for example, bereavement (Shaver & Fraley, 2008) or the many investigations of the ways in which romantic pair bonds serve attachment-related functions (Mikulincer & Shaver, 2007) as inherently any less "developmental" in orientation than, say, research on the legacy of early life course attachment-related experiences or the normative course of the development of attachments, it is of course the latter issues that tend to be the preoccupation of developmental psychology as a discipline. Second, we wish to note clearly at the outset that we believe that the graduate student interested in seriously engaging this domain of empirical inquiry would be well advised to follow up this chapter by reading (1) more comprehensive narrative reviews, such as those provided in the chapters of the *Handbook of Attachment* (Cassidy & Shaver, 2008), and (2) the meta-analyses (i.e., quantitative reviews) described throughout this chapter.

This chapter is divided into six sections. In the first, we explore the historical roots of attachment theory. Second, we describe Bowlby's normative account of the emergence of attachment relationships in the first months and years of life. Third, we describe individual differences in the quality of attachment relationships in infancy, childhood, and adulthood, as well as their assessment. Fourth, the primary hypotheses of attachment theory are explicated and briefly evaluated in terms of current evidence. Fifth, we demarcate the boundaries of the phenomenon of attachment relationships, in particular suggesting some ways in which aspects of the theory have been occasionally overextended or misunderstood. Finally, we conclude by noting what we believe to be some important future directions for attachment research in developmental psychology based on emerging lines of evidence.

HISTORICAL OVERVIEW

Questions regarding the legacy of early interpersonal experiences with primary caregivers have long been of great interest and, indeed, predate the origins of a formal developmental science. One of the first psychologists to formalize claims about the developmental significance of experiences in infancy for later personality development was, of course, the Austrian neurologist Sigmund Freud. Through his clinical method of psychoanalysis, Freud reasoned that many of the psychological problems that he was studying in adulthood had their origins in infancy. For example, Freud was the first to suggest that a strong tie between the mother and infant exists and influences personality development, for better or for worse (Freud, 1905). Because Freud focused mainly on adults suffering from psychological disorders, important flaws in his theory stemmed from the absence of prospective, longitudinal evidence from infancy, as well as his own apparent ambivalence, ultimately, about whether adult psychological adaptation and disorder are based in real or imagined interpersonal supports and challenges in the early life course (see Thompson & Goodman, Chapter 1, this volume).

The next major explanatory framework regarding the child's ties to caregivers came by way of Drive Reduction theory, which was proposed by Clark Hull in the 1940s. According to the drive reduction account, human behavior can be explained in terms of satisfying basic physical needs. Supporters of drive reduction theory claimed that humans have physical needs—including hunger and the need for contact comfort—that create tension, which in turn motivates people to reduce the tension by satisfying their needs. As applied to infant development, drive reduction theorists explained that the bond between mother and infant exists because the mother fulfills the infant's needs, and because the mother serves this role, the infant loves the mother in return (Bowlby, 1969/1982). In this view, the infant–caregiver *relationship* was a decidedly secondary drive.

In his seminal work, *Attachment and Loss: Attachment* (1969/1982), John Bowlby went a long way toward refuting the claims of drive reduction theory, asserting that it did not adequately explain the origin of the mother–infant relationship and mother–infant behavior. As evidence against drive reduction, Bowlby employed Harry Harlow's work with rhesus monkeys. Harlow and his colleagues (e.g., Harlow & Zimmerman, 1959; Harlow, 1961) had designed several controlled experiments in which they tested drive reduction theory's claim that one of the main contributors to the mother–infant connection is the food the mother provides her infant. In one now classic experiment, Harlow separated new-born rhesus macaques from their mothers and left each one alone with both a wire-framed "mother" that provided food and a terry-cloth "mother" that did not provide milk (the experiment also used counterbalanced conditions). According to a drive reduction account, primates should have preferred the wire-framed "mother" because it provided food. Contrary to this claim, Harlow found that the young macaques spent the majority of time with the terry-cloth "mother," even when it did not provide food, and went to the wire-framed surrogate only for nourishment (Harlow & Zimmerman, 1959). Bowlby (1969/1982) believed that this result, along with similar findings from Harlow's subsequent experiments with nonhuman primates, provided clear evidence that infants do not form a bond with their mothers solely because they provide sustenance.

Drawing on work from his own research, as well as insights from ethology, cognitive psychology, evolution, and cybernetics, Bowlby (1969/1982, 1973, 1980) proposed an alternative account to explain the mother–infant bond, which he called attachment theory. Importantly, however, the groundwork for Bowlby's theory of attachment was laid early in Bowlby's career in his clinical observations of delinquent boys, more than half of whom had experienced significant periods of maternal separation during their first 5 years of life (Bowlby, 1944), and in his collaboration with James Robertson, a psychiatric social worker who had previously conducted work observing children before, during, and after a stay away from home at residential nurseries or hospitals that lacked a stable mother substitute (Robertson, 1962). Robertson and Bowlby embarked on a systematic study that incorporated observations—a relatively new psychological method that Bowlby believed was critical to psychological research—on the influence of children's separation from their mothers on personality development. From this work, Bowlby, Robertson, and Rosenbluth (1952) described three stages of children's response to separation from the mother: (1) protest, (2) despair, and (3) detachment.

Bowlby claimed that children react so predictably and strongly to separation from their mothers due to the intercoordination of several behavioral control systems that, when activated, tend to result in proximity to the mother as a predictable outcome. He believed that humans, like other animals, have instinctive behaviors, and he thought of these as a characteristic set of behaviors that are performed by the individual in a particular environment. In turn, he proposed that such behavioral control systems follow a pattern that leads to a predictable result that enhances reproductive fitness. In terms of the mother–child relationship, when a child is separated from his or her mother (i.e., the environmental cue), the child will instinctively either protest the separation or, if able, follow his or her mother (i.e., instinctive behavioral response) and, typically, regain proximity to her (i.e., predictable result). Alternatively, when proximity is not regained, the child will likely go through the preceding three stages of behavior, described in Bowlby and Robertson's work (Bowlby et al., 1952).

To explain the presence of this behavioral control system in humans and the importance of proximity to the mother for the child, Bowlby, like other ethologists, believed that the behavioral system must be examined with respect to the environment in which it evolved. Drawing from examples of our closest genetic relatives as a means of understanding the environment in which humans evolved, Bowlby explained mother–infant behavior through examples provided in the ethological work on primates. Research on multiple primate species showed that they recognize their mothers within the first weeks of life. Furthermore, once primates begin to recognize their mothers, each of these species begin to direct certain types of behaviors, which Bowlby termed attachment behaviors, such as clinging, sucking, and calling out, specifically toward the caregiver. Not only were these attachment behaviors directed toward the mothers (typically, their primary caregivers) preferentially, but they were also triggered by specific events, either when a threat was present or the infant was separated from the mother. Bowlby theorized that these behavioral patterns—apparent not only in primates but also in human infants—could be explained by the environment in which humans evolved. Proximity to a caregiver would have been important for our ancestors because it promoted survival. As such, behaviors that promoted infant proximity to the mother would have been naturally selected for through evolution (Bowlby, 1969/1982).

In addition to being important to infant survival, Bowlby also believed that early infant attachment continued to influence behavior throughout development. He theorized that the behavioral systems that infants employ to maintain proximity to primary caregivers develop into control systems in which the goal of proximity is maintained but different plans of achieving proximity are compared with respect to the current environment on the basis of their feasibility in achieving the goal of proximity. Based on the then state-of-the-art research and theory in cognitive psychology, Bowlby believed that the only way these complex control systems could develop was through cognitive maps—more commonly referred to by attachment researchers as internal working models (IWMs), or representations of attachment. Bowlby believed that such cognitive maps were crucial to an individual's ability to transmit, store, and manipulate information that would be useful in making predictions about how best to achieve the goal of proximity. He believed that we carry these cognitive maps that are formed through repeated attachment-related behavioral interactions with us into novel situations in which they are employed to inform expectations for and behavior in future attachment-relevant interactions (Bowlby, 1969/1982). Before we examine the issue of *individual differences* in the *content* of individuals' internal working models, however, in the next section we discuss the normative emergence of attachment relationships in infancy and beyond.

ATTACHMENT THEORY AS A NORMATIVE ACCOUNT OF HUMAN DEVELOPMENT

One of the hallmarks of Bowlby's (1969/1982) theory of attachment is universality. According to attachment theory, essentially all infants are born with the building blocks that develop into the attachment behavioral system, and thus all infants have the ability to form an attachment relationship with a primary caregiver. The normative developmental course of attachment was proposed by Bowlby in the first book of his trilogy (Bowlby, 1969/1982) and comprises four distinctive phases (see Marvin & Britner, 2008). The first phase is defined by the presence of attachment behaviors that are not directed toward any person in particular. In the second phase, attachment behaviors are directed toward one, and sometimes more, attachment figure(s). Maintenance of proximity to one or more attachment figure(s) via approach and behavioral signals characterizes the third phase. Finally, in the fourth stage, a goal-corrected partnership is established. Although Bowlby (1969/1982) characterized attachment development as comprising distinct phases, he emphasized that the boundary between one phase and the next is blurred.

Phase 1: Orientation and Signals with Limited Discrimination of Figure

During the first phase of attachment development, Bowlby (1969/1982) proposed that the beginnings of the attachment behavioral system could be observed in the ways in which infants responded to stimuli. Bowlby (1969/1982) claimed that all infants tend to respond to stimuli in ways that will increase the likelihood of continued contact with humans, and thus all infants display behaviors that elicit caregiving behavior from adults. This observation is integral to Bowlby's theory of attachment because it highlights the dyadic nature of the attachment relationship. Said another way, infant attachment behavior cannot be understood without reference to the caregiver's behavior. Importantly, from shortly after the infant's birth until about 8–12 weeks, the infant has little control over his or her surroundings. Although an infant is equipped with behaviors that elicit caregiving, such signals are not fully developed and are directed toward a variety of people, including strangers. Therefore, much of the first phase in the development of the attachment relationship and the maintenance of the infant's proximity to the attachment figure are determined by the infant's attachment figure (e.g., the attachment figure's response to infant crying).

Phase 2: Orientation and Signals Directed toward One (or More) Discriminated Figure(s)

Throughout the first few years of the infant's life, the responsibility of maintaining proximity to the attachment figure slowly becomes more evenly distributed between the caregiver and the child, and eventually the child comes to take over more responsibility for maintaining proximity. The beginnings of this process are observable in the second developmental phase of attachment relationships, which lasts until the infant is about 6–9 months of age. In this phase, three distinct changes occur: (1) the simple attachment behaviors in Phase 1 become incorporated into chain-linked behavior systems, which the infant begins to exert some control over; (2) the range of stimuli that initiate and terminate attachment behaviors becomes restricted; and (3) the infant begins to initiate social interactions with the primary caregiver preferentially. Thus, in Phase 2, the maintenance of proximity is still largely the role of the caregiver.

Phase 3: Maintenance of Proximity to a Discriminated Figure by Means of Locomotion as Well as Signals

During the third phase of normative attachment development, which begins around 6–9 months and lasts until around 3 years, is the period during which, most attachment researchers believe, the infant has become attached to his or her attachment figure in a qualitative sense. Although the infant focuses his or her attachment behaviors on the caregiver in Phase 2, it is not until Phase 3 that distinct organizational changes in behavior centered on the attachment figure occur. The balance between all of these new developments (e.g., locomotion, cognitive skills, exploration desire) in the third phase of attachment development culminates in what Ainsworth (1967) termed the "hallmark" of infant attachment: the infant's use of the attachment figure as a secure base from which to explore the environment and a safe haven to retreat to in times of threat.

Phase 4: Formation of Goal–Corrected Partnership

The final phase in the development of the attachment relationship is the formation of a goal-corrected partnership between the infant and caregiver. As Bowlby (1969/1982) described it, the goal-corrected partnership is characterized by the child's ability to maintain proximity to the attachment figure through a burgeoning goal-corrected system with a primitive cognitive map, or representation of the child, the caregiver, and the environment. The defining characteristics of the child's goal-corrected system are that the primary caregiver is internalized as a separate object and that plans to achieve and maintain proximity to the caregiver can be weighed against one another using the child's developing cognitive map. This phase of attachment development is perhaps the least studied phase, and therefore many claims about the nature of the infant–caregiver relationship during this period of development remain speculative.

INDIVIDUAL DIFFERENCES IN ATTACHMENT

Attachment in Infancy

Issues related to the normative course of attachment relationships in general receive modest empirical attention. In contrast, the literature on attachment relationships, at least in developmental psychology, is thoroughly focused on questions related to the origins, correlates, and consequences of individual differences in the quality of these relationships or their embodied representations. By far, the most well-studied set of individual differences related to attachment relationships concerns variation in the quality of such relationships in infancy, particularly as assessed by the Strange Situation procedure, an observational laboratory tool designed by Bowlby's close collaborator Mary Ainsworth (Ainsworth et al., 1978).

The genius of the Strange Situation—an approximately 20-minute, structured parental separation and reunion procedure originally developed for 12- to 18-month-olds—is that it was designed to activate the key behavioral systems that operate under threatening attachment-related conditions (stranger presence, maternal absence) and that it focuses not on the cataloguing of discrete attachment behaviors (e.g., protest on separation) but on the *organization* of these behaviors when a caregiver is present (the quality of secure-base behaviors) and on reunion after moderately stressful separations (the quality of safe-haven behaviors). Thus a key question for a Strange Situation coder is not whether a given child shows distress when separated from a primary caregiver but whether such attachment-related distress is *effectively alleviated* on the return of his or her caregiver. One of the key contributions of this early work, albeit based on a small cohort of children, was Ainsworth's demonstration via extensive home observations that the individual differences observed in the laboratory Strange Situation mapped onto individual differences in the parenting such infants experienced in more naturalistic environments.

Beginning with studies in Uganda (Ainsworth, 1967) and the first American study of attachment-related individual differences (conducted in Baltimore, Maryland; Ainsworth et al., 1978), Ainsworth and her colleagues importantly established (1) that the majority of infants observed in the Strange Situation procedure effectively used their caregivers as a secure base of operations when the caregiver was present (e.g., competently explored toys located at a distance from the caregiver in the laboratory even after a stranger entered) and (2) that their distress on separation was effectively relieved by the caregiver's return both after a first separation (when the child was briefly left by the primary caregiver with a stranger) and after a second, more stressful parental separation (when the child was briefly left alone). Moreover, Ainsworth also identified variations on these behavioral themes: A relatively large minority of infants ignored their caregivers on reunion (a pattern Ainsworth termed anxious-*avoidance*), and a small minority of infants showed a kind of behavioral ambivalence in which they simultaneously signaled the desire for proximity yet were not effectively soothed by contact comfort from their caregivers (variously referred to as anxious-*ambivalence* or anxious-*resistance*).

In many respects, this early work by Ainsworth—and subsequent research conducted with Everett Waters's Attachment Q-Set (AQS; Waters & Deane, 1985) for characterizing early life course secure base behavior in naturalistic settings such as the home—has scaled up quite well. Most critically, a large amount of data collected through to the present has made it clear that avoidant and resistant behaviors can be reliably identified in a minority of infants across cultures (although occasionally with less or greater representation of avoidance or resistance) and that the majority of infants seem to share effective relationships with their primary caregivers characterized by their ability to use their caregivers as a secure base of operations and as a safe haven in times of uncertainty (van IJzendoorn & Sagi-Schwartz, 2008).

On the other hand, the standard conceptualization of attachment-related individual differences in infancy has met with some ultimately generative challenges over the years. First, as noted by Mary Main and her colleagues (Main & Hesse, 1990; Main & Solomon, 1986, 1990), a subset of infants (particularly those living under high stress or abusive conditions), in addition to showing secure, resistant, or avoidant behaviors in the Strange Situation procedure, also display momentary but striking anomalous behaviors suggesting a "breakdown" or *disorganization* of their attachment-related strategies. As examples, upon reunion during the Strange Situation, some infants strike their caregivers, adopt a "frozen" posture, or show admixtures of resistant and avoidant behaviors that make them difficult to classify using the original Ainsworth system. Indeed, such individuals originally were labeled A/Cs by coders who could not determine whether such cases ought to be categorized as avoidant (A in the Strange Situations coding system) or resistant (C in the Strange Situation coding system; secure infants are labeled B). Just as important, of course, is Main and Hesse's (1990) explanation for "disorganized/disoriented" behaviors. In contrast to the origins of the so-called "organized" categories (i.e., avoidant, secure, resistant), which are presumed by many to result from variation in sensitivity, Main and colleagues suggested that disorganized infants are faced with an irresolvable dilemma—the very individuals that such infants are evolutionarily adapted to seek out under threatening circumstances are, in fact, the source of their greatest fear.

A second challenge to the validity of the standard view of individual differences in infant attachment security came more recently with the taxometric and principal components analyses (PCAs) published by Chris Fraley and Susan Spieker (2003) based on one of the largest studies of the Strange Situation procedure published to date (the NICHD Study of Early Child Care and Youth Development; original $N = 1,364$). Fraley and Spieker's work is probably best known in the field for using taxometric techniques (e.g., Meehl, 1995) to examine the distributional properties of individual differences in attachment and finding that variation in attachment security appeared most compatible with a model in which individual differences in security are continuously rather than categorically distributed.

However, we would argue that a more conceptually important aspect of Fraley and Spieker's (2003) study is not yet as well appreciated. In addition to presenting taxometric analyses, Fraley and Spieker (2003) conducted one of the first PCAs of the rating scales used by Strange Situation coders to classify participants into attachment groups. Importantly, they found evidence that attachment-related individual differences appear to vary along two modestly correlated axes—one of attachment-related avoidance and a second of attachment-related anxiety (the latter a combination of indicators of resistance and disorganization).

This result is critically important because these PCA analyses suggest that the current categorical system might be misrepresenting a key aspect of individual differences in infant attachment security. More specifically, the current conceptualization implies that avoidance and resistance are polar opposites, whereas the evidence demonstrates that a given infant can be *simultaneously* high or low on both avoidance and anxiety or high on one dimension but low on the other. Furthermore, the fact that disorganization and resistance loaded on the same factor in this study calls into question their empirical distinctiveness. Combined with taxometric and PCA evidence from studies of self-reported attachment style (Fraley & Waller, 1998) and of the Adult Attachment Interview (AAI; Roisman, Fraley, & Belsky, 2007), we caution that the conclusions of older studies might need to be reevaluated in light of emerging evidence that attachment-related variation, as measured via diverse methods in infancy and adulthood, appears to reflect two modestly correlated dimensions of attachment-related avoidance and anxiety (for additional discussion, see Roisman, 2009).

Attachment in Childhood

Bowlby (1969/1982) proposed that the function of the attachment system in middle childhood changes from maintaining proximity to the attachment figure to being aware of the availability of the attachment figure. As mentioned previously, middle childhood is believed to mark a decline in the frequency and intensity of attachment behaviors. Specifically, fewer conditions will elicit the activation of attachment behaviors, and greater means of terminating attachment behavior are available to the child and attachment figure (Bowlby, 1969/1982).

According to attachment theory (Bowlby, 1969/1982), the transition of the function of the attachment system from proximity to the attachment figure to availability of the attachment figure is facilitated by the child's developing cognitive skills and the burgeoning ability to internalize early attachment experiences in the form of representations. Children's representations of early attachment experiences with each caregiver are believed to cohere into one generalized model of attachment relationships. Thus, in contrast to the specific attachment relationships that infants develop with primary caregivers, in middle childhood these relationships are believed to begin to combine into the child's general representation of attachment relationships.

Attachment research has focused on assessing attachment behavior in infancy, as already discussed, with the Strange Situation Procedure (Ainsworth et al., 1978) and in early childhood with either the Modified Strange Situation Procedure (MSSP; Cassidy & Marvin, 1992; Main & Cassidy, 1988) or the AQS (Posada, Waters, Crowell, & Lay, 1995). The MSSP is similar to the Strange Situation, except that the caregiver and child are separated for longer durations, a manipulation that is believed to induce separation anxiety in the child. As with the Strange Situation, in the MSSP, children's separation and reunion behavior is generally coded categorically using the same categories (A, B, C, or D for disorganized) based on the child's ability to use the caregiver as a secure base and safe haven. The AQS differs from the Strange Situation and MSSP in that observations are conducted in the home for 2–3 hours or longer. Based on these observations, 90 cards reflecting aspects of secure-base behavior, or a balance between exploration and proximity seeking, are sorted into nine piles based on whether the cards are or are not characteristic of the child's observed behavior. The sort is then compared with a prototypical sort to assess attachment security continuously.

Although the MSSP and the AQS have been successful in assessing attachment behavior in early childhood, some attachment researchers have begun to focus on assessing the transition from specific attachment relationships to the formation of generalized attachment representations in middle childhood. Because this area of attachment research is still developing, there is no dominant conceptual or methodological approach to measuring attachment in middle childhood (Kerns, 2008).

The lack of unity within the field has resulted in various methods of assessing children's attachment representations, ranging from prompted storytelling to family picture drawing, and various conceptualizations of attachment security, ranging from variation on continuous assessments of security to variation in specific patterns of attachment. The diverse approach to assessing attachment representations in middle childhood has been beneficial in that multiple measures allow researchers to thoroughly test the construct in a variety of ways. Conversely, the proliferation of assessments has also presented some challenges in that the conceptual rationale for the measures is often not well developed, resulting in ambiguity about how attachment is conceptualized. Similarly, researchers have primarily focused on assessment creation, leading to the relative lack of validity testing for many of the new assessments (Kerns, 2008; for a review, see Dwyer, 2005).

Among the assessments of children's attachment representations, the three most commonly used and well-known assessments include (1) picture response procedures, the most common being the Separation Anxiety Test (SAT; Klagsbrun & Bowlby, 1976), in which children describe how the child in the pictures feels and how she or he will respond; (2) doll-play scenarios, the most common being Inge Bretherton's Attachment Story Completion Task (ASCT; Bretherton, Ridgeway, & Cassidy, 1990), which children complete both verbally and by using dolls engaged in attachment-relevant stories; and (3) family drawings (e.g., Kaplan & Main, 1986), in which children draw a family portrait. Whereas the ASCT and the family-drawing task employ categorical coding systems similar to that for the Strange Situation, the SAT is coded based on a classification system focused on children's emotional openness and ability to describe constructive solutions to the attachment-related problems depicted.

All of these measures assess and classify children's representations of attachment in slightly different ways. Very little research has focused on the discriminant validity of the assessments, and no study has incorporated more than one of these measures in conjunction with earlier measures of attachment behavior in infancy or early childhood in order to determine how the measures' operationalizations of attachment representations compare in terms of having their roots in early attachment behavior (Kerns, 2008). Although this area of attachment research has produced many potentially useful measures of children's attachment representations, more research focused on the validity of the measures must be conducted before any conclusive statements can be made on the nature of children's attachment representations, how these representations develop in middle childhood, and how they may influence children's concurrent and future behavior.

Attachment in Adulthood

Until recently, most attachment research in developmental psychology with adolescents and adults has employed a semistructured interview, the AAI, about early attachment-related experiences to assess adults' states of mind with respect to attachment (Bakermans-Kranenburg & van IJzendoorn, 2009; Hesse, 2008; Main & Goldwyn, 1998). This measure was developed for the purpose of predicting infant attachment security in the Strange Situation (Ainsworth et al., 1978) from parents' narratives about their early attachment-related experiences. Specifically, AAI coding focuses on the coherence of adults' narratives; that is, their ability to talk about their early attachment-related experiences in an internally consistent manner without becoming emotionally overwhelmed (Hesse, 2008). As such, adult attachment-related variation is assessed with the AAI primarily in terms of *how* adults talk about their early experiences rather than *what* adults say about the nature of their childhood experiences (see Roisman, Fortuna, & Holland, 2006; Roisman, Padrón, Sroufe, & Egeland, 2002).

Paralleling the Strange Situation procedure, individuals are typically classified by trained coders into one of three primary categories that reflect the coherence of the discourse they produce. The majority of adults, described as *secure-autonomous*, freely and flexibly evaluate their childhood experiences, whether described as supportive or difficult in nature. In contrast, a smaller, although substantial, number of adults are described as *dismissing*. Dismissing individuals defensively distance themselves from the emotional content of the interview by normalizing harsh early memories, for example, or by idealizing their caregivers. Least common are *preoccupied* adults, who are unable to discuss their childhoods without becoming overwhelmed by their prior relationship experiences (see Hesse, 2008, for more details). In addition to classifying adults into one of these three mutually exclusive groups, coders also categorize individuals as *unresolved* if their discourse becomes disorganized while talking about loss or abuse experiences.

Recently, another measure known as the Attachment Script Assessment (ASA; Waters & Rodrigues-Doolabh, 2004), which focuses on adults' representations of early attachment-related experiences, has been increasingly used by researchers in developmental psychology. This measure incorporates the advancements made in cognitive psychology concerning how similarities across a class of experiences are internalized and mentally represented in the form of schemas or scripts (Waters & Waters, 2006). Specifically, researchers in cognitive psychology have found that through repetition of similar events, individuals develop a script that guides future behavior within similar events (Nelson, 1986; Schank, 1999). The ASA was developed to assess adults' access to a "secure base" script, which involves an adult's ability to generate narratives from sets of words in which attachment-related threats are recognized, competent help is provided, and the problem is resolved. Similar to the AAI, attachment variation is assessed based on adults' ability to tell coherent attachment-relevant narratives—also referred to as an access to a secure-base script—as opposed to adults' general ability to tell good stories.

Given the similarity between the AAI and the ASA in their emphasis on producing coherent attachment-relevant narratives (whether they are about one's autobiographical experiences, as in the AAI, or generic attachment narratives, as in the ASA), it is not surprising that, at least in preliminary studies based on relatively modest samples, adults' coherence as measured in the AAI is highly correlated with adults' access to a secure-base script as measured in the ASA (r's ranged from .50 to .60; Waters & Waters, 2006). Not only do these two measures share conceptual convergence, but there is increasing evidence that they also share empirical convergence in that they similarly predict outcomes such as infant attachment security (Bost et al., 2006; Veríssimo & Salvaterra, 2006) and physiological reactivity in the face of attachment-related threats (Groh & Roisman, 2009). It remains to future research, however—particularly focused on the childhood and adolescent antecedents of adult attachment-related variation as assessed using the ASA—to determine whether the ASA serves as a rough proxy for the AAI, which is, of course, a much more costly measure to administer, transcribe, and reliably code.

ATTACHMENT RESEARCH IN DEVELOPMENTAL PSYCHOLOGY: HYPOTHESES AND EVIDENCE

Although many new scholars assume that Bowlby's theory provides a straightforward set of testable hypotheses, we argue that it—not unlike many psychological theories—offers instead more of a generative framework for considering the developmental significance of relationships that involve safe-haven and secure-base functions. In this section, we describe the key hypotheses that have emerged in the field of developmental psychology based on this framework and briefly evaluate the evidence for each. A few important caveats attach to this discussion. First, in this section, we draw extensively from what we believe to be highly effective language used by van IJzendoorn and Sagi-Schwartz (2008) in their review of the cross-cultural evidence for the viability of attachment theory as a universal account of human development to describe the primary hypotheses of attachment research. Second, although we draw, where possible, on quantitative syntheses of the literature, it is worth noting at the outset that attachment research, at least in terms of data relevant to the early life course, is de facto a literature primarily about *mother*–child relationships. The relative neglect of father–child relationships (but see, e.g., Brown, McBride, Shin, & Bost, 2007) has some serious implications in terms of the state of knowledge in the field, as we detail later. Finally, as stated earlier, we suspect that a social-personality or clinical psychologist would see additional empirical questions as equally or even more central to adjudicating Bowlby's theory than the hypotheses explored herein. Nonetheless, in the interest of introducing attachment theory and research *from the perspective of developmental psychology*, we introduce and evaluate evidence for the hypotheses most central to the interests of developmental scientists.

The Universality Hypothesis

The basis of all other hypotheses about attachment is what van IJzendoorn and Sagi-Schwartz (2008) refer to as the *universality hypothesis*. As discussed earlier, Bowlby argued that infants are born biologically prepared to develop attachment relationships with their primary caregivers. The consequence of this claim is clear: that humans—except in the most extreme circumstances—do not differ from one another in terms of whether or not they have attachment relationships with primary caregivers in the early life course or even in the strength of these relationships, but rather vary with respect to the *quality* of the attachment relationships they share with their caregivers. Note that the paradox of how children can form (albeit disproportionately insecure) attachment relationships with abusive parents is in part resolved when one considers the literature on disorganized attachments discussed earlier.

What is the evidence for the universality hypothesis? To be sure, it is difficult to reject the claim that essentially all children over the course of the first year of life (and beyond) engage in attachment behaviors that are preferentially directed toward those adults who are most predictably available to them. Such evidence has been clearly documented cross-culturally (see van IJzendoorn & Sagi-Schwartz, 2008). However, we would nonetheless make the observation that it is not entirely clear that the field has settled on a straightforward way to evaluate precisely whether a given relationship is an attachment relationship. For example, we know of no straightforward way of determining with certainty whether a given person is a "primary caregiver" in judging whether it is appropriate to include such a caregiver in a study of the Strange Situation, a problem especially for studies of father–child attachment.

The Normativity Hypothesis

A second key claim is that a majority of attachment relationships will be *secure*. This hypothesis, although remarkably consistent with evidence across all cultures in which individual differences in security have been examined (van IJzendoorn & Sagi-

Schwartz, 2008), is also not above critique. For example, Simpson and Belsky (2008) have described insecure attachments (avoidance and resistance in particular) as local adaptations to challenging interpersonal circumstances that maximize reproductive fitness. Using this perspective as a point of departure, one could theoretically imagine a cultural context in which insecurity was the norm, in part because it maximized fitness. On the other hand, such a cultural context has yet to be documented.

The Antecedents Hypotheses

Regarding hypotheses about the *antecedents* of security, a strong claim can be made that virtually all such hypotheses, at least from within attachment scholarship, tend to emphasize environmentally mediated and, particularly, interpersonal processes that give rise to secure versus insecure attachments. An especially influential account, often referred to as the *sensitivity hypothesis*, is that secure relationships largely result from sensitive exchanges between caregiver and child, characterized by awareness of and prompt responsiveness to the attachment-related needs of children. In contrast, it is quite literally textbook to claim that different forms of insecurity (e.g., avoidance vs. resistance) are largely the result of distinctive forms of insensitive caregiving (by one influential account, rejection vs. inconsistent responsivity, respectively; Weinfield, Sroufe, Egeland, & Carlson, 2008).

On the broad point about the environmentally mediated origins of (in)security, the data would seem highly consistent with the standard view, at least as it applies to the development of infant–caregiver attachments. As we discuss in more detail later, behavior- and molecular-genetic studies have been largely unsuccessful in unearthing evidence for either anonymous (i.e., heritable) or specific (i.e., molecular) genetic involvement in the secure–insecure distinction or in promoting "organized" manifestations of insecurity (i.e., avoidance and resistance). On the other hand, although meta-analytic evidence (De Wolff & van IJzendoorn, 1997) has resulted in clear evidence that parental sensitivity and infant attachment security are correlated, the magnitude of this effect has been far less than overwhelming ($r = .24$ based on meta-analytic $N = 1,099$). More critical from our perspective is that we know of no meta-analytic evidence that different forms of insecurity are clearly differentiated as a function of parental behavior, although we suspect that such effects might well be easier to document if individuals were scaled on separate assessments of attachment-related avoidance and resistance, rather than using coding systems that, it seems incorrectly (Fraley & Spieker, 2003), view avoidance and resistance as mutually incompatible (see earlier discussion).

What complicates the literature on the antecedents of (infant) security greatly, however, is the rather clear-cut meta-analytic (van IJzendoorn, 1995) evidence for the robust intergenerational transmission of attachment (in)security, as documented with the aid of Main's previously described AAI (Main & Goldwyn, 1998). Beyond demonstrating convincingly that individuals who coherently talk about their childhood experiences (secure/autonomous caregivers) are more likely to have secure infants, there is even evidence in this literature for a rough matching between parental and child *in*security in that dismissing adults are at greater risk for developing avoidant relationships with their infants, whereas preoccupied caregivers are at heightened risk for developing resistant attachments with their progeny. Moreover, this intergenerational link has proven robust to many potential threats to the validity of the claim for a caregiver-driven, environmental mediation of the effect, including evidence that such intergenerational associations hold when AAIs are administered prebirth (Fonagy, Steele, & Steele, 1991) and when such studies are conducted with dyads that are not biologically related (Dozier, Stovall, Albus, & Bates, 2001). The juxtaposition of remarkably strong continuity in (in)security across generations (meta-analytic $r \sim .45$; van IJzendoorn, 1995), combined with an unclear behavioral mechanism, is generally referred to as the "transmission gap," a term first coined by Marinus van IJzendoorn (1995) that we discuss in greater detail later.

The Stability and Lawful Change Hypotheses

Some of the more challenging aspects of Bowlby's theory to examine empirically are those hypotheses that necessarily require prospective, longitudinal data to address (for an overview of such studies, see Grossmann et al., 2006). As such, the literature on the stability in attachments to adulthood and lawful change (i.e., theoretically consistent change in security over time) emerged only relatively recently and can be dated to about 2000, when a bundled set of three papers (Hamilton, 2000; Waters, Merrick, Treboux, Crowell, & Albersheim, 2000; Weinfield, Sroufe, & Egeland, 2000), in addition to a stand-alone paper by Lewis, Feiring, and Rosenthal (2000), were published in the same volume of the journal *Child Development*. Although the data presented in these papers (and subsequent reports) are occasionally characterized as "mixed" in terms of their evidence for stability, a meta-analysis by Fraley (2002) currently provides the most comprehensive data on this topic, yielding evidence for modest, though significant, stability in security from infancy to young adulthood. The issue of lawful change, in contrast, is more complicated, particularly by the limitations of the literature described next. Some studies (e.g., Weinfield et al. 2000), for example, provide evidence that negative and positive attachment-related change roughly tracks changes in the caregiving context. However, we caution that too few such reports exist to reach confident conclusions.

More generally, two important caveats apply in interpreting the literature on stability and lawful change over the longer term. First, by most standards, the total number of individuals studied from infancy to young adulthood in such investigations is quite modest. For example, we estimate (see Roisman & Haydon, 2011) that only about 750 AAIs have been administered to individuals who have been tracked prospectively from infancy (not all of whom were observed in the Strange Situation or another attachment-specific procedure) and that nearly half of those data have yet to appear in peer-reviewed outlets. Second, the literature itself is predicated on what would seem to be a highly childhood-centric notion that the key test of stability in security should involve the prediction from infant assessments of security (such as the Strange Situation procedure) to measures administered in adulthood (such as the AAI). Given that Bowlby primarily argued that adult IWMs were tolerably accurate representations of earlier experiences, the current focus on attachment-related stability of individual differences from infancy to young adulthood might eventually be viewed as an error of emphasis. Not unrelated to this point is that, to the extent that attachment theory makes any prediction of the stability of very early patterns of (in)security, Bowlby's prediction is quite vague—that of nonzero stability (Fraley, 2002). Few studies have arrayed the kind of data necessary to address each of these outstanding concerns, although an age-17.5-year attachment assessment of the NICHD Study of Early Child Care cohort (current $N \sim 1,000$) will be well positioned to advance the state of the science in this area.

The Competence Hypothesis

The final key hypothesis in attachment research in developmental psychology is variously referred to as the secure-base (Rothbaum, Weisz, Pott, Miyake, & Morelli, 2000) or competence (van IJzendoorn & Sagi-Schwartz, 2008) hypothesis. Although a number of important longitudinal studies focused on this family of hypotheses exist, the Minnesota Longitudinal Study of Parents and Children (Sroufe et al., 2005), a study originally of 267 elevated-risk mothers and their (now 34-year-old) children, clearly looms largest in terms of its impact on the field. A complete accounting of the results of this study—let alone the broader literature—could and indeed does fill volumes (e.g., Cassidy & Shaver, 2008; Grossmann et al., 2006; Sroufe et al., 2005). Nonetheless, broadly speaking, studies of the implications of attachment-related variation tend to focus on the prediction of three distinct outcomes: (1) interpersonal functioning, particularly in the context of peer interactions (e.g., Erickson, Sroufe, & Egeland, 1985; Schneider, Atkinson & Tardif, 2001) and, in the later life course, functioning in romantic relationships (Roisman, Collins, Sroufe, & Egeland, 2005); (2) externalizing problems (Fearon et al., 2010); and (3) internalizing problems (e.g., Bosquet & Egeland, 2006). In general, the literature can be read to generally support the conventional wisdom that secure individuals are more interpersonally effective and at lower risk for experiencing psychopathology. However, several limitations of this literature should be noted.

First, to our knowledge, only two reasonably comprehensive meta-analyses exist with respect to the literature on implications of attachment-related individual differences. In the first, Schneider and colleagues (2001) meta-analytically examined links between attachment security and peer functioning, finding that such associations were small to moderate in magnitude but larger for middle childhood and adolescent peer relations than for early childhood peer relationships. Similarly, Fearon et al. (2010) also found meta-analytic evidence for small effects of attachment insecurity and disorganization in the prediction of externalizing problems. However, in this latter study, findings were moderated by child sex: Effects were larger for boys. (As an aside, the interpretation of this effect is made quite challenging given the relative scarcity of father–child attachment data in the literature. Specifically, it is not clear whether it is attributable to security per se or to a presently undetectable effect of security vis-à-vis the opposite-sex caregiver.) Second, as noted by van IJzendoorn and Sagi-Schwartz (2008), the cross-cultural evidence for the competence hypothesis is clearly the leanest of any of the hypotheses of attachment theory—not due to the piling up of null findings in the literature but to the absence of data either way given the great difficulty of conducting relevant longitudinal studies.

ATTACHMENT RELATIONSHIPS: BOUNDARIES OF THE PHENOMENON

As should now be clear, fundamentally the attachment behavioral system regulates the maintenance of proximity to primary caregivers. However, perhaps the most important insight into the developmental significance of the organization of attachment-related behaviors is the recognition that such relationships are as much intimately tied to *autonomy* promotion (i.e., via a secure base) as they are to the provision of a safe haven when faced with environmental threats. Indeed, one of the seemingly paradoxical elements of attachment relationships is that, when well functioning (i.e., "secure"), they simultaneously support the ability to confidently explore the object world—via secure-base behavior—and provide a means of escaping (otherwise overwhelming) challenges via the safe haven. Although it is tempting, then, to think of less well-functioning attachment relationships as reflecting dysfunctions either in terms of their secure-base or safe-haven elements, attachment theorists (e.g., Weinfield et al., 2008) instead conceptualize such "anxious" attachment relationships as local *adaptations* to suboptimal caregiving contexts that maximize proximity.

In describing what attachment relationships are—typically enduring interpersonal contexts that adaptively regulate safe-haven and secure-base behavior in both ordinary and threatening environments (Waters & Cummings, 2000)—it seems equally important to address ways in which concepts and claims in attachment research and theory have been overextended and/or misunderstood. Perhaps most amenable to distortion are: (1) how crucially the theory views the significance of early interpersonal experiences, (2) the unproductive conflation of theories of maternal bonding (e.g., Klaus et al., 1972; Klaus & Kennel, 1976) with attachment theory, and (3) the debate about the degree to which attachment-related individual differences overlap with individual differences developed within alternative systems for understanding human variability (i.e., temperament). We explore each of these in turn.

First, it should be emphasized, as Bowlby did, that attachment theory offers a fundamentally probabilistic account of the implications of early attachment-related experiences (see also Sroufe, 1997). Bowlby was clear that, among adults, the embodiment of early interpersonal experiences (i.e., IWMs) were "tolerably accurate" reflections of prior experience that are capable of sometimes significant (i.e., apparently qualitative) change. Perhaps one source of confusion on this point derives from Sroufe's suggestion that early experience has some "special" significance; as, in this often-quoted passage: "earlier patterns may again become manifest in certain contexts, in the face of further environmental change, or in the face of certain critical developmental issues. While perhaps latent, and perhaps never even to become manifest again in some cases, the earlier pattern is not gone" (Sroufe, Egeland, & Kreutzer, 1990, p. 1364). However, as formalized in the mathematical models developed by Fraley and his associates (Fraley, 2002; Fraley & Brumbaugh, 2004), it is clear that the empirical implications of such a prototype model—if it, in fact, accurately reflects the reality of development—is merely that the causal association between security measured early in the life course and later assessments should reach a nonzero predictive value over time. On the other hand, it is of interest that the attachment-theory-inspired notion that early experience might have some unique (i.e., *incremental*) developmental significance remains entirely consistent with relevant data (Fraley, 2002; Fraley & Roisman, 2010).

A second misunderstanding of attachment theory, not unrelated to the first focused on the incorrect assumption that attachment theory is a deterministic theory about relationships, is that the terms *attachment* and *bonding* are equivalent. Briefly, the term *bonding* emerged from a—for a time—very influential theory developed by Klaus, Kennel, and their associates (e.g., Klaus & Kennel, 1976) claiming that parental contact with a newborn is absolutely essential in allowing maternal caregivers to properly "bond" with their progeny. Although preliminary research with an elevated-risk cohort supported this theory, subsequent research failed to replicate the initial findings (e.g., Myers, 1984; Svedja, Campos, & Emde, 1980).

One legacy of the work on bonding has been the occasional conflation of "bonding theory" with the concepts and propositions of attachment theory. Although many of the distinctions between bonding and attachment theory are perhaps obvious to the reader, we note nonetheless that: (1) bonding is a deterministic and attachment is a probabilistic theory; (2) bonding reflects psychological processes specific to the *adult's* emotional connection to his or her newborn child that are presumed to come online very quickly after birth, whereas much of attachment theory concerns itself with the way in which infants gradually organize their own attachment-related behaviors around the availability and responsiveness of their primary caregivers—whether biologically related or not—over the first year of life and beyond; and (3) in contrast to bonding, which references a broadly defined sense of emotional connection to and investment in one's newborn, attachments specifically reference behaviors, emotions, and cognitions that support secure-base and safe-haven dynamics within parent–child and (some) romantic relationships.

One final issue of some relevance in terms of the boundaries of attachment has been a long-standing, but at this point largely resolved, question of whether individual differences in attachment and those associated with temperament (and other aspects of incipient personality) are essentially redundant (summarized well by Mangelsdorf & Frosch, 1999, and Vaughn, Bost, & van IJzendoorn, 2008). For example, one line of argument, championed most notably by Jerome Kagan, suggested that highly avoidant infants are merely temperamentally fearless, whereas resistant infants are temperamentally difficult. In fact, the distinctiveness of attachment- and temperament-related constructs was in large part clarified conceptually in the 1980s (see Sroufe, 1985). For example, although it is not well known outside of attachment scholarship, secure infants are actually further subcategorized as B1s, B2s, B3s, and B4s as a function of how difficult these children find parental separation and therefore how much time they require to settle on reunion with their caregivers in the Strange Situation. In other words, secure babies represent the full range of what might be conceptualized as temperamental difficulty.

More empirically oriented work in this area has tended to fall into three categories: (1) studies examining the correlation between attachment-related variation and various temperament constructs (which themselves derive from several conceptual "families"), (2) studies of twins examining whether individual differences in security are heritable, and thereby perhaps influenced by the same putatively endogenous influences on temperament; and (3) newer molecular genetic studies examining whether "usual suspect" risk or differential susceptibility alleles (Belsky, Bakermans-Kranenburg, & van IJzendoorn, 2007) are correlated with either security versus insecurity generally or with specific forms of insecurity (i.e., disorganization).

Such work is rather straightforward to summarize in aggregate. First, the most complete narrative summaries of the links between attachment and temperament (Mangelsdorf & Frosch, 1999; Vaughn et al., 2008) have revealed scant evidence that security versus insecurity is associated with measures of temperamental variation, a null result that seems to hold across methods of assessment of temperamental variation. However, it is worth noting also that: (1) temperamental and attachment-related variation often make unique and interactive contributions to child development and (2) assessments of temperament and attachment security tend to be more highly correlated over development (Vaughn et al., 2008). On the other hand, relevant quantitative (meta-analytic) reviews of the link between temperament and attachment constructs do not as yet exist and, as with most of the attachment literature, the main conclusions of this literature might well be more nuanced than is currently apparent if infants were to be scaled on continuous metrics of attachment-related avoidance and anxiety (resistance–disorganization), as per Fraley and Spieker (2003). The anxiety dimension, for example, may be alternatively conceptualized as a measure of attachment-related distress, which might well have some basis in temperamental variation.

In terms of the behavior-genetic work, there are now several twin studies (Bakermans-Kranenburg, van IJzendoorn, Bokhorst, & Schuengel, 2004; Bokhorst et al., 2003; Fearon et al., 2006; O'Connor & Croft, 2001; Roisman & Fraley, 2008; Ricciuti, 1993) that are relevant to whether individual differences might have some genetic basis. Briefly, twin studies (one of two major classes of behavior-genetic research designs used with humans, the other being the adoption design) typically contrast the similarity of monozygotic (MZ; identical, who share 100% of their species-specific genetic complement in common with one another) with (typically same-sex) dizygotic (DZ; fraternal, who share on average 50% of their species-specific genetic complement in common with one another) twins on a given outcome (e.g., attachment security). Evidence that there is differential similarity within dyads by zygosity (MZ similarity > DZ similarity) provides direct evidence of a *correlation* between genetic relatedness and individual differences on some outcome and indirect evidence that genetic variation—in aggregate and in some distal manner—influences variability on the outcome of interest. In contrast, if co-twins show similarity on an outcome that is not accounted for by differences in similarity between MZs and DZs, such effects are termed *shared environmental* effects (anonymous nongenetic processes that result in individuals in the same home showing convergent outcomes). Finally, whatever variance is left over is termed the *nonshared environmental* effect (anonymous nongenetic processes that result in dissimilarity within families, a component that includes measurement error).

Results in the behavior-genetic literature related to attachment security in the early life course are remarkably consistent. With the exception of an early study that used a nonstandard assessment of attachment security (Finkel & Matheny, 2000), no evidence has yet emerged that MZ twins are significantly more similar than DZs on assessments of mother–child (Bokhorst et al., 2003) or father–child attachment (Bakermans-Kranenburg et al., 2004). Such univariate results were recently replicated in the large, nationally representative Early Childhood Longitudinal Study—Birth Cohort (Roisman & Fraley, 2008) and two independent studies that reported bivariate behavior-genetic analyses (Fearon et al., 2006; Roisman & Fraley, 2008) have further provided no evidence that the *correlation* between parental sensitivity and attachment security is genetically mediated. In contrast, all of these studies have revealed considerable evidence for both shared and nonshared environmental contributions to attachment (in)security.

Molecular-genetic work in this area has been quite similar in terms of its implications for genetic involvement in the genesis of attachment-related variation, at least in infancy. Much of the work in this area focuses on a variable number tandem repeat (VNTR) referred to as DRD4, a polymorphism that influences dopaminergic functioning that most commonly involves either four or seven repeats. Although a set of association and transmission studies based on a Hungarian cohort (Lakatos et al., 2000, 2002) seemed to implicate the DRD4 7+ repeat variant in increasing the risk for disorganization, particularly in interaction with a -521 T (versus C) promoter polymorphism, subsequent attempts to replicate this effect have failed to yield evidence that these genetic variations, in interaction (i.e., via epistasis) or on their own, increase risk for disorganization (see Bakermans-Kranenburg & van IJzendoorn, 2004). That said, several studies now have been published suggesting that specific genetic diatheses, combined with the "trigger" of attachment-relevant environmental stressors, increases risk for attachment disorganization (for a review, see Bakermans-Kranenburg & van IJzendoorn, 2007). In sum, there is little evidence for genetic or temperamental involvement in the genesis of security, although disorganization might be an exception, at least when genetic susceptibilities and environmental triggers co-occur.

THE FUTURE OF ATTACHMENT RESEARCH

As we hope is clear from the foregoing discussion, attachment theory and research have made profound and generative contributions to modern developmental science. Nonetheless, we believe that there remain significant challenges and important, though somewhat underexamined, issues in this area. We conclude, therefore, by touching on an admittedly incomplete set of issues that we believe merit attention moving forward.

First, as we have noted in several places in this chapter, the results of PCAs of large amounts of data on attachment-related individual differences pose some serious questions about the latent structure of attachment. In sum, we believe that data from diverse measures of attachment-related individual differences used to assess attachment-related individual differences across the life course (e.g., the Strange Situation procedure, self-reports of attachment style, and the AAI) are yielding increasing evidence that such variation reflects two modestly correlated axes: one of attachment-related avoidance and a second assessing attachment-related anxiety. Assuming that data drawn from large samples continues to substantiate this tentative conclusion, two issues remain. First, if avoidance and anxiety are not polar opposites but mutually compatible (and distinctive) aspects of attachment-related individual differences, the field would be wise to revisit its conclusions that have relied on the traditional systems for understanding the latent structure of (in)security. For example, it could be that parental sensitivity (especially to distress) is more strongly implicated in the development of attachment-related avoidance than of attachment-related anxiety, whereas parental intrusiveness (vs. autonomy promotion) might show the opposite pattern. Similarly, and perhaps more important, we suspect it likely that by scaling individuals separately in terms of avoidance and anxiety, it will become more straightforward to document evidence for the distinctive correlates of avoidance versus anxiety. Finally—as a separate endeavor—it is of interest whether avoidance and anxiety, if empirically distinctive, are each distributed categorically or continuously in the population. Although the results of such future taxometric analyses do not have the potential to undermine any particular hypothesis of attachment theory (which is formally indifferent to the way in which individual differences in security are distributed; Waters & Beauchaine, 2003), such analyses might radically restructure how attachment researchers discuss and conceptualize the nature of the individual differences so central to attachment research as an empirical science.

A second area in need of continued engagement is the "transmission gap" (van IJzendoorn, 1995). As was the case 15 years ago, two empirically derived facts remain rather clear: (1) the intergenerational transmission of attachment security is demonstrably strong in magnitude and not easily dismissed to methodological critiques and (2) observed parental sensitivity (at least in the relatively low-stress contexts in which it is typically assessed) accounts for only a small proportion of the observed continuity of (in)security across generations. We acknowledge that there is the inclination on the part of some in the field to conclude that the latter result is largely attributable to the brief assessments we in the field tend to use to measure parental sensitivity. However, one alternative possibility, suggested by Thompson (1997) and others (Goldberg, Grusec, & Jenkins, 1999), is that individual differences in attachment should be most clearly manifested in behavior when an individual is faced with stressors that challenge or otherwise activate the attachment behavioral system. Consistent with this hypothesis, some emerging evidence suggests that parental sensitivity to distress may be more strongly predictive of infant attachment security than sensitivity to nondistress (McElwain & Booth-LaForce, 2006). Similarly, we (Groh & Roisman, 2009) have begun a program of research specifically focused on whether the transmission gap can, in part, be explained by patterns of parental physiological activation when caregivers are faced with attachment-related challenges.

A third major area in need of attention in attachment research is the nonshared environment. Our view is that perhaps attachment researchers have celebrated too much the results from behavior-genetic studies for shared and nonshared environmental (but not particularly strong genetic) influences on the development of attachment security (Fearon et al., 2006; Roisman & Fraley, 2008). Although we are convinced that the role of child genetic contributions to variation in attachment security in infancy is indeed minimal (that is, if the logic of the twin study can be counted on), it may well be that twin studies overestimate the role of the shared environment on the development of attachment-related individual differences among nontwins. For example, studies conducted in the early life course (van IJzendoorn et al., 2000) and adolescence (Kiang & Furman, 2007)—though not especially numerous—actually find rather modest evidence that attachment security strongly "runs in families," with waning convergence between nontwin siblings with age. Said another way, it would appear that the nonshared environment (e.g., parental differential treatment, differential timing of stressful events) plays a particularly central, though largely undocumented, role in the development of security. The fact that (nontwin) siblings tend not to be all that similar in terms of the quality of their attachment relationships to the (same) primary caregiver is not, in fact, inconsistent with evidence of (strong) intergenerational transmission (van IJzendoorn, 1995) or of (more modest) within-person stability in security (Fraley, 2002). However, it does suggest that attachment researchers would be well advised to conduct more work leveraging family systems research designs (i.e., sampling multiple children per family) to examine the specific nonshared processes that account for the observed differences in security within families (but see van IJzendoorn et al., 2000).

Fourth and finally—and this is an area in which much progress is beginning to be made—attachment researchers must fully reconcile nature and nurture in our science. As we have discussed previously, the early framing of such issues (particularly in the late 1970s and 1980s) was to view such forces as inherently in opposition (viz.: Are temperament and individual differences in security redundant?). Today, it is clear that one key way in which progress can be made in terms of perhaps the most vexing issue in attachment research—identifying what the IWM is, exactly, and how is it embodied—is by leveraging neurobiological methods and theory that have the potential to add both constraints to (e.g., is a given model biologically plausible?) and evidence for (in patterns of context-specific autonomic, electroencephalographic, and fMRI activation) particular conceptualizations of the IWM (Coan, 2008). Similarly, gene-×-environment studies are already providing hints as to how, for example, the child's genome might influence the way in which attachment-related inputs are perceived and the degree to which attachment-related experiences influence the later course of development.

To be sure, there are many other areas in need of careful empirical attention in the coming years, including outstanding individual-differences questions such as the role of distal stressors and/or more proximal attachment-related challenges in "activating" underlying attachment-related models (Kobak, 2002; Roisman, 2009), as well as remaining questions regarding the normative development of attachment, such as those that would yield a more careful mapping of the normative shifts in attachment-related "targets" across key developmental transitions (i.e., the transferring of primary attachments from parental caregivers to romantic partners in young adulthood) and the complementary restructuring of relevant attachment-related hierarchies (Kobak, Rosenthal, Zajac, & Madsen, 2007). Our expectation is that the scholarly engagement of these (and other) unanswered questions will make the next decade of attachment research as intellectually stimulating and illuminating as the last five have been.

SUGGESTED READINGS

Bowlby, J. (1982). *Attachment and loss: Vol. 1. Attachment.* New York: Basic Books. (Original work published 1969)

Cassidy, J., & Shaver, P. R. (Eds.). (2008). *Handbook of attachment: Theory, research, and clinical applications* (2nd ed.). New York: Guilford Press.

Fraley, R. C., & Spieker, S. J. (2003). Are infant attachment patterns continuously or categorically distributed? A taxometric analysis of Strange Situation behavior. *Developmental Psychology, 39*, 387–404.

Roisman, G. I., & Fraley, R. C. (2008). A behavior-genetic study of parenting quality, infant attachment security, and their covariation in a nationally representative sample. *Developmental Psychology, 44*, 831–839.

van IJzendoorn, M. (1995). Adult attachment representations, parental responsiveness, and infant attachment: A meta-analysis on the predictive validity of the Adult Attachment Interview. *Psychological Bulletin, 117*, 387–403.

REFERENCES

Ainsworth, M. D. S. (1967). *Infancy in Uganda: Infant care and the growth of attachment.* Baltimore, MD: Johns Hopkins Press.

Ainsworth, M. D. S., Blehar, M. C., Waters, E., & Wall, S. (1978). *Patterns of attachment: A psychological study of the Strange Situation.* New York: Erlbaum.

Bakermans-Kranenburg, M. J., & van IJzendoorn, M. H. (2004). No association of the dopamine D4 receptor (DRD4) and -521 C/T promoter polymorphisms with infant attachment disorganization. *Attachment and Human Development, 6*, 211–218.

Bakermans-Kranenburg, M. J., & van IJzendoorn, M. H. (2007). Research review: Genetic vulnerability or differential susceptibility in child development: The case of attachment. *Journal of Child Psychology and Psychiatry, 48*, 1160–1173.

Bakermans-Kranenburg, M. J., & van IJzendoorn, M. H. (2009). The first 10,000 adult attachment interviews: Distributions of adult attachment representations in clinical and non-clinical groups. *Attachment and Human Development, 11*, 223–263.

Bakermans-Kranenburg, M. J., van IJzendoorn, M. H., Bokhorst, C. L., & Schuengel, C. (2004). The importance of shared environment in infant–father attachment: A behavioral genetic study of the Attachment Q-sort. *Journal of Family Psychology, 18*, 545–549.

Belsky, J., Bakermans-Kranenburg, M. J., & van IJzendoorn, M. H. (2007). For better and for worse: Differential susceptibility to environmental influences. *Current Directions in Psychological Science 16*, 300–304.

Bokhorst, C. L., Bakermans-Kranenburg, M. J., Fearon, R. M., van IJzendoorn, M. H., Fonagy, P., & Schuengel, C. (2003). The importance of shared environment in mother–infant attachment security: A behavioral genetic study. *Child Development, 74*, 1769–1782.

Bosquet, M., & Egeland, B. (2006). The development and maintenance of anxiety symptoms from infancy through adolescence in a longitudinal sample. *Development and Psychopathology, 18*, 517–550.

Bost, K. K., Shin, N., McBride, B. A., Brown, G. L., Vaughn, B. E., Coppola, G., et al. (2006). Maternal secure base scripts, children's attachment security, and mother–child narrative styles. *Attachment and Human Development, 8*, 241–260.

Bowlby, J. (1944). Forty-four juvenile thieves: Their characters and home life. *International Journal of Psycho-Analysis, 25*, 19–52, 107–127.

Bowlby, J. (1982). *Attachment and loss: Vol. 1. Attachment.* New York: Basic Books. (Original work published 1969)

Bowlby, J. (1973). *Attachment and loss: Vol. 2. Separation: Anxiety and anger.* New York: Basic Books.

Bowlby, J. (1980). *Attachment and loss: Vol. 3. Loss: Sadness and depression.* New York: Basic Books.

Bowlby, J., Robertson, J., & Rosenbluth, D. (1952). A two-year-old goes to the hospital. In R. S. Eisler, A. Freud, H. Hartmann, & E. Kris (Eds.), *Psychoanalytic study of the child* (Vol. 7, pp. 82–94). New York: International Universities Press.

Bretherton, I., Ridgeway, D., & Cassidy, J. (1990). Assessing internal working models of the attachment relationship: An attachment story completion task for 3-year-olds. In M. Greenberg, D. Cicchetti, & E. M. Cummings (Eds.), *Attachment in the preschool years: Theory, research, and intervention* (pp. 273–308). Chicago: University of Chicago Press.

Brown, G. L., McBride, B. A., Shin, N., & Bost, K. K. (2007). Parenting predictors of father–child attachment security: Interactive effects of father involvement and fathering quality. *Fathering, 5*, 197–219.

Cassidy, J., & Marvin, R. S., with the MacArthur Attachment Working Group. (1992). *Attachment organization in preschool children: Coding guidelines* (4th ed.). Unpublished manuscript, University of Virginia.

Cassidy, J., & Shaver, P. R. (Eds.). (2008). *Handbook of attachment: Theory, research, and clinical applications* (2nd ed.). New York: Guilford Press.

Coan, J. A. (2008). Toward a neuroscience of attachment. In J. Cassidy & P. R. Shaver (Eds.), *Handbook of attachment: Theory, research, and clinical applications* (2nd ed., pp. 241–265). New York: Guilford Press.

De Wolff, M. S., & van IJzendoorn, M. H. (1997). Sensitivity and attachment: A meta-analysis on parental antecedents of infant attachment. *Child Development, 68*, 571–591.

Dixon, W. E. (2002). 20 studies that revolutionized child psychology. *Society for Research in Child Development: Developments, 45*(2), 1–4.

Dozier, M., Stovall, K. C., Albus, K. E., & Bates, B. (2001). Attachment for infants in foster care: The role of caregiver state of mind. *Child Development, 72*, 1467–1477.

Dwyer, K. M. (2005). The meaning and measurement of attachment in middle and late childhood. *Human Development, 48*, 155–182.

Erickson, M. F., Sroufe, L. A., & Egeland, B. (1985). The relationship between quality of attachment and behavior problems in preschool in a high-risk sample. *Monographs of the Society for Research in Child Development, 50*, 147–166

Fearon, R. P., Bakermans-Kranenburg, M. J., van IJzendoorn, M. H., Lapsley, A., & Roisman, G. I. (2010). The significance of insecure attachment and disorganization in the development of children's externalizing behavior: A meta-analytic study. *Child Development, 81*, 435–456.

Fearon, R. M. P., van IJzendoorn, M. H., Fonagy, P., Bakermans-Kranenburg, M. J., Schuengel, C., & Bokhorst, C. L. (2006). In search of shared and nonshared environmental factors in security of attachment: A behavior-genetic study of the association between sensitivity and attachment security. *Developmental Psychology, 42*, 1026–1040.

Finkel, D., & Matheny, A. P., Jr. (2000). Genetic and environmental influences on a measure of infant attachment security. *Twin Research, 3,* 242–250.

Fonagy, P., Steele, H., & Steele, M. (1991). Maternal representations of attachment during pregnancy predict the organization of infant–mother attachment at one year of age. *Child Development, 62,* 891–905.

Fraley, R. C. (2002). Attachment stability from infancy to adulthood: Meta-analysis and dynamic modeling of developmental mechanisms. *Personality and Social Psychology Review, 6,* 123–151.

Fraley, R. C., & Brumbaugh, C. C. (2004). A dynamical systems approach to understanding stability and change in attachment security. In W. S. Rholes & J. A. Simpson (Eds.), *Adult attachment: Theory, research, and clinical implications* (pp. 86–132). New York: Guilford Press.

Fraley, R. C., & Roisman, G. I. (2010). *The legacy of early experiences in development: Formalizing alternative models of how early experiences are carried forward over time.* Manuscript under review.

Fraley, R. C., & Spieker, S. J. (2003). Are infant attachment patterns continuously or categorically distributed? A taxometric analysis of Strange Situation behavior. *Developmental Psychology, 39,* 387–404.

Fraley, R. C., & Waller, N. G. (1998). Adult attachment patterns: A test of the typological model. In J. A. Simpson & W. S. Rholes (Eds.), *Attachment theory and close relationships* (pp. 77–114). New York: Guilford Press.

Freud, S. (1905). Three essays on the theory of sexuality. In J. Strachey (Ed., & Trans.), *The standard edition of the complete psychological works of Sigmund Freud* (Vol. 7). London: Hogarth Press.

Goldberg, S., Grusec, J. E., & Jenkins, J. M. (1999). Confidence in protection: Arguments for a narrow definition of attachment. *Journal of Family Psychology, 13,* 475–483.

Groh, A. M., & Roisman, G. I. (2009). Adults' autonomic and subjective responses to infant vocalizations: The role of secure base script knowledge. *Developmental Psychology, 45,* 889–893.

Grossmann, K. E., Grossmann, K., & Waters, E. (Eds.). (2006). *Attachment from infancy to adulthood.* New York: Guilford Press.

Hamilton, C. E. (2000). Continuity and discontinuity of attachment from infancy through adolescence. *Child Development, 71,* 690–694.

Harlow, H. F. (1961). The development of affectional patterns in infant monkeys. In B. M. Foss (Ed.), *Determinants of infant behavior* (Vol. 1). New York: Wiley.

Harlow, H. F., & Zimmerman, H. R. (1959). Affectional responses in the infant monkey. *Science, 130,* 421–432.

Hesse, E. (2008). The Adult Attachment Interview: Protocol, method of analysis, and empirical studies. In J. Cassidy & P. R. Shaver (Eds.), *Handbook of attachment: Theory, research, and clinical applications* (2nd ed., pp. 552–598). New York: Guilford Press.

Kaplan, N., & Main, M. (1986). *A system for the analysis of children's family drawings in terms of attachment.* Unpublished manuscript, University of California, Berkeley.

Kerns, K. A. (2008). Attachment in middle childhood. In J. Cassidy & P. R. Shaver (Eds.), *Handbook of attachment: Theory, research, and clinical applications* (2nd ed., pp. 366–382). New York: Guilford Press.

Kiang, L., & Furman, W. (2007). Representations of attachment to parents in adolescent sibling pairs: Concordant or discordant? *Child and Adolescent Development, 117,* 73–89.

Klagsbrun, M., & Bowlby, J. (1976). Responses to separation from parents: A clinical test for young children. *British Journal of Projective Psychology and Personality Study, 21,* 7–27.

Klaus, M. H., Jerauld, J. R., Kreger, N., McAlpine, W., Steffa, M., & Kennel, J. H. (1972). Maternal attachment: Importance of the first postpartum days. *New England Journal of Medicine, 286,* 460–473.

Klaus, M. H., & Kennel, J. H. (1976). *Maternal-infant bonding.* St. Louis, MO: Mosby.

Kobak, R. (2002). Building bridges between social, development, and clinical psychology. *Attachment and Human Development, 4,* 216–222.

Kobak, R., Rosenthal, N., Zajac, K., & Madsen, S. (2007). Adolescent attachment hierarchies and the search for an adult pair bond. *New Directions in Child Development: Adolescent Attachment, 117,* 57–72.

Lakatos, K., Nemoda, Z., Toth, I., Ronai, Z., Ney, K., & Sasvari-Szekely, M. (2002). Further evi-dence for the role of the dopamine D4 receptor (DRD4) gene in attachment disorganization: Interaction of the exon III 48–bp repeat and the 521 C/T promoter polymorphisms. *Molecular Psychiatry, 7*, 27–31.

Lakatos, K., Toth, I., Nemoda, Z., Ney, K., Sasvari-Szekely, M., & Gervai, J. (2000). Dopamine D4 receptor (DRD4) gene polymorphism is associated with attachment disorganization in infants. *Molecular Psychiatry, 5*, 633–637.

Lewis, M., Feiring, C., & Rosenthal, S. (2000). Attachment over time. *Child Development, 71*, 707–720.

Main, M., & Cassidy, J. (1988). Categories of response to reunion with the parent at age 6: Predict-able from infant attachment classifications and stable over a 1–month period. *Developmental Psychology, 24*, 415–426.

Main, M., & Goldwyn, R. (1998). *Adult Attachment Rating and Classification Systems, Version 6. 0*. Unpublished manuscript, University of California, Berkeley.

Main, M., & Hesse, E. (1990). Parents' unresolved traumatic experiences are related to infant dis-organization attachment status: Is frightened and/or frightening parental behavior the linking mechanism? In M. Greenberg, D. Cicchetti, & E. Cummings (Eds.), *Attachment in the pre-school years: Theory, research, and intervention* (pp. 161–182). Chicago: University of Chicago Press.

Main, M., Kaplan, N., & Cassidy, J. (1985). Security in infancy, childhood, and adulthood: A move to the level of representation. In I. Bretherton & E. Waters (Eds.), Growing points of attach-ment theory and research. *Monographs of the Society for Research in Child Development, 50*(1 & 2), 66–104.

Main, M., & Solomon, J. (1986). Discovery of an insecure, disorganized/disoriented attachment pat-tern: Procedures, findings, and implications for the classification of behavior. In M. Yogman & T. B. Brazelton (Eds.), *Affective development in infancy* (pp. 95–124). Norwood, NJ: Ablex.

Main, M., & Solomon, J. (1990). Procedures for identifying infants as disorganized/disoriented during the Ainsworth Strange Situation. In M. T. Greenburg, D. Cicchetti, & E. M. Cum-mings (Eds.), *Attachment in the preschool years* (pp. 121–160). Chicago: University of Chicago Press.

Mangelsdorf, S., & Frosch, C. (1999). Attachment and temperament: One construct or two? In H. Reese (Ed.), *Advances in child development and behavior* (Vol. 27, pp. 181–220). New York: Academic Press.

Marvin, R. S., & Britner, P. A. (2008). Normative development: The ontogeny of attachment. In J. Cassidy & P. R. Shaver (Eds.), *Handbook of attachment: Theory, research, and clinical appli-cations* (2nd ed., pp. 269–294). New York: Guilford Press.

McElwain, N. L., & Booth-LaForce, C. (2006). Maternal sensitivity to infant distress and nondis-tress as predictors of infant–mother attachment security. *Journal of Family Psychology, 20*, 247–255.

Meehl, P. E. (1995). Bootstraps taxometrics: Solving the classification problem in psychopathology. *American Psychologist, 50*, 266–275.

Mikulincer, M., & Shaver, P. R. (2007). *Attachment in adulthood: Structure, dynamics, and change*. New York: Guilford Press.

Myers, B. J. (1984). Mother–infant bonding: The status of this critical-period hypothesis. *Develop-mental Review, 4*, 240–274.

Nelson, K. (1986). *Event knowledge: Structure and function in development scripts and narratives*. Mahwah, NJ: Erlbaum.

O'Connor, T. G., & Croft, C. M. (2001). A twin study of attachment in preschool children. *Child Development, 72*, 1501–1511.

Posada, G., Waters, E., Crowell, J. A., & Lay, K. L. (1995). Is it easier to use a secure mother as a secure base? Attachment Q-sort correlates of the Adult Attachment Interview. *Monographs of the Society for Research in Child Development, 60*(2–3, Serial No. 244), 133–145.

Ricciuti, A. E. (1993). Child–mother attachment: A twin study. *Dissertation Abstracts Interna-tional, 54*, 3364.

Robertson, J. (Ed.). (1962). *Hospitals and children: A parent's-eye view*. New York: International Universities Press.

Roisman, G. I. (2009). Adult attachment: Toward a rapprochement of methodological cultures. *Current Directions in Psychological Science, 18*, 122–126.

Roisman, G. I., Collins, W. A., Sroufe, L. A., & Egeland, B. (2005). Predictors of young adults' representations of and behavior in their current romantic relationship: Prospective tests of the prototype hypothesis. *Attachment and Human Development, 7*(2), 105–121.

Roisman, G. I., Fortuna, K., & Holland, A. (2006). An experimental manipulation of retrospectively defined earned and continuous attachment security. *Child Development, 77*, 59–71.

Roisman, G. I., & Fraley, R. C. (2008). A behavior-genetic study of parenting quality, infant attachment security, and their covariation in a nationally representative sample. *Developmental Psychology, 44*, 831–839.

Roisman, G. I., Fraley, R. C., & Belsky, J. (2007). A taxometric study of the Adult Attachment Interview. *Developmental Psychology, 43*, 675–686.

Roisman, G. I., & Haydon, K. C. (2011). Earned-security in retrospect: Emerging insights from longitudinal, experimental, and taxometric investigations. In D. Cicchetti & G. I. Roisman (Eds.), *The origins and organization of adaptation and maladaptation: Minnesota symposia on child psychology* (Vol. 36). New York: Wiley.

Roisman, G. I., Padrón, E., Sroufe, L. A., & Egeland, B. (2002). Earned-secure attachment status in retrospect and prospect. *Child Development, 73*, 1204–1219.

Rothbaum, R., Weisz, J., Pott, M., Miyake, K., & Morelli, G. (2000). Attachment and culture: Security in Japan and the U. S. *American Psychologist, 55*, 1093–1104.

Schank, R. (1999). *Dynamic memory revisited.* Cambridge, UK: Cambridge University Press.

Schneider, B. H., Atkinson, L., & Tardif, C. (2001). Child–parent attachment and children's peer relations: A quantitative review. *Developmental Psychology, 37*, 86–100.

Shaver, P. R., & Fraley, R. C. (2008). Attachment, loss, and grief: Bowlby's views and current controversies. In J. Cassidy & P. R. Shaver (Eds.), *Handbook of attachment: Theory, research, and clinical applications* (2nd ed., pp. 48–77). New York: Guilford Press.

Simpson, J. A., & Belsky, J. (2008). Attachment theory within a modern evolutionary framework. In J. Cassidy & P. R. Shaver (Eds.), *Handbook of attachment: Theory, research, and clinical applications* (2nd ed., pp. 131–157). New York: Guilford Press.

Sroufe, L. A. (1985). Attachment classification from the perspective of infant–caregiver relationships and infant temperament. *Child Development, 56*, 1–14.

Sroufe, L. A. (1997). Psychopathology as an outcome of development. *Development and Psychopathology, 9*, 251–268.

Sroufe, L. A., Egeland, B., Carlson, E. A., & Collins, W. A. (2005). *The development of the person: The Minnesota study of risk and adaptation from birth to adulthood.* New York: Guilford Press.

Sroufe, L. A., Egeland, B., & Kreutzer, R. (1990). The fate of early experience following developmental change: Longitudinal approaches to individual adaptation in childhood. *Child Development, 61*, 1363–1373.

Svedja, M. J., Campos, J. J., & Emde, R. N. (1980). Mother–infant "bonding": Failure to generalize. *Child Development, 51*, 775–779.

Thompson, R. (1997). Sensitivity and security: New questions to ponder. *Child Development, 68*, 595–597.

van IJzendoorn, M. (1995). Adult attachment representations, parental responsiveness, and infant attachment: A meta-analysis on the predictive validity of the Adult Attachment Interview. *Psychological Bulletin, 117*, 387–403.

van IJzendoorn, M. H., Moran, G., Belsky, J., Pederson, D., Bakermans-Kranenburg, M. J., & Fisher, K. (2000). The similarity of siblings' attachment to their mother. *Child Development, 71*, 1086–1098.

van IJzendoorn, M. H., & Sagi-Schwartz, A. (2008). Cross-cultural patterns of attachment: Universal and contextual dimensions. In J. Cassidy & P. R. Shaver (Eds.), *Handbook of attachment: Theory, research, and clinical applications* (2nd ed., pp. 880–905). New York: Guilford Press.

Vaughn, B. E., Bost, K. K., & van IJzendoorn, M. H. (2008). Attachment and temperament: Additive and interactive influences on behavior, affect, and cognition during infancy and childhood. In J. Cassidy & P. R. Shaver (Eds.), *Handbook of attachment: Theory, research, and clinical applications* (2nd ed., pp. 192–216). New York: Guilford Press.

Veríssimo, M., & Salvaterra, F. (2006). Maternal secure-base scripts and children's attachment security in an adopted sample. *Attachment and Human Development, 8,* 261–273.

Waters, E., & Beauchaine, T. P. (2003). Are there really patterns of attachment?: Comment on Fraley and Spieker (2003). *Developmental Psychology, 39,* 417–422.

Waters, E., & Cummings, E. M. (2000). A secure base from which to explore close relationships. *Child Development, 71,* 164–172.

Waters, E., & Deane, K. E. (1985). Defining and assessing individual differences in attachment relationships: Q-methodology and the organization of behavior in infancy and early childhood. *Monographs of the Society for Research in Child Development, 50,* 41–65.

Waters, E., Merrick, S., Treboux, D., Crowell, J., & Albersheim, L. (2000). Attachment security in infancy and early adulthood: A twenty-year longitudinal study. *Child Development, 71,* 684–689.

Waters, H. S., & Rodrigues-Doolabh, L. (2004). *Manual for decoding secure base narratives.* Unpublished manuscript, State University of New York, Stony Brook.

Waters, H. S., & Waters, E. (2006). The attachment working models concept: Among other things, we build script-like representations of secure base experiences. *Attachment and Human Development, 8,* 185–198.

Weinfield, N. S., Sroufe, L. A., & Egeland, B. (2000). Attachment from infancy to early adulthood in a high-risk sample: Continuity, discontinuity, and their correlates. *Child Development, 71,* 695–702.

Weinfield, N. S., Sroufe, L. A., Egeland, B., & Carlson, E. (2008). Individual differences in infant–caregiver attachment: Conceptual and empirical aspects of security. In J. Cassidy & P. R. Shaver (Eds.), *Handbook of attachment: Theory, research, and clinical applications* (2nd ed., pp. 78–101). New York: Guilford Press.

6

Families, Parenting, and Discipline

George W. Holden
Brigitte Vittrup
Lisa H. Rosen

John B. Watson (1878–1958), the founder of the psychological school of behaviorism, was also one of the fathers of parenting research as a consequence of two pioneering contributions. First, he conducted experimental research on infants in an effort to answer questions about the role of the environment. This work included his famous conditioning study of emotional reactions in Little Albert (Horowitz, 1992). More important, largely based on extrapolations from that study, he developed a child-rearing philosophy described in the first book intended for parents that focused on children's emotional health, *The Psychological Care of Infant and Child* (Watson, 1928; see also Thompson & Goodman, Chapter 1, this volume).

That book, dedicated "to the first mother who brings up a happy child," addressed several of the current key issues in the area of social development and the family. Phrased as questions, these include: What role does the environment play in a child's adjustment? To what degree do parents affect their children's development? and Can a single child-rearing behavior (for Watson it was indulgent coddling of an infant) have long-term negative consequences? Although Watson was both controversial and extremist in his views, he did stimulate research into these questions with work that is continuing almost 100 years later (Horowitz, 1992).

The word *parenting* is derived from the Latin verb *parere*, meaning "to bring forth." Indeed, the core task for parents is bringing a healthy child forward through time by guiding that child along positive developmental trajectories so he or she becomes a competent adult in a particular cultural context. Many tasks are inherent in that process, as we describe, and the scientific understanding of that task continues to change and become more refined.

Child rearing occurs mostly in the context of a family. A central characteristic of families is their structure, defined as the individuals who make up the family unit. In turn, that family composition affects the quality of parenting. Given the changing structure and characteristics of families in the United States, intrafamilial interactional processes are being affected.

One key interactional process and a salient aspect of child rearing is discipline. Indeed, the types of disciplinary practices used are often regarded as defining features of how a child is reared. The use of particular disciplinary techniques is influenced by many factors that include parents' beliefs and cultural background, as well as the child's age and behavioral characteristics. Discipline is frequently studied by psychologists and others because it is regarded as a potent interactional domain in promoting the child's self-regulation. At the same time, if misapplied, it can negatively affect children. In fact, the ways in which parents discipline their children are increasingly being viewed as an ethical issue, and it has become a matter of international political concern. These topics are the focus of this chapter.

SETTING THE STAGE

Changing Structure of Families

Ontogeny, or an individual's development across the lifespan, occurs in contexts. Ecological theories of development (e.g., Bronfenbrenner & Morris, 2006) remind us that individuals are embedded in multiple layers of contexts (e.g., immediate surroundings, neighborhood, urban or rural setting, state, country, geographical region) and that each layer can affect development. The most immediate context involves a child's interactions with others. It is now well established that the structure of the family—whether it contains one or two parents and the presence of siblings—can have significant impact on parenting and, in turn, the child's socioemotional adjustment (e.g., Demo & Acock, 1996).

In contemporary United States society, there is now much more variation in the family structure than there was in 1960, when 91% of U.S. children were raised in two-parent families (Federal Interagency Forum on Child and Family Statistics, 2008). Today, 32% of children live in mother-headed households, and 3% of children live with only their fathers. These statistics differ dramatically by race and ethnicity: 23% of white children live with a single mother, compared with 65% of black children and 37% of Hispanic children (Annie E. Casey Foundation, 2009).

Single parenthood may be the result of separation or divorce, of never having been married, or, in relatively rare cases (i.e., 2%), of the death of a spouse. Divorce often leads to single parenthood: 16–35% of marriages end within the first 10 years, the time period in which children are most likely to be born. Although the incidence of divorce has leveled off, over the past 20 years or so, there has been a steady increase in the number of unmarried women who become mothers (Martin, Kochanek, Strobino, Guyer, & MacDorman, 2005).

Family structure has multiple repercussions for both parents and children. For example, being raised by a single parent typically means spending long hours at day care and living in lower income neighborhoods. Children in single-parent homes are exposed to greater stress, particularly if the child has experienced parental conflict, separation, and divorce. This stress is then manifested in children's mental health and behavioral problems (Strohschein, 2005). Stress also affects parents' mental health and negatively affects the quality of child rearing (Deater-Deckard, 2004).

Cultural Diversity between Families

Research into families over the past decade has also clearly documented the role of another type of diversity in families in the United States—as a consequence of ethnic, racial, or cultural background. Investigations of minority groups and how their child-rearing practices are affected by their living circumstances, ethnic or cultural identities, and, for immigrants, their degree of assimilation into the dominant culture, now appear with regularity in the literature. Cultural differences can be found in parental child rearing goals, as well as practices. For example, Chinese American, African American, and Mexican American mothers value tradition and conformity, as well as achievement, more than European American mothers do (Suizzo, 2007). Immigrant families newly arrived in the United States bring their values from their home countries (Hernandez, Denton, & Macartney 2008), such as, in the case of Chinese immigrants, an orientation toward physical closeness, family relatedness, and interdependence (Rothbaum et al., 2000; see also Weisner, Chapter 15, this volume).

Diversity in parenting can be even more apparent when cultural influences based on country of origin are considered. Child rearing from a cross-cultural perspective reveals a wide range of differences, as well as similarities. Subtle interactional differences, as well as larger variations in child-rearing values, goals, and behaviors, have been identified (Bornstein & Lansford, 2010).

The two types of diversity in families identified here—that of family structure and ethnic, racial, and and cultural background—point to the need to recognize the context in which the parenting is occurring. That is not to say that other forms of family diversity do not affect family functioning. For example, the religiosity of the parents, the biological or adoptive status of the children, and the sexual orientation of the parents each have been shown to affect child-rearing practices. It is all of these characteristics that, in combination with child attributes, form the fabric of the interactions that we call parenting.

WHAT IS PARENTING?

Child rearing represents a complex domain of behavior that is surprisingly challenging to characterize and quantify. It consists of a large constellation of cognitions (e.g., values, goals, attitudes), behaviors (affection, disciplinary practices, communication), and emotions (joy, pride, irritability, anger). Over the years, investigators have proposed various ways of parsing the nature of child rearing. Four terms are particularly useful for differentiating the nature of child rearing: *tasks*, *dimensions*, *style*, and *practices*.

One way to think about the nature of child rearing is to identify the different *tasks* involved. Bradley (2007) enumerated six fundamental tasks. First and foremost, parents must *provide safety and sustenance* to their children if they are to survive. Second, to promote their children's psychological health, parents need to *give socioemotional support*. This task involves various actions, the most prominent of which is providing love, warmth, and encouragement. Third, rearing children requires supplying *adequate stimulation and instruction*. Even neonates need stimulation to avoid boredom. As the child grows, this task becomes more important and includes providing appropriate instruction. *Surveillance* or *monitoring* the child, is a fourth basic task. This task consists of knowing where children are and what their activities are, as well as assessing how they are developing. A fifth task, *providing structure*, refers to the presence of family routines, organization, and discipline in the child's life. Some children have chaotic lives with little discipline and structure, in contrast to others who follow firm schedules and must adhere to strict behavioral standards. Finally, *providing social connectedness* (to family, friends, and others) represents parents' sixth task. Through this process, children become social actors in their environment. Each of these six tasks comprises multiple behaviors.

Orthogonal to but transcending many of those tasks are the *dimensions* of parenting. Three of the fundamental elements were specified by Skinner, Johnson, and Snyder (2005). The first is *responsiveness*, which also has been referred to as warmth or emotional availability. Attachment theorists believe that this caregiving dimension is the most important (e.g., Bowlby, 1988). A second dimension is referred to as *structure* because it captures the extent to which a parent sets limits, controls or disciplines, and has expectations about the child. The third dimension is *autonomy support*. Parents who support children's autonomy do not coerce but, rather, respect children and encourage expressions of individuality.

The ways in which those dimensions come together have been labeled parenting *style*. According to Darling and Steinberg (1993), parenting styles are based on attitudes toward the child that are then communicated to the child and create an emotional climate. Picture a warm parent who engages in some control but at the same time respects the child's individuality. Now consider a depressed parent who is incapable of being responsive. Both parents perform many of the same child-rearing tasks and may engage in the same behaviors on each dimension (e.g., responding, disciplining), but stylistically they do it in very different ways. Those differences are captured by the concept of parenting style.

The fourth child-rearing element is *practices*, or the actual behaviors engaged in. How do parents discipline or express warmth? What specific behaviors does the parent engage in to promote the child's autonomy or feelings of connectedness to the parent? These are the types of questions that focus on specific child-rearing behaviors.

Although these four terms are useful for thinking about the nature of parenting, those terms are not informative about why parents engage in particular behaviors or styles. To address why parents engage in a behavior or a behavioral style, it is helpful to consider the motives behind child rearing. Such motives are conceptualized as child-rearing goals.

Parenting as Goal-Oriented Behavior

Parents engage in child rearing with an obvious long-term goal in mind—assisting the child to become a competent adult. This concept has long been studied under the label of *socialization*. As defined by Maccoby (2007), "socialization refers to processes whereby naïve individuals are taught the skills, behavior patterns, values, and motivations needed for competent functioning in the culture in which the child is growing up" (p. 13). The notion of socialization captures the goal orientation—parents have at least one eye focused on the future.

Socialization practices are culture-specific, as mentioned previously. Parents from

Eastern countries raise their children to be interdependent and family-oriented, in contrast to Western parents, who promote independence in their children (Bornstein & Lansford, 2010). Cultural beliefs and values about socialization are not border-bound but are imported by immigrant families and continue to affect their behavior (Suizzo, 2007).

Beyond recognizing how socialization is affected by cultural child-rearing traditions, researchers are increasingly identifying different parenting practices. Based on individual goals, values, and circumstances, it is now apparent that parents engage in domain-specific socialization practices. For example, there is now evidence that parents differentially socialize their children in the domains of gender, cognition, emotion, prosocial development, religious beliefs, physical activity, health behavior and coping with stress, political beliefs, positive affect, and, for minority parents, race awareness (see Grusec & Hastings, 2007 for chapters on many of these topics).

How Best to Study Parenting

Given the complexity inherent in parenting behavior, as well as its differing conceptualizations, how should child rearing be studied? The answer, in short, is in multiple ways. Since systematic parenting research began in early 20th century, seven distinct approaches to the study of child rearing can be identified (Holden, 2010). The oldest approach consists of studying *parenting traits*. That method is described in more detail later. However, researchers have also studied parent–child relations through six other approaches. The *social learning* approach seeks to understand parents from the perspective of learning principles. This approach focuses on parents as agents whose main function lies in dispensing rewards or punishments. The *social-address* approach considers parental behavior as being determined by the cultural or subcultural (i.e., socioeconomic status) locale in which the parent resides. The *child-effects* method is utilized to understand how children's behavior or characteristics elicit different parental behavior. The *momentary-process* approach examines the role that subtle and fleeting behaviors have in influencing behavior, such as what occurs when a parent reacts emotionally to a child's misbehavior. A sixth approach focuses on *parental social cognition* and how it relates to parental behavior. It began with the study of parental attitudes but has expanded to include beliefs and knowledge, perceptions and attributions, expectations, and other types of parental thinking. The newest method involves using *structural equation modeling*. Large longitudinal datasets are analyzed to examine how variables mediate or moderate relations between parental characteristics and child outcomes.

Due to its prominence among the approaches and its utility in identifying characteristics of parents associated with positive child outcomes, we next describe the parenting-trait approach in some detail. The approach, sometimes called "parenting styles," began in the 1940s and continues to be popular. Although more than 20 different parenting-trait schemes have been studied (Holden & Miller, 1999), the best-known example of this typological approach is Baumrind's model (Baumrind, 1971, 2005). Her work highlighted two fundamental child-rearing dimensions: warmth and structure. Warmth refers to the degree to which parents are responsive, supportive, and sensitive to the needs and feelings of their children. Structure, or demandingness, concerns the extent to which parents attempt to control and have expectations about their children's behavior. From these two dimensions, Baumrind distinguished three basic child-rearing styles: authoritative, authoritarian, and permissive.

These styles tie nicely into the three fundamental child-rearing dimensions discussed earlier. *Authoritative* parenting is characterized by high degrees of both warmth and structure. These parents are accepting and responsive to their children but they hold and communicate clear expectations for mature child behavior. Authoritative parents use firm and consistent discipline when necessary, sharing their reasoning with their children. They encourage discussion and grant age-appropriate autonomy to their children. In contrast, authoritarian parents are demanding and rigid without taking into consideration their children's desires or point of view. They do not negotiate and are reluctant to grant autonomy. In contrast to both groups, permissive parents make few demands or expectations. They are loving and supportive but very lenient, and fail to set behavioral limits. Instead, children of permissive parents are given considerable decision-making power and autonomy at an early age, such as what to eat or when to go to bed.

A fourth category of parenting traits was subsequently identified. Labeled "rejecting/neglecting" (or uninvolved) these parents are characterized by low levels of warmth, and structure, and had few expectations (Baumrind, 2005; Maccoby & Martin, 1983). They may also actively reject their children or may neglect their responsibilities as caregiver.

A wide range of child outcomes has been examined as a function of the different parenting styles. The results have been remarkably similar: authoritative parenting is associated with positive outcomes, such as competent social functioning and academic success. In contrast, both authoritarian and permissive parenting styles (as well as rejecting/neglecting) have been linked to a variety of children's problems, including aggression, depression, delinquency, and diminished social competence (e.g., Steinberg & Silk, 2002).

Although a great deal has been learned by applying Baumrind's parenting-trait framework, several criticisms have been levied against this approach. As noted by Baumrind herself (1971), not all parents can be categorized into one of the parenting styles. Another limitation is that the role of fathers was not appreciated in Baumrind's longitudinal study of families. Parental behavior is also not monolithic: child-rearing behavior differs across context, children, and time. Further, researchers have noted that when child outcomes are examined as a function of parenting style, the effect size is often small (e.g., Lamborn, Mounts, Steinberg, & Dornbusch, 1991), and the relations might be quite complex, varying as a function of gender and race. Indeed, there is a need to scrutinize how these different types of parents rear their children. Nevertheless, the approach has been useful in linking child-rearing patterns to children's behavioral outcomes.

Controversies: Who Is the Causal Agent?

The fundamental controversy in child-rearing research is who—or what—causes differences in children. Watson had a simplistic view of causation—he espoused a unidirectional effect from parent to child. That belief resulted in his oft-cited quote: "Give me a dozen healthy infants and the environment of my choice, and I will give you a banker, baker, and yes, even a beggar and a criminal" (Watson, 1926, p. 10). The controversy about whom or what causes effects on children has seen many manifestations at the levels of parenting trait, socialization agent, and specific behavior.

At the level of parenting traits, Baumrind's views about parental influence were challenged. Her longitudinal study provided support for the view that parents with authoritative styles had children who subsequently showed greater competence than children of other parents. However, Catherine Lewis (1981) argued that Baumrind had it backward and that the observed relations could be accounted for by children's characteristics. More compliant and competent children elicit different behavior from their parents; a parent need not use coercion or harsh disciplinary strategies (i.e., authoritarian behavior) with an obedient and easygoing child. In contrast, difficult children will not respond to reasoning and therefore elicit more—and harsher—discipline. Consequently, Lewis and others (e.g., Kerr, Stattin, Biesecker, & Ferrer-Wreder, 2003) argued for recognizing child effects when considering the determinants of parental behavior and its potential effects.

The same fundamental controversy over causality of parental behavior resurfaced provocatively in the mid-1990s. In an effort to reconcile behavioral genetics data with other research findings, Harris (1995) proposed that the environment—but not the socialization provided by parents—was indeed important in influencing development. Rather than parental nurturance being the important feature of the environment, she crafted a case for the view that peer influence during adolescence had powerful and enduring effects. Parental influence, she argued, has diminished by the teen years, and peers trump whatever lingering parental control remains.

Not surprisingly, this thesis elicited a variety of heated rebuttals, both in the popular and in the scholarly literature. Although Harris's recognition that peers can influence youths is undoubtedly true, a number of her arguments were criticized on such grounds as her limited review of the research, problems in her use and interpretation of behavioral genetics data, and omission of the recognition that parents can affect peer involvement (e.g., Collins, Maccoby, Steinberg, Hetherington, & Bornstein, 2000). Nevertheless, Harris (1995) did skillfully provide an example of the causality controversy concerning who the most important socialization agents for children are.

A final example of this continuing controversy over effects occurs at the level of a specific child-rearing behavior. The dispute involves the practice of physical punishment, most commonly manifested as slapping and spanking. Although the origins of this controversy are unknown, some readers of the Bible believe that the practice is advocated in the Book of Proverbs in the Old Testament. Given that philosophers such as John Locke (1693/1699) took strong positions against the practice, there is no doubt that the practice is, by far, the longest standing child-rearing controversy.

Although research into the practice had periodically been associated with negative child outcomes, it was not until Gershoff (2002a) conducted a meta-analysis of 88 studies that the overwhelming direction of the evidence became apparent. When tabulating the effects of physical punishment (primarily operationalized as spanking), the data were remarkably consistent. Spanking children was associated with 1 positive effect (that of immediate compliance) but 10 negative outcomes, including decreased moral internalization, mental health, quality of the parent–child relationship and an increased likelihood of aggression, antisocial behavior, and risk of child as well as partner abuse. Ironically, child aggression, the very reason why parents often spank, is the most common unintended consequence (Gershoff, 2002a).

The results from the review were challenged by some scholars (e.g., Baumrind, Larzelere, & Cowan, 2002). They raised methodological issues about shortcomings in the research: the research was largely limited to correlational studies, children's characteristics (i.e., difficultness) need to be controlled for in order to rule out child effects, the fact that neighborhoods and race/ethnicity can moderate the effects, and the possibility that abusive parents were included in the analyses. More recent carefully designed studies have addressed most of these concerns (except for the lack of experimental studies) and continue to find negative effects associated with physical punishment (e.g., Berlin et al., 2009).

These controversies attest to the importance of examining the topic of discipline. As the central ingredient of parental structure, discipline is one of the two major constructs of child-rearing research (attachment is the other; see Roisman & Groh, Chapter 5, this volume). The popularity of research into the construct is revealed by the number of instruments developed to measure it. According to one review, 55 questionnaires and 22 interviews have been developed to measure the construct (Locke & Prinz, 2002). Next we examine how parental use of discipline changes with the child's development from infant through adolescence and some of the variables linked to the frequency and ways it is expressed.

DISCIPLINE

The word *discipline* has multiple meanings and connotations. As a verb, it is defined as the training of a child to ensure proper behavior. More commonly, the word is used synonymously with punishment. When parents are asked to identify common discipline methods, they typically mention punishment with a focus on punitive techniques, such as slapping a hand, scolding, spanking, or withdrawal of privileges (Michels, Pianta, & Reeve, 1993). However, parents' role in training involves much more than simply dispensing disciplinary techniques.

At the core of child training is the teaching of right from wrong so that the child will develop into a well-adjusted and self-regulated individual. This process requires children to internalize parental behavioral prescriptions for their conduct. According to Grusec and Goodnow (1994), this behavior change occurs in two steps. First, the child must accurately interpret the parents' intended message. Then, in order for that change to be long-lasting, children need to accept the parental message and adopt it as their own. The way those steps are enacted change with development and vary widely across families.

Infants and Toddlers

When does this training begin? The earliest form of discipline consists of management of the infant through the structuring of routines. Parents determine, in conjunction with the infant's temperament and needs, a regular schedule of feeding and sleeping. Before long, as infants begin to initiate contact with the environment, and especially when they become mobile, parents then must set limits and create safe areas for the infant to explore. This necessitates parental childproofing of the environment and anticipatory or proactive parenting to reduce the likelihood that the infant will come into contact with potentially dangerous objects.

Childproofing and other parental preventative behaviors can never completely stop a child from engaging in behaviors the parent does not like. Undesired behaviors, but nonetheless developmentally appropriate actions, include touching prohibited objects, crying, grabbing and pinching, and putting objects in mouths. Some parents will interpret those behaviors as requiring correction before habits are formed. The evidence indicates that even before infants can crawl, many parents are attempting to eliminate undesired behaviors. In a national sample, 32% of parents with infants ages

4–9 months reported that they engaged in verbal punishment (i.e., yelling), and 6% had begun the use of physical punishment by spanking the infants (Regalado, Sareen, Inkelas, Wissow, & Halfon, 2004). Although information about the infants' transgressions was not reported, it is likely the source of the discipline consisted of such offenses as fussing, crying, and reaching for objects. By 12 months of age, more than one-third of parents participating in a longitudinal study admitted to using some form of coercive discipline, in addition to diverting, reasoning, ignoring, and even negotiating (Vittrup, Holden, & Buck, 2006). Coercive discipline included yelling (36%), slapping hands (21%), threatening (19%), removing toys or objects (18%), spanking (14%), and using time-out (12%; see Figure 6.1). Although parents may believe that early discipline is necessary for proper socialization, given infants' limited cognitive abilities, as well as their physiological responses to being spanked or slapped, these early disciplinary behaviors are potentially damaging for the child's physiological and emotional development (Bugental, Martorell, & Barraza, 2003).

Toddlerhood, with its increased mobility, curiosity, and desire for mastery of the environment, requires constant supervision to prevent unintentional injury and inevitably elicits more frequent discipline (Morrongiello, Klemencic, & Corbett, 2008). Although parents are trying to protect and teach their children to comply with paren-

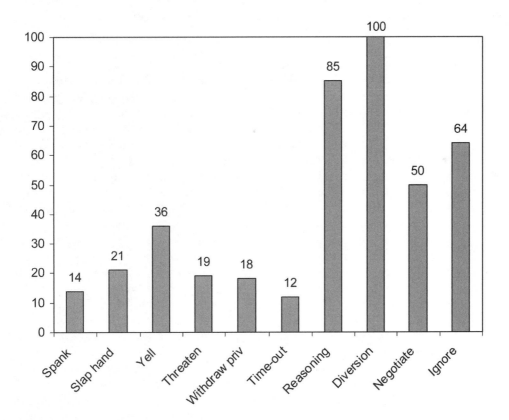

FIGURE 6.1. Percent of parents who had used various discipline methods by the time their children were 12 months old. Withdraw priv = withdrawal of privileges. Data from Vittrup, Holden, and Buck (2006).

tal instructions, their toddlers are operating under very different principles. One- to three-year-olds are oriented toward exploring and mastering the environment, as they experiment with autonomy. This inevitably results in parent–toddler conflicts, defiant reactions, and discipline (Dix, Stewart, Gershoff, & Day, 2007).

How parents respond to these expressions of autonomy has behavioral repercussions for the children. Ineffective or inappropriate parental discipline is likely to result in the development of behavior problems. In a cross-sectional study of more than 2,000 Dutch toddlers and preschoolers, the emergence of aggressive, oppositional, and/or overactive syndrome problems could be seen (van Zeigl et al., 2006). For example, 25% of the mothers of 12-month-olds reported that their children displayed at least one-third of the externalizing behavior problems listed on the widely used Child Behavior Checklist. The incidence of externalizing problems was higher with 24- and 36-month-olds. That study provides good evidence that the label of "terrible 2s" can be accurate but may be applicable well before 24 months.

Parents typically respond to increasing toddler noncompliance and autonomy experimentation with the strategy of asserting their power. This "power assertion" is commonly manifested in yelling and using physical force. In the Vittrup et al. (2006) longitudinal study, by 24 months about 81% of the parents reported yelling in anger at their children, 45% of the parents reported spanking, and about 31% reported slapping the children's hands. The rates of parental use of harsh and punitive discipline typically increase when the children are 36 months old (e.g., Vittrup et al., 2006).

Preschoolers

By the time children are 4 years old, they have experienced considerable physical, cognitive, and emotional regulation growth. Their attention span is longer, memory is better, receptive and productive language abilities are expanded, and their logical abilities have improved considerably from just a year or two earlier. Preschoolers can now identify and express emotions, but they do not yet fully understand them and therefore are unable to fully control their emotions. Consequently, reasoning and the use of logical consequences with preschoolers becomes a much more effective tool for managing child behavior. Although 85% of parents reported that they reasoned with their 12-month-old children, by the time they are preschoolers, all parents are reporting that they commonly use that technique (see Figure 6.1; Vittrup et al., 2006).

Preschoolers continue to engage in acts of noncompliance; however, they are more skillful in asserting their autonomy. Direct defiance tends to decrease in frequency and is replaced with simple refusal and negotiation. In a longitudinal study, Kuczynski and Kochanska (1990) found that the best predictor of 5-year-olds' responses to parental power assertion was the type of strategy used by the mothers during the toddler years. The most successful strategies included verbal reprimands and positive reinforcement of desired behavior. On the other hand, physical punishment was associated with passive noncompliance.

One of the reasons discipline changes with child age is due to parental cognitions: Parents expect more mature behavior from their preschoolers than they had expected earlier (Dix, Ruble, & Zambarano, 1989). However, children's desire for autonomy and their inability to fully control their emotions and behavior run counter to this expectation. Consequently, a number of investigators have found that the use of punitive discipline peaks when children are between the ages of 3 and 5 years old. In the Vittrup et al. (2006) longitudinal study, it was discovered that when asked about discipline practices in the past week, 59% of parents of 4-year-olds reported having spanked, and almost all parents reported having yelled, threatened, used time-outs, or taken away privileges. Straus (2001) found that at least 90% of parents use physical punishment by the time their children are 3–4 years old. Verbal punishment, consisting of scolding, yelling, or derogating the child, is even more common, and 91% of parents admit to yelling at their children by the time they are 19–35 months old (Regalado et al., 2004).

Discipline Errors with Young Children

Harsh discipline, typically operationalized as yelling, threatening, and frequent use of physical punishment, is problematic for a number of reasons. Parents who rely on harsh and punitive disciplinary practices do not promote the development of the children's ability to regulate their emotions and behavior. Rather, the harsh discipline reflects inappropriate regulatory behavior and elicits negative emotional arousal in the child (Scaramella & Leve, 2004). Parents who use physical punishment to obtain compliance find that as children grow in size and become more defiant, they have to increase the intensity of the coercion to obtain the same results. By escalating the intensity of their punitive discipline, a pattern of escalation that some children will match, parents engage in "coercive cycles" (Patterson, 1982). These hostile and angry interactions are characterized by both parents' and children's attempts to force the other to acquiesce. To that end, negativity and physical aggression escalate before someone (often the parent) gives in. Children thus learn to use and are reinforced for using this type of behavior pattern (Eddy, Leve, & Fagot, 2001).

Coercive cycles lead to a variety of problems in children, such as peer aggression, delinquency, and antisocial behavior (Patterson, DeBaryshe, & Ramsey, 1989), and reflect one of the more serious discipline mistakes that parents of young children make. However, parents make a number of other discipline errors. These mistakes include being inconsistent in use of discipline, giving in to the child, inadvertently reinforcing undesired behaviors, and failing to reinforce desired behaviors (O'Leary, 1995). Other errors can be identified by observing a parent engaged in discipline. Some parents make the mistake of being overreactive to children's minor misdeeds, being too verbal when admonishing children, or being too lax in applying discipline (Arnold, O'Leary, Wolff, & Acker, 1993).

These discipline errors have a variety of determinants. For some parents, it is a lack of knowledge about appropriate child-rearing practices. Other parents may subscribe to inappropriate beliefs about discipline, may be stressed, or may be unable to adequately regulate emotional reactions of frustration and anger (Regalado et al., 2004).

School-Age Children

By the time children reach school age, they have a well-developed theory of mind, so they are now able to take others' perspectives and become less egocentric in thought (Wellman, Cross, & Watson, 2001). Their thinking becomes more logical, and they are able to better remember. Parents can now also explain to children the consequences of their behavior and expect to be understood, thus making reasoning a more effective discipline method.

With children's emerging cognitive and social competencies, the nature of discipline changes. Parents of 8-year-olds report using such techniques as reasoning, limit setting, withdrawing privileges, reprimands, yelling, and experiencing logical consequences. However, school-age children are not immune from physical punishment, though its use drops precipitously during this developmental period (Straus, 2001).

By the age of 6 years, children have developed nuanced views about the disciplinary methods used on them. When interviewing children about their views of videotaped disciplinary vignettes, Vittrup and Holden (2010) found that 6- to 10-year-old children consider reasoning to be the most fair and most effective method for long-term behavior change, whereas spanking was regarded as least effective. The children generally perceived reasoning to have pedagogic value in that it included teaching a message to the child. On the contrary, they believed that the power of spanking lay mainly in its fear factor, and they recognized that children might quickly forget the parent's discipline message because spanking did not possess the same instructive quality as reasoning did.

Although physical punishment wanes during the school years, one way that some parents attempt to discipline and control their children is through psychological control. This type of control refers to "control attempts that intrude into the psychological and emotional development of the child" (Barber, 1996, p. 3296). Psychological control, then, includes behaviors such as calling into question the child's feelings, limiting verbal expression, inducing guilt, and withdrawing love (Barber, Maughan, & Olsen, 2005). Parents who use psychological control attempt to manipulate the child's thinking processes or emotions in an effort to constrain their children. For example, parents may manipulate their child by making him or her feel guilty or, alternatively, by communicating that their affection is contingent on whether the child follows parental orders.

During the school years, children's verbal misbehavior becomes more common. Children are now able to better distinguish between truth and lies, and parents assume that this ability will lead them to lie less frequently. However, the opposite appears to be true: Wilson, Smith, and Ross (2003) reported that in their naturalistic observation, 4-year-olds lied once every 2 hours, but by the age of 6 this had increased to about once every 1½. Whereas young children tend to lie as a way of experimenting with their new cognitive abilities, older children mainly lie to cover up transgressions. Parents often recognize that the cover-up is in fact a lie and dispense a consequence for the transgression; however, they often do not punish the accompanying lie, and thus children learn that there are no real adverse consequences for the lies. This is likely the reason that lying continues.

Similarly, as children develop better understanding of empathy and the dynamics of social relationships, they may begin to tell "white lies" to spare a friend's feelings. Thus lying may develop into a successful strategy, and research shows that unless parents curb it prior to the age of 7, it is likely to continue. The recommended child-rearing strategy for decreasing the frequency of lying is not to punish the child but rather to ask children to promise to tell the truth and that if they do so, it will make their parents very happy (Talwar & Lee, 2008). Children seek to please their parents, and if they learn that honesty—above and beyond good behavior—is valuable to their parents, then they are more likely to stop the fabrications.

Because schoolchildren are spending considerable amounts of time away from home—either at school or with peers—"parenting from afar" is now necessary. If parents have established rules and limits during the earlier years, and if the children have internalized their parents' morals, this transition will be much easier. Children who are intrinsically motivated to follow their parents' rules and behave appropriately are easier to "manage" compared with children who rely on threats of punishment to remind them not to misbehave (Gordon, 1989).

Child aggression continues to be a problem with some children and has been linked to family and child characteristics, as well as disciplinary problems. In a recent study of more than 1,500 children ages 6–12 years, the key risk variables included both family structure features and child characteristics (Joussemet et al., 2008). Having a young mother, being reared in a single-parent household, being a boy, and having a reactive temperament were all determinants of more aggressive child behavior.

Adolescence

Adolescence has been referred to by G. Stanley Hall, one of the forefathers of developmental research, as a "period of storm and stress" (1904, p. xiii), and stereotypes of the difficult adolescent abound. The common perception of adolescents as moody and confrontational often makes parents wary of the teenage years. Indeed, adolescence can present new challenges to families, as this is a period of many transitions. The preadolescent and adolescent years bring substantial physical, hormonal, and cognitive change.

Adolescence brings adjustments to the parent–child relationship as adolescents begin to spend less time with parents and more time with peers (Steinberg & Silk, 2002). Conflict within the parent–adolescent relationship is often perceived as the norm; however, empirical research indicates that conflict declines in frequency across adolescence and that the majority of families do not experience extreme levels of conflict. Contrary to popular beliefs, the majority of families successfully navigate through adolescence (D'Angelo & Omar, 2003).

Parents are able to help guide their children through adolescence, but in order to do so effectively they must continue to monitor, supervise, and exert some control over their adolescent while at the same time encouraging autonomy (Goossens, 2006). Research into the adolescent years reveals that appropriate parental control continues to be associated with positive developmental outcomes, as it helps adolescents learn that their behavior must be congruent with society's norms (Steinberg & Silk, 2002). Of course, the nature of parental control during adolescence is quite different from that manifested earlier in the child's life. As we discuss next, the key characteristics of effective control during adolescence have changed from those of childhood. However, disciplinary techniques that were previously ineffective, including physical punishment and psychological control, continue to be ineffective with teens and relate to behavior problems.

Effective Discipline

Parents differ markedly in the extent to which they attempt to control their adolescents' behavior. Some parents set strict limits with their adolescents, whereas other parents are lax. Overall, limit setting tends to decrease across the adolescent years as teenagers seek, and are given, greater autonomy (Barber, Maughan, & Olsen, 2005). That does not mean that effective parents have relinquished control over their teenagers. Rather, the form of control is modified and shifts to one of a supervisory nature.

At the level of parental traits, authoritative parenting has often been linked with higher levels of adolescent competence and school success. Adolescent children of authoritative mothers report higher levels of self-esteem and life satisfaction and lower levels of depression (Milevsky, Schlechter, Netter, & Keehn, 2007). Fewer problem behaviors, including lower levels of school misconduct, substance use, and delinquency, are also associated with this style of parenting (Adamczyk-Robinette, Fletcher, & Wright, 2002). Adolescents from authoritative homes report the most positive academic outcomes, as indexed by measures such as grade point average and orientation to school (Lamborn et al., 1991; Spera, 2005).

In terms of specific child-rearing practices, two key behaviors are limit setting and monitoring. By this developmental stage, adolescents desire that their individuality be respected and that they be given autonomy. Some adolescents seek to rebel against or at least test authority figures. They enjoy "pushing the limits" of what parents consider acceptable behavior through experimentation and association with problematic peers (Harris, 1995). Consequently, limit setting involves informing adolescents that they cannot engage in particular activities or go out with certain individuals or that they need to return home by a certain hour.

Another hallmark of effective discipline during the adolescent years is appropriate monitoring. Monitoring refers to "a set of correlated parenting behaviors involving attention to and tracking of the child's whereabouts, activities, and adaptations" (Dishion & McMahon, 1998, p. 61). Parental knowledge of their children's activities and companions becomes increasingly important during adolescence, as teenagers spend less time with their parents and more time with their peers in unsupervised activities. Monitoring serves a protective function against delinquent behavior, whereas lower levels of surveillance are associated with greater sexual risk taking, substance use, and arrests (DiClemente et al., 2001; Jacobson & Crockett, 2000). Intervention studies have shown that teaching parental monitoring skills can help reduce risky behaviors in adolescence (Wu et al., 2003).

Although researchers have typically defined parental monitoring as a set of parenting behaviors, many investigations have not measured parenting behaviors directly but instead have assessed parental knowledge about their adolescents (Crouter & Head, 2002). Kerr and Stattin (2003) pointed out that parental knowledge of adolescents requires that the teens reveal information to their parents. Some adolescents freely volunteer information about their activities and companions, but others may engage in information management and edit what information they share or even actively attempt to deceive their parents. Teenage girls are more likely to share information with parents than boys are (Smetana, 2008). Further, parents can create an environment that promotes adolescent disclosure by behaving in a warm and responsive fashion (Smetana, 2008). Thus monitoring is not simply a parental behavior but rather a function of the reciprocal, bidirectional relationship process involving disclosure of information to the parent.

Limit setting and monitoring serve a protective function. Parental limit setting and control were found to be associated with lower increases in externalizing problems over time (Galambos, Barker, & Almeida, 2003). Similarly, setting limits and monitoring also help protect adolescents from engaging in high-risk behaviors such as truancy and substance use (Steinberg & Silk, 2002).

Ineffective Discipline

Parents of adolescents are prone to engage in two ineffective types of discipline. The first mistake is to continue to use physical punishment and other forms of coercion.

Although physical discipline is more common at earlier ages, some parents continue to use corporal punishment during adolescence. As many as 40–50% of adults report that they were physically punished at least once during their adolescence (Straus, 2001; Turner & Muller, 2004). As was the case with younger children, physical discipline in adolescence is associated with both internalizing and externalizing problems (Bender et al., 2007). Further, the frequency with which corporal punishment is experienced during adolescence predicts internalizing problems during the college years (Turner & Muller, 2004). The effects of physical punishment appear to carry forward into adulthood; the experience of corporal punishment during adolescence is associated with increased risk of depression, suicidal ideation, substance use, and child abuse in adulthood (Straus, 2001).

The other problematic parenting practice is the use of psychological control. This disciplinary practice is intended to manipulate the youth into complying with the parent's wishes. Although the practice may be effective in achieving the parent's goals, it comes with a cost. Psychological control is associated with negative self-perceptions and internalizing problems in adolescents (Barber, 1996).

The Nature of Effective Discipline across Childhood

So how can one best summarize the nature of effective discipline across the childhood and adolescent years? It helps to remember parents' overriding socialization goal: to guide a child to develop into a competent member of society. As is evident from the preceding descriptions, the form that the discipline takes must change along with the developing child. Children's temperament, emotions, memory processes, reasoning skills, language development, and sense of right and wrong all contribute to their behavioral regulation. Other factors also affect their behavior, such as the quality of their relationship with their parents, their parents' child-rearing style, and their reactions to the particular parental discipline practice used.

To better comprehend how children react to discipline and, in turn, appreciate the nature of its effectiveness, Gershoff (2002b) constructed a three-step model of children's reactions to discipline. Although she developed it to account for how parental physical punishment affects preschool children's short-term and long-term processing and outcomes, the model applies to other disciplinary techniques and other ages of children as well. As we show, the child's perception of the misdeed and appropriateness of the parental response is central to her model.

The central part of the model begins with a parent's response to a child. The child then reacts to the parent's action with, in some cases, an initial physiological (e.g., pain) and emotional (e.g., fear or anger) reaction. Those responses represent the initial phase of child reactions. Note that only some types of disciplinary responses will initiate those initial reactions—such as spanking or verbal punishment (yelling, hostile or negative comments). If a physiological response is elicited, that initiates a variety of biological (e.g., hormonal) and central nervous system changes as a response to the stress (Bugental, Olster, & Martorell, 2003).

The second step, occurring within seconds, consists of the child engaging in some initial cognitive processing. Why did I get punished? Was I at fault? Was the punishment appropriate? Those types of appraisals are affected by whether the cognitions are "hot" due to angry reactions or not. Hot cognitions may short-circuit the initial appraisal process and result in defiance. In contrast, "cold" processing of an event is more apt to lead to compliance (Dix et al., 2007).

The third step of the model is the most important, because it concerns the long-term cognitive processing of the event and subsequent adjustment. In this phase, children process the event with more detachment from the incident. Here considerations including prior observational learning, external versus internal attributions, and social information processing inform the child's reactions to the prior incident. This long-term cognitive processing will then lead to the long-term child outcomes and ties into Grusec and Goodnow's (1994) model of internalization mentioned earlier. Children who interpret the parent's disciplinary message accurately (i.e., that their behavior was out of line and therefore the parent was reasonable in trying to prohibit it) will be more likely to adopt that standard of behavior for themselves. However, if the child incorrectly interprets the message or rejects the message, the child will not change his or her behavior.

In several different ways this model is helpful for thinking about discipline and its effects. First, it reveals a serious shortcoming of the child discipline literature: Most of the work is based on the perspective of parents or other adults, such as teachers. Only a handful of studies have assessed discipline from the child's or adolescent's perspective (e.g., Dobbs & Duncan, 2004; Ritchie & Ritchie, 1981; Vittrup & Holden, 2010). As the model makes clear, children's perceptions are critical, because ultimately the effectiveness of the discipline depends on how the child has cognitively processed it. In the long term, the child's good behavior reflects internal motivation to behave appropriately in the absence of a parent (Grusec & Goodnow, 1994).

Another reason that it is important to collect children's perspectives is that people interpret events differently, and this is particularly true when there are major developmental differences between individuals. For example, parents tend to describe their spanks as "gentle" and "loving," whereas their children may report them as a "hard" or "very hard" hit (Dobbs & Duncan, 2004, p. 376). The children in this study also revealed that their parents were usually angry when they spanked, whereas parents tend to report that they spank only when they are calm. Such discrepancies in reports can dramatically affect the understanding of the dynamics operating during disciplinary encounters.

Children's reports about spanking reveal that most children think the practice is ineffective in promoting behavior change. One of the first studies that collected children's perspectives about spanking found that less than one-third of the children thought it was an effective disciplinary technique (Ritchie, Paine, & Tourelle, 1980). The children revealed that after a spanking, they were more likely to feel angry and revengeful rather than guilty about their misbehavior. In a subsequent study with older children, Ritchie and Ritchie (1981) determined that many adolescents viewed withdrawal of privileges as a more severe form of discipline than spanking and thus more effective. However, the children acknowledged that they preferred to be spanked because it was over quickly. Almost 30 years later and on a different continent, similar views about spanking were reported by 6- to 10-year-old children (Vittrup & Holden, 2010).

Why isn't physical punishment more effective? Part of the reason is that it is not applied in the correct way. This problem can be seen when considering spanking from the perspective of operant conditioning. One of the basic mechanisms of learning is through a stimulus–response process in which behaviors are rewarded, ignored, or punished. The pioneer of learning processes, Thorndike (1932), in his "law of effect," recognized that rewarded behavior recurs. Thus children engage in appropriate behavior when such behavior is rewarded either extrinsically or intrinsically. Conversely, ignored or punished behaviors are less likely to recur.

According to the learning theorist Domjan (2005), animal studies have revealed that effective punishment requires four conditions. The punishment must occur after every transgression, the punishment must happen immediately after the transgression, the punishment should occur without warning, and, at least initially, it should be delivered with high intensity. However, in evaluating reports of spankings, it is clear that parents do not administer spanking in the prescribed ways necessary for it to be effective. Mothers do not spank consistently in response to the same misdeeds, they sometimes do not spank immediately after misbehavior but wait until they are in a private location, they warn children in advance, and they don't spank hard (e.g., Vittrup et al., 2006).

As these examples of problems in administering spankings illustrate, focusing on eliminating undesired child behaviors is an approach destined to fail. Parents are not always around when children misbehave—especially as children get older and spend more time away from home. If a child misbehaves at school or day care, the parents often are not notified until the child is picked up, and thus discipline is delayed. Similarly, parents may not be aware that a misdeed has occurred (such as when a child bullies another child or a teenager surreptitiously drinks alcohol). This is part of the reason why reliance on discipline will not be successful.

Instead of basing the parent–child relationship on power and control, a much more effective orientation is one that is centered on mutual respect, cooperation, and appropriate levels of autonomy support (Maccoby, 2007). Through the fostering of positive, warm relationships, children will grow up to feel a sense of connection with and support from parents. Along with reducing attempts to discipline, these efforts will result, ironically, in improved child behavior and reduced stress on the parent. In turn, families will be happier, the topic we next address.

Discipline in the Context of the Family

As indicated previously, children are reared with two parents in 65% of families in the United States (Annie E. Casey Foundation, 2009). Whether there are one or two parents present affects the nature of the relationship between parents and children. As Leve and Fagot (1997) found, based on observations as well as questionnaires, single parents (both mothers and fathers) tended to get more irritable and angry with their children compared with married parents. This was likely a reflection of the stress they were under, although stress was not assessed. However, there was also another discipline-related difference due to structure. Single parents tended to adopt a positive, problem-solving orientation to child management, in contrast to the two-parent families, who established discipline-oriented styles. Presumably, the single parents sought to reduce family stress by facilitating positive, cooperative, and mature child behavior.

There are other ways that the presence of a second parent changes the disciplinary context. First, the father may use different disciplinary techniques than the mother. For example, in a study of 106 married parents of preschoolers, 64% of the fathers reported a power-assertive disciplinary style, in contrast to the 65% of mothers who indicated a reasoning-based disciplinary style (Hart, DeWolf, Wozniak, & Burts, 1992). This gender difference likely varies by culture. For example, Chinese parents showed a somewhat different pattern, as reported by adolescents. Although fathers tended to be harsher disciplinarians, it was the mothers who engaged in higher levels of control (Shek, 2005). In addition, economically disadvantaged Chinese fathers engaged in less control and had poorer relations with their children than did the middle-class fathers.

A second effect of having two parents as potential disciplinary agents concerns the ways and extent to which the parents work together or antagonistically. This is known as coparenting. Coparenting in the area of discipline is believed to be particularly important for children's functioning. Indeed, in order for child guidance and discipline to be maximally effective, parents need to present a "united front," because it shows consistency and predictability. However, a very different dynamic is established if the nondisciplining parent privately undermines the other parent's discipline (McHale et al., 2002). In these types of situations, the child's self-regulatory capacities can be compromised (e.g., Brody, Stoneman, Smith, & Gibson, 1999).

As the foregoing description of discipline across the developmental years highlights, child misbehavior and disciplining children are sources of stress, both for the parents and for the family system. At the same time, disciplining children can be a cause of conflict between couples. Given that parenting and child-rearing attitudes are transmitted through generations, many people subscribe to the same attitudes and strategies that their own parents held and used (e.g., Holden, Thompson, Zambarano, & Marshall, 1997). As such, partner conflict over child-rearing issues—most prominently related to discipline—are common (Feinberg, 2003). Parental disagreement over child rearing—often over discipline-related issues—is a predictor of marital conflict and lack of satisfaction (Jouriles et al., 1991). In turn, marital conflict has been linked to negative child and adolescent outcomes, such as behavior problems, diminished self-esteem, and poor social skills, especially when undermining occurs (Buehler & Gerard, 2002; Feinberg, 2003).

If child discipline is potentially a contentious issue for married couples, it is even more so after parents separate or divorce. Discipline in these situations is particularly problematic for two reasons. First, children are likely to react to the disruption and change with behavior problems. Thus divorcing parents typically face behavior problems in their children that are responded to with discipline. Second, child-rearing disagreements in general, and disciplinary issues in particular, remain a source of continuing conflict between the divorced parents. This conflict is often driven by the tendency of noncustodial fathers to adopt permissive and indulgent parenting practices (Hetherington & Stanley-Hagan, 2002).

Another type of family structure variable that can affect discipline and its efficacy is the presence of siblings. Families with two or more children give rise to a novel phenomenon: evaluating how they are parented in comparison with their siblings, or what is labeled "differential treatment" by parents. Differential treatment, whether it is actual or perceived, has been recognized to occur in discipline, as well as in areas such as affection, time spent with children and chores. Differential use of discipline has been observed in parents of toddlers and preschoolers, school-age children, and adolescents, as a series of studies by McHale and her colleagues, as well as others, have shown (e.g., McHale, Updegraff, Shanahan, Crouter, & Killoren, 2005). Generally, older siblings are disciplined more than younger siblings. How differential treatment affects children differs across age but largely depends on the child's perception of the fairness of the treatment (McHale, Updegraff, Jackson-Newsom, Tucker, & Crouter, 2000).

In sum, parent–child disciplinary interactions are affected by the context. One of the central attributes of the context is the family structure—composed of the number of parents and children. A second type of attribute is the socioeconomic and cultural context. Discipline is affected by both of these attributes in several ways. For example, stress on the parents can directly affect family functioning and discipline. These attributes can also indirectly affect discipline and its effectiveness because they are mediated by the children's perceptions of them.

THE POLITICS OF DISCIPLINE

The ways in which parents discipline their children represent an unusual topic in social development because it is not just of academic interest. More than any other topic in the field, discipline of children crosses over into the public arena, because it concerns their ethical treatment. Is it acceptable to use harsh discipline with children? Is it okay to hit or spank a child? What about slapping? These questions reflect the nature of the ongoing international controversy over the use of physical punishment. The debate consists of an amalgamation of psychological, cultural, and philosophical issues.

One side of the debate is represented by the prominent sociologist Murray Straus. He has researched the consequences of spanking on children and youths for the past two decades. His studies, in addition to many others, show that physical punishment of children is detrimental to their social competence, mental health, and even their cognitive development. In fact, he considers the practice tantamount to child abuse. Furthermore, he argues that physical punishment is both a reflection of and contributes to a cultural orientation of violence (Straus, 2001).

At the other end of the continuum are conservative Christian authors such as James Dobson (2004) and John Rosemond (1994), who essentially ignore the empirical research evidence. Instead, they rely on a different source of authority—the Bible. Based primarily on five proverbs found in the Old Testament that refer to the "rod of correction," they argue that physical punishment is necessary to teach obedience and respect for parents. In line with learning theory, Dobson (2004) argued that spankings should cause pain; otherwise, it will not be a deterrent to future misbehaviors. Despite the scientific evidence to the contrary (e.g., Gershoff, 2002a), he maintains that corporal punishment makes children less aggressive and teaches them to live in harmony with authority.

Other researchers have challenged the quality of the evidence, as we mentioned earlier (Baumrind et al., 2002; Larzelere & Kuhn, 2005). For example, they mention the child-effects argument: Difficult children will elicit spanking, and thus their behavior causes spanking. They also point out that when spanking is perceived by children as a normative practice, then the negative effects are mediated. Indeed, some studies find that in African American families, use of corporal punishment is linked to adolescent competence (e.g., Deater-Deckard & Dodge, 1997). Based on these concerns and findings, Baumrind wrote "a blanket injunction against disciplinary spanking by parents is not scientifically supportable" (1996, p. 828).

Despite Baumrind's views, many countries have enacted bans on physical punishment. The earliest ban involved outlawing corporal punishment of children in the school system. Poland enacted the ban in 1783—perhaps due to the influence of John Locke's book published 90 years earlier. To date, more than 100 countries have followed suit and prohibited school corporal punishment. However, no such ban exists in the United States. Nevertheless, 30 states have passed legislation to prohibit school corporal punishment (Gershoff, 2008).

More controversial than banning corporal punishment in schools is outlawing parents' spanking their own children in their own homes. Sweden was the first country to enact this legislation in 1979 in an effort to draw attention to the problem of spanking and to precipitate, on a national scale, a change in child-rearing practices and attitudes. Subsequently, 28 countries have adopted similar bans, with Poland, Tunisia, and Kenya being the most recent nations to prohibit all corporal punishment of children (Global Initiative to End All Corporal Punishment of Children, 2010).

In contrast to those nations that have enacted a ban, physical punishment in the United States continues to be widely supported by the public. In a national poll conducted in 2004, 71% of respondents believed that spanking is an important socialization method (see Gershoff, 2008). In addition to those positive attitudes toward physical punishment, the United States is a country in which individualism, independence, and adult rights and liberties are valued and government intrusion into the lives of families is viewed with contempt. Parents do not want to be told how to rear their children by the government or anyone else. In the past few years, attempts to introduce bills in state legislatures in California, Massachusetts, Minnesota, and Texas relating to physical punishment of children have met with considerable criticism and opposition. Nevertheless, as judged by the continued appearance of articles in newspapers and magazines and on the Internet, the issue continues to be hotly contested.

These types of articles continue to feed the controversy in the United States, as well as giving conflicting advice. Parents who seek advice about discipline from pediatricians, magazines, the Internet, or books discover incompatible advice and have difficulty in discerning the consensus view about discipline methods. In addition, some parents hold strong attitudes—either pro or con—on the topic and have held these attitudes well before their children were born (Holden et al., 1997). Attitudes toward physical punishment in turn influence behavior. Parental attitudes toward spanking when children are 6 months old remained stable over several years and correlated significantly with later reported spanking (Vittrup et al., 2006). Thus parents' orientation toward physical punishment is often based on deep-seated beliefs transmitted across generations and related to personal experiences. Parenting books and articles are often ineffectual in their efforts to sway opinion. For these reasons, it is likely that the debate over the use of physical punishment with children will continue in the United States well into this century.

DIRECTIONS FOR FUTURE RESEARCH

Considerable strides have been made in better understanding the nature of discipline, its determinants, and how it affects children. This knowledge has been achieved by studying parent–child relations from multiple approaches, ranging from correlating parenting traits with child outcomes to examining momentary processes of compliance and defiance. Insights have also been gained from assessing the child's point of view, as well as examining the role of contextual variables. Those approaches set the stage for future research into discipline and family functioning. Three directions appear to be most promising.

Although the study of parenting styles has been helpful in revealing general relations between child rearing and children's outcomes, we now need to continue to "unpack" parenting styles. Dissecting parenting styles into constituent dimensions and behaviors—otherwise known as disaggregating parenting—is necessary to further our understanding of the unique contributions of specific parenting behaviors and how these behaviors interact. Parental control was the strongest predictor of behavior problems, whereas acceptance–involvement was a stronger predictor of psychosocial development (Gray & Steinberg, 1999).

The second direction involves better understanding of the processes involved in discipline and internalization from the child's perspective and how those processes change over development. More investigations into children's reactions to discipline are needed to reveal how children process contentious interactions and the variables that mediate or moderate that process. Going beyond children's cognitive reactions to look at physiological reactions to both negative and positive interactions is also a promising research direction for process-oriented research (Bugental, Olster, et al., 2003).

The third direction involves the continued efforts to put discipline into context. This means recognizing the multiple contexts within which the interactions occur. The most immediate context is the parent–child relationship. How does the quality of the relationship, including attachment or feelings of connectedness, relate to the parent's child management behavior and children's acceptance of that? Furthermore, how does the nature of parental socialization goals affect their controlling and disciplining? The family structure and relationships between other family members represent another type of context and require further explication. The neighborhood, socioeconomic status, and race or ethnicity provide yet a third layer of context. Finally, there is a need to continue investigating disciplinary techniques as they relate to socioeconomic and cultural influences. The ways in which each of these contextual layers influences disciplinary behavior, as well as how they interrelate, merit more investigation.

CONCLUSION

Much has been learned about how parents bring forth children with regard to discipline. Although training children remains a fundamental parental role, it must be done appropriately. Ironically, the research increasingly is revealing that a reliance on discipline is not the way to rear competent, healthy, and well-regulated children. Rather, promoting positive and cooperative parent–child relationships will not only be much more effective but will also avoid the potential problems that have been linked to physical punishment. After all, John B. Watson recognized that in 1928 when he concluded "I have tried punishment ... [and it has] proved wholly ineffective" (p. 139).

SUGGESTED READINGS

Bornstein, M. H. (2002). *Handbook of parenting* (Vols. 1–5). Mahwah, NJ: Erlbaum.

Bugental, D. B., & Grusec, J. E. (2006). Socialization processes. In N. Eisenberg, W. Damon, & R. M. Lerner (Eds.), *Handbook of child psychology: Vol. 3, Social, emotional, and personality development* (6th ed., pp. 366–428). Hoboken, NJ: Wiley.

Grusec, J. E., & Hastings, P. D. (2007). *Handbook of socialization: Theory and research.* New York: Guilford Press.

Holden, G. W. (2010). *Parenting: A dynamic perspective.* Los Angeles: Sage.

Kuczynski, L. (Ed.). (2003). *Handbook of dynamics in parent–child relations.* Thousand Oaks, CA: Sage.

REFERENCES

Adamczyk-Robinette, S., Fletcher, A. C., & Wright, K. (2002). Understanding the authoritative parenting–early adolescent tobacco use link: The mediating role of peer tobacco use. *Journal of Youth and Adolescence, 31,* 311–318.

Annie E. Casey Foundation. (2009). *2009 kids count: Data book.* Baltimore: Author.

Arnold, D. S., O'Leary, S. G., Wolff, L. S., & Acker, M. M. (1993). The Parenting Scale: A measure of dysfunctional parenting in discipline situations. *Psychological Assessment, 5,* 137–144.

Barber, B. K. (1996). Parental psychological control: Revisiting a neglected construct. *Child Development, 67,* 3296–3319.

Barber, B. K., Maughan, S. L., & Olsen, J. A. (2005). Patterns of parenting across adolescence. *New Directions for Child and Adolescent Development, 108,* 5–16.

Baumrind, D. (1971). Current patterns of parental authority. *Developmental Psychology, 4,* 1–103.

Baumrind, D. (1996). A blanket injunction against disciplinary use of spanking is not warranted by the data. *Pediatrics, 98,* 828–831.

Baumrind, D. (2005). Patterns of parental authority and adolescent autonomy. *New Directions for Child and Adolescent Development, 108,* 61–69.

Baumrind, D., Larzelere, R. E., & Cowan, P. A. (2002). Ordinary physical punishment: Is it harmful? Comment on Gershoff (2002). *Psychological Bulletin, 128,* 580–589.

Bender, H. L., Allen, J. P., McElhaney, K. B., Moore, C. M., Davis, S. M., Kelly, H. O., et al. (2007). Use of harsh physical discipline and developmental outcomes in adolescence. *Development and Psychopathology, 19,* 227–242.

Berlin, L. J., Ispa, J. M., Fine, M. A., Malone, P. S., Brooks-Gunn, J., Brady-Smith, C., et al. (2009). Correlates and consequences of spanking and verbal punishment for low-income white, African American, and Mexican American toddlers. *Child Development, 80,* 1403–1420.

Bornstein, M. H., & Lansford, J. E. (2010). Parenting. In M. H. Bornstein (Ed.), *Handbook of cultural developmental science* (pp. 259–277). New York: Psychology Press.

Bowlby, J. (1988). *A secure base: Parent–child attachment and healthy human development.* New York: Basic Books.

Bradley, R. H. (2007). Parenting in the breach: How parents help children cope with developmentally challenging circumstances. *Parenting: Science and Practice, 7,* 99–148.

Brody, G. H., Stoneman, Z., Smith, T., & Gibson, N. M. (1999). Sibling relationships in rural African American families. *Journal of Marriage and Family, 61,* 1046–1057.

Bronfenbrenner, U., & Morris, P. (2006). The ecology of developmental processes. In W. Damon & R. Lerner (Eds.), *Handbook of child psychology* (6th ed., Vol. 1, pp. 993–1028). New York: Wiley.

Buehler, C., & Gerard, J. M. (2002). Marital conflict, ineffective parenting, and children's and adolescents' maladjustment. *Journal of Marriage and Family, 64,* 78–92.

Bugental, D. B., Martorell, G. A., & Barraza, V. (2003). The hormonal costs of subtle forms of infant maltreatment. *Hormones and Behavior, 43,* 237–244.

Bugental, D. B., Olster, D. H., & Martorell, G. A. (2003). A developmental neuroscience perspective on the dynamics of parenting. In L. Kuczynski (Ed.), *Handbook of dynamics in parent–child relations* (pp. 25–48). Thousand Oaks, CA: Sage.

Collins, W. A., Maccoby, E. E., Steinberg, L., Hetherington, E. M., & Bornstein, M. H. (2000). Contemporary research on parenting: The case for nature and nurture. *American Psychologist, 55,* 218–232.

Crouter, A. C., & Head, M. R. (2002). Parental monitoring and knowledge of children. In M. H. Bornstein (Ed.), *Handbook of parenting: Vol. 3. Being and becoming a parent* (2nd ed., pp. 461–483). Mahwah, NJ: Erlbaum.

D'Angelo, S. L., & Omar, H. A. (2003). Parenting adolescents. *International Journal of Adolescence Medicine and Health, 15,* 11–19.

Darling, N., & Steinberg, L. (1993). Parenting style as context: An integrative model. *Psychological Bulletin, 113,* 487–496.

Deater-Deckard, K. (2004). *Parenting stress.* New Haven, CT: Yale University.

Deater-Deckard, K., & Dodge, K. A. (1997). Externalizing behavior problems and discipline revisited: Nonlinear effects and variation by culture, context, and gender. *Psychological Inquiry, 8*, 161–175.

Demo, D. H., & Acock, A. C. (1996). Family structure, family process, and adolescent well-being. *Journal of Research on Adolescence, 6*, 457–488.

DiClemente, R. J., Wingood, G. M., Crosby, R., Sionean, C., Cobb, B. K., Harrington, K., et al. (2001). Parental monitoring: Associations with adolescents' risk behaviors. *Pediatrics, 107*, 1363–1368.

Dishion, T. J., & McMahon, R. J. (1998). Parental monitoring and the prevention of child and adolescent problem behavior: A conceptual and empirical formulation. *Clinical Child and Family Psychology Review, 1*, 61–75.

Dix, T., Ruble, D. N., & Zambarano, R. J. (1989). Mothers' implicit theories of discipline: Child effects, parent effects, and the attribution process. *Child Development, 60*, 1373–1391.

Dix, T., Stewart, A. D., Gershoff, E. T., & Day, W. H. (2007). Autonomy and children's reactions to being controlled: Evidence that both compliance and defiance may be positive markers in early development. *Child Development, 78*, 1204–1221.

Dobbs, T., & Duncan, J. (2004). Children's perspectives on physical discipline: A New Zealand example. *Child Care in Practice, 10*, 367–379.

Dobson, J. (2004). *The new strong-willed child: Birth through adolescence*. Carol Stream, IL: Tyndale House.

Domjan, M. (2005). *Essentials of conditioning and learning* (3rd ed.). Belmont, CA: Wadsworth/Thompson Learning.

Eddy, J. M., Leve, L. D., & Fagot, B. (2001). A replication and extension of Patterson's coercive model. *Aggressive Behavior, 27*, 14–25.

Federal Interagency Forum on Child and Family Statistics. (2008). *America's children in brief: Key national indicators of well-being*. Washington, DC: U.S. Government Printing Office.

Feinberg, M. (2003). The internal structure and ecological context of coparenting: A framework for research and intervention. *Parenting: Science and Practice, 3*, 95–131.

Galambos, N. L., Barker, E. T., & Almeida, D. M. (2003). Parents do matter: Trajectories of change in externalizing and internalizing problems in early adolescence. *Child Development, 74*, 578–594.

Gershoff, E. (2002a). Corporal punishment by parents and associated child behaviors and experiences: A meta-analytic and theoretical review. *Psychological Bulletin, 128*, 539–579.

Gershoff, E. (2002b). Corporal punishment, physical abuse, and the burden of proof: Reply to Baumrind, Larzelere, and Cowan (2002), Holden (2002), and Parke (2002). *Psychological Bulletin, 128*, 602–611.

Gershoff, E. (2008). *Report on physical punishment in the United States: What research tells us about its effects on children*. Columbus, OH: Center for Effective Discipline.

Global Initiative to End All Corporal Punishment of Children. (2010). *Ending legalized violence against children: Global Report 2010*. Nottingham, UK: Author.

Goossens, L. (2006). The many faces of adolescent autonomy: Parent–adolescent conflict, behavioral decision-making, and emotional distancing. In S. Jackson & L. Goossens (Eds.), *Handbook of adolescent development* (pp. 135–153). New York: Psychology Press.

Gordon, T. (1989). *Teaching children self-discipline*. New York: Random House.

Gray, M. R., & Steinberg, L. (1999). Unpacking authoritative parenting: Reassessing a multidimensional construct. *Journal of Marriage and Family, 61*, 574–587.

Grusec, J. E., & Goodnow, J. J. (1994). Impact of parental discipline methods on the child's internalization of values: A reconceptualization of current points of view. *Developmental Psychology, 30*, 4–19.

Grusec, J. E., & Hastings, P. D. (Eds.). (2007). *Handbook of socialization: Theory and research*. New York: Guilford Press.

Hall, G. S. (1904). *Adolescence: Its psychology and its relations to physiology, anthropology, sociology, sex crime, religion, and education* (Vols. 1–2). New York: Appleton.

Harris, J. R. (1995). Where is the child's environment: A group socialization theory of development. *Psychological Review, 102*, 458–489.

Hart, C. H., DeWolf, D. M., Wozniak, P., & Burts, D. C. (1992). Maternal and paternal disciplinary styles: Relations with preschoolers' playground behavioral orientations and peer status. *Child Development, 63*, 879–892.

Hernandez, D. J., Denton, N. A., & Macartney, S. E. (2008). Children in immigrant families: Looking to America's future. *Social Policy Report, 22,* 3–22.

Hetherington, E. M., & Stanley-Hagan, M. (2002). Parenting in divorced and remarried families. In M. H. Bornstein (Ed.), *Handbook of parenting: Vol. 3. Being and becoming a parent* (pp. 287–316). Mahwah, NJ: Erlbaum.

Holden, G. W. (2010). *Parenting: A dynamic perspective.* Los Angeles: Sage.

Holden, G. W., & Miller, P. C. (1999). Enduring and different: A meta-analysis of the similarity in parents' child rearing. *Psychological Bulletin, 125,* 223–254.

Holden, G. W., Thompson, E. E., Zambarano, R. J., & Marshall, L. A. (1997). Child effects as a source of change in maternal attitudes toward corporal punishment. *Journal of Social and Personal Relationships, 14,* 481–490.

Horowitz, F. D. (1992). John B. Watson's legacy: Learning and environment. *Developmental Psychology, 28,* 360–367.

Jacobson, K. C., & Crockett, L. J. (2000). Parental monitoring and adolescent adjustment: An ecological perspective. *Journal of Research on Adolescence, 10,* 65–97.

Jouriles, E. N., Murphy, C. M., Farris, A. M., Smith, D. A., Richters, J. E., & Waters, E. (1991). Marital adjustment, parental disagreements about child rearing, and behavior problems in boys: Increasing the specificity of the marital assessment. *Child Development, 62,* 1424–1433.

Joussemet, M., Vitaro, F., Barker, E. D., Côté, S., Nagin, D. S., Zoccolillo, M., et al. (2008). Controlling parenting and physical aggression during elementary school. *Child Development, 79,* 411–425.

Kerr, M., & Stattin, H. (2003). Parenting of adolescents: Action or reaction? In A. C. Crouter (Ed.), *Children's influence of family dynamics: The neglected side of family relationships* (pp. 121–151). Mahwah, NJ: Erlbaum.

Kerr, M., Stattin, H., Biesecker, G., & Ferrer-Wreder, L. (2003). Relationships with parents and peers in adolescence. In R. M. Lerner, M. A. Easterbrooks, & J. Mistry (Eds.), *Handbook of psychology: Developmental psychology* (pp. 395–415). Hoboken, NJ: Wiley.

Kuczynski, L., & Kochanska, G. (1990). Development of children's noncompliance strategies from toddlerhood to age 5. *Developmental Psychology, 26,* 398–408.

Lamborn, S. D., Mounts, N. S., Steinberg, L., & Dornbusch, S. M. (1991). Patterns of competence and adjustment among adolescents from authoritative, authoritarian, indulgent, and neglectful families. *Child Development, 62,* 1049–1065.

Larzelere, R., & Kuhn, B. (2005). Comparing child outcomes of physical punishment and alternative discipline tactics: A meta-analysis. *Clinical Child and Family Psychology Review, 8,* 1–37.

Leve, L. D., & Fagot, B. I. (1997). Gender-role socialization and discipline processes in one- and two-parent families. *Sex Roles, 36,* 1–21.

Lewis, C. (1981). The effects of parental firm control: A reinterpretation of findings. *Psychological Bulletin, 90,* 547–563.

Locke, J. (1699). *Some thoughts concerning education* (4th ed.). London: A. & J. Churchill. (Original work published 1693)

Locke, L. M., & Prinz, R. J. (2002). Measurement of parental discipline and nurturance. *Clinical Psychology Review, 22,* 895–929.

Maccoby, E. E. (2007). Historical overview of socialization research and theory. In J. E. Grusec & P. D. Hastings (Eds.), *Handbook of socialization: Theory and research* (pp. 13–41). New York: Guilford Press.

Maccoby, E. E., & Martin, J. A. (1983). Socialization in the context of the family: Parent–child interaction. In P. H. Mussen (Series Ed.) & E. M. Hetherington (Vol. Ed.), *Handbook of child psychology: Vol. 4. Socialization, personality, and social development* (4th ed., pp. 1–101). New York: Wiley.

Martin, J., Kochanek, K. D., Strobino, D. M., Guyer, B., & MacDorman, M. F. (2005). Annual summary of vital statistics—2003. *Pediatrics, 115,* 619–634.

McHale, J., Khazan, I., Erera, P., Rotman, T., DeCourcey, W., & McConnell, M. (2002). Coparenting in diverse family systems. In M. H. Bornstein (Ed.), *Handbook of parenting* (2nd ed., Vol. 3, pp. 75–108). Mahwah, NJ: Erlbaum.

McHale, S. M., Updegraff, K. A., Jackson-Newsom, J., Tucker, C. J., & Crouter, A. C. (2000).

When does parents' differential treatment have negative implications for siblings? *Social Development, 9,* 149–172.

McHale, S. M., Updegraff, K. A., Shanahan, L., Crouter, A. C., & Killoren, S. E. (2005). Siblings' differential treatment in Mexican American families. *Journal of Marriage and Family, 67,* 1259–1274.

Michels, S., Pianta, R. C., & Reeve, R. E. (1993). Parent self-reports of discipline practices and child acting-out behaviors in kindergarten. *Early Education and Development, 4,* 139–144.

Milevsky, A., Schlechter, M., Netter, S., & Keehn, D. (2007). Maternal and paternal parenting styles in adolescents: Associations with self-esteem, depression, and life satisfaction. *Journal of Child and Family Studies, 16,* 39–47.

Morrongiello, B. A., Klemencic, N., & Corbett, M. (2008). Interactions between child behavior patterns and parent supervision: Implications for children's risk of unintentional injury. *Child Development, 79,* 627–638.

O'Leary, S. (1995). Parental discipline mistakes. *Current Directions in Psychological Science, 4,* 11–13.

Patterson, G. R. (1982). *Coercive family process.* Eugene, OR: Castalia.

Patterson, G. R., DeBaryshe, B. D., & Ramsey, E. (1989). A developmental perspective on antisocial behavior. *American Psychologist, 44,* 329–335.

Regalado, M., Sareen, H., Inkelas, M., Wissow, L. S., & Halfon, N. (2004). Parents' discipline of young children: Results from the National Survey of Early Childhood Health. *Pediatrics, 113,* 1952–1958.

Ritchie, J., Paine, H., & Tourelle, L. (1980). Sex differences in physical punishment: The children's view. In J. Ritchie (Ed.), *Psychology of women: Research record III* (pp. 104–136). Hamilton, New Zealand: University of Waikato.

Ritchie, J., & Ritchie, J. (1981). *Spare the rod.* Sydney, Australia: Allen & Unwin.

Rosemond, J. (1994). *To spank or not to spank: A parent's handbook.* Kansas City, MO: Andrews & McMeel.

Rothbaum, F., Pott, M., Azuma, H., Miyake, K., & Weisz, J. (2000). Trade-offs in the study of culture and development: Theories, methods, and values. *Child Development, 71,* 1159–1161.

Scaramella, L. V., & Leve, L. D. (2004). Clarifying parent–child reciprocities during early childhood: The Early Childhood Coercion model. *Clinical Child and Family Psychology Review, 7,* 89–107.

Shek, D. T. L. (2005). Perceived parental control processes, parent–child relational qualities, and psychological well-being in Chinese adolescents with and without economic disadvantage. *Journal of Genetic Psychology, 166,* 171–188.

Skinner, E., Johnson, S., & Snyder, T. (2005). Six dimensions of parenting: A motivational model. *Parenting: Science and Practice, 5,* 175–235.

Smetana, J. G. (2008). "It's 10 o'clock: Do you know where your children are?": Recent advances in understanding parental monitoring and adolescents' information management. *Child Development Perspectives, 2,* 19–25.

Spera, C. (2005). A review of the relationship among parenting practices, parenting styles, and adolescent school achievement. *Educational Psychology Review, 17,* 125–146.

Steinberg, L., & Silk, J. (2002). Parenting adolescents. In M. Bornstein (Ed.), *Handbook of parenting: Vol. 1. Children and parenting* (2nd ed., pp. 103–133). Mahwah, NJ: Erlbaum.

Straus, M. (2001). *Beating the devil out of them.* New Brunswick, NJ: Transaction.

Strohschein, L. (2005). Parental divorce and child mental health trajectories. *Journal of Marriage and Family, 67,* 1286–1300.

Suizzo, M.-A. (2007). Parents' goals and values for children: Dimensions of independence and interdependence across four U.S. ethnic groups. *Journal of Cross-Cultural Psychology, 38,* 506–530.

Talwar, V., & Lee, K. (2008). Social and cognitive correlates of children's lying behavior. *Child Development, 79,* 866–881.

Thorndike, E. L. (1932). *The fundamentals of learning.* New York: Columbia University, Teachers College.

Turner, H. A., & Muller, P. A. (2004). Long-term effects of child corporal punishment on depressive symptoms in young adults: Potential moderators and mediators. *Journal of Family Issues, 25,* 761–782.

van Zeijl, J., Mesman, J., Stolk, M. N., Alink, L. R. A., van IJzendoorn, M. H., Bakermans-Kranenburg, M. J., et al. (2006). Terrible ones?: Assessment of externalizing behaviors in infancy with the Child Behavior Checklist. *Journal of Child Psychology and Psychiatry, 47,* 801–810.

Vittrup, B., & Holden, G. W. (2010). Children's assessments of corporal punishment and other disciplinary practices: The role of age, race, SES, and exposure to spanking. *Journal of Applied Developmental Psychology, 31,* 211–220.

Vittrup, B., Holden, G. W., & Buck, M. (2006). Attitudes predict the use of physical punishment: A prospective study of the emergence of disciplinary practices. *Pediatrics, 117,* 2055–2064.

Watson, J. B. (1926). What the nursery has to say about instincts. In C. A. Murchison, M. Bentley, & K. Dunlap (Eds.), *Psychologies of 1925: Powell lectures in psychological theory* (pp. 1–35). Worcester, MA: Clark University.

Watson, J. B. (1928). *Psychological care of infant and child.* New York: Norton.

Wellman, H. M., Cross, D., & Watson, J. (2001). Meta-analysis of theory-of-mind development: The truth about false belief. *Child Development, 72,* 655–684.

Wilson, A. E., Smith, M. D., & Ross, H. S. (2003). The nature and effects of young children's lies. *Social Development, 12,* 21–45.

Wu, Y., Stanton, B. F., Galbraith, J., Kaljee, L., Cottrell, L., Li, X., et al. (2003). Sustaining and broadening intervention impact: A longitudinal randomized trial of 3 adolescent risk reduction approaches. *Pediatrics, 111,* e32–e38.

7

Peer Relations as a Developmental Context

William M. Bukowski
Duane Buhrmester
Marion K. Underwood

There is no lack of evidence that peer relations matter. We can look first at the comments that centenarians made when they were asked to explain the secrets to living for more than 100 years. One of the most frequently mentioned secrets for having a long life of health and happiness was the importance of having good friends. As a second example, the son of one of us (W.M.B.) looked into his child care classroom one day and then refused to go in. He declared, "I am going home." When asked to explain his decision, the boy stated his reason emphatically: his best friend was absent. Without his friend, there was apparently no other reason to justify his further presence on this day. A third form of evidence for the importance of friends comes from one of the best-selling series of books of all time: the Harry Potter series. On the surface they seem to be mere fantasy stories of magic, wizardry, and adventure. After all, Harry is forced to deal with all sorts of challenges, games, and tasks that are far beyond the day-to-day experiences that children have today or have ever had. There is no doubt that in these stories Harry and his two companions, Hermione and Ron, have experiences that most children cannot even imagine. Nevertheless, even the "muggles" among us will recognize that the power of the stories about Harry Potter comes from their depictions of what it is like to go through the many challenges of growing up in the company of one's friends.

At every point in the life cycle—old age, preschool, and school age—peer relations provide an important context for development. Starting at a young age, we live in a peer-rich world. Young children spend large amounts of time in the presence of their agemates. Interaction with peers occurs in classrooms, in after-school activities, in neighborhood playgrounds, and via electronic media. Adolescents and adults typically share the most basic activities and experiences of their lives—work, play, recreation, and romance—with persons of their own age. Older persons often share the later years of their lives with their friends, especially if their spouses have died and if their families live far away.

The importance of the peer system has not been lost on developmental psychologists (Hartup & Stevens, 1997). For over a century psychologists have developed theories and conducted empirical studies to identify and understand the features and effects of children's and adolescents' experiences with their peers. The findings from their studies have provided convincing evidence of the significant role that peers play in development (see Bukowski, Brendgen & Vitaro, 2007). Experiences with peers are associated with the good (e.g., happiness, health, school achievement, and multiple aspects of well-being) and the not so good (e.g., aggression, depressed affect, school dropout, and drug use). In this chapter we show how peer relations affect development in both positive and negative ways during childhood and adolescence.

WHY STUDY PEER RELATIONS?

Peer relations have been implicated in multiple developmental processes. Peers are mentioned in the best known theoretical accounts of development, and there is an impressive database regarding the association between indices of competent functioning with peers and subsequent well-being. In the following sections we point to different perspectives on and motivators for research on peer relations. From one point of view, the peer domain is seen as a context in which the basic mechanisms of social learning processes account for behavioral change. A second perspective recognizes that the peer domain constitutes a social "world" whose processes and effects are distinct from the social world that includes adults. Accordingly, it provides unique and important opportunities for development. A third motivation or perspective regarding peer relations is data driven. It emphasizes the empirical evidence that functioning with peers in childhood is a strong, if not the strongest, predictor of adult adjustment. In a final section we discuss the need to see peer relations as a multilevel system.

Opportunities for Social Learning and Experiences

One of the simplest motivations for research on peer relations has to do with time and amount of contact. The peer domain is a primary social world for children and adolescents. Even preschool children can spend large amounts of time with their peers. The classroom and schoolyard, neighborhood playgrounds, summer camps, sports teams, and specialty performance classes (e.g., dancing, singing, and playing a musical instrument in a band or orchestra) are largely peer-based activities. This vast amount of contact with peers provides multiple opportunities for fundamental socialization experiences. In their interactions with each other, humans, like other social animals, are known to affect each other via two basic processes of social learning. First, it has been known for several decades that peers reward and punish each other for various forms of positive and negative behavior (see Hartup, Glazer, & Charlesworth, 1966). Second, peers imitate each other. Given their similarity and proximity to each other, they are natural role models for each other (Hartup & Coates, 1967). Via these basic forms of social learning, peers "shape" each other along multiple dimensions of behavior, from aggression to altruism.

As part of their time together and in their contact with each other, children offer each other particular forms of experience. These experiences can be affective or behavioral, and they can be positive, negative, or neutral. Positive experiences include opportunities for acceptance, companionship, and intimacy (Furman & Buhrmester, 1985). Another form of positive experience can be protection against negative experiences such as victimization, exclusion, and rejection (see Davies, 1984; Hodges, Malone & Perry, 1997). An example of a neutral form of experience is exploration. Promoting each other's involvement in new activities is a key component to peer-based processes such as play and collaborative learning (Azmitia & Montgomery, 1993) . It can also be part of the initiation into or encouragement of drug use and other forms of risk (Grosbras et al., 2007). Each of these forms of positive, negative, and neutral experience that come from contact with peers is given further treatment in the remainder of this chapter.

A Unique Social World of Potential Equality

It is not just time, however, that matters. Children also provide each other with unique experiences that derive from the potential for equality in their relationships. Whereas interaction between children and their parents, teachers, and other adults is typically marked by inequalities of competence and power, interactions between peers is, almost by definition, more likely to be characterized by equality. The significance of this distinction between their hierarchical, or "vertical," interactions with adults and their more egalitarian, or "horizontal," interactions with peers comes in the larger number of opportunities for experiences of negotiation, co-construction, and affection based on an equal footing. Piaget (1932) pointed to the importance of peer *interaction*, especially peer discourse, conflict resolution, and negotiation, as critically important for the development of higher levels of operational thinking, especially in the social domain. Piaget argued that interaction with peers provided opportunities for children to explore and negotiate conflicting ideas, discuss different points of view, and find ways of reconciling differences between them. For Piaget these opportunities for co-construction with peers were an important context for adaptive development, especially in regard to the understanding of others' internal states, including thoughts, emotions, and intentions.

Vygotsky (1978) also emphasized the importance of co-construction with peers. He proposed that via cooperation and by taking advantage of each other's particular forms of expertise, children can resolve problems that neither would be capable of alone (Doise & Mugny, 1984; Golbeck, 1998). By fitting into the upper range of of one's friend's competence, a child can stimulate the friend's level of functioning and cognitive development (Hartup, 1996).

Aside from their effects on cognitive development, children's experiences with peers have also been identified as important experiences underlying emotional development and adjustment. A point of theoretical convergence between the views of a set of sociologists known as the symbolic interactionists and those of the American psychiatrist Harry Stack Sullivan (1953) is the claim that that people define themselves according to how they believe they are perceived by others. According to the symbolic interactionists, one's recognition of how one is perceived and treated by others forms the basis not only of the self-concept but also of how one perceives others. Mead

(1934) claimed that exchanges among peers that involve cooperation, competition, conflict, and/or friendly discussion afford opportunities for learning about the self and for understanding others.

Sullivan (1953) was particularly interested in the experience of peer relations during pre- and early adolescence. Sullivan described these close relationships as relations between "chums" or coequals. Sullivan theorized that relationships with coequals at this time of the lifespan were the first true interpersonal experiences based on reciprocity and exchange between equals. He claimed that the effect of these was to promote a sense of well-being due to the opportunities that they provided for self-validation. Sullivan believed that the positive experiences of having a "chum" could be so powerful as to allow an early adolescent to overcome "warps" that may have resulted from prior family experiences. He also argued that the experience of being isolated from the group during this period would lead early adolescents to have concerns about their adequacy and their acceptability as a desirable peer. Accordingly, Sullivan (1953) proposed that children and early adolescents who are incapable of creating a place for themselves within the peer group would develop enduring feelings of inferiority and a sense of psychological distress.

Empirical Evidence of the Association between Childhood Peer Relations and Adult Adjustment

Consistent with Sullivan's theory, a large number of studies have shown that measures of functioning among peers during childhood and early adolescence are associated with measures of externalizing and internalizing during adulthood. Results of prospective longitudinal studies provide evidence of the negative effects of problematic peer relations during childhood and early adolescence. These negative outcomes cover a wide range of subsequent adjustment problems, including aspects of criminality, school dropout, admissions to psychiatric hospitals, dishonorable discharges from military service, and unemployment (Parker & Asher, 1987). Peer rejection in particular is known to be associated with subsequent externalizing problems, including delinquency, conduct disorder, attentional difficulties, and substance abuse (Kupersmidt & Coie, 1990), and internalizing problems across the lifespan, including low self-esteem, anxiety problems, loneliness, and depressive symptoms (Kraatz-Keily, Bates, Dodge, & Pettit, 2000; Sandstrom, Cillessen, & Eisenhower, 2003). There is evidence also that children who have less than positive relations with peers are vastly more likely to fail a subsequent grade (Ollendick, Weist, Borden, & Greene, 1992), have more trouble adjusting after a school transition (Coie, Lochman, Terry, & Hyman, 1992), and show a higher risk of subsequent absenteeism (DeRosier, Kupersmidt, & Patterson, 1994). Friendlessness in childhood has been shown to be a particular risk factor for multiple forms of maladjustment problems in adulthood (Bagwell, Newcomb, & Bukowski, 1998).

Peer Relations as a Multilevel Experience

Either explicitly or implicitly, any theory that is aimed at explaining a phenomenon needs to provide a description of what the phenomenon is. Providing a description of what peer relations consist of is not easy, as they include a wide range of features and experiences. These experiences not only come in different forms, but they also occur at different levels of social complexity, specifically the individual, interaction, relationship, and group levels (Hinde, 1987). Events and processes at each level are distinct from events and processes at other levels, even as they are constrained and influenced by them. The level of the *individual* refers to the characteristics and tendencies that children bring to their involvement with peers. These include social skills, typical modes of social behavior (e.g., aggression or withdrawal), temperaments and patterns of physiological response to arousal, social perceptions and cognitions, and social needs. The level of the *interaction* includes what children actually do with each other. This would include play, talk, participation in self- or adult-structured activities, and activities in schools. The shared experience of interactions provides the basis for *relationships*. Relationships are enduring patterns of interaction between two children that are organized around particular themes, roles, or shared views maintained by the two relationship partners. Friendship is the most common form of relationships for persons of all ages. Each of these three levels is situated in a *group* context. Groups consist of set of individuals who are organized by structural characteristics (i.e., the children in a classroom) or by affective ties or common activities or interests. The dynamics and structural properties of groups can be at least partially distinct from the experiences that group members have at lower levels of social complexity.

Summary

Peer relations research has been seen in the literature on social development for over 100 years (Monroe, 1898). This enduring interest in understanding what peer relations are and with how these experiences affect development comes from at least three sources. First is the status of the peer group as a social context that affords the basic forms of socialization experience, such as rewards and modeling. Second is the body of theoretical accounts that ascribe functional developmental significance to the opportunity for "coequal" interaction between peers. Well-known theorists such as Piaget, Vygotsky, and Sullivan have argued that peer relations are a critical context for cognitive and emotional development. A third source is the extensive database showing that measures of functioning among peers during childhood and adolescence are powerful predictors of subsequent adjustment and well-being. Risk status for externalizing problems, internalizing problems, and academic difficulties has been shown to be associated with problematic peer relations in childhood and adolescence. Individually and together, these perspectives show that peer relations are essential to development, as they provide the context for the acquisition of critical skills needed for adequate functioning during adulthood. In the next three sections, we describe the features and effects of peer relations during three developmental periods—specifically, early childhood, the school-age period, and adolescence.

EARLY CHILDHOOD: PLAY AND BASIC SKILLS

Many young children gleefully join the world of their peers as soon as they have the opportunity to be around other children. Few other interactions match the level of ecstatic joy of preschool-age children greeting each other and running off to play cops and robbers or hide and seek or pretending to be married. Researchers' efforts to capture the excitement of early peer interactions have been shaped by the settings in which young children have been observed (Howes & Lee, 2006). Early studies of preschool peer relations were conducted in laboratory nursery schools where children were taken a few mornings a week for a socialization experiences with peers. These peer experiences were important, as children were spending most of their time at home being cared for by their mothers, perhaps in the company of their siblings. As more women joined the workforce, researchers had opportunities to observe infants, toddlers, and preschoolers who were spending whole days together. "The nursery school experience might be compared to a date, while the childcare experience is more like living together" (Howes & Lee, 2006, p. 137). Not surprisingly, young children's interactions seem more sophisticated when they have opportunities to interact all day, sometimes for years.

Beginning in infancy, children form relationships with their peers, as well as their caregivers, and seem to follow a similar developmental sequence in generating these relationships (Hay, 1985). Initially, infants are able to identify peers as possible social partners; at about 6 months of age, they smile and make nondistressed vocalizations toward other infants (Vandell, Wilson, & Buchanan, 1980). Next they begin to communicate with peers. By about 6 months of age, they begin to direct vocalizations, smiles, gestures, and touches toward other infants (Vandell et al., 1980). In the second year, infants begin to engage in simple patterns of interactions involving cooperative games and conflict episodes (Hay, 1985). By 18 months to 2 years of age, children begin to modify their behaviors in response to partners (Hay, 1985). Even 18-month-olds are more likely to separate from their mothers and go to a different room to play with toys in the presence of an unfamiliar peer (Gunnar, Senior, & Hartup, 1984), and 25-month-olds in Soviet child care centers were less likely to cry in the presence of a stranger when a peer was present (Ispa, 1981). Infants as young as 6 months establish patterns of interaction that are distinct to particular relationships (Hay, Nash, & Pederson, 1981), and toddlers form distinct relationships with patterns of contingent interactions that are distinct from what would be predicted by either partner's interactions with other peers (Ross & Lollis, 1989). Together these experiences promote the development of a concept of the other and of the relationship (Hay, 1985).

Theoretical Perspectives on Early Childhood Peer Relations

Theorists have viewed peer relations in early childhood as limited by children's cognitive development (Selman, 1980). In part this claim may arise from an overreliance on young children's verbal reports instead of observations of their ongoing interactions with well-acquainted peers (Howes, 1996). Sullivan (1953) characterized toddlers and preschoolers as being strongly motivated by the need to have peers to play with them (Buhrmester, 1996). On the basis of children's interview responses, young children expect friends to play with them and to stay close by (Bigelow, 1977), and they view friendships in terms of momentary interactions determined by proximity and liking to do similar activities (Selman, 1980). Naturalistic observations of preschoolers at play yield a much richer picture of early relationship processes, all of which serve the central goal of this developmental period—coordinated play (Gottman, 1986).

Preschool Play

Toddler play features much gleeful repetition, often having to do with gross motor activities, and can be characterized as "more bodily joyful than toyful" (Lokken, 2000, p. 174). From observations of children from infancy through preschool, Howes and Matheson (1992) developed a peer play scale that describes the sequence in which children develop increasingly sophisticated forms of play: parallel play, parallel aware play, simple social play, complementary and reciprocal play, cooperative social pretend play, and complex social pretend play. More than half of children younger than 2 engage in pretend play, and pretend play episodes involve an average of 3.1 strategies (behaviors such as imitation, joining, and verbal recruitment; Howes, 1985).

Naturalistic observations of older preschoolers getting to know one another and playing together with friends suggest that coordinated play requires establishing common ground and successful escalation of affect and activities and is supported by amity, skills in information exchange, conflict management, and the willingness to engage in early forms of self-exploration (Gottman, 1986). Preschoolers who "hit it off" develop a "me-too climate of acceptance," in which they can engage in shared fantasy play, often around themes of growth or transformation or related to working out fears (Gottman, 1986, p. 195). In the following example, Billy (age 4) and Jonathan (age 3) are playing a fantasy game in a tub of water.

B: And I hate sharks. But I love to eat sardines.

J: I love to eat shark.

B: Yeah, but they're so big!

J: But we can cut their tail.

B: But what happens if we cut them to two?

J: It would bite us, it would swim, and we would have to run. Run very fast, run to our homes.

B: Yeah, but ummm ...

J: By the trees. Mr. Shark bited the door down and we would have to run way in the forest.

B: Yeah, but ... if he bited all the trees down.

J: And then we would have to shoot him. Yeah, and the shark is poison.

B: But pink is. Red is, yellow is.

B: Yeah, but people are too. What happened if the shark ate us?

J: We would have to bite him, on his tongue.

B: Yeah, what happened if we bite him so far that we made his tongue metal?

J: Yeah.

B: Then he couldn't have breaked out of metal.

J: He can eat metal open. Sharks are so strong they can even bite metal.

B: Yes.

J: How about concrete? Concrete could make it? (Gottman, 1986, p. 161)

In this exchange, we see the two boys confront the fear of sharks and enjoy negotiating the details of the best way to manage shark attacks with glee and excitement, some discord, but also a fairly high rate of agreement. This level of amity may have been facilitated by the fact that these two children were of the same gender.

From the start of the toddler period, children prefer playing mostly with peers of the same gender, especially in child care or preschool settings (Serbin, Moller, Gulko, Powlishta, & Colburne, 1994). Observational studies show that 50–60% of 3- to 6-year-old children's interactions are with peers of the same gender, that 70–80% of the variance in play partner choice is predicted by gender, and that frequency of same-gender play is consistent across time (Martin & Fabes, 2001). Children may develop strong preferences for same-gender peers because boys and girls develop different play styles due to gender differences in physiological and emotional arousal (Fabes, 1994), because girls withdraw from boys because of boys' more rough style of play (Maccoby, 1998), because preschool children are more reinforced by peers and teachers for same-gender behavior (Fagot, 1994), or because they have developed solid concepts of gender that lead them to prefer children who are "like me" (Martin, 1994).

The widespread observation of gender segregation is so striking that experts have suggested that girls and boys grow up in separate gender cultures in same-gender groups in which they socialize each other in different interaction styles and different expectations for relationships (Maccoby, 1998). In support of this theory, observations of preschool peers show that for boys, playing with other boys predicts increases in forceful, rough-and-tumble style of play, whereas for girls, playing more with girls predicts decreases in activity level and aggression and playing more near adults (Martin & Fabes, 2001). As powerful as gender segregation seems to be in child-care or group contexts, it is important to remember that other-gender interactions do occur. Even in preschool classrooms, children move in and out of same- and other-gender interactions to some degree (Martin, Fabes, Hanish, & Hollenstein, 2005). Still, the vast majority of interactions between peers in group settings are with same-gender peers, which likely has a great impact on children's activities and the friendships they form in preschool. (See Leaper & Bigler, Chapter 12, this volume.)

Individual Differences and Early Childhood Peer Relations

Whereas research on young children's peer interactions has often focused on descriptions of the behavior of typically developing children, research on older children's peer relationships has examined the functions that peer relations might serve and origins and outcomes of individual differences (Howes, 1996). This section reviews research on preschool children's friendships, social networks, and status in the larger peer group and considers the relations between each level of the peer system and children's psychological adjustment.

Friendships

Children seem to show strong preferences for playing with particular peers long before they can talk about friendship (Howes, 1996). In one observational study of friendships in child-care classrooms for infants, toddlers, and preschoolers, friendship was defined as mutual preference for interaction, complementary and reciprocal play, and shared positive affect (Howes, 1983). When friendship is defined in behavioral terms, even infants and toddlers are observed to have friends, and 75% of preschoolers had a friend (Howes, 1983). Toddler friendships persist across time (Howes, 1988, 1996). Preschool friendships may serve some of the same functions as older children's friendships: companionship, intimacy, and mutual affection (Howes, 1996). Being able to form reciprocal friendships in preschool relates to children's affective social competence and skills in sending emotional signals and in regulating emotional experiences (Dunsmore, Noguchi, Garner, Casey, & Bhullar, 2008). Even preschoolers have "best friends"; having a best friend in a sample of 3- to 7-year-olds was related to being female and to being high on prosocial behavior (Sebanc, Kearns, Hernandez, & Galvin, 2007).

Many friendships in preschool settings are between children of the same gender; other-gender friendships decrease as children move into preschool (Howes & Phillipsen, 1992). Although other-gender friendships may "go underground" at school, they may continue in neighborhoods and other settings (Gottman, 1986). Young children who establish other-gender friendships before the preschool period continue to interact with these other-gender friends at school; "for children enrolled in child care as infants, early friendships were more powerful than gender segregation" (Howes & Phillipsen, 1992, p. 241).

In addition to offering opportunities for companionship and, at times, high glee, early friendships are important opportunities for young children to learn and practice important skills. Over the course of a school year, pairs of young children in stable friendships showed the greatest increases in complexity of play (Howes, 1983), and children who engaged in more sophisticated play were more prosocial and less aggressive (Howes & Phillipsen, 1992). Preschoolers are more likely to respond to another child's crying if that child is a friend (Howes & Farver, 1987). Conflicts between friends are frequent but are more likely to be resolved by compromise and mutual disengagement and more likely to be followed by continued interaction than conflicts between nonfriends (Hartup, Laursen, Stewart, & Eastenson, 1988). Being able to form friendships in early childhood relates to positive adjustment for children (Hay, Payne, & Chadwick, 2004).

Peer Groups and Social Networks

Even as early as preschool, group interactions may shape individuals in important ways (Boivin, Vitaro, & Poulin, 2005). As children move through the preschool years, boys' social networks seem to increase in size, whereas girls' social networks become smaller (Benenson, 1994). Although most research on peer group homophily (the tendency of children to interact with others similar to them) and peer group influence has been conducted with older samples, the few studies available suggest that even young children tend to spend time with children who are similar to them on important characteristics. For example, preschool children interact with peers who are similar to them on aggression, whether aggression (defined as name-calling, teasing, and physical harm; Farver, 1996) is measured by observations by teacher ratings (Snyder, Horsch, & Childs, 1997), or by peer nominations (van den Oord, Rispens, Goudena, & Vermande, 2000).

Remember also that boys interact primarily with groups of other boys and that boys' same-gender play predicts increases in aggression and activity level, whereas girls play mostly with other girls and same-gender play predicts decreases in aggression and activity level (Martin & Fabes, 2001). The consequences of playing with same-gender peers may be especially profound for children who are at risk because of temperamental arousability. For highly arousable girls, play with same-gender peers predicted a decrease in behavior problems, whereas for highly arousable boys, play with same-gender peers predicted an increase in behavior problems (Fabes, Shepard, Guthrie, & Martin, 1997).

Peer Status

In addition to having friends and playing in groups, preschoolers also develop status within their classroom-based peer groups. Status for preschoolers typically refers to the extent to which they have more or less positive social standing with peers. Pre-schoolers' social status has often been measured by sociometric interviews in which young children are asked to look at pictures of classmates and identify other children whom they do and do not like (Asher, Singleton, Tinsley, & Hymel, 1979).

Sociometric studies reveal that some preschool children experience more glee and acceptance with peers than others. Preschoolers who are well liked by peers are more prosocial (Ladd, Price, & Hart, 1988). Children disliked by preschool classmates score higher on physical and relational aggression (Crick, Casas, & Mosher, 1997). However, even in preschool, the relation between aggressive behavior and peer rejection may be complex and may depend on other characteristics of the child. Preschoolers characterized as bistrategic—high on aggression but also high on prosocial ways of controlling resources—were actually preferred by peers and were viewed by teachers as more morally mature (Hawley, 2003). The relation between social withdrawal and peer status may be similarly complex (see Rubin, Coplan, & Bowker, 2009, for a review). Quiet, solitary, constructive play by preschoolers has been viewed as harmless (Rubin, 1982) and perhaps a behavioral indicator of social uninterest (Rubin & Asendorph, 1993) but also as a possible tactic for young children coping with social wariness (Henderson, Marshall, Fox, & Rubin, 2004). Social withdrawal may be associated with being disliked by peers, especially for boys (Coplan, Gavinski-Molina, Lagace-Seguin, & Wichmann, 2001).

For young children, forming successful relationships with peers is an incredible accomplishment that requires considerable skill in joint attention, causal understanding, imitation, language, and emotion regulation (Hay et al., 2004). Although many young children are able to form relationships and interact smoothly in groups, some are not, and even preschool peer relations may well have a "darker side" (Hartup, 2003). Peer difficulties in preschool can be remarkably stable (Howes & Phillipsen, 1998). Peer problems in early childhood likely result from and predict poor psychological adjustment (Hay et al., 2004). However, in seeking to understand the causes and consequences of peer problems, it is important to remember that for many young children, early peer interactions are sources of fun, companionship, and even high glee. In the words of Hay et al. (2004), "it is time for psychologists and psychiatrists to turn their attention once again to the serious study of fun" (p. 100).

PEER RELATIONS IN THE SCHOOL–AGE PERIOD: EXPANSION AND FOCUS

Although the school-age years are often portrayed as a period of latency (i.e., not much more than a quiet time between the rapid changes of childhood and those of adolescence), it is actually a period of much change and consolidation. It is a time of increased activity with peers and an expansion of the peer group beyond contexts that are close to the family or selected by it. During early childhood, peer interactions make up about 10% of a child's social time; by age 10 this amount is more than 30% (Rubin, Bukowski & Parker, 2006). Beyond the increase in time spent together, the features of peer interaction change, and peer relationships take on a heightened significance. These changes are both quantitative and qualitative as the purpose of many peer-based experiences change. Moreover, the effects of peer relations change. In this section we show how peer interaction changes during the school-age period, and then we discuss how relationships change.

What Do Peers Do with Each Other?

During the school-age period the level of negative behavior between peers does not differ much from early childhood, but the forms of negative behavior do (see Dodge, Coie, & Lynam 2006). Indirect forms of aggression, such as verbal and relational aggression (insults, derogation, threats, gossip), increase as direct physical aggression decreases. The purpose of aggression changes also. Compared with preschoolers, the aggressive behavior of 6- to 12-year-olds is less frequently aimed at object possession and more likely to be directed at others. The frequency of "mock" or "nonliteral" aggression, such as rough-and-tumble play, appears to fit a U-shaped developmental function (Pellegrini, 2002). Although this form of play makes up 5% of preschoolers' social activities, it makes up 10–17% during the early school-age years and then decreases to about 5% by age 12 (Humphreys & Smith, 1984).

Increases in positive forms of interaction during the school-age years tend to be small (Eisenberg, Fabes & Spinrad, 2006). Modest increases can be seen in heightened levels of generosity, helpfulness, or cooperation that children engage in with their peers. In parallel, by middle childhood, increases are found in the frequencies of games with or without formal rules. In these latter activities, children's interactions with peers are highly coordinated, involving both positive (cooperative, prosocial) and negative (competitive, agonistic) forms of behavior (Rubin, Fein, & Vandenberg, 1983).

One form of interaction that becomes much more frequent during the school-age years is conversation (Zarbatany, Hartmann, & Rankin, 1990). Peers like to talk to each other, whether in a face-to-face context, over the old-fashioned telephone, or via more modern communication devices such as mobile phone and Internet-based systems. One component of this more frequent amount of conversation is an increased frequency of gossip (Eder & Enke, 1991; Kuttler, Parker, & La Greca, 2002; Parker & Gottman, 1989). Gossip provides a means of sharing information about group dynamics and activities and of establishing positions in the group hierarchy. There is evidence that most school-age children recognize talk about a nonpresent peer as a form of gossip, and they recognize that it can be inaccurate and injurious (Kuttler et al. 2002).

The dark side of peer interaction in the school-age period is manifested in bullying and victimization (Espelage, Bosworth, & Simon, 2000; Olweus, 1993). Bullying refers to repeated acts of either verbal or physical aggression aimed at particular peers (i.e., victims). Bullying makes up a substantial portion of the aggression that occurs in the peer group (Olweus, 1993). The aspect of bullying that distinguishes it from other forms of aggressive behavior is its specific aim at a particular peer. Bullying is directed at certain peers, and victims compose up to 10% of the school population (NICHD Early Child Care Research Network, 2001; Olweus, 1984; Perry, Kusel, & Perry, 1988). Bullies are known to have particular tendencies, including relatively weak control over their aggressive impulses and a tolerance for aggressive behavior (Olweus, 1993). They are known to use force without emotion and to do so outside of the ongoing flow of interaction among peers (Perry, Perry, & Kennedy, 1992).

It is known that victims tend to show particular characteristics also. Two well-known "risk" indicators for being victimized are elevated scores on measures of aggression and of social withdrawal (Olweus, 1978; Perry et al., 1988). Nearly every study that has assessed the association between aggressiveness and victimization has revealed a positive correlation (e.g., Camodeca, Goossens, Terwogt, & Schuengel, 2002; Hanish & Guerra, 2000, 2004; Hodges et al., 1997; Snyder et al., 2003). The findings regarding aggression appear to be culturally invariant.

Victimization has been shown to be positively associated with aggression in samples drawn from North American, Southern Asian (Khatri & Kupersmidt, 2003) and East Asian (Schwartz, Farver, Chang, & Lee-Shin, 2002; Xu, Farver, Schwartz, & Chang, 2003) samples.

It is important to recognize that victimization can occur at multiple levels of social complexity (Graham & Juvonen, 2000; Schafer, Werner, & Crick, 2002), including the dyad (Crick & Nelson, 2002) and the group (Bukowski & Sippola, 2001). Two sets of ideas explain why aggression and social withdrawal are associated with victimization. One idea distinguishes between the processes related to withdrawal and aggression (Olweus, 1993). It claims that withdrawn children are victimized because they are easy and nonthreatening prey and are unlikely to retaliate when treated badly, whereas aggressive children are victimized because their irritating behavior provokes negative reactions from others. Another view uses a single model to explain victimization (Bukowski & Sippola, 2001). It claims that children victimize peers who do not promote the basic group goals of coherence, harmony, and evolution. According to this view, aggressive and withdrawn children do not promote these positive aspects of group functioning, and as a result they are victimized.

Peer Relations as Affective Experiences

Aside from the behaviors that make up the peer interactions, the peer experiences of school-age children have an affective component that involves liking and disliking. As in early childhood, the patterns of peer interactions during the school-age years are largely determined by these forms of affect. Children are known to spend vastly more time with the peers they like than with those they dislike (Bukowski & Hoza, 1989). A repercussion of this pattern is that children who are more disliked than liked (i.e., those who are rejected; Newcomb & Bukowski, 1983) have many fewer opportunities for interaction than children who are more liked than disliked (i.e., are "popular"). The characteristics of rejected children in the school-age period are roughly the same as those of disliked preschool children. They show high rates of reactive and poorly regulated aggression and/or tend to be withdrawn or uninvolved with others. Neither of these factors is likely to promote a child's attractiveness to the other children who make up the peer group.

Relationships

One of the most pronounced changes in relationships during middle childhood concerns children's understanding of what defines *friendship*. Although even young children recognize that friendship consists of reciprocity and shared affect, it is not until the school-age years that friendship is perceived to have an enduring quality that transcends the present moment. Whereas young school-age children (7-year-olds) see friendship in terms of rewards and costs (i.e., friends are individuals who are interesting or rewarding to be with), older children (10-year-olds) see the importance of shared social values and perceptions for friendship (Bigelow, 1977). They recognize that friendship involves loyalty and dedication. These older children also possess more intimate knowledge of their friends (Berndt, 2002) and think about their friends in a more differentiated and integrated manner (Peevers & Secord, 1973).

The experience of friendship changes during the school-age years also. At this time friendship choices become more stable, and they are more likely to be reciprocated in middle childhood than at earlier ages, perhaps as a result of the more positive and abstract qualities that are ascribed to friendship at this time (Berndt & Hoyle, 1985). Friendship also takes on important functions and forms of significance in regard to affect and experience. During this time friendless children are more likely to be lonely and victimized by peers (Boulton, Trueman, Chau, Whitehand, & Amatya, 1999; Brendgen, Vitaro, & Bukowski, 2000; Kochenderfer & Ladd, 1996). Moreover friendship can protect at risk children from being victimized (Hodges et al. 1997), and it can reduce the negative effects associated with victimization (Hodges, Boivin, Vitaro, & Bukowski, 1999). Friendship has been shown to also reduce the negative impact of being from a nonoptimal (e.g., either rigid, chaotic, or enmeshed) family (Gauze, Bukowski, Aquan-Assee, & Sippola, 1996). These findings confirm Sullivan's (1953) claim that friendship can be a security system for older school-age children.

These effects are likely due to the features that emerge in friendship during the school-age years. Newcomb and Bagwell (1995) have shown that children are more likely to behave in positive ways with friends than with nonfriends or to ascribe positive characteristics to their interactions with friends. They reported specifically that in their interactions with friends, relative to interactions with nonfriends, children show more affective reciprocity and emotional intensity and enhanced levels of emotional understanding. Although there are no differences between friends and nonfriends in the frequency of conflict, there is ample evidence that friends and nonfriends resolve conflicts in different ways. Friends tend to resolve conflicts in a way that will preserve or promote the continuity of their relationship (Laursen, Finkelstein, & Townsend Betts, 2001). It is likely that this style of conflict resolution is associated with the conception at this age that friendship is an enduring experience.

In addition to the friendships they form, children can also form *antipathies*, or relationships based on mutual disliking (Hartup & Abecassis, 2002). Overall, the frequency of antipathies is rare, but it is known to vary across classrooms (Abecassis, Hartup, Haselager, Scholte, & Van Lieshout, 2002). In some classrooms as many as 58% of the children participate in an enemy relationship. Just as friendship is distinct from being liked, antipathies are distinct from being disliked (Hodges & Card, 2003). The effects of antipathy are not clear (Abecassis, 2003). Children who are in antipathy relationships show higher levels of depressed affect than those shown by other children, and the presence of a mutual antipathy appears to exacerbate the effect of other negative experiences. Perhaps a benefit of being in an antipathy relationship is the opportunity to gain a clearer sense of the cost of being disliked and perhaps also a clearer sense of self as children recognize the features that they like and dislike in others.

ADOLESCENCE: THE INTENSIFICATION OF FRIENDSHIP

The central feature in the development of peer relationships during adolescence is the increased significance of friendship as teens establish autonomy from parents. Adolescents in the United States spend more time interacting with friends than with parents (Csikszentmihalyi & Larson, 1984), and they report relying as much on friends as on parents for closeness and support during middle and late adolescence (Furman & Buhrmester, 1992). Friendships also become closely linked to adolescents' psychological well-being and development.

We have seen already that the nature of friendship undergoes important changes across preschool and middle childhood, although some features remain constant. During adolescence, friends become collaborators in a quest to understand themselves and validate one another. Sullivan argued that adolescent friendships satisfy needs of *intimacy* and *consensual validation* (Buhrmester & Furman, 1986). Adolescents describe friendship more abstractly in terms of interpersonal dynamics, such as loyalty/commitment ("we trust each other, he is always there for me") and intimacy ("I can tell her anything, she understands me"), and in terms of compatible personalities ("we like the same things"). Although these changes in conceptions of friendship partially reflect cognitive growth from concrete to formal operational thought (Selman, 1981), they also parallel changes in interactions that researchers have directly observed. Gottman (1986) observed that adolescent friendships (ages 13–17) are even more talk-focused, with *joint self-exploration* being the focal concern. Confidential self-disclosure and gossip are used not only to build solidarity but also to explore and evaluate similarities and differences between oneself and peers, as well as how one stacks up against abstract ideals. Numerous questionnaire studies confirm that there are significant increases in intimate self-disclosure between friends across middle and late adolescence (see Buhrmester & Prager, 1995; McNelles & Connolly, 1999).

Scholars also find interesting differences between boys' and girls' friendships (Rose & Rudolph, 2006) in middle adolescence. Girls more often than boys define friendship in terms of intimacy and supportiveness, especially during middle adolescence (McDougall & Hymel, 2007). Observational studies find that girls spend more time talking to each other than boys do (Moller, Hymel, & Rubin, 1992), whereas questionnaire studies consistently find that female friends report greater intimate self-disclosure than male friends do during middle and late adolescence but not necessarily during childhood (Buhrmester & Prager, 1995; Rose & Rudolph, 2006). Recently, however, scholars have begun to question the two cultures/worlds theory (Thorne, 1993; Underwood, 2004; Zarbatany, McDougall, & Hymel, 2000). They are concerned that the two cultures/worlds framework exaggerates stereotypic differences between boys' and girls' friendships, when, in fact, the core features of their friendships are highly similar: for both sexes, mutual liking and spending enjoyable time together are the most important features of friendship. Moreover, the magnitude of sex differences is generally not large compared with variability within sexes, suggesting that there is more overlap than differences in the nature of boys' and girls' friendships. Thus it is misleading to suggest that all boys' friendships are fundamentally different from all girls' friendships.

Starting in late elementary school, adolescents report an increasing number of other-gender friendships (Connolly, Furman, & Konarski, 2000). Whereas Sullivan (1953) suggested that these relationships might be motivated by emergent sexual needs, more recent studies find that adolescents report that other-gender friendships are not necessarily sexually motivated and that they have many of the same features of same-gender friendships (McDougall & Hymel, 2007). Although other-gender friendships start in childhood as less close and intense than same-gender friendships, they become increasingly intimate across middle and late adolescence (Sharabany, Gershoni, & Hofman, 1981). Dexter Dunphy's (1963) ethnographic research on Australian youths paints a slightly different picture of the function of other-gender friendships. He suggested that there is a progression across adolescence, starting with networks of same-gender friends he called cliques, moving to an intermingling of boys' and girls' cliques in larger crowds, which culminates during late adolescence by moving to smaller, mixed-gender cliques that often include romantic couples. Dunphy, therefore, contended that mixed-gender friendships scaffold the development of romantic relationships by providing a social context in which males and females can meet and start dating. Recent studies support this view (Connolly et al., 2000) and further suggest that cross-gender friendships help prepare adolescents for romantic relationships by fostering better understanding of gender differences in interests, interaction styles, and expectations for romance (Connolly, Craig, Goldberg, & Pepler, 2004).

Determinants of Friendship in Adolescence

Researchers have sought to understand the factors that determine the number of friends that youths have, the qualities of their friendships, and the characteristics of the peers with whom they are friends. A sizable minority of adolescents—perhaps 25%—have no peers who claim them as friends. Why? Because a basic requirement of friendship is that peers like each other, many of the factors that determine peer-group acceptance and rejection also play a role in friendship formation. Similar to the correlates of peer-group status, chronic friendlessness is associated with aggressiveness and lack of prosocial skills (Wojslawowicz Bowker, Rubin, Burgess, Booth-Laforce, & Rose-Krasnor, 2006) and especially with social timidity, sensitivity, and withdrawal (Parker & Seal, 1996).

So what factors determine whether any two adolescents become friends? At a fundamental level, peers must have contact with each other in order for friendships to get started, a condition scholars refer to as *propinquity*. Youths become friends with peers whom they are frequently around in a classroom, neighborhood, sports team, or religious groups. Most often the structure of youths' social contacts is stratified and segregated demographically, so that a youth's pool of potential friends is likely to include peers who are similar to him or her in terms of race, ethnicity, education, and economic characteristics (Kandel, 1978; Savin-Williams & Berndt, 1990).

Beyond the similarity created by societal structures, youths are also motivated to make friends with peers based on *similarity* in terms of their interests, abilities, preferences, and social reputations (Aboud & Mendelson, 1998). Scholars use the term *homophily* to denote the tendency of "birds of a feather" to "flock together" in term of friends having similar characteristics (Kandel, 1978; Prinstein & Dodge, 2008). Research has shown that friends, compared with nonfriends, tend to be more similar to each other in terms of a wide range of characteristics, including academic performance (Epstein, 1983), levels of aggression and deviance (Cairns, Cairns, Neckerman, Gest, & Gariépy, 1988; Dishion, Patterson, Stoolmiller, & Skinner, 1991), substance use (Kandel, 1978; Urberg, Chen, & Shyu, 1991), and even levels of psychological problems, such as depressive symptoms and shyness (Haselager, Hartup, van Lieshout, & Riksen-Walraven, 1998; Hogue & Steinberg, 1995).

Although similarity can bring peers to the doorstep of a potential friendship, adolescents must exercise certain *social skills* in order to build and maintain a mutually satisfying friendship (Buhrmester, 1996; Samter, 2003). Although considerable research has identified the skills associated with being accepted or rejected by childhood peer groups, researchers have only begun to identify the skills that are unique to dyadic friendship during adolescence. Scholars generally assume that social skills can be thought of in terms of the interpersonal tasks involved in building and maintaining satisfying relationships (Asher & McDonald, 2009; Dodge, McClaskey, & Feldman, 1985) and that the skills unique to friendship likely change with age in concert with the changing expectations and core interactional processes of friendships. For example, one study found that skills in initiating relationships, appropriate self-disclosure, and providing emotional support become more strongly associated with friendship quality during adolescence as compared with childhood (Buhrmester, 1990). Youths who are more skilled at handling these friendship tasks are able to make higher quality friendships as they move from elementary school to junior high school, which is known to be a difficult social transition (Aikins, Bierman, & Parker, 2005).

In addition to whether youths are good or bad at certain skills, qualitative differences in behavioral and attachment-security *styles* also affect the qualities of friendships. Aggressive adolescents' friendships are more conflicted, less supportive, and of shorter length than typical youths' friendships (Coie et al., 1999; Grotpeter & Crick, 1996), whereas shy/withdrawn youths' friendships are less fun and less supportive (Rubin, Wojslawowicz, Rose-Krasnor, Booth-Laforce, & Burgess, 2006). Adolescents with secure attachment styles report that their friendships are of higher quality than those with insecure styles (Furman, 2001; Zimmermann, 2004). Also, friends who both have secure styles show better connection with each other and similar conversational patterns when they are observed interacting than do pairs in which one or both of the friends are insecure (Weimer, Kerns, & Oldenburg, 2004).

Friends' Influence

Early in this chapter, we discussed Sullivan's (1953) well-known view that peers, and especially close friends, make sizable contributions to the course of children's development. In general terms, he suggested that with age, peers increasingly affect how youths think and feel about themselves on a daily basis. Sullivan also argued that there are interpersonal challenges uniquely faced in friendship that are not present in relationships with parents, and thus friendships are the formative context in which youths normatively gain certain social knowledge and skills. For example, it is not until close friends open up and confide to one another their private insecurities and dreams that they must assume the role of intimate support providers. Finally, Sullivan thought that experiences with friends can, at times, undo lessons learned in earlier parent–child relationships. For example, a close, supportive friendship can show adolescents that people can be trustworthy and caring even if their parents were unavailable or rejecting.

There is little doubt that experiences with friends affect youths' emotional lives. By gathering detailed information about adolescents' activities and moods over the course of a week, Larson and Richards (1991) found that highs and lows of moods directly paralleled the events that transpired with peers. On the positive side, the emotional high point of a week for many teenagers was Saturday night, when they went out with friends. At the same time, being home alone on the weekend can be a lonely low point of the week.

Numerous other studies have found that more enduring aspects of youths' emotional well-being and behavioral adjustment are correlated with the number and quality of youths' friendships. For example, loneliness is especially tied to peer relations. Youths who are friendless or have low-quality friendships have been found to be chronically lonely (Parker & Asher, 1993; Renshaw & Brown, 1993) and have lower self-esteem (Berndt, 2002; Keefe & Berndt, 1996). Friendships that are characterized by conflict and unbalanced affections are associated with depressive symptoms, especially among girls (Prinstein, Borelli, Cheah, Simon, & Aikins, 2005; Selfhout, Branje, & Meeus, 2009). Youths whose friendships involve more arguments and hostility also tend to evidence more disruptive and aggressive behavioral problems in school (Dunn, 2004; Poulin, Dishion, & Haas, 1999).

We should not, however, automatically interpret such correlations as indicating that friendship experiences causally shape adolescent characteristics. As all introductory psychology students are taught, correlation does not necessarily mean causation. In some cases, a correlation may reflect a reverse direction of cause. For example, the similarity between friends may be a selection effect rather than a consequence of the sustained interaction between the friends (Vitaro, Boivin, & Bukowski, 2009). In other cases, correlations reflect reciprocal or transactional causes across time. For instance, levels of adolescents' interpersonal skills are correlated with having friendships that are more supportive in quality (Buhrmester, 1990). Here prosocial skills likely alternate between being a cause and a consequence of friendship: Skills enhance a child's effectiveness in forming friendships, and, in turn, reinforcing experiences within friendships improve the adolescent's level of competence (Barry & Wentzel, 2006). In still other cases, a correlation may be due to a "third variable" that causally shapes both friendship experiences and youths' dispositions. For example, because children who are not accepted by the peer group are also less likely to have high-quality friendships, correlations between friendship and child outcomes may be caused by low group status rather than friendship per se (Vitaro et al., 2009).

There is clear-cut evidence that friendships affect subsequent adolescent outcomes, but *the effects can be positive or negative*. On the positive side, having friends can help adolescents avoid potential adjustment problems. For example, longitudinal studies have found that having at least one close friend during early and middle adolescence reduced the risk of depressive symptoms during young adulthood, even after accounting for levels of depressive symptoms during adolescence (Bagwell, Schmidt, Newcomb, & Bukowski, 2001; Pelkonen, Marttunen, & Aro, 2003). Friendships also seem capable of "undoing" negative effects resulting from unfortunate experiences in the family. Sullivan (1953) argued that positive friendships in preadolescence can offset the damage created by abusive or neglecting parents. Recent evidence seems to confirm this. Many studies show that cold and conflicted relationships with parents put children at increased risk for subsequent externalizing and internalizing problems outside the family. However, among children from at-risk families, those that have high-quality friendships end up developing fewer problems than those who are friendless or have low-quality friendships (Bukowski, Motzoi, & Meyer, 2009). Thus friendship can "buffer" children against problems that they were otherwise expected to develop.

The evidence is less clear, however, as to whether positive features of friendship contribute directly to more positive adolescent outcomes. For instance, Sullivan's (1953) theory argues that intimate friendships during early adolescence validate a child's sense of personal worth, and thus researchers have expected to find that friendship intimacy is associated with the growth of an increasingly positive sense of self-esteem (Berndt, 2004). Carefully conducted longitudinal studies, however, have found limited support for this view. Although higher levels of self-esteem are correlated with better quality friendships at any point in time, there is little indication that friendship quality predicts *changes* (either for the better or worse) in self-esteem across time (Keefe & Berndt, 1996). This is a good example of the axiom that correlation does not necessarily equal causation. Researchers remain puzzled by the fact that friendship quality is correlated with, but does not apparently cause, changes in self-esteem (Bukowski et al., 2009).

There is much stronger evidence that friendships precipitate changes in problematic outcomes (Vitaro et al., 2009). It is important to note, however, that it is the *characteristics of the friend*, in terms of his or her attitudes and interaction styles, that seem to be most responsible for changing the course of a youth's development. Numerous studies have documented that adolescents whose friends are disruptive and aggressive become increasingly disruptive and aggressive themselves across time (Dishion et al., 1991). This causal effect was experimentally demonstrated by a study intended to prevent at-risk adolescent boys from developing more serious conduct problems. Participants were randomly assigned to several types of treatment, one of which involved learning self-regulation skills in small groups that included other boys who were also at risk (because they, too, showed early signs of disruptive behavior). This small-group treatment backfired. Rather than preventing conduct problems, 1 and 3 years later teachers reported that the boys who had been in these groups had more, rather than fewer, conduct problems compared with the control group (Dishion, McCord, & Poulin, 1999). Why? A careful analysis of video recordings of the small-group treatment sessions revealed that the boys had engaged in what the researchers called "deviance training"; that is, the boys (who were already inclined to be disruptive) reinforced each other through laughter and nonverbal feedback whenever someone in the group broke the rules or used inappropriate language (Dishion, Spracklen, Andrews, & Patterson, 1996). Indeed, there may even be benefits in at-risk youths not having friends, at least in terms of preventing conduct problems, because they often befriend other deviant peers. For example, disruptive and rejected children have been found to become less delinquent and aggressive if they did not have friends (Vitaro, Brendgen, & Wanner, 2005; Kupersmidt, Burchinal, & Patterson, 1995).

But not all friends have "bad" characteristics, so having friends with "good" characteristics should also, at least in theory, "rub off" on adolescents. Indeed, there is some, although more limited, evidence of such positive effects of friends. For instance, one study found that teenagers' school involvement and grades improved over the course of a school year if they started out with friends who were high versus low achievers (Berndt & Keefe, 1995). Thus the effect of friends' characteristics can be either positive or negative, depending on the nature of the friends' characteristics (Berndt, 1999).

There are also cases in which friends simultaneously have both positive and negative effects. Take the interesting case of "corumination" among friends. Corumination occurs when friends disclose their problems to one another, but then repeatedly go over and over the details of the problem and their feelings about them (Rose, 2002). This is most common among girls' friendships. The positive effect of such discussions is that it makes the friends feel greater intimacy and support in their relationships. The negative effect of corumination is that it results in girls perseverating on their problems, which has the effect of increasing their anxiety and depression across time (Rose, Carlson, & Waller, 2007). Similarly, although having a deviant friend may increase a youth's own level of deviance, the friendship also provides needed companionship, acceptance, and validation that can prevent feelings of loneliness and isolation (Brendgen et al., 2000). In both these examples, the benefit of friendship is that it satisfies social needs, whereas the cost comes from picking up maladaptive habits from the friend.

SUMMARY/WHAT'S NEXT?

This chapter shows that research on the features and effects of peer relations has a rich and enduring place in the social developmental literature. Theory about peer relations refers to a rich set of constructs and processes that occur at multiple levels of social complexity and that involve several forms of action, including behavior, cognition, affect, and the "self." In spite of this rich history, however, many basic questions about peer relations remain unanswered or even unasked. Some of these issues are related to process, whereas others have to do with variations in effects across individuals and with "where" peer relations happen. Two process-oriented issues appear to be especially pressing. One concerns the presumption that experiences with peers are antecedent to "outcomes" such as depressed affect and measures of the self. There is a need to consider whether affect and the self can be "determinants" of peer experiences, as well as being outcomes. Work on these questions would be especially useful if it were framed according to processes of attraction, as well as processes of influence. A second process-oriented question concerns the circumstances in which peer influence is most likely to happen. Research on peer influence has typically considered whether it happens and how individual change is influenced by friend characteristics. There is also a need to know whether some individuals (e.g., those with low self-esteem or who come from a minority background) are more likely to be influenced by peers than are others.

"Where" questions deserve attention, also. Peer relations occur in particular places. There is evidence already that the "place" where peer relations occur matters (Chen, French, & Schneider, 2006). Nevertheless, little is known about how the specific characteristics of particular places affect what peer experiences consist of and how they affect development. Most studies so far have been satisfied with identifying place effects and have not tried to explain the reasons that account for them. This type of research is needed. The "places" that need to be studied are diverse—classrooms, neighborhoods, urban versus rural locations, socioeconomic circumstances, and, of course, the electronic village of cyberspace. Knowing how peer relations function in each of these contexts will add to our understanding of what peer experience is and how it influences well-being and adjustment.

ACKNOWLEDGMENTS

Work on this chapter was supported by grants from the Social Sciences and Humanities Research Council of Canada and from the National Institutes of Health (R01 MH 63076, K02 MH73616, and R01 HD60995). The authors are grateful to Dominique Paiement for her careful bibliographic assistance and to Gillian Labrie.

SUGGESTED READINGS

Buhrmester, D., & Furman, W. (1987). The development of companionship and intimacy, *Child Development, 58,* 1101–1113.

Bukowski, W. M., & Adams, R. (2005). Peer relations and psychopathology: Markers, mechanisms, mediators, moderators, and meanings. *Journal of Clinical Child and Adolescent Psychology, 34,* 3–10.

Roseth, C. J., Johnson, D. W., & Johnson, R. T. (2008). Promoting early adolescents' achievement

and peer relationships: The effects of cooperative, competitive, and individualistic goal structures. *Psychological Bulletin, 134,* 223–246.

Rubin, K. H., Bukowski, W. M., & Parker, J. G. (2006). Peer interactions, relationships, and groups.
In W. Damon (Series Ed.) & N. Eisenberg (Vol. Ed.), *Handbook of child psychology* (6th ed.,
pp. 571–645). New York: Wiley.

Underwood, M. K., Galen, B. R., & Paquette, J. A. (2001). Top ten challenges for understanding
gender and aggression in children: Why can't we all just get along? *Social Development, 10,*
248–266.

REFERENCES

Abecassis, M. (2003). I hate you just the way you are: Exploring the formation, maintenance and
need for enemies. In E. Hodges & N. Card (Eds.), *Enemies and the darker side of peer relation*
(pp. 5–22). New York: Jossey-Bass.

Abecassis, M., Hartup, W. W., Haselager, G. J. T., Scholte, R. H. J., & Van Lieshout, C. F. M.
(2002). Mutual antipathies and their significance in middle childhood and adolescence *Child
Development, 73,* 1543–1556.

Aboud, F., & Mendelson, M. (1998). Determinants of friendship selection and quality: Developmental
perspectives. In W. M. Bukowski, A. F. Newcomb, & W. W. Hartup (Eds.), *The company they keep:
Friendship in children and adolescence* (pp. 87–112). New York: Cambridge University Press.

Aikins, J., Bierman, K., & Parker, J. (2005). Navigating the transition to junior high school: The
influence of pre-transition friendship and self-system characteristics. *Social Development,
14*(1), 42–60.

Asher, S., & McDonald, K. (2009). The behavioral basis of acceptance, rejection, and perceived
popularity. In K. H. Rubin, W. M. Bukowski, & B. Laursen (Eds.), *Handbook of peer interactions, relationships, and groups* (pp. 232–248). New York: Guilford Press.

Asher, S. R., Singleton, L. C., Tinsley, B. R., & Hymel, S. (1979). A reliable sociometric measure for
preschool children. *Developmental Psychology, 15,* 443–444.

Azmitia, M., & Montgomery, R. (1993). Friendship, transactive dialogues, and the development of
scientific reasoning. *Social Development, 2,* 202–221.

Bagwell, C., Newcomb, A. F., & Bukowski, W. M. (1998). Preadolescent friendship and rejection as
predictors of adult adjustment. *Child Development, 69,* 140–153.

Bagwell, C., Schmidt, M., Newcomb, A., & Bukowski, W. (2001). Friendship and peer rejection as
predictors of adult adjustment. In D. W. Nagle & C. A. Erdley (Eds.), *The role of friendship in
psychological adjustment* (pp. 25–49). San Francisco: Jossey-Bass.

Barry, C., & Wentzel, K. (2006). Friend influence on prosocial behavior: The role of motivational
factors and friendship characteristics. *Developmental Psychology, 42*(1), 153–163.

Benenson, J. F. (1994). Ages four to six years: Changes in the structures of play networks of girls and
boys. *Merrill–Palmer Quarterly, 40,* 478–487.

Berndt, T. (1999). Friends' influence on students' adjustment to school. *Educational Psychologist,
34*(1), 15–28.

Berndt, T. (2002). Friendship quality and social development. *Current Directions in Psychological
Science, 11,* 7–10.

Berndt, T. (2004). Children's friendships: Shifts over a half-century in perspectives on their development and their effects. *Merrill–Palmer Quarterly, 50*(3), 206–223.

Berndt, T. J., & Hoyle, S. G. (1985). Stability and change in childhood and adolescent friendships.
Development Psychology,21, 1007–1015.

Berndt, T., & Keefe, K. (1995). Friends' influence on adolescents' adjustment to school. *Child Development, 66*(5), 1312–1329.

Bigelow, B. J. (1977). Children's friendship expectations: A cognitive-developmental study. *Child
Development, 48,* 246–253.

Boivin, M., Vitaro, F., & Poulin, F. (2005). Peer relationships and the development of aggressive
behavior in early childhood. In R. E. Tremblay, W. W. Hartup, & J. Archer (Eds.), *Developmental origins of aggression* (pp. 376–397). New York: Guilford Press.

Boulton, M. J., Trueman, M., Chau, C., Whitehand, C., & Amatya, K. (1999). Concurrent and longitudinal links between friendships and peer victimization: Implications for befriending interventions. *Journal of Adolescence, 22*, 461–466.

Brendgen, M., Vitaro, F., & Bukowski, W. (2000). Deviant friends and early adolescents' emotional and behavioral adjustment. *Journal of Research on Adolescence, 10*(2), 173–189.

Buhrmester, D. (1990). Friendship, interpersonal competence, and adjustment in preadolescence and adolescence. *Child Development, 61*, 1101–1111.

Buhrmester, D. (1996). Need fulfillment, interpersonal competence, and the developmental contexts of early adolescent friendships. In W. M. Bukowski, A. F. Newcomb, & W. W. Hartup (Eds.), *The company they keep: Friendship in childhood and adolescence* (pp. 158–185). New York: Cambridge University Press.

Buhrmester, D., & Furman, W. (1986). The changing functions of friendship in childhood: A neo-Sullivanian perspective. In V. J. Derlega & B. A. Winstead (Eds.), *Friendship and social interaction* (pp. 43–62). New York: Springer-Verlag.

Buhrmester, D., & Prager, K. (1995). Patterns and functions of self-disclosure during childhood and adolescence. In K. J. Rotenberg (Ed.), *Disclosure processes in children and adolescents* (pp. 10–56). New York: Cambridge University Press.

Bukowski, W. M., Brendgen, M., & Vitaro, F. (2007). Peers and socialization: Effects on externalizing and internalizing problems. In J. E. Grusec & P. D. Hastings (Eds.), *Handbook of socialization: Theory and research* (pp. 355–381). New York: Guilford Press.

Bukowski, W., & Hoza, B. (1989). Popularity and friendship: Issues in theory, measurement, and outcome. In T. J. Berndt & G. W. Ladd (Eds.), *Peer relationships in child development* (pp. 15–45). Oxford, UK: Wiley.

Bukowski, W., Motzoi, C., & Meyer, F. (2009). Friendship as process, function, and outcome. In K. H. Rubin, W. M. Bukowski, & B. Laursen (Eds.), *Handbook of peer interactions, relationships, and groups* (pp. 217–231). New York: Guilford Press.

Bukowski, W. M., & Sippola, L. K. (2001). Groups, individuals, and victimization: A view of the peer system. In J. Juvonen & S. Graham (Eds.), *Peer harassment in school: The plight of the vulnerable and victimized* (pp. 355–377). New York: Guilford Press.

Cairns, R., Cairns, B., Neckerman, H., Gest, S., & Gariépy, J. (1988). Social networks and aggressive behavior: Peer support or peer rejection? *Developmental Psychology, 24*(6), 815–823.

Camodeca, M., Goossens, F. A., Terwogt, M. M., & Schuengel, C. (2002). Bullying and victimization among school-age children: Stability and links to proactive and reactive aggression. *Social Development, 11*, 332–345.

Chen, X., French, D., & Schneider, B. (2006). *Peer relationships in cultural context.* New York: Cambridge University Press.

Coie, J., Cillessen, A., Dodge, K., Hubbard, J., Schwartz, D., Lemerise, E., et al. (1999). It takes two to fight: A test of relational factors and a method for assessing aggressive dyads. *Developmental Psychology, 35*(5), 1179–1188.

Coie, J. D., Lochman, J. E., Terry, R., & Hyman, C. (1992). Predicting early adolescent disorder from childhood aggression and peer rejection. *Journal of Consulting and Clinical Psychology, 60*, 783–792.

Connolly, J., Craig, W., Goldberg, A., & Pepler, D. (2004). Mixed-gender groups, dating, and romantic relationships in early adolescence. *Journal of Research on Adolescence, 14*(2), 185–207.

Connolly, J., Furman, W., & Konarski, R. (2000). The role of peers in the emergence of heterosexual romantic relationships in adolescence. *Child Development, 71*(5), 1395–1408.

Coplan, R. J., Gavinski-Molina, M. H., Lagace-Seguin, D., & Wichmann, C. (2001). When girls versus boys play alone: Gender differences in the associates of nonsocial play in kindergarten. *Developmental Psychology, 37*, 464–474.

Crick, N. R., Casas, J. F., & Mosher, M. (1997). Relational and overt aggression in preschool. *Developmental Psychology, 33*(4), 589–600.

Crick, N. R., & Nelson, D. A. (2002). Relational and physical victimization within friendship: Nobody told me there'd be friends like these. *Journal of Abnormal Child Psychology, 30*, 599–607.

Csikszentmihalyi, M., & Larson, R. (1984). *Being adolescent: Conflict and growth in the teenage years.* New York: Basic Books.

Davies, B. (1982). *Life in the classroom and playground.* Oxford, UK: Routledge.

DeRosier, M., Kupersmidt, J., & Patterson, C. (1994). Children's academic and behavioral adjustment as a function of the chronicity and proximity of peer rejection. *Child Development, 65,* 1799–1813.

Dishion, T., McCord, J., & Poulin, F. (1999). When interventions harm: Peer groups and problem behavior. *American Psychologist, 54*(9), 755–764.

Dishion, T., Patterson, G., Stoolmiller, M., & Skinner, M. (1991). Family, school, and behavioral antecedents to early adolescent involvement with antisocial peers. *Developmental Psychology, 27*(1), 172–180.

Dishion, T., Spracklen, K., Andrews, D., & Patterson, G. (1996). Deviancy training in male adolescent friendships. *Behavior Therapy, 27*(3), 373–390.

Dodge, K. A., Coie, J. D., & Lynam, D. (2006). Aggression and antisocial behavior in youth. In W. Damon (Series Ed.) & N. Eisenberg (Vol. Ed.), *Handbook of child psychology: Vol. 3. Social, emotional, and personality development* (6th ed., pp. 719–788). New York: Wiley.

Dodge, K., McClaskey, C., & Feldman, E. (1985). Situational approach to the assessment of social competence in children. *Journal of Consulting and Clinical Psychology, 53*(3), 344–353.

Doise, W., & Mugny, G. (1984). *The social development of the intellect.* Oxford, UK: Pergamon Press.

Dunn, J. (2004). *Children's friendships: The beginning of intimacy.* Malden, MA: Blackwell.

Dunphy, D. (1963). The social structure of urban adolescent peer groups. *Sociometry, 26,* 230–246.

Dunsmore, J. C., Noguchi, R. J. P., Garner, P. W., Casey, E. C., & Bhullar, N. (2008). Gender specific linkages of affective social competence with peer relations in preschool children. *Early Education and Development, 19,* 211–237.

Eder, D., & Enke, J. L. (1991). The structure of gossip: Opportunities and constraints on collective expression among adolescents. *American Sociological Review, 56,* 494–508.

Eisenberg, N., Fabes, R. A., & Spinrad, T. L. (2006). Prosocial development. In W. Damon (Ed.), *Handbook of child psychology: Vol. 3. Social, emotional, and personality development.* (5th ed.). New York: Wiley.

Epstein, J. (1983). The influence of friends on achievement and affective outcomes. In J. Epstein & N. Karweit (Eds.), *Friends in school* (pp. 177–200). New York: Academic Press.

Espelage, D. L., Bosworth, K., & Simon, T. R. (2000). Examining the social context of bullying behaviors in early adolescence. *Journal of Counseling and Development, 78,* 326–333.

Fabes, R. A. (1994). Physiological, emotional, and behavioral correlates of gender segregation. In C. Leaper (Ed.), *Childhood gender segregation: Causes and consequences* (pp. 19–34). San Francisco: Jossey-Bass.

Fabes, R. A., Shepard, S. A., Guthrie, I. K., & Martin, C. L. (1997). Roles of temperamental arousal and gender-segregated play in young children's social adjustment. *Developmental Psychology, 33,* 693–702.

Fagot, B. I. (1994). Peer relations and the development of competence in boys and girls. In C. Leaper (Ed.), *Childhood gender segregation: Causes and consequences* (pp. 53–66). San Francisco: Jossey-Bass.

Farver, J. M. (1996). Aggressive behavior in preschoolers' social networks: Do birds of a feather flock together? *Early Childhood Research Quarterly, 11,* 333–350.

Furman, W. (2001). Working models of friendships. *Journal of Social and Personal Relationships, 18*(5), 583–602.

Furman, W., & Buhrmester, D. (1985). Children's perceptions of the personal relationships in their social networks. *Developmental Psychology, 21,* 1016–1022.

Furman, W., & Buhrmester, D. (1992). Age and sex differences in perceptions of networks of personal relationships. *Child Development, 63,* 103–115.

Gauze, C., Bukowski, W. M., Aquan-Assee, J., & Sippola, L. K. (1996). Interactions between family environment and friendship and associations with self-perceived well-being during early adolescence. *Child Development, 67,* 2201–2216.

Golbeck, S. L. (1998). Peer collaboration and children's representation of the horizontal surface of liquid. *Journal of Applied Developmental Psychology, 19,* 571–592.

Gottman, J. (1986). The world of coordinated play: Same- and cross-sex friendship in young children. In J. M. Gottman & J. G. Parker (Eds.), *Conversations with friends: Speculations on affective development* (pp. 139–190). New York: Cambridge University Press.

Graham, S., & Juvonen, J. (2000). *Peer harassment in school*. New York: Guilford Press.

Grosbras, M.-H., Jansen, M., Leonard, G., McIntosh, A., Osswald, K., Poulsen, C., et al. (2007). Neural mechanisms of resistance to peer influence in early adolescence. *Journal of Neuroscience, 27*, 8040–8045.

Grotpeter, J., & Crick, N. (1996). Relational aggression, overt aggression, and friendship. *Child Development, 67*(5), 2328–2338.

Gunnar, M., Senior, K., & Hartup, W. W. (1984). Peer presence and the exploratory behavior of 18- and 30-month-old children. *Child Development, 35*, 1103–1109.

Hanish, L. D., & Guerra, N. G. (2000). Predictors of peer victimization among urban youth. *Social Development, 9*, 521–543.

Hanish, L. D., & Guerra, N. G. (2004). Aggressive victims, passive victims, and bullies: Developmental continuity or developmental change? *Merrill–Palmer Quarterly, 50*, 17–38.

Hartup, W. W. (1996). The company they keep: Friendships and their developmental significance. *Child Development, 67*, 1–13.

Hartup, W. W. (2003). Toward understanding mutual antipathies in childhood and adolescence. *New Directions in Child and Adolescent Development, 102*, 111–123.

Hartup, W. W., & Abecassis, M. (2002). Friends and enemies: Their significance in child development. In P. Smith & C. Hart (Eds.), *Handbook of social development* (pp. 285–307). London: Blackwell.

Hartup, W. W., & Coates, B. (1967). Imitation of a peer as a function of reinforcement from the peer group and rewardingness of the model. *Child Development, 38*, 1003–1016.

Hartup, W. W., Glazer, J. A., & Charlesworth, R. (1967). Peer reinforcement and sociometric status. *Child Development, 38*, 1017–1024.

Hartup, W. W., Laursen, B., Stewart, M. I., & Eastenson, A. (1988). Conflict and the friendship relations of young children. *Child Development, 59*, 1590–1600.

Hartup, W. W., & Stevens, N. (1997). Friendships and adaptation in the life course. *Psychological Bulletin, 121*, 355–370.

Haselager, G., Hartup, W., van Lieshout, C., & Riksen-Walraven, J. (1998). Similarities between friends and nonfriends in middle childhood. *Child Development, 69*(4), 1198–1208.

Hawley, P. H. (2003). Strategies of control, aggression, and morality in preschools: An evolutionary perspective. *Journal of Experimental Child Psychology, 85*, 213–235.

Hay, D. F. (1985). Learning to form relationships in infancy: Parallel attainments with parents and peers. *Developmental Review, 5*, 122–161.

Hay, D. F., Payne, A., & Chadwick, A. (2004). Peer relations in childhood. *Journal of Child Psychology and Psychiatry, 45*, 84–108.

Henderson, H. A., Marshall, P. J., Fox, N. A., & Rubin, K. H. (2004). Psychophysiological and behavioral evidence for varying forms and functions of nonsocial behaviors in preschoolers. *Child Development, 75*, 251–263.

Hinde, R. A. (1987). *Individuals, relationships and culture*. Cambridge: Cambridge University Press.

Hodges, E., Boivin, M., Vitaro, F., & Bukowski, W. (1999). The power of friendship: Protection against an escalating cycle of peer victimization. *Developmental Psychology, 35*(1), 94–101.

Hodges, E. V. E., & Card, N. A. (Eds.). (2003). *Enemies and the darker side of peer relations*. San Francisco: Jossey-Bass.

Hodges, E. V. E., Malone, M. J., & Perry, D. G. (1997). Individual risk and social risk as interacting determinants of victimization in the peer group. *Developmental Psychology, 33*, 1032–1039.

Hogue, A., & Steinberg, L. (1995). Homophily of internalized distress in adolescent peer groups. *Developmental Psychology, 31*(6), 897–906.

Howes, C. (1983). Patterns of friendship. *Child Development, 54*, 1041–1053.

Howes, C. (1985). Sharing fantasy: Social pretend play in toddlers. *Child Development, 56*, 1253–1258.

Howes, C. (1988). Peer interaction of young children. *Monographs of the Society for Research in Child Development* (Serial No. 217).

Howes, C. (1996). The earliest friendships. In W. M. Bukowski, A. F. Newcomb, & W. W. Hartup (Eds.), *The company they keep: Friendship in childhood and adolescence* (pp. 66–86). New York: Cambridge University Press.

Howes, C., & Farver, J. (1987). Toddler's responses to the distress of their peers. *Journal of Applied Developmental Psychology, 8,* 441–452.

Howes, C., & Lee, L. (2006). Peer relations in young children. In L. Balter & C. S. Tamis-LeMonda (Eds.), *Child psychology: A handbook of contemporary issues* (pp. 135–151). New York: Psychology Press.

Howes, C., & Matheson, C. C. (1992). Sequences in the development of competent play with peers: Social and social pretend play. *Child Development, 28,* 961–974.

Howes, C., & Phillipsen, L. (1992). Gender and friendship: Relationships within peer groups of young children. *Social Development, 1,* 230–242.

Howes, C., & Phillipsen, L. (1998). Continuity in children's relations with peers. *Social Development, 7,* 340–349.

Humphreys, A., & Smith, P. K. (1987). Rough-and-tumble play, friendship, and dominance in school children: Evidence of continuity and change with age. *Child Development, 58,* 201–212.

Ispa, J. (1981). Peer support among Soviet day care toddlers. *International Journal of Behavioral Development, 4,* 255–269.

Kandel, D. B. (1978). Homophily, selection, and socialization in adolescent friendships. *American Journal of Sociology, 84*(2), 427–436.

Keefe, K., & Berndt, T. (1996). Relations of friendship quality to self-esteem in early adolescence. *Journal of Early Adolescence, 16*(1), 110–129.

Khatri, P., & Kupersmidt, J. B. (2003). Aggression, peer victimization, and social relationships among Indian youth. *International Journal of Behavioral Development, 27*(1), 87–95.

Kochenderfer, B., & Ladd, G. (1996). Peer victimization: Cause or consequence of school maladjustment? *Child Development, 67,* 1305–1317.

Kraatz-Keily, M., Bates, J. E., Dodge, K. A., & Pettit, G. S. (2000). A cross-domain analysis: Externalizing and internalizing behaviors during 8 years of childhood. *Journal of Abnormal Child Psychology, 28,* 161–179.

Kupersmidt, J., Burchinal, M., & Patterson, C. (1995). Developmental patterns of childhood peer relations as predictors of externalizing behavior problems. *Development and Psychopathology, 7*(4), 825–843.

Kupersmidt, J. B., & Coie, J. D. (1990). Preadolescent peer status, aggression, and school adjustment as predictors of externalizing problems in adolescence. *Child Development, 61,* 1350–1362.

Kuttler, A. F., Parker, J. G., & La Greca, A. M. (2002). Developmental and gender differences in preadolescents' judgments of the veracity of gossip. *Merrill–Palmer Quarterly, 48,* 105–132.

Ladd, G. W., Price, J. M., & Hart, C. H. (1988). Predicting preschoolers' peer status from their playground behaviors. *Child Development, 59,* 986–992.

Larson, R., & Richards, M. (1991). Daily companionship in late childhood and early adolescence: Changing developmental contexts. *Child Development, 62*(2), 284–300.

Laursen, B. (1996). Closeness and conflict in adolescent peer relationships: Interdependence with friends and romantic partners. In W. M. Bukowski, A. F. Newcomb, & W. W. Hartup (Eds.), *The company they keep: Friendship in childhood and adolescence* (pp. 186–210). New York: Cambridge University Press.

Laursen, B., Bukowski, W., Aunola, K., & Nurmi, J. (2007). Friendship moderates prospective associations between social isolation and adjustment problems in young children. *Child Development, 78*(4), 1395–1404.

Laursen, B., Finkelstein, B., & Townsend Betts, N. (2001). A developmental meta-analysis of peer conflict resolution. *Developmental Review, 21*(4), 423–449.

Lokken, G. (2000). Tracing the social style of toddler peers. *Scandinavian Journal of Educational Research, 44,* 163–176.

Maccoby, E. E. (1998). *The two sexes: Growing up apart, coming together.* Cambridge, MA: Harvard University Press.

Martin, C. L. (1994). Cognitive influences on the development and maintenance of gender segregation. In C. Leaper (Ed.), *Childhood gender segregation: Causes and consequences* (pp. 35–52). San Francisco: Jossey-Bass.

Martin, C. L., & Fabes, R. A. (2001). The stability and consequences of young children's same-sex peer interactions. *Developmental Psychology, 37,* 431–446.

Martin, C. L, Fabes, R. A., Hanish, L. D., & Hollenstein, T. (2005). Social dynamics in the preschool. *Developmental Review, 25,* 299–327.

McDougall, P., & Hymel, S. (2007). Same-gender versus cross-gender friendship conceptions: Similar or different? *Merrill-Palmer Quarterly, 53*(3), 347–380.

McNelles, L., & Connolly, J. (1999). Intimacy between adolescent friends: Age and gender differences in intimate affect and intimate behaviors. *Journal of Research on Adolescence, 9*(2), 143–159.

Mead, G. H. (1934). *Mind, self, and society* (Charles W. Morris, Ed.). Chicago: University of Chicago Press.

Moller, L., Hymel, S., & Rubin, K. (1992). Sex typing in play and popularity in middle childhood. *Sex Roles, 26*(7), 331–353.

Monroe, W. S. (1898). Social consciousness in children. *Psychological Review, 5,* 68–70.

Newcomb, A., & Bagwell, C. (1995). Children's friendship relations: A meta-analytic review. *Psychological Bulletin, 117*(2), 306–347.

Newcomb, A. F., & Bukowski, W. M. (1983). Social impact and social preference as determinants of children's peer group status. *Developmental Psychology, 19,* 856–867.

NICHD Early Child Care Research Network. (2001). Child care and children's peer interaction at 24 and 36 months: The NICHD Study of Early Child Care. *Child Development, 72,* 1478–1500.

Ollendick, T. H., Weist, M. D., Borden, M. G., & Greene, R. W. (1992). Sociometric status and academic, behavioral, and psychological adjustment: A five-year longitudinal study. *Journal of Consulting and Clinical Psychology, 60,* 80–87.

Olweus, D. (1978). *Aggression in the schools: Bullies and whipping boys.* Oxford, UK: Hemisphere.

Olweus, D. (1984). Stability in aggressive and withdrawn, inhibited behavior patterns. In R. M. Kaplan, V. J. Konecni, & R. W. Novaco (Eds.), *Aggression in children and youth* (pp. 104–136). The Hague: Nijhoff.

Olweus, D. (1993). *Bullying at school: What we know and what we can do.* Oxford, UK: Blackwell.

Parker, J., & Asher, S. (1993). Friendship and friendship quality in middle childhood: Links with peer group acceptance and feelings of loneliness and social dissatisfaction. *Developmental Psychology, 29*(4), 611–621.

Parker, J. G., & Asher, S. R. (1987). Peer relations and later personal adjustment: Are low-accepted children at risk? *Psychological Bulletin, 102,* 357–389.

Parker, J. G., & Gottman, J. M. (1989). Social and emotional development in a relational context: Friendship interaction from early childhood to adolescence. In T. J. Berndt & G. W. Ladd (Eds.), *Peer relations in child development* (pp. 95–131). New York: Wiley.

Parker, J., & Seal, J. (1996). Forming, losing, renewing, and replacing friendships: Applying temporal parameters to the assessment of children's friendship experiences. *Child Development, 67*(5), 2248–2268.

Peevers, B. H., & Secord, P. F. (1973). Developmental changes in attribution of descriptive concepts to persons. *Journal of Personality and Social Psychology, 27,* 120–128.

Pelkonen, M., Marttunen, M., & Aro, H. (2003). Risk for depression: A six-year follow-up of Finnish adolescents. *Journal of Affective Disorders, 77,* 41–51.

Pellegrini, A. D. (2002). Rough-and-tumble play from childhood through adolescence: Development and possible functions. In P. K. Smith & C. H. Hart (Eds.), *Blackwell handbook of childhood social development* (pp. 438–453). London: Blackwell.

Perry, D. G., Kusel, S. J., & Perry, L. C. (1988). Victims of peer aggression. *Developmental Psychology, 24,* 807–814.

Perry, D. G., Perry, L., & Kennedy, E. (1992). Conflict and the development of antisocial behavior. In C. Shantz & W. W. Hartup (Eds.), *Conflict in child and adolescent development.* New York: Cambridge University Press.

Piaget, J. (1932). *The moral judgment of the child.* Glencoe, IL: Free Press.

Poulin, F., Dishion, T., & Haas, E. (1999). The peer influence paradox: Friendship quality and deviancy training within male adolescent friendships. *Merrill–Palmer Quarterly, 45*(1), 42–61.

Prinstein, M. J., Borelli, J. L., Cheah, C. S. L., Simon, V. A., & Aikins, J. W. (2005). Adolescent girls' interpersonal vulnerability to depressive symptoms: A longitudinal examination of reassurance-seeking and peer relationships. *Journal of Abnormal Psychology, 114,* 676–688.

Prinstein, M., & Dodge, K. (2008). Current issues in peer influence research. In M. J. Prinstein & K. A. Dodge (Eds.), *Understanding peer influence in children and adolescents* (pp. 3–13). New York: Guilford Press.

Renshaw, P., & Brown, P. (1993). Loneliness in middle childhood: Concurrent and longitudinal predictors. *Child Development, 64*(4), 1271–1284.

Rose, A. (2002). Co-rumination in the friendships of girls and boys. *Child Development, 73*(6), 1830–1843.

Rose, A., Carlson, W., & Waller, E. (2007). Prospective associations of co-rumination with friendship and emotional adjustment: Considering the socioemotional trade-offs of co-rumination. *Developmental Psychology, 43*(4), 1019–1031.

Rose, A., & Rudolph, K. (2006). A review of sex differences in peer relationship processes: Potential trade-offs for the emotional and behavioral development of girls and boys. *Psychological Bulletin, 132*(1), 98–131.

Ross, H. S., & Lollis, S. P. (1989). A social relations analysis of toddler peer relationships. *Child Development, 60,* 1082–1091.

Rubin, K. H. (1982). Nonsocial play in preschoolers: Necessarily evil? *Child Development, 533,* 651–657.

Rubin, K. H., & Asendorph, J. (Eds.). (1993). *Social withdrawal, inhibition, and shyness in childhood*. Hillsdale, NJ: Erlbaum.

Rubin, K. H., Bukowski, W. M., & Parker, J. G. (2006). Peer interactions, relationships and groups. In W. Damon (Series Ed.) & N. Eisenberg (Vol. Ed.), *Handbook of child psychology* (6th ed., pp. 571–645). New York: Wiley.

Rubin, K. H., Coplan, R. J., & Bowker, J. C. (2009). Social withdrawal in childhood. *Annual Review of Psychology, 60,* 141–171.

Rubin, K. H., Fein, G., & Vandenberg, B. (1983). Play. In P. H. Munsen (Series Ed.) & E. M. Hetherington (Vol. Ed.), *Handbook of child psychology: Vol. 4. Socialization, personality and social development* (pp. 693–774). New York: Wiley.

Rubin, K., Wojslawowicz, J., Rose-Krasnor, L., Booth-LaForce, C., & Burgess, K. (2006). The best friendships of shy/withdrawn children: Prevalence, stability, and relationship quality. *Journal of Abnormal Child Psychology, 34*(2), 143–157.

Samter, W. (2003). Friendship interaction skills across the life-span. In J. O. Greene & B. R. Burleson (Eds.), *Handbook of communication and social interaction skills* (pp. 637–684). Mahwah, NJ: Erlbaum.

Sandstrom, M. J., Cillessen, A. H. N., & Eisenhower, A. (2003). Children's appraisal of peer rejection experiences: Impact on social and emotional adjustment. *Social Development, 12,* 530–550.

Savin-Williams, R., & Berndt, T. (1990). Friendship and peer relations. In S. Feldman & G. Elliott (Eds.), *At the threshold: The developing adolescent* (pp. 277–307). Cambridge, MA: Harvard University Press.

Schafer, M., Werner, N. E., & Crick, N. R. (2002). A comparison of two approaches to the study of negative peer treatment: General victimization and bully/victim problems among German schoolchildren. *British Journal of Developmental Psychology, 20,* 281–306.

Schwartz, D., Farver, J. M., Chang, L., & Lee-Shin, Y. (2002). Victimization in South Korean children's peer groups. *Journal of Abnormal Child Psychology, 30,* 113–125.

Sebanc, A. M., Kearns, K. T., Hernandez, M. D., & Galvin, K. B. (2007). Predicting having a best friend in young children: Individual characteristics and friendship features. *Journal of Genetic Psychology, 168,* 81–95.

Selfhout, M. H. W., Branje, S. J. T., & Meeus, W. H. J. (2009). Developmental trajectories of perceived friendship intimacy, constructive problem solving, and depression from early to late adolescence. *Journal of Abnormal Child Psychology, 37*(2), 251–264.

Selman, R. L. (1980). *The growth of interpersonal understanding: Developmental and clinical analyses*. New York: Academic Press.

Selman, R. (1981). The child as a friendship philosopher. In S. R. Asher & J. M. Gottman (Eds.), *The development of children's friendships* (pp. 242–272). New York: Cambridge University Press.

Serbin, L. A., Moller, L. C., Gulko, J., Powlishta, K. K., & Colburne, K. A. (1994). The emergence of gender segregation in toddler playgroups. In C. Leaper (Ed.), *Childhood gender segregation: Causes and consequences* (pp. 7–18). San Francisco: Jossey-Bass.

Sharabany, R., Gershoni, R., & Hofman, J. (1981). Girlfriend, boyfriend: Age and sex differences in intimate friendship. *Developmental Psychology, 17*(6), 800–808.

Snyder, J., Brooker, M., Patrick, M. R., Snyder, A., Schrepferman, L., & Stoolmiller, M. (2003). Observed peer victimization during early elementary school: Continuity, growth, and relation to risk for child antisocial and depressive behavior. *Child Development, 74*, 1881–1898.

Snyder, J., Horsch, E., & Childs, J. (1997). Peer relationships of young children: Affiliative choices and the shaping of aggressive behavior. *Journal of Clinical Child Psychology, 26*, 145–156.

Sullivan, H. S. (1953). *The interpersonal theory of psychiatry.* New York: Norton.

Thorne, B. (1993). *Gender play: Girls and boys in school.* New Brunswick, NJ: Rutgers University Press.

Underwood, M. K. (2004). Gender and peer relations: Are the two gender cultures really all that different? In J. B. Kupersmidt & K. A. Dodge (Eds.), *Children's peer relations: From developmental science to intervention to policy* (pp. 21–36). Washington, DC: American Psychological Association.

Urberg, K., Cheng, C., & Shyu, S. (1991). Grade changes in peer influence on adolescent cigarette smoking: A comparison of two measures. *Addictive Behaviors, 16*(1), 21–28.

van den Oord, E. J. C. G., Rispens, J., Goudena, P. P., & Vermande, M. (2000). Some developmental implications of structural aspects of preschoolers' relations with classmates. *Journal of Applied Developmental Psychology, 21*, 616–639.

Vandell, D. L., Wilson, K. S., & Buchanan, N. R. (1980). Peer interaction in the first year of life: An examination of its structure, content, and sensitivity to toys. *Child Development, 51*, 481–488.

Vitaro, F., Boivin, M., & Bukowski, W. M. (2009). The role of friendship in child and adolescent psychosocial development. In K. Rubin, W. M. Bukowski, & B. Laursen (Eds.), *Handbook of peer interactions, relationships, and groups* (pp. 568–588). New York: Guilford Press.

Vitaro, F., Brendgen, M., & Wanner, B. (2005). Patterns of affiliation with delinquent friends during late childhood and early adolescence: Correlates and consequences. *Social Development, 14*(1), 82–108.

Vygotsky, L. S. (1978). *Mind in society: The development of higher psychological processes.* Cambridge, MA: Harvard University Press.

Weimer, B., Kerns, K., & Oldenburg, C. (2004). Adolescents' interactions with a best friend: Associations with attachment style. *Journal of Experimental Child Psychology, 88*(1), 102–120.

Wojslawowicz Bowker, J., Rubin, K., Burgess, K., Booth-LaForce, C., & Rose-Krasnor, L. (2006). Behavioral characteristics associated with stable and fluid best friendship patterns in middle childhood. *Merrill–Palmer Quarterly, 52*(4), 671–693.

Xu, Y., Farver, J., Schwartz, D., & Chang, L. (2003). Identifying aggressive victims in Chinese children's peer groups. *International Journal of Behavioral Development, 27*(3), 243–252.

Zarbatany, L., Hartmann, D. P., & Rankin, D. B. (1990). The psychological functions of preadolescent peer activities. *Child Development, 61*, 1067–1980.

Zarbatany, L., McDougall, P., & Hymel, S. (2000). Gender-differentiated experience in the peer culture: Links to intimacy in preadolescence. *Social Development, 9*(1), 62–79.

Zimmermann, P. (2004). Attachment representations and characteristics of friendship relations during adolescence. *Journal of Experimental Child Psychology, 88*(1), 83–101.

8

Romantic Relationships in Adolescence

Jennifer Connolly
Caroline McIsaac

One need only spend a few minutes in a high school, at the mall, or listening to popular music to be reminded that romantic relationships are a defining feature of the adolescent years. Yet romantic involvements are a totally new social enterprise for youths, challenging them to express their emerging feelings of passion, love, and sexuality in the more familiar world of peer experiences. Even though the vast majority of adolescent dating relationships do not endure past the high school years, these initial experiences are important first steps in the journey toward establishing a loving romantic partnership in adulthood. Tracking this progression provides important insights into how the core components of love—passion, intimacy, and commitment—develop in young people, regardless of their genders, sexual orientations, or cultural backgrounds.

We begin the chapter by defining adolescent romantic relationships and outlining the prevalence and patterns of dating experiences. Next we discuss the major theories that guide current developmental research on romantic relationships. This provides us with a useful foundation to introduce the notion that romantic development unfolds in a series of stages. We then turn our discussion to three key questions: How do adolescents describe their romantic relationships in terms of such qualities as intimacy, sexuality, and conflict? How do adolescents' romantic relationships fit into the connections that they have already established with family and friends? and finally, How do romantic relationships affect adolescents' mental health? We conclude by highlighting some burning issues and providing suggestions for future research.

SETTING THE STAGE:
DEFINING ROMANTIC RELATIONSHIPS

What is a romantic relationship? This is a complex question to answer, because romantic relationships can differ considerably from person to person and also within one relationship over the duration of the couple's time together. Broadly speaking, romantic relationships entail three component features—passion, intimacy, and commitment—that may be present in varying degrees in different relationships (Sternberg, 1986). Passionate attraction and sexual desire are the sine qua non of romantic relationships. Without these elements, the relationship is just a friendship, not one of romantic status (Connolly, Craig, Goldberg, & Pepler, 1999). Equally important, romantic relationships are mutually acknowledged close connections between two people. These intimate bonds are facilitated by companionable interactions, as well as the sharing of personal thoughts and feelings. When these intimate and passionate moments are sustained, romantic commitments emerge such that a couple makes a deliberate and mutual decision to be exclusive and to remain together into the future. There is good evidence that the elements of passion, intimacy, and commitment are present in all romantic relationships regardless of the age of the partners, even though enduring commitments are not as characteristic of young adolescents' relationships and emerge later in the developmental life stage (Connolly et al., 1999).

Moving from abstract ideas about the core features of love to the concrete world of teen experiences, it is necessary for researchers to define what is meant by a "romantic relationship" in a way that young people can recognize and respond to. Researchers most often use terms such as *boyfriend* or *girlfriend* to solicit information from an adolescent about whether or not he or she is part of a romantic couple. Yet some researchers have questioned the value of using these formal terms because the language that teens use when speaking to each other is often quite informal and part of the slang terminology of the popular culture. Although slang may help researchers connect with particular groups of adolescents, there is a risk to this practice, because teen language is often highly changeable and localized to specific communities and peer groups; what works in one setting, at one time, may not work in another. Therefore, there is a general consensus that asking teens about their "boyfriends and girlfriends" is the most practical approach, even though these terms may not be the ones used by youths themselves (Furman & Hand, 2006).

An important definitional issue is distinguishing between dating activities and romantic relationships. Although youths who are in a formalized romantic relationship with one another may go to the movies or to a party, these activities can also be done by adolescents who do not have boyfriends or girlfriends and may, in fact, be an important context for them to spend time with other teens to whom they are romantically attracted. In this chapter, we refer to romantic relationship status when the focus is on the connection between the two partners and to dating or romantic activities when the focus is on the content of their interactions and the couple status is less certain.

PREVALENCE AND COMMON FEATURES

Objective information on the frequency with which adolescents have romantic relationships has been greatly aided by data gathered as part of the ADD–Health Longitudinal Survey, which is a large-scale, nationally representative study of youth in the United States. Utilizing the question "Have you had a special romantic relationship with anyone in the last 18 months?" the ADD–Health data show that romantic relationships are common during adolescence and that the frequency of youths reporting them steadily increases with age (Carver, Joyner, & Udry, 2003). Approximately 25% of 12-year-olds, 50% of 15-year-olds, and 70% of 18-year-olds report having a romantic relationship, either currently or within the preceding 18 months. Most teenagers report more than one romantic relationship during their adolescent years; in fact, four is the modal number of romantic relationships experienced (Connolly & McIsaac, 2009).

Because many youths have several relationships in their adolescent years, a key point is to consider the length of these relationships. Not surprisingly, adolescent romantic relationships are time-limited (Carver et al., 2003). Youths under the age of 14 years typically report relationships of a few weeks' duration and rarely report durations of longer than 4 months (Carver et al., 2003; Connolly & Johnson, 1996; Feiring, 1996; Shulman & Scharf, 2000). Romantic relationships become more enduring with age. Sixteen-year-olds typically report that their relationships last for 6 months, and 18-year-olds typically report that their relationships endure for 1 year or more. These duration changes are likely due to an increasing capacity to maintain intimate relationships (Connolly & Johnson, 1996). Duration differences may also relate to the difficulty of tracking the "official" beginnings of relationships (Carver et al., 2003). This is especially challenging for younger adolescents, as the shorter durations they report may stem from the fact that they have fuzzy boundaries between romantic and nonromantic relationships.

Relationship Breakups

In light of the short duration of relationships, one might suspect that breakups would be both common and frequent during adolescence. Indeed, there is evidence that relationship terminations occur frequently across the full spectrum of the adolescent years (Connolly & McIsaac, 2009). Paralleling the age-related increase in romantic relationships, the number of youths reporting a breakup also increases with age. Whereas less than half of 11- to 13-year-olds report the experience of a breakup, almost all 20- to 25-year olds do so. At the same time, the likelihood of reporting a recent breakup (i.e., within the last 12 months) decreases with age. The less frequently occurring romantic dissolutions of older adolescents likely reflects their increased skill in sustaining relationships, as well as selecting compatible romantic partners with whom the relationship is more likely to endure. Adolescents give many reasons for the ending of a romantic relationship. Generally, though, relationships end when adolescents no longer feel that the partner provided the "emotional spark" of a passionate relationship and that they no longer had fun together, shared intimate feelings, or even felt sexually attracted to each other (Connolly & McIsaac, 2009).

Boys versus Girls

Although boys and girls generally report comparable frequencies of romantic relationships, there are some notable differences between them. For instance, in early adolescence, more boys than girls report having a current romantic relationship (Connolly, Craig, Goldberg, & Pepler, 2004; Longmore, Manning, & Giordano, 2001). That being said, those girls who do report a romantic relationship indicate a longer duration than the boys, a pattern that continues across the adolescent years (Carver et al., 2003; Shulman & Scharf, 2000). There is also evidence to suggest that parenting practices differentially influence the romantic experiences of early adolescents. Girls, relative to boys, are more intensely supervised, and this restricts their participation in romantic activities (Kan, McHale, & Crouter, 2008). New patterns take shape in mid- to late adolescence as girls now become more likely than boys to report a romantic relationship (Carver et al., 2003). Although the reason for this trend is unknown, it is possible that girls' desire to be in a relationship can be fulfilled once the limits imposed by parental supervision decline. In middle adolescence, the trend for girls to date older boys also emerges (Carver et al., 2003), a pattern that continues across the lifespan.

Race and Ethnic Influences

Current research suggests that adolescents from different ethnic groups may not be the same in their likelihood of engaging in romantic relationships. Although white teens generally do not differ from teens of African, Caribbean, or Latino background in terms of romantic experiences, Asian Americans are significantly less likely than all of these ethnic groups to report a current romantic partner (Carver et al., 2003; Connolly et al., 2004; Lau, Markham, Lin, Flores, & Chacko, 2009). This difference is attributed to cultural variation in the acceptability of adolescent dating within different cultures, with collectivist societies favoring a later onset of romantic experiences than societies with an individualistic belief system.

Sexual Minority Youths

Roughly 5% of adolescents report same-sex romantic attractions, or sexual-minority orientations (Carver et al., 2003; Russell & Consolacion, 2003), and these youths have as many romantic experiences as their heterosexual peers. This research has shown us that sexual-minority youths have very fluid romantic attractions and date opposite-sex partners, as well as same-sex ones (Russell & Consolacion, 2003). This fluidity is especially true of sexual-minority girls and reflects gender differences in the quest for a stable gender identity as gay or lesbian (Glover, Galliher & Lamere, 2009).

THEORIES OF ROMANTIC RELATIONSHIPS

Two theories guide much of the research on adolescent romantic relationships, namely, attachment theory and developmental-contextual theory. These perspectives have a common interest in understanding how teens become more knowledgeable and skilled in romantic relationships over time. Both of these perspectives also are interested in how the personal characteristics of individual teenagers interact with features of their social environment to ultimately determine the kinds of romantic relationships they will experience. Yet these perspectives differ in the relative weight they give to these facets: attachment theory puts more emphasis on the personal beliefs and expectations that individuals have about close relationships, even if these beliefs are outside of the individual's conscious awareness, whereas developmental-contextual theories put more emphasis on teens' experiences in relationships, especially with friends and family.

Romantic Attachment Theory

Romantic attachment theorists suggest that the function of romantic relationships is to provide adolescents and adults with the safe haven and secure base that they first experienced as infants and young children with their parents (Hazan & Shaver, 1987). These relationship functions begin to transfer from parents to romantic partners during the adolescent period, a movement that is motivated by adolescents' emerging desire to have these needs met by a person to whom they are sexually attracted. As with their parental relationships, adolescents may differ in the types of attachments they form with their romantic partners (Collins & Sroufe, 1999). Some adolescents will form a secure attachment to their romantic partners, meaning that they will trust them for support in times of stress and to be emotionally available on a consistent basis. Other adolescents will form insecure romantic attachments to their partners. Although the way that these adolescents will express their insecurity can vary, insecurity generally implies that they will be uncomfortable turning to their partners for support. Both secure and insecure expectations of relationships are shaped by the attachments that teens had with their parents when they were children, as well as the more recent experiences that they have with friends and other people whom they may have dated (Furman & Simon, 1999).

Developmental–Contextual Theory

Developmental-contextual theorists shift the focus away from the expectations individuals have about relationships to consider how these individuals may have been influenced by the interconnected set of social systems in which they grew up. The renowned scholar, Urie Bronfenbrenner, first proposed the general idea that individuals are influenced by different layers of their social environment, from their more immediate experiences with friends and family all the way to the broader messages that they receive from the sociocultural groups to which they belong (Bronfenbrenner, 1979). Developmental-contextual theories rely on Bronfenbrenner's ideas in that they argue that romantic relationships are shaped by processes in the family and the peer group, as well as by cultural beliefs about the nature of love, the correct age at which to begin dating, and the roles that males and females should play in romantic relationships.

STAGES OF ROMANTIC DEVELOPMENT

Regardless of whether their ideas about romance are based on attachment theory or on developmental-contextual theory, researchers of adolescent relationships have been united in their goal of accounting for the progression of romantic involvements across the teenage years. Contemporary scholars address this issue by positing a series of stages through which romantic relationships evolve to reach their mature form.

The first of these stage models was proposed by Furman and Wehner (1994). They outlined a behavioral systems theory to account for how romantic relationships progressively evolve to fulfill all of the functions of a traditional attachment relationship, namely intimacy and caretaking, as well as the emerging need for sexuality. Furman and Wehner are also credited with highlighting the affiliative function of adolescent romance, arguing that companionship and the sharing of pleasurable time together lies at the crux of dating during this stage of life. These scholars outlined four stages through which adolescents pass: (1) *simple interchanges* between opposite-sex peers that are motivated by pubertal maturation; (2) *casual dating* in short-term partnerships that fulfills early and middle adolescents' needs for affiliation and passionate feelings; (3) *stable relationships* in which older adolescents' needs for intimacy are met alongside those of sexuality and affiliation; and (4) *committed relationships* in which young adults are more able to be caretakers for all of their partner's emotional needs.

B. Bradford Brown (1999), in contrast, proposed a developmental-contextual model of adolescent relationships in which adolescents' growing need to learn more about themselves as people, as opposed to their need to form close relationships, is the key motivator of the progression of romantic experiences. Brown argues that a central challenge of adolescence is to create an integrated self-image that includes the romantic self. The romantic self-image entails both a group-based identity formed by the romantic norms of a peer crowd and a self-based identity that adolescents define independently of their social group. Brown outlines four phases through which this romantic identity develops: (1) the *initiation phase*, in which peers provide norms for romantic relationships and define the boundaries for spending time with the opposite sex; (2) the *status phase* wherein adolescents prize those romantic relationships that enhance their social positions in the peer group; (3) the *affection phase*, in which adolescents become more open to the individual expression of affectionate needs and are less tied to group values; and (4) the *bonding phase*, in which adolescents and young adults come to select partners who complement their own personalities, goals, and styles of relating.

We have also proposed a developmental-contextual theory of adolescent romantic stages (Connolly et al., 2004; Connolly & Goldberg, 1999). We believe that adolescents' inner drive to realize *both* intimacy and identity needs is what motivates their participation in more advanced forms of romance over time. What's more, romantic involvements provide the key context for these needs to be achieved because the passionate and sexual feelings awoken by puberty lead teens to realize that they can no longer have all of their intimacy and identity needs met by their parents and friends. We have also outlined four stages of romance: (1) the *infatuation stage,* wherein younger teens have the opportunity to explore their romantic passions by discussing them with peers or by personal fantasy or preoccupation; (2) the *affiliative stage*, in which socially skilled peers initiate the formation of mixed-gender peer groups in early adolescence and spark group dating; (3) the *intimate stage*, in which middle adolescents participate in dyadic romantic relationships that have a life outside of the peer group, and include more mature forms of intimacy; and (4) the *committed stage*, in which older adolescents begin to balance the closeness they have established with an exclusive partner with their need for personal expression and identity.

In the past decade, many researchers have examined the staging of romantic relationships during adolescence, and their findings support the ideas outlined here. In contrast to the models that delineate four stages, however, the evidence points to three romantic stages.

Stage 1: Entry into Romantic Attractions and Affiliations in Early Adolescence

Empirical data confirm that the first stage of romantic development is triggered by puberty (Dornbusch et al., 1981; Friedlander, Connolly, Pepler, & Craig, 2007; Smolak, Levine, & Gralen, 1993). During the age range of 11–13 years, adolescents become intensely interested in matters of romance, and this topic dominates conversations with friends (Eder, 1993), as well as internal fantasies (Tuval-Mashiach, Walsh, Harel, & Shulman, 2009). Crushes and shared infatuations become new ways of joining with same-sex friends, even if there is little actual interaction with the object of the teens' affection. This new, shared interest in romance moves adolescents away from having only same-sex friendships, as is typically the case throughout childhood, toward the formation of mixed-gender peer groups in which there is an opportunity to connect with romantically attractive others (Connolly et al., 2004). In the middle school years, more than 80% of students report activities such as going to the movies, sports activities, dances, and parties with groups of boys and girls (Connolly et al., 2004; Meier & Allen, 2009). These activities gently advance romantic development because they bring both genders into social situations in which romantic attractions are possible but not obligatory. These initial cross-gender interactions are, however, dictated as much by status as by personal chemistry, as youths popular with their same-sex peers socialize with popular other-sex peers (Bukowski, Sippola, & Hoza, 1999) and are the first in the peer group to initiate romantic relationships (Carlson & Rose, 2007).

Stage 2: Exploring Romantic Relationships in Middle Adolescence

Two forms of involvement are evident in the second stage of romantic development, roughly spanning the middle adolescent period of 14–16 years of age. First, casual dating emerges as an important form of romantic involvement. These connections are short-lived and last only a few months (Feiring, 1996; Seiffge-Krenke, 2003). The second form of involvement during this exploratory stage is "dating in groups," in which the casual romantic connections that youths form are embedded in a peer context (Connolly, Furman, & Konarski, 2000; Kuttler, La Greca, & Prinstein, 1999). Essentially, the mixed-gender peer networks that were formed in early adolescence become increasingly populated by teen couples. At this time, dating activities complement, rather than replace, time spent with friends because both occur in the context of the peer group. Friends can be the "brokers" of dating by conveying their friend's romantic attraction and confirming whether or not this is reciprocated. Romantic participation in middle adolescence is heavily linked to social status in the peer group, and high-status youths are more likely to be involved in dating activities than their lower-status classmates (Franzoi, Davis, & Vasquez-Suson, 1994).

Stage 3: Consolidating Dyadic Romantic Bonds in Late Adolescence

The final stage of romantic involvement typically occurs at the end of the high school years and concerns the formation of dyadic romantic relationships. At this time, romantic relationships are rooted in strong emotional bonds and resemble the couple relationships of adulthood. These bonds often last for a year or more, and adolescents describe them as serious, exclusive, and highly rewarding in terms of companionship and emotional support (Connolly & Johnson, 1996; Furman & Buhrmester, 1992; Seiffge-Krenke, 2003; Shulman & Scharf, 2000). This newfound romantic maturity coincides with adolescents' decreasing level of involvement in larger peer groups and greater attention to the quality of their couple relationships (Kuttler & La Greca, 2004). Yet increasing involvement with a romantic partner can also interfere with adolescents' need to maintain a separate sense of self, and, at this stage, adolescents struggle with questions of identity, a struggle that continues to characterize the romantic bonds of adulthood.

Gender and Romantic Stages

Boys and girls do not differ much in the trajectories of their romantic stages (Carver et al., 2003; Connolly et al., 2004; Meier & Allen, 2009), and once the transition from same-sex to mixed-sex social contexts has been made, boys and girls follow very similar pathways to romantic relationships. Nonetheless, there are some differences in the romantic roles adopted by boys and girls. Girls typically preside over the social settings that allow romantic interests to flourish in the early adolescent years as they initiate the cross-gender contacts that eventually lead to larger mixed-gender peer groups (Connolly, Furman, & Konarski, 2000; Feiring, 1999). Once these mixed-gender groups have been created, boys then take the lead in connecting with girls in more direct romantic ways by initiating dates (Jackson, Jacob, Landman-Peeters, & Lanting, 2001; Pellegrini & Long, 2007). Once dating has been initiated, girls again seem to dictate the quality of the relationship. Because girls learn a lot about how to share personal feelings and offer support in their childhood best-friendships, they are in a better position than boys, who learn more about competition and how to maintain high status and respect in their childhood peer groups, to shape the emotional tone of the relationship (McIsaac, Connolly, McKenney, Pepler, & Craig, 2008).

Intraindividual Differences in Romantic Stages

Stage theory presents a normative picture of romantic development in that it strives to describe the most typical experiences of most individuals within a given age group at any given time. Although this focus is very useful, it is also necessary to note that it can obscure many of the important changes that may be occurring for individual adolescents. For example, some teens may experiment with forms of romance from different levels of involvement, even though most of their romantic experiences are in line with what stage theories would consider to be typical for their age. Research from our lab has shown that younger teens often cycle between mixed-gender affiliations and group dating (Connolly et al., 2004), whereas older teens cycle between exploratory or casual relationships and more serious, stable pairings (Dhariwal, Connolly, Paciello, & Caprara, 2009).

Interindividual Differences in Romantic Stages

Researchers also note that participation in romantic relationships can vary among individuals of the same age, whether in the timing of their participation or in the types of activities in which they engage (Collins, 2003). In terms of romantic timing, younger adolescents who form romantic partnerships ahead of their agemates are known as "early starters" (Neemann, Hubbard, & Masten, 1995; Zimmer-Gembeck, Siebenbruner, & Collins, 2001), whereas older adolescents who have not yet entered into romantic relationships are often known as "late bloomers" (Caspi, Elder, & Bem, 1988). Girls' early entry into dating has been the focus of much research because it is thought to put them at risk for various mental health challenges. There has been almost no research into late bloomers, even though there may be social and emotional challenges for these youths as well. We return to a discussion of the adjustment implications of atypical timing in a later section and focus here on what is known about the predictors of early entry into romance.

Early Starters

As previously discussed, the most typical romantic activity for early adolescents is socializing in mixed-gender peer groups. Nonetheless, approximately 15–20% of youths between the ages of 11 and 13 years report a current romantic relationship, and up to 35% of youths in this age range report having some previous experience in a romantic partnership (Carver et al., 2003; Connolly et al., 2004). Consistent with this accelerated trend, early-starting youths experience a larger number of romantic dissolutions and more frequent partner turnover than their relatively on-time counterparts (Zimmer-Gembeck et al., 2001). There is also some evidence that early entry into relationships places adolescents on a trajectory of ongoing involvement with different partners, rather than just a single relationship at one point in time (Neeman et al., 1995; Raley, Crissey & Muller, 2007).

Early dating is most consistently predicted by early pubertal maturation (Ellis & Garber, 2000; Magnusson, Stattin, & Allen, 1985; Phinney, Jensen, Olsen, & Cundick, 1990). These findings refer especially to adolescent girls, and the links between puberty and early dating are less consistent for boys (Susman et al., 1985). Other predictors of early dating are found in the family. Insecure attachment and lax parental supervision have both been linked to early dating (Cooper, Shaver, & Collins, 1998; Friedlander et al., 2007). Youths from divorced families also tend to become involved in romantic relationships at younger ages than do youths whose parents remain together (Cavanagh, Crissey, & Raley, 2008). Finally, peer-group dynamics may give rise to early dating, as associating with older peers is a risk for starting romantic relationships at young age, likely because these peers model more advanced forms of dating involvement (Friedlander et al., 2007; Stattin & Magnusson, 1990).

CHARACTERISTICS OF ADOLESCENT ROMANTIC RELATIONSHIPS

As previously noted, mature romantic relationships entail three components: passion, intimacy, and commitment (Sternberg, 1986). Developmental researchers have been guided by this tripartite model, and early in the evolution of the scientific study of adolescent romance, it was used as a foundation for describing the characteristics of these relationships (Connolly et al., 1999). These early studies uncovered both similarities in and differences between the romantic bonds of adolescents and adults. Like adults, teens view their romantic relationships as passionate and intimate; however, unlike adults, teens do not consider commitment to be a valued attribute of their relationships (Feiring, 1996). Also differently from adults, companionship, with or without emotional intimacy, is a highly prioritized component of boyfriend–girlfriend relationships in adolescence (Connolly et al., 1999). In the next sections we describe what is known about these key characteristics of romantic relationships in adolescence.

Passion

Feelings of intense love, attraction, and longing for another person are the essence of romantic passion (Connolly & Goldberg, 1999; Tuval-Mashiach et al., 2008), and it is the passionate component of romantic relationships that distinguishes these bonds from close connections with friends and family at any age. Although the passionate attractions of early adolescents typically remain at the level of fantasy and do not translate into an actual relationship, these feelings can both enhance and complicate romantic couplings later in development. Being in love with a specific person involves pleasurable physiological, cognitive, and behavioral experiences; however, this increased arousal and preoccupation with another can also contribute to sleeplessness, distractibility, excessive reassurance seeking, and concern about possible rejection or betrayal for both boys and girls (Brand, Luethi, von Planta, Hatzinger & Holsboer-Trachsler, 2007; Larson, Clore, & Wood, 1999).

Most people might intuitively think that passion is the spark for sexual behaviors in adolescence, but surprisingly the overlap of sexuality and passion has only recently become a topic of interest to developmentalists (Zimmer-Gembeck & Helfand, 2008). Rather, researchers who study sexual development have mostly focused on the age at which most teens become sexually active, especially with regard to sexual intercourse, and have not considered the relationship status of the sexual partners. The small amount of data that we do have tell us that most teens' sexual activities occur with someone they are dating and, by the middle of adolescence, about half of established couples report having sex with one another (Cavanagh, 2007). As might be expected, sexual activities become more intense with age; younger teens most often engage in light sexual behaviors, such as hugging, holding hands, or kissing, whereas older teens often expand the sexual component of their relationship to include more intimate behaviors (Manning, Giordano, & Longmore, 2006; Williams, Connolly & Cribbie, 2008).

Adolescent boys and girls differ in the extent to which sexuality is a key motivator of their romantic experiences (Cavanagh, 2007; Feiring, 1996). Boys' ideal romantic relationships often include a significant sexual component, whereas girls' ideal romantic relationships are more focused on emotional intimacy and companionship, with partners engaging in affectionate forms of sexuality such as hugging and cuddling. These idealized conceptions of romantic relationships reflect the social norms that boys and girls follow with regard to sexual codes of conduct that are enforced by same-gender peer groups. For girls, it is permissible to engage in sexual activity so long as it is accompanied by emotional closeness and occurs within the context of a stable and long-term partnership (O'Sullivan & Meyer-Bahlburg, 2003). Girls who are sexually active outside of these parameters are typically condemned by their same-sex peers (i.e., labeled with derogatory terms) and experience a marked decrease in their social standing. In contrast, male norms center on the stereotype of heightened masculinity. Adolescent boys encourage each other to actively pursue purely sexual encounters with girls (Tolman, Spencer, Harmon, Rosen-Reynoso, & Striepe, 2004). However, more recent research suggests that the personal values of many boys, outside of the peer context, lean more toward personal compatibility and the desire to get to know better someone to whom they are romantically attracted (Smiler, 2008).

Intimacy

Adolescents consider their romantic relationships to be among the most supportive and caring of all their personal connections (Adams, Laursen & Wilder, 2001; Connolly & Johnson, 1996; Laursen & Williams, 1997; Seiffge-Krenke, 2000, 2003; Shulman & Scharf, 2000). They show their intimacy by encouraging one another and communicating loving sentiments, disclosing personal feelings, developing a sense of honesty and trust. By the end of adolescence, boyfriends and girlfriends ascend to the top of the hierarchy of close relationships in terms of the perceived level of intimacy and support that they offer, surpassing both parents and friends (Adams et al., 2001; Furman & Buhrmester, 1992; Laursen & Williams, 1997; Meeus, Branje, van der Valk, & de Wiede, 2007; Seiffge-Krenke, 2000). More sophisticated expressions of intimacy among older adolescents are attributed to their increased skill in managing close relationships in ways that address the unique emotional needs of each partner. How romantic intimacy is experienced also varies with gender. Girls generally view their romantic relationships as more intimate than boys do, a finding consistent with girls' greater sensitivity to close relationships of all kinds (Connolly & Johnson, 1996; Haugen, Welsh, & McNulty, 2008).

Affiliation, that is, spending time together in activities that are mutually enjoyable, is a central facet of intimacy for adolescent romance, and companionship is a principal motivator for romantic couplings at this age (Connolly et al., 1999; Feiring, 1996). Time spent with a romantic partner increases with age, alongside more emotional forms of intimacy (Furman & Buhrmester, 1992). The intertwining of affiliation and emotional intimacy is likely not coincidental, as shared time is in large part a precursor to deepening closeness. However, affiliation is an important relationship attribute in its own right, and adolescents of all ages point to a lack of companionship with a romantic partner as the primary reason for ending a relationship (Connolly & McIsaac, 2009). Unlike emotional intimacy, there are no gender differences in romantic affiliation (Carver et al., 2003; Connolly & Johnson, 1996; Seiffge-Krenke, 2003).

CONFLICT IN ADOLESCENT ROMANTIC RELATIONSHIPS

Conflict occurs when partners have different perspectives and expectations of each other or the relationship. Developmentalists are especially interested in studying conflict because of the dual role it can play in the functioning of the relationship: When conflict negotiation is handled through compromise and active listening, it can bring partners together and increase their sense of closeness (Shulman, 2003; Simon, Kobielski, & Martin, 2008); but when conflict is handled by using coercion and threats, it can be very destabilizing and has the potential to escalate an interaction to the point of physical aggression (O'Leary & Slep, 2003). Adolescent romantic partners do have conflicts with one another, especially over issues such as jealousy, trust, betrayal, and neglect (McIsaac et al., 2008); however, they tend to disagree less often with each other than they do with other members of their social network, especially their parents (Furman & Shomaker, 2008). The frequency of conflict between romantic partners increases with age, following the same pattern as intimacy (Shulman, Tuval-Mashiach, Levran, & Anbar, 2006). This overlap is likely not a coincidence, as relationship partners must be sufficiently close to become aware of differences in their expectations. Also, partners must be invested enough in the relationship to want to negotiate the issue rather than avoid it, downplay it, or break up.

Adolescent boys and girls do not differ from one another in their reports of the amount of conflict that occurs in their romantic relationships (Furman & Buhrmester, 1992). Yet, they do differ in their preferred ways of negotiating the conflict, with girls reporting more compromise and boys reporting more confrontation (Feldman

& Gowen, 1998). A very intriguing study by Shute and Charlton (2006) shows that boyfriends and girlfriends sometimes negotiate conflict with one another in ways that are more typical of the other gender; boys use more compromise with a girlfriend than they do with a friend, and girls use more overt anger with a boyfriend than they do with a friend. It is possible that boyfriends and girlfriends imitate the conflict style of the opposite gender in order to help their partner "get the message" and make the conflict negotiation proceed more smoothly, thus avoiding a breakup.

CONNECTIONS BETWEEN PARENTS, FRIENDS, AND ROMANTIC PARTNERS

Romantic relationships are part and parcel of young people's social mosaic, and these involvements are connected to the structure and quality of their ties with family members and friends. A key question for scholars, from both the attachment and developmental-contextual perspectives, is to explain how close relationships shape the ways that adolescents function in their romantic involvements. Irrespective of the aforementioned differences between these two theoretical traditions, both support the idea that relationships with parents and friends can influence romantic relationships in positive and negative ways. We summarize here what is known about the independent and joint contributions of parents and friends to romantic relationships.

Parental Influences

Numerous pathways exist through which parents influence their adolescent children's romantic involvements. First, attachment theory tells us that parents provide an emotional base for young people on which to build other relationships (Furman & Wehner, 1994). Hence the quality of the emotional bond between adolescents and their parents should be predictive of the closeness and support that adolescents experience in their romantic partnerships—a prediction that has generally been upheld (Laursen, Furman, & Mooney, 2006; Seiffge-Krenke, Shulman, & Klessinger, 2001; Smetana & Gettman, 2006). What's more, the results of two longitudinal studies suggest that the quality of the parent–child relationship in childhood as well as in adolescence contributes to the level of trust and emotional expression in the romantic bonds of young adults (Mayseless & Scharf, 2007; Roisman, Madsen, Hennighausen, Sroufe, & Collins, 2001). A recent line of evidence also suggests that the quality of the relationship that adolescents have with their mothers and fathers is more or less influential on their romantic partnerships at different points in development, especially among girls (Scharf & Mayseless, 2008). Mother–daughter relationships are most salient in the mid-adolescent years, whereas fathers influence their daughters more once they get older. This pattern may be due to the changing nature of romance; greater intimacy with a romantic partner is sought in the late teen years, and fathers may serve as prototypes for their daughters as they strive to create these more mature relationships with a partner.

Parental interactions also forecast how boys and girls will manage conflict with a romantic partner. Several studies show that adolescents use the same strategies to solve problems with their romantic partners as they do with their parents, be it compromise, avoidance, or coercion (Martin, 1990; Reese-Weber & Bartle-Haring, 1998; Reese-Weber & Kahn, 2005). How mothers and fathers solve problems in their own relationship with one another is also an important determinant of how teens will handle fights with their boyfriends and girlfriends. Adolescents whose parents have an antagonistic marital relationship are more likely than other teens to be hostile with a romantic partner (Scharf & Mayseless, 2001; Stocker & Richmond, 2007). Attachment theory would suggest that this occurs because interparental conflict shapes adolescents' expectations about romantic relationships. Supporting this idea, adolescent girls who were exposed to episodes of hostility between their parents were more likely than other girls to have insecure romantic attachments, which, in turn, increased their risk for engaging in unsafe sexual activities and becoming overly preoccupied with dating (Steinberg, Davila, & Fincham, 2006).

A consideration of family conflict leads inevitably to a discussion about the effects of divorce. There is emerging evidence that family dissolutions cast a shadow on adolescents' romantic development. Teens from divorced families hold less favorable views about committed romantic relationships than do youths whose families are still intact, and they also report lower levels of intimacy in their romantic partnerships (Giuliani, Iafrate, & Rosnati, 1998; van Schaick & Stolberg, 2001). The more family transitions that teens go through, the more upheavals they seem to report in their own romantic relationships. Youths who live in single-parent homes or in a blended family report more frequent romantic partner turnover in adolescence than youths from stable family backgrounds (Cavanagh et al., 2008). Developmental psychologists have yet to settle on an explanation for the differences between youths from intact and dissolved families; however, the transmission of insecure working models of attachment is a strong candidate.

Certain styles of parenting are thought to be more useful than others in terms of fostering healthy romantic development in adolescence. Authoritative parenting styles, which involve balancing supervision and monitoring with encouragement and supportive dialogue about the adolescent's emerging desire to explore connections outside of the family, are most predictive of positive romantic experiences in the teen years (Auslander, Short, Succop, & Rosenthal, 2009; Kan et al., 2008). Parenting practices that support adolescents' growing wish for independence have also been connected to teens' level of comfort with expressing their true opinions to their romantic partners (Taradash, Connolly, Pepler, Craig, & Costa, 2001). Adolescents who grow up in homes in which closeness does not suffer because family members disagree on a particular issue likely feel more secure about opening up to their romantic partners, even if their opinions are different. Even though encouraging independence is linked to social success in adolescence, parents must still do so within the context of rules and expectations about romantic relationships. Parents who insist that their teen inform them about the happenings in their romantic lives are more successful than parents who restrict the romantic activities of their children or prescribe codes of conduct (Madsen, 2008).

Friend Influences

As previously discussed, peers are the single most important conduit of romantic development in adolescence. Further attesting to the significance of peers, available research suggests that quality of the relationships that adolescents have with their friends, be they positive or negative, predicts the quality of their relationships with romantic partners. The level of closeness, trust, and openness that adolescents have with their friends is mirrored by comparable qualities in their romantic relationships (Connolly

& Johnson, 1996; Kuttler & LaGreca, 2004; Laursen et al., 2006; Seiffge-Krenke, 2000; Shulman & Scharf, 2000). Autonomy with friends also appears to generalize; adolescents who feel confident expressing their differing views with their friends do this with their romantic partners as well (Taradash et al., 2001). Turning to negative qualities, hostility, argumentativeness, and feelings of irritation are also correlated between friends and dating couples (Furman, Simon, Shaffer, & Bouchey, 2002; Kuttler & LaGreca, 2004; Stocker & Richmond, 2007). Adolescents who bully their peers are also more likely to be aggressive toward a romantic partner and to participate in relationships that are characterized by an unequal balance of power (Connolly, Pepler, Craig, & Taradash, 2000).

Given these strong links between friends and romantic partners, one may well ask the question of whether the flow of influence can move the other way, namely, whether romantic involvements influence friendships. Although the available information is rather sparse, it does seem that the pattern of influence can be bidirectional. For example, mirroring the way friends create opportunities for romantic partner contacts, there is evidence that extensive romantic involvements lead to expanded peer networks, although sometimes the contact is with deviant peers (Lonardo, Giordano, Longmore, & Manning, 2009). Romantic involvements can also have negative effects on close friendships, as the time spent with a romantic partner may lead to neglect of the friend and ensuing feelings of jealousy (Roth & Parker, 2001). Clearly, an important task for adolescents is learning to balance the competing demands of friends and romantic partners in ways that promote harmony and agreement in the two social contexts.

Joint Contributions of Parents and Friends

Parents and friends create overlapping contexts of social influence within which romantic development occurs. Sometimes these influences are conjoint, meaning that families and friends seemingly work together to effect romantic development in a similar way, thereby amplifying the overall outcome. Laursen and his colleagues (2006) uncovered a pattern of influence that provides a good example of conjoint effects. Adolescents in their study could be clustered into groups based on the levels of support they perceived from their mothers, their best friends, and their romantic partners. Teens who indicated high levels of support in all three relationships considered themselves to be more competent at handling romantic interactions than other groups of teens. Following a similar process, Stocker and Richmond (2007) found that friends and family can also have a conjoint effect on romantic relationships that is negative. Hostility within these social spheres jointly contributed to coercive patterns of conflict within adolescent couples.

Scholars have also considered whether families and friends exert more or less influence on romantic relationships at different points of development. We call this pattern a primacy effect to reflect the fact that one relationship type dominates over the other. Research generally supports the idea that friends hold a primary position of influence over the romantic relationships of adolescents, even though the qualities of friendships and parent–teen relationships tend to be closely related (Furman et al., 2002). This finding matches the prediction of attachment theorists that the provision of security and emotional safety is transferred from friends to romantic partners in adolescence, having made the earlier transition from parents to friends (Furman & Wehner, 1994). Primacy effects of parental relationships begin to take shape in the period of emerging adulthood. Having a secure attachment to a parent in infancy predicts similar beliefs about one's romantic relationship partner in adulthood, thus showcasing the importance of having early relationship experiences that are positive and close to long-term social successes (Simpson, Collins, Tran, & Haydon, 2007). The primacy effect of parents may emerge at this point in development because young people's acquisition of more refined romantic skills presumably makes them more capable of initiating and maintaining romantic relationships without the direct support of their friends.

ROMANTIC RELATIONSHIPS AND WELL-BEING

We have argued in this chapter that romantic relationships are both normative and developmentally beneficial for teens. Having a romantic relationship is associated with enhanced self-esteem, popularity, social acceptance, and feelings of competence in managing day-to-day interactions with friends and dating partners (Grover, Nangle, & Zeff, 2005). Yet despite these benefits, romantic relationships are also associated with negative social and health outcomes. The explanation for these coexisting positive and negative effects is not known (Furman, Low, & Ho, 2009). However, considerable advances have been made in understanding how and why youths' romantic relationships might place them at risk for mental health problems, especially depression and delinquency.

Depression

Intuitively speaking, romantic relationships make people happy and should therefore protect them from feelings of loneliness, despair, and isolation that so often spark episodes of depression. This association is true among adults; however, the connection between depression and romantic relationships is less straightforward in adolescence (Davila, 2008). Joyner and Udry (2000) were the first to report the rather perplexing finding that adolescents, and especially girls, with a romantic relationship are more depressed than adolescents who are not dating. Curious about this nonintuitive finding, researchers have strived to identify the circumstances under which having a romantic relationship may be depressogenic for young people. We now highlight the central developmental and individual factors that seem to increase the risk of depression among adolescents who have romantic relationships.

First, the timing of romantic relationships is important to consider, as it appears that depressive symptoms are more common for teens, and especially girls, who participate in couple dating by the age of 12 years (Compian, Gowen, & Hayward, 2004; Natsuaki, Biehl, & Ge, 2009). Whether these psychological problems are due only to the early timing of their romantic experiences is not entirely clear. For instance, young adolescent girls who start dating early often come from families with more conflict and instability, and these family struggles may amplify their experience of emotional distress well before their dating relationships even get started (Doyle, Brendgen, Markiewicz, & Kamkar, 2003). Davila and her colleagues (2009) have also found that girls who are *already* feeling depressed tend to seek out romantic relationships more than other girls, perhaps as a way of alleviating their low mood. Regardless of their emotional state, romantic relationships are likely challenging for young teens, as life has not yet prepared them to handle all of the ups and downs of the dating world, including managing the pressures of whether or not to engage in sexual activity. Some recent research suggests that it is sexual activity, rather than the romantic relationship itself, that accounts for increased levels of depression among early-starting girls (Monahan & Lee, 2008).

Second, the expectations that adolescents have for their romantic relationships can place them at risk for depression. An insecure working model of romantic attachment has been linked to depressive symptoms among girls in both the early and late adolescent period (Davila, Steinberg, Kachadourian, Cobb, & Fincham, 2004). Insecure attachments are problematic, as many youths with this style of attachment are intensely drawn to relationships; but soon after they enter into them, they experience significant distress because they are unable to fully trust their partners or view themselves as worthy of love (Davila et al., 2004). A related relationship expectation, known as rejection sensitivity, also puts adolescents at risk for maladjustment when they begin dating. Adolescents who are *rejection sensitive* anxiously expect to be rejected by their boyfriends or girlfriends, which in turn causes them to overreact to just the slightest hint of rejection, even if this was not the original intention of their partner (Downey, Bonica, & Rincón, 1999). It is not surprising that being overly sensitive to romantic rejection is connected to depression for both boys and girls (Harper, Dickson, & Welsh, 2006).

A third explanation for the link between romantic relationships and depression concerns the negative interactions that may be going on between the partners. Being in a relationship that is marked by constant criticism, contempt, defensiveness, and emotional withdrawal is distressing enough for experienced adults, let alone teens who are new to the world of dating! Depressive symptoms, as well as other internalizing problems such as anxiety, are frequently reported by adolescents whose relationships are characterized by fights, a lack of mutual support, and unequal decision-making power (Galliher, Rostosky, Welsh, & Kawaguchi, 1999; La Greca & Harrison, 2005; Reese-Weber & Marchand, 2002). The volatile nature of low-quality romantic relationships such as these presumably makes them more prone to breakup, a stressful event that in and of itself can set in motion the feelings of worthlessness, abandonment, and despair that underlie depressive disorders (Monroe, Rohde, Seeley, & Lewinsohn, 1999; Rizzo, Daley, & Gunderson, 2006). Breakups are especially difficult when they are initiated by the partner and when there is an established pattern of unstable relationships and frequent partner turnovers (Connolly & McIsaac, 2009; Davies & Windle, 2000).

Delinquency

Similar to the patterns noted for depression, breaking rules and acting out are more common among adolescents who begin romantic relationships at a young age. Early-starting boys and girls report higher rates of aggression, bullying, school problems, alcohol and drug use, and risky sexual behaviors than teens who follow a more gradual course of romantic development (Friedlander et al., 2007; Haynie, Giordano, Manning, & Longmore, 2005). Increased rates of delinquency among early starters may have something to do with the partners whom they end up dating (Stattin & Magnusson, 1990; Young & D'Arcy, 2005). Because there are relatively few teens in their own age group who are interested in couple relationships, early starters look to older groups of youths for potential dating partners. Almost by default, younger teens are left to date deviant partners because older teens who are functioning well are probably not romantically interested in someone who is much younger.

When romantic relationships become more typical in middle adolescence, peers continue to play a role in predicting delinquency. Even though friends can provide a great deal of comfort and support when working through the ups and downs of dating, they can also influence adolescents to engage in minor acts of delinquency and health-risk behaviors with their romantic partners (Dishion & Piehler, 2007). These negative outcomes are more likely for youths who are "overinvolved" in relationships, meaning that they participate in lots of casual relationships with different partners over a relatively short period of time (Davies & Windle, 2000). In addition, youths who are friends with delinquent teens are more likely to break rules themselves and also to date others who do the same (Lonardo et al., 2009). These findings speak to the notion of homophily, which refers to the idea that "birds of a feather flock together," a concept that can be applied to romantic partners, as well as friends (Simon, Aikins, & Prinstein, 2008; see also Bukowski, Buhrmester, & Underwood, Chapter 7, this volume).

FUTURE DIRECTIONS

Developmental research on adolescent romantic relationships has come a long way since the field first began in the mid-1990s. From a rather uninformed starting point, a substantial literature on this topic has now emerged. Our understanding of adolescent romance has improved in all of the areas that we summarized in this chapter, providing a foundation for further meaningful examination of adolescent romantic relationships. We now outline several directions for future research that we consider essential for the ongoing advancement of this area of social development.

The theories we currently have about romantic development need to do a better job of accounting for the diverse social experiences that young people have growing up, well before they contemplate dating, as these background factors may set them up for radically different kinds of romantic trajectories. A good start to this endeavor would be to consider how teens enter into relationships even if they do not have mixed-gender peer groups. Youths who have historically lacked cross-gender friendships, be this due to social rejection, poor mental or physical health, or cultural or familial prohibitions, may nonetheless become involved in dating at some later point in their development, and yet our current theories do not speak to this process at all. Acknowledging different starting points for romantic development might begin to shed light on the experiences of *late bloomers*, a group that has been woefully understudied. Although delaying relationships might pose a long-term challenge to the socioemotional development of some of these youths, largely because late bloomers will have had fewer opportunities to practice and refine their romantic skills before they enter adulthood, the prolonging of romantic onset may also be a beneficial strategy for those youths who choose to focus their energies on school, sports, or volunteer activities. Theories that propose alternate paths to mature and fulfilling romantic relationships would be of great assistance in teasing apart the different outcomes associated with late-blooming youths, as well as other issues related to off-time involvements more generally.

Continuing with our theme of understanding variation in adolescent romance, we suggest that researchers pay more attention to the romantic experiences of youths who come from different, and especially non-Western, cultures. Few studies compare the developmental timetables, relationship qualities, and patterns of peer and family influence that might exist between adolescents from different cultural groups.

Such comparisons would no doubt be challenging from a methodological perspective, because of the need to determine the best way for researchers to systematically ask about romantic relationship status and participation in cross-sex and dating activities in different ethnocultural contexts, and yet considering the meaning of romance in different cultural contexts will allow researchers to better understand those aspects of romance that are primarily shaped by context and those that are universal.

The scientific study of adolescent romance would be greatly benefited by tracking the progression of a single relationship across its complete life cycle, from initiation to dissolution. Most researchers study romantic relationships when they first get going, or once the couple has been established; only rarely have they considered what happens when adolescents terminate their relationships. Yet breakups can have a powerful impact on adjustment, and the ways in which adolescents make sense of these stressful events may be important predictors of well-being and future participation in relationships. Aside from learning about romantic dissolutions, a life-cycle focus would also allow researchers to explore how the quality of a single relationship strengthens or changes as partners adjust to one another's emotional needs and cues. This approach would be particularly helpful in deepening our understanding of how gender may shape these partner effects. Adolescent boys and girls bring very different skills and expectations to their romantic involvements, and understanding how they each learn to connect with their opposite-sex partners has important implications for the promotion of healthy relationships.

It is now evident that romantic relationships are embedded in a broader set of peer and family connections and that those social contexts are mutually influential. At present, however, most research has examined the influence of families, peers, or friends on romantic development. We still need to learn more about how an adolescent's romantic experiences might influence the quality of other relationships. For example, how do romantic relationships alter the nature of the parent–child interaction, especially around issues of autonomy and independence? Likewise, we need to examine the renegotiations that occur in a close friendship once one friend enters into a serious romantic partnership. Finally, the influence that romantic partners have on each other is quite unexplored.

We conclude our suggestions for future research by commenting that romantic relationships are part of adolescents' emerging developmental assets. When romantic experiences are paced with the competencies of the adolescent and embedded in a social context that both supports and regulates appropriate involvement, romantic relationships are healthy and beneficial. Consistent with our new understanding of the importance of focusing our attention on the positive aspects of youth development rather than on "deficits" in their functioning, it is critical for researchers to share what we know about positive romantic development with youths and also with the adults who support them in multiple contexts.

SUGGESTED READINGS

Carver, K., Joyner, K., & Udry, J. R. (2003). National estimates of adolescent romantic relationships. In P. Florsheim (Ed.), *Adolescent romantic relations and sexual behavior: Theory, research, and practical implications* (pp. 23–56). Mahwah, NJ: Erlbaum.

Collins, W. A. (2003). More than myth: The developmental significance of romantic relationships during adolescence. *Journal of Research on Adolescence, 13,* 1–24.

Connolly, J. A., & McIsaac, C. (2009). Romantic relationships in adolescence. In R. Lerner & L. Steinberg (Eds.), *Handbook of adolescent psychology* (3rd ed., pp. 104–151). Hoboken, NJ: Wiley

Davila, J. (2008). Depressive symptoms and adolescent romance: Theory, research, and implications. *Child Development Perspectives*, 2, 26–31.

Furman, W., Brown, B. B., & Feiring, C. (Eds.). (1999). *The development of romantic relationships in adolescence*. New York: Cambridge University Press.

Seiffge-Krenke, I. (2003). Testing theories of romantic development from adolescence to young adulthood: Evidence of a developmental sequence. *International Journal of Behavioral Development*, 27, 519–531.

Shulman, S. Tuval-Mashiach, R., Levran, E., & Anbar, S. (2006). Conflict resolution patterns and longevity of adolescent romantic couples: A 2-year follow-up study. *Journal of Adolescence*, 29, 575–588.

REFERENCES

Adams, R. E., Laursen, B., & Wilder, D. (2001). Characteristics of closeness in adolescent romantic relationships. *Journal of Adolescence, 24*, 353–363.

Auslander, B. A., Short, M. B., Succop, P. A., & Rosenthal, S. L. (2009). Associations between parenting behaviors and adolescent romantic relationships. *Journal of Adolescent Health, 45*, 98–101.

Brand, S., Luethi, M., von Planta, A., Hatzinger, M., & Holsboer-Trachsler, E. (2007). Romantic love, hypomania, and sleep pattern in adolescents. *Journal of Adolescent Health, 41*, 69—76.

Bronfenbrenner, U. (1979). *The ecology of human development*. Cambridge, MA: Harvard University Press.

Brown, B. B. (1999). "You're going out with who?": Peer group influences on adolescent romantic relationships. In W. Furman, B. B. Brown, & C. Feiring (Eds.), *The development of romantic relationships in adolescence* (pp. 291–329). New York: Cambridge University Press.

Bukowski, W. M., Sippola, L. K., & Hoza, B. (1999). Same and other: Interdependency between participation in same—and other—sex friendships. *Journal of Youth and Adolescence, 28*, 439–459.

Carlson, W., & Rose, A. J. (2007). The role of reciprocity in romantic relationships in middle childhood and early adolescence. *Merrill–Palmer Quarterly, 53*, 262–290.

Carver, K., Joyner, K., & Udry, J. R. (2003). National estimates of adolescent romantic relationships. In P. Florsheim (Ed.), *Adolescent romantic relations and sexual behavior: Theory, research, and practical implications* (pp. 23–56). Mahwah, NJ: Erlbaum.

Caspi, A., Elder, G. H., & Bem, D. J. (1988). Moving away from the world: Life-course patterns of shy children. *Developmental Psychology, 24*, 824—831.

Cavanagh, S. E. (2007). The social construction of romantic relationships in adolescence: Examining the role of peer networks, gender, and race. *Sociological Inquiry, 77*, 572–600.

Cavanagh, S. E., Crissey, S. R., & Raley, R. K. (2008). Family structure history and adolescent romance. *Journal of Marriage and Family, 70*, 698–714.

Collins, W. A. (2003). More than myth: The developmental significance of romantic relationships during adolescence. *Journal of Research on Adolescence, 13*, 1–24.

Collins, W. A., & Sroufe, L. A. (1999). Capacity for intimate relationships: A developmental construction. In W. Furman, B. B. Brown, & C. Feiring (Eds.), *The development of romantic relationships in adolescence* (pp. 125–147). New York: Cambridge University Press .

Compian, L., Gowen, L. K., & Hayward, C. (2004). Peripubertal girls' romantic and platonic involvement with boys: Associations with body image and depression symptoms. *Journal of Research on Adolescence, 14*, 23–47.

Connolly, J., Craig, W., Goldberg, A., & Pepler, D. (1999). Conceptions of cross-sex friendships and romantic relationships in early adolescence. *Journal of Youth and Adolescence, 28*, 481–494.

Connolly, J., Craig, W., Goldberg, A., & Pepler, D. (2004). Mixed-gender groups, dating, and romantic relationships in early adolescence. *Journal of Research on Adolescence, 14*, 185–207.

Connolly, J., Furman, W., & Konarski, R. (2000). The role of peers in the emergence of heterosexual romantic relationships in adolescence. *Child Development, 71*, 1395–1408.

Connolly, J. A., & Goldberg, A. (1999). Romantic relationships in adolescence: The role of friends and peers in their emergence and development. In W. Furman, B. B. Brown, & C. Feiring (Eds.), *The development of romantic relationships in adolescence* (pp. 266–290). New York: Cambridge University Press.

Connolly, J. A., & Johnson, A. M. (1996). Adolescents' romantic relationships and the structure and quality of their close interpersonal ties. *Personal Relationships, 3*, 185–195.

Connolly, J. A., & McIsaac, C. (2009). Romantic dissolutions in adolescence: Problems with independence and interdependence. *Journal of Adolescence, 32*, 1209–1223.

Connolly, J., Pepler, D., Craig, W., & Taradash, A. (2000). Dating experiences of bullies in early adolescence. *Child Maltreatment, 5*, 299–310.

Cooper, M. L., Shaver, P. R., & Collins, N. L. (1998). Attachment styles, emotion regulation, and adjustment in adolescence. *Journal of Personality and Social Psychology, 74*, 1380–1397.

Davies, P. T., & Windle, M. (2000). Middle adolescents' dating pathways and psychosocial adjustment. *Merrill–Palmer Quarterly, 46*, 90–118.

Davila, J. (2008). Depressive symptoms and adolescent romance: Theory, research, and implications. *Child Development Perspectives, 2*, 26–31.

Davila, J., Steinberg, S. J., Kachadourian, L., Cobb, R., & Fincham, F. (2004). Romantic involvement and depressive symptoms in early and late adolescence: The role of a preoccupied relational style. *Personal Relationships, 11*, 161–178.

Davila, J., Stroud, C. B., Starr, L. R., Miller, M. R., Yoneda, A., & Hershenberg, R. (2009). Romantic and sexual activities, parent–adolescent stress, and depressive symptoms among early adolescent girls. *Journal of Adolescence, 32*, 909–924.

Dhariwal, A., Connolly, J., Paciello, M., & Caprara, G. V. (2009). Adolescent peer relationships and emerging adult romantic styles: A longitudinal study of youth in an Italian community. *Journal of Adolescent Research, 24*(5), 579–600.

Dishion, T. J., & Piehler, T. F. (2007). Peer dynamics in the development and change of child and adolescent problem behavior. In A. S. Masten (Ed.), *Multilevel dynamics in developmental psychopathology: Pathways to the future* (pp. 151–180). Mahwah, NJ: Erlbaum.

Dornbusch, S. M., Carlsmith, M., Gross, R. T., Martin, J. A., Jennings, D., Rosenberg, A., et al. (1981). Sexual development, age, and dating: A comparison of biological and social influences upon one set of behaviors. *Child Development, 52*, 179–185.

Downey, G., Bonica, C., & Rincón, C. (1999). Rejection sensitivity and adolescent romantic relationships. In W. Furman, B. Brown, & C. Feiring (Eds.), *The development of romantic relationships in adolescence* (pp. 148–174). New York: Cambridge University Press.

Doyle, A. B., Brendgen, M., Markiewicz, D., & Kamkar, K. (2003). Family relationships as moderators of the association between romantic relationships and adjustment in early adolescence. *Journal of Early Adolescence, 23*, 316–340.

Eder, D. (1993). "Go get ya a French!": Romantic and sexual teasing among adolescent girls. In D. Tannen (Ed.), *Gender and conversational interaction* (pp. 17–31). New York: Oxford University Press.

Ellis, B. J., & Garber, J. (2000). Psychosocial antecedents of variation in girls' pubertal timing: Maternal depression, stepfather presence, and marital and family stress. *Child Development, 71*, 485–501.

Feiring, C. (1996). Concepts of romance in 15-year-old adolescents. *Journal of Research on Adolescence, 6*, 181–200.

Feiring, C. (1999). Other-sex friendship networks and the development of romantic relationships in adolescence. *Journal of Youth and Adolescence, 28*, 495–512.

Feldman, S. S., & Gowen, L. K. (1998). Conflict negotiation tactics in romantic relationships in high school students. *Journal of Youth and Adolescence, 27*, 691–717.

Franzoi, S. L., Davis, M. H., & Vasquez-Suson, K. A. (1994). Two social worlds: Social correlates and stability of adolescent status groups. *Journal of Personality and Social Psychology, 67*, 462–473.

Friedlander, L. J., Connolly, J. A., Pepler, D. J., & Craig, W. M. (2007). Biological, familial, and peer influences on dating in early adolescence. *Archives of Sexual Behavior, 36*, 821–830.

Furman, W., & Buhrmester, D. (1992). Age and sex differences in perceptions of networks of personal relationships. *Child Development, 63,* 103–115.

Furman, W., & Hand, L. S. (2006). The slippery nature of romantic relationships: Issues in definition and differentiation. In A. C. Crouter, & A. Booth (Eds.), *Romance and sex in adolescence and emerging adulthood: Risks and opportunities* (pp. 171–178). Mahwah, NJ: Erlbaum.

Furman, W., Low, S., & Ho, M. J. (2009). Romantic experience and psychosocial adjustment in middle adolescence. *Journal of Clinical Child and Adolescent Psychology, 38,* 75–90.

Furman, W., & Shomaker, L. B. (2008). Patterns of interaction in adolescent romantic relationships: Distinct features and links to other close relationships. *Journal of Adolescence, 31,* 771–788.

Furman, W., & Simon, V. A. (1999). Cognitive representations of adolescent romantic relationships. In W. Furman, B. Brown, & C. Feiring (Eds.), *The development of romantic relationships in adolescence* (pp. 75–98). New York: Cambridge University Press.

Furman, W., Simon, V. A., Shaffer, L., & Bouchey, H. A. (2002). Adolescents' working models and styles for relationships with parents, friends, and romantic partners. *Child Development, 73,* 241–255.

Furman, W., & Wehner, E. (1994). Romantic views: Toward a theory of adolescent romantic relationships. In R. Montemayor, G. R. Adams, & T. P. Gullotta (Eds.), *Personal relationships during adolescence* (Vol. 6, pp. 168–195). Thousand Oaks, CA: Sage.

Galliher, R. V., Rostosky, S. S., Welsh, D. P., & Kawaguchi, M. C. (1999). Power and psychological well-being in late adolescent relationships. *Sex Roles, 40,* 689–710.

Giuliani, C., Iafrate, R., & Rosnati, R. (1998). Peer-group and romantic relationships in adolescents from intact and separated families. *Contemporary Family Therapy: An International Journal, 20*(1), 93–105.

Glover, J. A., Galliher, R. V., & Lamere, T. G. (2009). Identity development and exploration among sexual minority adolescents: Examination of a multidimensional model. *Journal of Homosexuality, 56,* 77–101.

Grover, R. L., Nangle, D. W., & Zeff, K. R. (2005). The measure of adolescent heterosocial competence: Development and initial validation. *Journal of Clinical Child and Adolescent Psychology, 34*(2), 282–291.

Harper, M. S., Dickson, J. W., & Welsh, D. P. (2006). Self-silencing and rejection sensitivity in adolescent romantic relationships. *Journal of Youth and Adolescence, 35,* 459–467.

Haugen, P. T., Welsh, D. P., & McNulty, J. K. (2008). Empathic accuracy and adolescent romantic relationships. *Journal of Adolescence, 31*(6), 709–727.

Haynie, D. L., Giordano, P. C., Manning, W. D., & Longmore, M. A. (2005). Adolescent romantic relationships and delinquency involvement. *Criminology: An Interdisciplinary Journal, 43*(1), 177–210.

Hazan, C., & Shaver, P. (1987). Romantic love conceptualized as an attachment process. *Journal of Personality and Social Psychology, 52,* 511–524.

Jackson, S., Jacob, M. N., Landman-Peeters, K., & Lanting, A. (2001). Cognitive strategies employed in trying to arrange a first date. *Journal of Adolescence, 24,* 267–279.

Joyner, K., & Udry, J. R. (2000). You don't bring me anything but down: Adolescent romance and depression. *Journal of Health and Social Behavior, 41,* 369–391.

Kan, M. L., McHale, S. M., & Crouter, A. C. (2008). Parental involvement in adolescent romantic relationships: Patterns and correlates. *Journal of Youth and Adolescence, 37,* 168–179.

Kuttler, A. F., & La Greca, A. M. (2004). Linkages among adolescent girls' romantic relationships, best friendships, and peer networks. *Journal of Adolescence, 27,* 395–414.

Kuttler, A. F., La Greca, A. M., & Prinstein, M. J. (1999). Friendship qualities and social–emotional functioning of adolescents with close, cross-sex friendships. *Journal for Research on Adolescence, 9,* 339–366.

La Greca, A. M., & Harrison, H. M. (2005). Adolescent peer relations, friendships, and romantic relationships: Do they predict social anxiety and depression? *Journal of Clinical Child and Adolescent Psychology, 34,* 49–61.

Larson, R., Clore, G. L., & Wood, G. (1999). The emotions and romantic relationships: Do they wreak havoc on adolescents? In W. Furman, B. Brown, & C. Feiring (Eds.), *The development of romantic relationships in adolescence* (pp. 19–49). New York: Cambridge University Press.

Lau, M., Markham, C., Lin, H., Flores, G., & Chacko, M. R. (2009). Dating and sexual attitudes in Asian-American adolescents. *Journal of Adolescent Research, 24,* 91–113.

Laursen, B., Furman, W., & Mooney, K. S. (2006). Predicting interpersonal competence and self-worth from adolescent relationships and relationship networks: Variable-centered and person-centered perspectives. *Merrill–Palmer Quarterly, 52,* 572–600.

Laursen, B., & Williams, V. A. (1997). Perceptions of interdependence and closeness in family and peer relationships among adolescents with and without romantic partners. In S. Shulman & W. A. Collins (Eds.), *Romantic relationships in adolescence: Developmental perspectives* (pp. 3–20). San Francisco: Jossey-Bass.

Lonardo, R. A., Giordano, P. C., Longmore, M. A., & Manning, W. D. (2009). Parents, friends, and romantic partners: Enmeshment in deviant networks and adolescent delinquency involvement. *Journal of Youth and Adolescence, 38,* 367–383.

Longmore, M. A., Manning, W. D., & Giordano, P. C. (2001). Preadolescent parenting strategies and teens' dating and sexual initiation: A longitudinal analysis. *Journal of Marriage and the Family, 63,* 322–335.

Madsen, S. D. (2008). Parents' management of adolescents' romantic relationships through dating rules: Gender variations and correlates of relationship qualities. *Journal of Youth and Adolescence, 37,* 1044–1058.

Magnusson, D., Stattin, H., & Allen, V. L. (1985). Biological maturation and social development: A longitudinal study of some adjustment processes from mid-adolescence to adulthood. *Journal of Youth and Adolescence, 14,* 267–283.

Manning, W. D., Giordano, P. C., & Longmore, M. A. (2006). Hooking up: The relationship contexts of "nonrelationship" sex. *Journal of Adolescent Research, 21,* 459–483.

Martin, B. (1990). The transmission of relationship difficulties from one generation to the next. *Journal of Youth and Adolescence, 19,* 181–200.

Mayseless, O., & Scharf, M. (2007). Adolescents' attachment representations and their capacity for intimacy in close relationships. *Journal of Research on Adolescence, 17,* 23–50.

McIsaac, C., Connolly, J. A., McKenney, K. S., Pepler, D., & Craig, W. (2008). Conflict negotiation and autonomy processes in adolescent romantic relationships, *Journal of Adolescence, 31,* 691–707.

Meeus, W. H. J., Branje, S. J. T., van der Valk, I., & de Wiede, M. (2007). Relationships with intimate partner, best friend, and parents in adolescence and early adulthood: A study of the saliency of the intimate partnership. *International Journal of Behavioral Development, 31,* 569–580.

Meier, A., & Allen, G. (2009). Romantic relationships from adolescence to young adulthood: Evidence from the National Longitudinal Study of Adolescent Health. *Sociological Quarterly, 50,* 308–335.

Monahan, K. C., & Lee, J. M. (2008). Adolescent sexual activity: Links between relational context and depressive symptoms. *Journal of Youth and Adolescence, 37,* 917–927.

Monroe, S. M., Rohde, P., Seeley, J. R., & Lewinsohn, P. M. (1999). Life events and depression in adolescence: Relationship loss as a prospective risk factor for first onset of major depressive disorder. *Journal of Abnormal Psychology, 108,* 606–614.

Natsuaki, M. N., Biehl, M. C., & Ge, X. (2009).Trajectories of depressed mood from early adolescence to young adulthood: The effects of pubertal timing and adolescent dating. *Journal of Research on Adolescence, 19,* 47–74.

Neemann, J., Hubbard, J., & Masten, A. S. (1995). The changing importance of romantic relationship involvement to competence from late childhood to late adolescence. *Development and Psychopathology, 7,* 727–750.

O'Leary, K. D., & Slep, A. M. S. (2003). A dyadic longitudinal model of adolescent dating aggression. *Journal of Clinical Child and Adolescent Psychology, 32,* 314–327.

O'Sullivan, L. F., & Meyer-Bahlburg, H. F. (2003). African American and Latina inner-city girls' reports of romantic and sexual development . *Journal of Social and Personal Relationships, 20,* 221–238.

Pellegrini, A. D., & Long, J. D. (2007). An observational study of early heterosexual interaction at middle school dances. *Journal of Research on Adolescence, 17,* 613–638.

Phinney, V. G., Jensen, L. C., Olsen, J. A., & Cundick, B. (1990). The relationship between early development and psychosexual behaviors in adolescent females. *Adolescence, 25,* 321–332.

Raley, R. K., Crissey, S., & Muller, C. (2007). Of sex and romance: Late adolescent relationships and young adult union formation. *Journal of Marriage and Family, 69,* 1210–1226.

Reese-Weber, M., & Bartle-Haring, S. (1998). Conflict resolution styles in family subsystems and adolescent romantic relationships. *Journal of Youth and Adolescence, 27,* 735–752.

Reese-Weber, M., & Kahn, J. H. (2005). Familial predictors of sibling and romantic-partner conflict resolution: Comparing late adolescents from intact and divorced families. *Journal of Adolescence, 28,* 479–493.

Reese-Weber, M., & Marchand, J. F. (2002). Family and individual predictors of late adolescents' romantic relationships. *Journal of Youth and Adolescence, 31,* 197–206.

Rizzo, C. J., Daley, S. E., & Gunderson, B. H. (2006). Interpersonal sensitivity, romantic stress, and the prediction of depression: A study of inner-city, minority adolescent girls. *Journal of Youth and Adolescence, 35,* 469–478.

Roisman, G. I., Madsen, S. D., Hennighausen, K. H., Sroufe, L. A., & Collins, W. A. (2001). The coherence of dyadic behaviour across parent–child and romantic relationships as mediated by the internalized representation of experience. *Attachment and Human Development, 3,* 156–172.

Roth, M. A., & Parker, J. G. (2001). Affective and behavioural responses to friends who neglect their friends for dating partners: Influences of gender, jealousy and perspective. *Journal of Adolescence, 24,* 281–296.

Russell, S. T., & Consolacion, T. B. (2003). Adolescent romance and emotional health in the United States: Beyond binaries. *Journal of Clinical Child and Adolescent Psychology, 32,* 499–508.

Scharf, M., & Mayseless, O. (2001). The capacity for romantic intimacy: Exploring the contribution of best friend and marital and parental relationships. *Journal of Adolescence, 24,* 379–399.

Scharf, M., & Mayseless, O. (2008). Late adolescent girls' relationships with parents and romantic partner: The distinct role of mothers and fathers. *Journal of Adolescence, 31,* 837–855.

Seiffge-Krenke, I. (2000). Diversity in romantic relations of adolescents with varying health status: Links to intimacy in close friendships. *Journal of Adolescent Research, 15,* 611–636.

Seiffge-Krenke, I. (2003). Testing theories of romantic development from adolescence to young adulthood: Evidence of a developmental sequence. *International Journal of Behavioral Development, 27,* 519–531.

Seiffge-Krenke, I., Shulman, S., & Klessinger, N. (2001). Adolescent precursors of romantic relationships in young adulthood. *Journal of Social and Personal Relationships, 18,* 327–346.

Shulman, S. (2003). Conflict and negotiation in adolescent romantic relationships. In P. Florsheim (Ed.), *Adolescent romantic relations and sexual behavior: Theory, research, and practical implications* (pp. 109–135). Mahwah, NJ: Erlbaum.

Shulman, S., & Scharf, M. (2000). Adolescent romantic behaviors and perceptions: Age- and gender-related differences, and links with family and peer relationships. *Journal of Research on Adolescence, 10,* 99–118.

Shulman, S., Tuval-Mashiach, R., Levran, E., & Anbar, S. (2006). Conflict resolution patterns and longevity of adolescent romantic couples: A 2-year follow-up study. *Journal of Adolescence, 29,* 575–588.

Shute, R., & Charlton, K. (2006). Anger or compromise?: Adolescents' conflict resolution strategies in relation to gender and type of peer relationship. *International Journal of Adolescence and Youth, 13,* 55–69.

Simon, V. A., Aikins, J. W., & Prinstein, M. J. (2008). Romantic partner selection and socialization during early adolescence. *Child Development, 79,* 1676–1692.

Simon, V. A., Kobielski, S. J., & Martin, S. (2008). Conflict beliefs, goals, and behavior in romantic relationships during late adolescence. *Journal of Youth and Adolescence, 37,* 324–355.

Simpson, J. A., Collins, W. A., Tran, S., & Haydon, K. C. (2007). Attachment and the experience and expression of emotions in romantic relationships: A developmental perspective. *Journal of Personality and Social Psychology, 92,* 355–367.

Smetana, J. G., & Gettman, D. C. (2006). Autonomy and relatedness with parents and romantic development in African American adolescents. *Developmental Psychology, 42,* 1347–1351.

Smiler, A. P. (2008). "I wanted to get to know her better": Adolescent boys' dating motives, masculinity ideology, and sexual behavior. *Journal of Adolescence, 31,* 17–32.

Smolak, L., Levine, M. P., & Gralen, S. (1993). The impact of puberty and dating on eating problems among middle school girls. *Journal of Youth and Adolescence, 22*, 355–368.

Stattin, H., & Magnusson, D. (1990). *Pubertal maturation in female development* (Vol. 2). Hillsdale, NJ: Erlbaum.

Steinberg, S. J., Davila, J., & Fincham, F. (2006). Adolescent marital expectations and romantic experiences: Associations with perceptions about parental conflict and adolescent attachment security. *Journal of Youth and Adolescence, 35*, 333–348.

Sternberg, R. J. (1986). A triangular theory of love. *Psychological Review, 93*, 119–135.

Stocker, C. M., & Richmond, M. K. (2007). Longitudinal associations between hostility in adolescents' family relationships and friendships and hostility in their romantic relationships. *Journal of Family Psychology, 21*, 490–497.

Susman, E. J., Nottelmann, E. D., Inoff, G. E., Dorn, L. D., Cutler, G. B, Loriaux, D.L., et al. (1985). The relation of hormone levels and physical development and social–emotional behavior in young adolescents. *Journal of Youth and Adolescence, 14*, 245–252.

Taradash, A., Connolly, J., Pepler, D., Craig, W., & Costa, M. (2001). The interpersonal context of romantic autonomy in adolescence. *Journal of Adolescence, 24*, 365–377.

Tolman, D., Spencer, R., Harmon, Y., Rosen-Reynoso, M., & Striepe, M. (2004). Getting close, staying cool: Early adolescent boys' experiences with romantic relationships. In N. Way & J. Chu (Eds.), *Adolescent boys: Exploring diverse cultures of boyhood* (pp. 235–255). New York: New York University Press.

Tuval-Mashiach, R., Walsh, S., Harel, S., & Shulman, S. (2008). Romantic fantasies, cross-gender friendships, and romantic experiences in adolescence. *Journal of Adolescent Research, 23*, 471–487.

van Schaick, K., & Stolberg, A. L. (2001). The impact of paternal involvement and parental divorce on young adults' intimate relationships. *Journal of Divorce and Remarriage, 36*, 99–122.

Williams, T., Connolly, J. A., & Cribbie, R. (2008). Light and heavy heterosexual activities of young Canadian adolescents: Normative patterns and differential predictors. *Journal of Research on Adolescence, 18*, 145–172.

Young, A. M., & d'Arcy, H. (2005). Older boyfriends of adolescent girls: The cause or a sign of the problem? *Journal of Adolescent Mental Health, 36*, 410–419.

Zimmer-Gembeck, M. J., & Helfand, M. (2008). Ten years of longitudinal research on U.S. adolescent sexual behavior: Developmental correlates of sexual intercourse and the importance of age, gender and ethnic background. *Developmental Review, 28*(2), 153–224.

Zimmer-Gembeck, M. J., Siebenbruner, J., & Collins, W. A. (2001). Diverse aspects of dating: Associations with psychosocial functioning from early to middle adolescence. *Journal of Adolescence, 24*, 313–336.

Part III

Social Behaviors

9

Aggression

Marion K. Underwood

A group of guys started teasing me in the locker room after practice and
pushed me up against the locker. I asked them to stop but they started
slapping me around and teasing me more. They spit on my equipment. They
acted like it was all a joke, but I was beat up pretty badly and it really hurt.

We would leave one girl out of our group on purpose nearly every day, just
because we were jerks and wanted to be mean. This happened to be my day.
All of my friends wouldn't talk to me, gave me nasty looks, and wouldn't
let me sit with them at lunch.
— *College students recalling peer maltreatment in middle school*
(in Rosen et al., 2011)

When children are angry with their peers or wish to pursue their social goals,
they may engage in aggressive behaviors that cause physical and social harm. Physical aggression emerges in the second year of life and is frequent during the early preschool period (Tremblay et al., 1999). Physical aggression decreases for most children
with development (Dodge, Coie, & Lynam, 2006). Social aggression is behavior that
harms others' friendships and social status by social exclusion, gossip, and friendship manipulation (Underwood, 2003). Social aggression emerges in the preschool
period (Crick, Casas, & Mosher, 1997; McNeilly-Choque, Hart, Robinson, Nelson,
& Olsen, 1996), may be normative at low levels in the elementary and early junior high
school years (Underwood, Galen, & Paquette, 2001), and decreases for most children
as they develop (Underwood, Beron, & Rosen, 2009). However, a few individuals follow high and rising trajectories for physical and social aggression, and high levels of
physical and social aggression in childhood predict negative outcomes in adolescence
and beyond (Dodge, Coie, et al., 2006; Crick, Ostrov, & Kawabata, 2007; Underwood, Beron, & Rosen, 2011).

This chapter provides an overview of the development of physical and social aggression. First, the chapter considers the challenging issues of definitions and subtypes. Next, aggression and gender are discussed. The remainder of the chapter is organized developmentally, presenting the research evidence for what we know about physical and social aggression in preschool, middle childhood, and adolescence. Each section begins with information about the typical forms and frequencies of aggression in each developmental period. Next, subsections present evidence for possible origins of individual differences and developmental outcomes associated with chronic aggression. The chapter ends with a discussion of prevention and intervention to reduce aggressive behavior in children and pressing questions for future research.

DEFINITIONS AND SUBTYPES

More than 200 definitions of aggression exist in the research literature, but they all share two features: (1) perpetrators must intend to harm and (2) victims must feel hurt (Harré & Lamb, 1983). These criteria hold for behaviors that cause social, as well as physical, harm (Crick, Bigbee, & Howes, 1996; Galen & Underwood, 1997; Underwood, 2003). These criteria also apply to reactive aggression, which is angry, impulsive, and motivated by frustration, as well as to instrumental aggression, which is more cool and deliberate and serves to achieve social goals (Dodge & Coie, 1987). Investigators have proposed numerous subtypes of aggression, perhaps in part because aggression is such a broad construct, and research has yielded conflicting findings on such basic issues as whether aggression is always done in anger or must always cause physical harm. Subtypes of aggression abound (Underwood et al., 2001) and include the following: antisocial versus prosocial (Sears, 1961), physical versus verbal (Buss, 1961), indirect versus direct (Buss, 1961; Bjorkqvist, Osterman, & Kaukiainen, 1992; Feshbach, 1969; Frodi, Macaulay & Thome, 1977), targeted versus targetless (Buss, 1961), instrumental versus hostile (Feshbach, 1964), attack versus defense (Feshbach, 1964), expressive (Maccoby & Jacklin, 1974), reactive versus proactive (Dodge & Coie, 1987), institutional (Bjorkqvist & Niemela, 1992), rational versus manipulative (Bjorkqvist, Osterman, & Kaukiainen, 1992), physical versus social (Cairns, Cairns, Neckerman, Gest, & Gariepy, 1988; Galen & Underwood, 1997; Paquette & Underwood, 1999), overt versus relational (Crick, 1996; Crick & Grotpeter, 1995; Crick et al., 1996), physical versus nonphysical (Rys & Bear, 1997), psychological versus physical (Capaldi & Crosby, 1997), and reputational as opposed to overt and relational (Prinstein & Cillessen, 2003).

Fully considering this dizzying array of subtypes is beyond the scope of this chapter. This chapter focuses on physical and social aggression. A wealth of empirical evidence suggests that physical aggression predicts negative outcomes for children (Dodge, Coie, et al., 2006). Studying social aggression holds promise for understanding anger and aggression among girls (Crick & Zahn-Waxler, 2003; Underwood, 2003). This chapter uses the term *social aggression* (instead of relational or indirect aggression) because social aggression is conceptualized as including all behaviors that do social harm, whether the behavior is direct or indirect, verbal or nonverbal (Archer & Coyne, 2005). Because the constructs of indirect, social, and relational aggression overlap and no consensus has emerged as to the best term, this chapter includes previous research on indirect and relational, as well as social, aggression, but I use the term *social aggression* throughout so as to avoid confusion.

Although physical aggression is strongly associated with other antisocial behaviors, such as delinquency and substance abuse (Dodge, Coie, et al., 2006), the focus here is squarely on aggression directed toward peers. This chapter attempts to tell a precise developmental story that will be more coherent if it emphasizes one class of behavior instead of diverse forms of rule breaking, and aggression itself is a broad construct.

AGGRESSION AND GENDER

Understanding aggression in childhood requires careful consideration of gender. Aggression is forbidden behavior often born of anger, and girls are socialized more strongly against overt expressions of anger than are boys from young ages (Underwood, 2003; Zahn-Waxler & Polanichka, 2004). Forms of aggression are related to gender stereotypes that preschoolers understand (Giles & Heyman, 2005), stereotypes that characterize boys as hitting and girls as gossiping and excluding.

Men and boys engage in more physical aggression than girls and women do (Dodge, Coie, et al., 2006), but some girls fight physically. Physically aggressive girls, though fewer in number, are at risk for many of the same negative outcomes as physically aggressive boys are (Underwood & Coie, 2004), and physically aggressive girls and boys follow similar developmental trajectories (Gorman-Smith & Loeber, 2005; Martino, Ellickson, Klein, McCaffrey, & Edelen, 2008).

Gender differences in other forms of aggression are less clear. Although girls engage in social aggression more than they do physical aggression (Osterman et al., 1998), this does not necessarily mean that girls are more socially aggressive than boys are. Perhaps because social aggression is so consistent with gender stereotypes of girls as backbiting, it has been tempting to assume that girls are more socially aggressive than boys are. Experts have made strong claims that girls and boys are equally aggressive but that their aggressive behavior takes different forms (Crick et al., 1999), that "girls manipulate and boys fight" (Bjorkqvist, Lagenspetz, & Kaukiainen, 1992, p. 117). However, gender differences in social aggression have been inconsistent and depend on the rater and the age of the children (Archer, 2004). A recent, exhaustive meta-analysis found that the gender difference in social aggression favoring girls, though significant, is so small as to be trivial and that gender does not moderate the relations between either form of aggression and adjustment (Card, Stucky, Sawalani, & Little, 2008). Though girls and boys may not differ significantly on frequency of social aggression, gender may relate to social aggression in even more important ways, such as the social processes by which it unfolds (Underwood, 2003). This review highlights how the social processes, functions, and consequences of aggressive behavior may differ for girls and boys.

PHYSICAL AGGRESSION IN THE PRESCHOOL YEARS

Physical aggression begins early in life. Mothers report that 80% of 17-month-olds engage in physical aggression, including taking things from others (74%), pushing (46%), biting (24%), kicking (24%), fighting (23%), threatening to hit (23%), and physically attacking (21%; Tremblay et al., 1999). Given that physical aggression seems to be so frequent as to be almost developmentally normative at this stage, the most important question to ask may be why most children desist in physical aggression as they mature (Tremblay et al., 1999). As Dodge (2006) has proposed, responding angrily to perceived provocation is universal, and thus "a basic task of life is to learn to behave non-aggressively" (p. 793).

Although many children engage in physical aggression in the second year of life, individuals follow different trajectories for physical aggression as they mature. Trajectory analyses of a large study of a nationally representative U.S. sample found five trajectory groups on the basis of mothers' reports of physical aggression from ages 2 through 9: very low (45%), low (25%), moderate but declining (12%), moderate (15%), and high (3%; NICHD Early Child Care Research Network, 2004). For the moderate and high groups, levels of physical aggression remained stable from ages 2 through 5, but declined slightly thereafter.

Origins and Explanations

Early individual differences in physical aggression may be linked to genetics and temperament. Behavioral geneticists estimate that childhood physical aggression is approximately 60% heritable (Moffitt, 2005). Molecular genetics research suggests that genetic vulnerabilities may moderate effects of children's life experiences to determine which children begin to engage in violence. Maltreated children who have low levels of monoamine oxidase A (MAOA) activity due to a polymorphism on the MAOA gene are more likely to develop aggressive, violent behaviors in adolescence and adulthood than maltreated children with high MAOA expression (Caspi et al., 2002). Genes may influence behavior by influencing structural features of the brain; the MAOA polymorphism relates to reduced volume in the amygdala and in the ventral prefrontal cortex, both of which have been shown to relate to antisocial behavior (Raine, 2008). Genes may also affect individual differences in aggression via temperament, that is, inherited personality characteristics evident early in life (Buss & Plomin, 1984). Several temperamental dimensions have been linked to emerging aggression in childhood: fearlessness, poor self-regulation, and irritability (Kingston & Prior, 1995; Lengua, West, & Sandler, 1998).

Parenting also influences which children continue or increase their physical aggression during the preschool years. Children following high developmental trajectories for aggression from ages 2 through 9 are more likely to come from lower-income families, to have less educated mothers, and to have parents who are observed to be less sensitive and responsive (NICHD, 2004). Parents who may be overwhelmed by their young child's difficult temperament and noncompliance may respond to the child's negative behaviors by engaging in coercive cycles, responding increasingly harshly to escalating noncompliance, then giving in to the child's demands, thereby reinforcing the intensely noncompliant behavior (Patterson, 1982). Parents' engagement in coercive cycles with children predicts aggression and antisocial behavior during childhood and adolescence (Patterson, 1986). Parents' use of physical discipline predicts higher levels of children's externalizing problems for European American children but lower levels of externalizing problems for African American children, perhaps because African American families understand physical discipline as protective and as a way of teaching (Lansford, Deater-Deckard, Dodge, Bates, & Pettit, 2004). More general parenting styles have also been linked to individual differences in early childhood aggression; parents who use an authoritarian style with low warmth and high punitiveness have young children who are higher on physical aggression with peers (Baumrind, 1989; Hart, DeWolf, & Burts, 1992; see also Holden, Vittrup, & Rosen, Chapter 6, this volume).

Gender likely also influences individual differences in aggression. From early in life, parents socialize girls more than boys to refrain from expressing anger overtly (see Zahn-Waxler & Polanichka, 2004, for a review). Gender differences are not evident in physical aggression during toddlerhood (Loeber & Hay, 1997), but they may emerge during the preschool years (Coie & Dodge, 1998) as children begin to interact with peers. Children begin to segregate by gender in the second year of life (Serbin, Moller, Gulko, Powlishta, & Colburne, 1994) and may start to socialize each other in different peer cultures (Maccoby, 1998). For boys, this may lead to greater encouragement for physical aggression. Time spent playing with same-gender peers predicts increases in gender-stereotyped behaviors, which for boys leads to increases in active, rough play (Martin & Fabes, 2001). Young children play with peers who have similar levels of physical aggression (Farver, 1996; Snyder, Horsch, & Childs, 1997). When boys and girls who have difficulty regulating emotions spend large amounts of time playing with other boys, their problem behaviors increase, including aggression (Fabes, Shepard, Guthrie, & Martin, 1997).

Girls may also desist in physical aggression because they know that girls are not supposed to fight, because they spend much time in the company of other girls who share this view, and because, when girls do aggress physically, they are unlikely to influence their peers. When observed in preschool classrooms, girls' physically aggressive behaviors are less likely to influence peers (Fagot & Hagan, 1985). For girls, the onset of gender labeling is related to decreased physical aggression with peers, but this relation is not observed for boys (Fagot, Leinbach, & Hagan, 1986). Preschool children understand that boys are likely to be more physically aggressive than girls (Giles & Heyman, 2005).

Developmental Consequences

Even in the preschool years, when physical aggression may be somewhat typical, high rates of physical aggression are related to peer difficulties. Observational evidence suggests that engaging in physical aggression is often immediately followed by rejecting behaviors from peers (Arnold, Hanrock, Ortiz, & Stowe, 1999). The rejecting behaviors convey dislike or exclusion and are similar to social aggression, but they may also be natural responses to being hurt by others. Peer nomination studies find that both physical and social aggression are related to peer rejection in preschool classrooms (Crick et al., 1997; see also Bukowski, Buhrmester, & Underwood, Chapter 7, this volume).

High levels of physical aggression in the preschool years also predict difficulties with the transition to kindergarten and elementary school. Children observed to be highly aggressive in preschool are more likely to be rejected by peers in kindergarten and to be viewed as hostile and aggressive by teachers (Ladd & Price, 1987; Ladd & Burgess, 1999). Peer rejection during the kindergarten year predicts negative perceptions of school, school avoidance, and lower levels of academic achievement by the end of the school year (Ladd, 1990).

However, person-centered analyses that examined groups of children following different developmental trajectories for physical aggression found that not all children who were aggressive in preschool had problems later (NICHD Early Child Care Research Network, 2004). Children with moderate levels of preschool aggression that had declined by age 5 were not at increased risk of social and academic problems in third grade, whereas those following the moderate but not decreasing or high trajectories were at higher risk of mother–child conflict, academic problems, lower social competence with peers and parents, and higher levels of behavior problems in third grade.

SOCIAL AGGRESSION IN THE PRESCHOOL YEARS

Social aggression emerges as early as age 3 (Crick et al., 1997; McNeilly-Choque et al., 1996). Statements that reflect typical forms of preschool social aggression include: "won't invite someone to their birthday party if they can't have their own way," "won't let a kid play in the group if they are mad at the kid," "tell other kids that they can't play with the group unless they do what the group wants them to do," and "won't listen to someone when they are mad at them, might even cover their ears" (Crick et al., 1997, p. 583). Few studies have examined growth and change in social aggression across the preschool period, but one longitudinal study of social aggression as assessed by maternal reports found that a subgroup high on social aggression increased in this behavior from age 4 to age 6 (Vaillancourt, Miller, Fagbemi, Cote, & Tremblay, 2007).

Origins and Explanations

Much less is known about the early developmental origins of individual differences in social aggression. Although few investigations have examined early biological factors that might contribute to growth in social aggression, one study found that stress reactivity as indexed by rises in cortisol across the child-care day was positively related to social aggression for both girls and boys (Dettling, Gunnar, & Donzella, 1999).

As has been found for physical aggression, early social aggression may be related to harsh parenting. For a sample of Russian preschoolers, social aggression as reported by teachers was negatively related to paternal responsiveness for boys and to maternal coercion for girls (Hart, Nelson, Robinson, Olsen, & McNeilly-Choque, 1998). A study with Chinese preschoolers found that children's social aggression as reported by teachers was related to parents' psychological control (Nelson, Hart, Yang, Olsen, & Jin, 2006).

Because engaging in most forms of social aggression requires the use of language, as children become more verbally sophisticated, they become more likely to engage in social aggression and less likely to aggress physically because the risk for punishment is great (Bjorkqvist, 1994). Interestingly, preschool children's skill in using language positively predicts engaging in social aggression as rated by teachers (Bonica, Arnold, Fisher, Zeljo, & Yershova, 2003).

Developmental Consequences

Researchers are only beginning to examine how social aggression in preschool relates to psychological adjustment. For both girls and boys, peer nominations of social aggression were related to peer rejection, but for boys, teacher-rated social aggression was positively related to peer acceptance (Crick et al., 1997). For girls only, teacher ratings of social aggression were positively correlated with teacher ratings of depression. Another preschool study found that observed proactive social aggression predicted peer rejection 4–5 months later (though reactive social aggression did not) and that both proactive and reactive social aggression predicted increases in student–teacher conflict (Ostrov & Crick, 2007).

PHYSICAL AGGRESSION IN MIDDLE CHILDHOOD

As children move through elementary school, most follow decreasing trajectories for physical aggression (Dodge, Coie, et al., 2006). However, a subgroup remains high and increases in physical aggression across this period (Broidy et al., 2003). In the Child Development Project that followed a U.S. sample from ages 6 through 12, 64% of boys followed a stable low trajectory for physical aggression as assessed by teacher ratings, 29% followed a stable moderate trajectory, and 7% followed a high and rising trajectory (Broidy et al., 2003).

Origins and Explanations

Early risk factors that contribute to growth in physical aggression in the preschool years likely continue to operate in middle childhood. Genes continue to influence brain structure in ways that may influence aggressive and antisocial behavior (Raine, 2008), genetic vulnerabilities continue to interact with life experiences to determine who becomes violent (Caspi et al., 2002), and children with difficult temperaments may continue to have their extreme noncompliance unintentionally reinforced by parents who get locked into coercive interchanges with children (Patterson, 1986). Children who engage in aggressive and other antisocial behaviors prior to adolescence have been characterized as "early starter" or "life-course-persistent" antisocial youths and are hypothesized to be at greater risk for antisocial behavior into adulthood (Moffitt, 1993; Moffitt et al., 2008; Patterson, DeBaryshe, & Ramsey, 1989).

Children's exposure to parents' marital conflict also confers risk for aggression and for other behavior problems (Parke et al., 2001). Parents' and 7- to 13-year-olds' reports of interparental conflict were related to children's aggression as rated by parents and teachers, and this relation was mediated by the child's having an aggressogenic cognitive style (endorsing aggression as an appropriate strategy for resolving conflicts; Marcus, Lindahl, & Malik, 2001). Children's behavior problems are likely most influenced by interparental conflicts that are intense or physical or that involve the silent treatment and withdrawal (Cummings, Davies, & Campbell, 2000). There may be same-gender modeling effects (Snyder, 1998), such that girls' aggression is more strongly related to mothers' negative conflict strategies and boys' aggression is more strongly related to fathers' use of coercive strategies.

Harsh, punitive parenting continues to confer risk for physical aggression during middle childhood. Mothers' use of power-assertive discipline is associated with first and fourth graders' endorsing negative strategies for resolving peer conflicts (Hart, Ladd, & Burleson, 1990). Physical discipline, even spanking alone, confers risk for physical aggression on the kindergarten playground (Strassberg, Dodge, Pettit, & Bates, 1994). A summer camp study with maltreated and comparison groups found that physical abuse predicted increases in physical aggression with peers for both girls and boys (Cullerton-Sen et al., 2008). Children whose parents physically abuse them are more likely to develop a hostile attribution bias, a tendency to view ambiguous social stimuli as hostile (Dodge, Bates, & Pettit, 1990), which in turn relates to a propensity for aggressive behavior because children retaliate against misperceived slights (Dodge, 2006).

Attributing hostile intent to others' challenging behaviors has been linked to reactive physical aggression in over 100 studies (Dodge, 2006). Many young children infer hostile intent from behaviors that cause them harm, but, via socialization, they are helped to make more benign attributions. However, some children may develop persistent hostile attribution biases as a result of neurological tendencies toward impulsivity and of socialization by the environment, including physical abuse, modeling of hostile attributions, insecure attachment, and growing up in a culture that emphasizes retaliation and defending one's honor (Dodge, 2006). Children's hostile attribution biases contribute to growth in physical aggression, even when controlling for parental harsh discipline and prior aggressive behavior (Dodge, Pettit, Bates, & Valente, 1995). Compelling evidence for a causal relation between hostile attribution biases and physical aggression comes from intervention studies that show that teaching children to make more positive attributions in the face of peer provocation results in decreases in aggressive behavior (Dodge, 2006; Hudley & Graham, 1993).

Just as in preschool, children's peers influence their tendencies to engage in physical aggression during middle childhood, when children care desperately about fitting in and getting along with their same-sex peer groups (Gottman & Mettetal, 1986). Early elementary students in classrooms with higher ratios of aggressive peers increase in their physical aggression across time (Kellam, Ling, Merisca, Brown, & Ialongo, 1998). Peer-group socialization of aggression, or any other behaviors, may operate via two mechanisms: Children may be drawn together in social groups because of their similarity on important characteristics, but once groups are formed, peers in groups may actively socialize each other to become more similar in behavior (Cairns & Cairns, 1994; Kindermann, 1993). Highly aggressive peers tend to form social groups with each other (Cairns et al., 1988; Espelage, Holt, & Henkel, 2003). Belonging to peer groups high in physical aggression predicts growth in physical aggression across the late-middle-childhood to early-adolescent age ranges, and peer socialization of aggression is stronger in high-status, visible groups (Ellis & Zarbatany, 2007; Espelage et al., 2003). As noted by Ellis and Zarbatany (2007), "The advantageous position enjoyed by central groups may encourage dominance-related skills that help maintain status and access to valued resources such as space, equipment, and attention from peers" (p. 1253).

Another likely influence on growth in physical aggression during middle childhood is media violence. Decades of research show that viewing aggression on television and in movies is related to aggressive behavior in children (Huesmann, Moise-Titus, Podolski, & Eron, 2003). Exposure to media violence likely contributes to short-term increases in aggression due to priming and to longer-term growth in aggression by offering daily opportunities for observational learning of cognitions that facilitate aggression (Huesmann, 1998). Viewing television violence from ages 6 through 10 predicted increased physical aggression in adulthood (Huesmann et al., 2003). Meta-analytic reviews have found that the correlation between exposure to media violence and children's aggression is .32, which means that watching violent media accounts for about 10% of the variance in childhood aggression (Paik & Comstock, 1994), one of the most robust effects in developmental psychology (Coie & Dodge, 1998). The relation between exposure to media violence and childhood aggression is comparable in magnitude to that between cigarette smoking and lung cancer (Bushman & Anderson, 2001). Some children are more susceptible to the effects of television violence than others, including children with parents who are rigid or indifferent and children with poor social relationships, poor psychological adjustment, and diagnoses of disruptive behavior disorders (Comstock, 2008).

Developmental Consequences

As greater numbers of children desist in physical aggression across the preschool and early elementary years, those who persist in fighting continue to suffer negative consequences. Children high on physical aggression are at risk for low academic achievement. Children following a high physical aggression trajectory from ages 2 through 9 had lower achievement test scores in third grade and were observed to have lower classroom engagement than children low on aggression, but many of these group differences disappeared when demographic characteristics such as ethnicity and family income were controlled (NICHD Early Child Care Research Network, 2004). Physically aggressive children may struggle with school because they enter kindergarten with poor school readiness. The frustration of not being academically successful may contribute to their aggression, either because their aggression leads them to be socially rejected and distracted from their academic work by their pain and frustration or because the same lack of skills and maturity contributes both to their resorting to aggression to solve peer problems and to their struggling with academic work (Coie & Krehbiel, 1984). From kindergarten through second grade, aggressive behavior is fairly stable and continues to be associated with peer dislike and problematic relationships with teachers (Ladd & Burgess, 1999). Aggression in elementary school predicts decreases in school engagement and academic achievement, and this relation is partially mediated by conflict with teachers (Stipek & Miles, 2008). Following a high physical aggression trajectory in childhood predicts dropping out of high school in adolescence (Kokko, Tremblay, Lacourse, Nagin, & Vitaro, 2006).

Engaging in physical aggression leads to peer rejection for many children (Coie, Belding, & Underwood, 1988). A pioneering study brought unacquainted children together in experimental play groups over the course of a week to observe the emergence of social status as sociometric nominations were collected after each day (Coie & Kupersmidt, 1983). By the third day, being physically aggressive in the play sessions was related to peer dislike.

Still, not all physically aggressive children are socially rejected by their peers. Whether a physically aggressive boy will be rejected by peers depends on whether he also has other desirable qualities (Rodkin, Farmer, Pearl, & Van Acker, 2000). In this study, two subgroups of popular boys were identified on the basis of teacher reports. One group was popular-prosocial (model) and was perceived by peers as nonaggressive, low on shyness, cool, athletic, leaders, and good students. Another subgroup was popular-antisocial (tough), and those boys were perceived by peers as antisocial, as well as cool and athletic, and perceived themselves as physically aggressive.

Whether aggression leads to peer rejection also depends on the context, on the degree to which the aggressive child's behavior is different from that of other children in the group. In a summer camp study, highly aggressive boys were disliked only when they were members of a group that included few aggressive children (Wright, Giammarino, & Parad, 1986). Similarly, a study of a large sample of first graders found that for boys, aggression was related to peer rejection only when the levels of classroom aggression were low; in classrooms with highly aggressive children, aggression and peer preference were positively correlated (Stormshak et al., 1999). However, for girls, there was less support for the person–group similarity hypothesis; physical aggressiveness was always negatively related to peer preference for girls, regardless of the aggressiveness of classroom peers.

Perhaps in part from a desire to affiliate with similar peers or because nonaggressive peers shrink from contact with some aggressive youths, aggressive children tend to join peer groups that engage in deviant behavior (Dishion, 2000). Deviant peer groups encourage high-risk youths to engage in increasing levels of deviant behavior (Dodge, Dishion, & Lansford, 2006), but it is important to remember that not all youths are equally influenced by antisocial peers (Dodge, 2008). The group most susceptible to deviant peer influence is boys who are already beginning to engage in antisocial behavior but are not firmly committed to the antisocial lifestyle (Dodge & Sherrill, 2006).

Children following high trajectories for physical aggression are at increased risk for other antisocial behaviors. For the NICHD Early Child Care Research Network (2004) sample, children in high-physical-aggression trajectory groups were at increased risk of symptoms of attention-deficit/hyperactivity disorder (ADHD) and oppositional defiant disorder (ODD), as well as externalizing symptoms on the Child Behavior Checklist, even after demographic and family factors were controlled. A comprehensive meta-analysis found that physical aggression was related to externalizing problems (emotion dysregulation, attention problems, delinquency, and conduct disorder), peer difficulties, and low prosocial behavior (Card et al., 2008). Membership in a high-trajectory group for physical aggression in childhood predicts violence in adolescence (Kokko et al., 2006).

SOCIAL AGGRESSION IN MIDDLE CHILDHOOD

Whereas most children decrease in physical aggression with maturity, some have suggested that they might increase in social aggression. This heterotypic continuity may arise because children are sophisticated enough to realize that they are much more likely to be punished for physical than for social aggression (Bjorkqvist, 1994). However, a direct test of this hypothesis with data from the National Longitudinal Survey of Youth in Canada (Tremblay et al., 1999) found little support for heterotypic continuity; children were consistent across time in their use of different forms of aggression, according to maternal reports (Vaillancourt, Brendgen, Boivin, & Tremblay, 2003).

Despite strong claims that social aggression increases across childhood and reaches its peak in preadolescence (Bjorkqvist et al., 1992; Cairns et al., 1988), little evidence is available for growth and change in social aggression during the middle childhood period. Many studies of social aggression rely on peer nominations that must be standardized within grade, and thus developmental differences cannot be examined (e.g., Crick & Grotpeter, 1995). Although some peer rating studies of social aggression suggest developmental increases from ages 8 to 11 (Bjorkqvist et al., 1992), data from the different age groups came from two separate studies, and statistical tests were not conducted to examine age differences. When interviewed yearly about their worst conflicts with peers, girls increased in reports of social manipulation from grades 4 through 7 (Cairns et al., 1988), but these narratives assessed victimization and not developmental change in individuals' social aggression.

A few recent longitudinal studies suggest that social aggression may remain stable or decrease slightly for most children during the elementary years. As with physical aggression, there appears to be a sizable subgroup (32%) that is high and rising on social aggression between ages 4 and 10 according to mothers' reports (Vaillancourt et al., 2007). However, this subgroup increased only between ages 4 and 6 and stayed stable in social aggression from ages 6 to 10. In an ongoing longitudinal study that assessed social aggression from age 9 to age 14 using teacher ratings, the sample overall declined in social aggression across time (Underwood et al., 2009). In this same longitudinal sample, the group following a higher developmental trajectory actually decreased from age 9 to age 14, but when trajectories were estimated jointly for social and physical aggression, there was a high and rising subgroup that increased in both social and physical aggression between grades 3 and 8.

Origins and Explanations

Although less is known about possible developmental origins of individual differences in social aggression, recent empirical evidence offers intriguing clues. A large twin study suggests weaker genetic effects for social than for physical aggression; heritability seemed to account for only 20% of the variance in social aggression as compared with 50–60% of the variance in physical aggression (Brendgen et al., 2005). Few studies have explored the relation between temperamental characteristics and social aggression, but one investigation found that lower levels of temperamental inhibition were related to being higher on a composite of social and physical aggression in grades 1, 3, and 5 (Park et al., 2005). Early evidence suggests that cardiac reactivity may relate differently to forms of aggressive conduct for girls and boys (Murray-Close & Crick, 2007). For girls only, heightened cardiac reactivity while discussing a social provocation was related to teacher ratings of social aggression with peers, whereas for boys only, lower cardiac reactivity was related to physical aggression.

Just as exposure to marital conflict relates to physical aggression, children's exposure to negative interparental conflict strategies relates to children's social aggression. Parents may model social aggression for children by triangulating them in parental disputes. In one study of children of divorced parents, the child's triangulation in the parents' marital disputes mediated the relation between postdivorce conflict and daughters' social aggression at school (Kerig, Brown, & Patenaude, 2001). Another study with children in the third and fourth grades found that for girls only, parents' reports of negative interpersonal conflict resolution strategies were related to girls' social and physical aggression as rated by teachers (Underwood, Beron, Gentsch, Galperin, & Risser, 2008). Exposure to negative interparental conflict strategies may be a predictor of social aggression only for girls due to the power of same-gender modeling (Snyder, 1998). Also, girls report feeling more caught between parents than boys do (Buchanan, Maccoby, & Dornbusch, 1991), so they may witness more relationship manipulation by parents.

Few studies have examined whether aversive parenting relates to social aggression in middle childhood. An important exception is a summer camp study with maltreated and comparison groups, which found that for girls only, having experienced sexual abuse predicted social aggression with peers (Cullerton-Sen et al., 2008). The authors suggested that "sexual abuse violates aspects of relationships, such as trust and intimacy, which are known to be associated with socially aggressive behavior patterns" (Cullerton-Sen et al., 2008, p. 1739).

Evidence for links between milder forms of aversive parenting and social aggression in school-age children has been more mixed. One investigation with 5- to 8-year-olds found that for girls only, maternal laxness relates to children's social aggression as reported by teachers (Brown, Arnold, Dobbs, & Doctoroff, 2007). For a sample of fourth graders, permissive parenting was related to social aggression at school as assessed by peer nominations (Sandstrom, 2007). Another investigation with children ages 9–10 found no relations between maternal and paternal authoritarian parenting and social and physical aggression as rated by teachers at school (Underwood et al., 2008). One possible explanation for these null findings may be that specific parenting processes may be more strongly related to children's social aggression than overall parenting styles, for example, parents' actively engaging in disparagement of peers (Sullivan, 1953) or failing to intervene or even positively reinforcing children's negative gossip and social exclusion.

Only a few studies have explored whether social information-processing variables may relate to social aggression. Two different studies with children in grades 3–6 found that children rated by peers as high on social aggression were more likely to attribute hostility and reported more distress when responding to hypothetical vignettes depicting ambiguous social provocation (Crick, 1995; Crick, Grotpeter, & Bigbee, 2002). However, social aggression seems less clearly related to how children evaluate the outcomes of aggressive behavior, another important information-processing step. Children's own level of social aggression with peers was unrelated to their evaluations of socially aggressive strategies in hypothetical vignettes, although girls evaluated social aggression more positively than boys did (Crick & Werner, 1999). Moral reasoning may also be related to social aggression; girls who referred to social convention (Is there a rule against it?) in making moral judgments about aggression scenarios were rated higher by teachers on social aggression than girls who used other approaches (Murray-Close, Crick, & Galotti, 2006).

By its very nature, social aggression requires the involvement of peers and is likely influenced by qualities of friendships and social networks. Children understand that engaging in social aggression sometimes means choosing to gain higher status with a group at the expense of a relationship with a particular peer (Delveaux & Daniels, 2000). Children high on social aggression have friendships that are higher on intimacy and exclusivity (Grotpeter & Crick, 1996), and growth in intimate self-disclosure between friends predicts growth in social aggression for girls only (Murray-Close, Ostrov, & Crick, 2007). A twin study found that both genetics and having a socially aggressive friend explained significant variance in each child's social aggression (Brendgen et al., 2008). In another study, for girls only, having friends high in social aggression predicted increases in social aggression from third to fourth grade (Werner & Crick, 2004). Belonging to a peer group in which the other members are high on social aggression predicts individuals' growth in social aggression over time for children in grades 6–8, especially if the particular group is high on status and centrality in the school community (Ellis & Zarbatany, 2007).

Television and movies are rife with depictions of social aggression, and media exposure to social aggression may contribute to individual differences in the extent to which children malign and exclude others. Animated Disney films contain an average of 9.23 incidents of social aggression per hour (Coyne & Whitehead, 2008). Consider also that children are likely viewing ample social aggression in programs intended for adults, including reality programs in which adults gleefully vote each other off the island or out of the house. Researchers are just beginning to examine how viewing social aggression in the media relates to children's social aggression with peers in real life. In one clever experimental study, children who viewed a video depicting social aggression evaluated a confederate more negatively, opted to give the confederate less money, and endorsed indirectly aggressive strategies in a hypothetical vignette more than children who saw a video with no aggression (Coyne, Archer, & Eslea, 2004). Children's self-reported viewing of British television programs high on social aggression predicted their social aggression as rated by peers at school, and girls rated by peers as high on social aggression watched television depicting social aggression more often than all other groups (Coyne & Archer, 2005).

Developmental Consequences

Engaging in high levels of social aggression also seems to confer risk for maladjustment in middle childhood. However, the relation between social aggression and peer status may be complex. On the one hand, peer nominations for social aggression are positively associated with peer rejection (Crick & Grotpeter, 1995), and some evidence suggests that the link between engaging in social aggression and peer rejection is stronger for girls than for boys (Rys & Bear, 1997). On the other hand, the sociometric group rated highest by peers on social aggression is actually the controversial group, defined by receiving many "like least" and "like most" nominations (Crick & Grotpeter, 1995). Successful deployment of social aggression requires at least some social connections and social influence to exclude, malign, and manipulate the friendships of others.

Research has yet to examine how engaging in social aggression is related to academic achievement. Educators are concerned that engaging in social aggression may relate to impaired academic performance for some students because the mental energy required to manipulate others might detract from academics (Talbott, 1997). However, other evidence suggests that social aggression is related to social intelligence (Kaukiainen et al., 1999), and thus socially aggressive children may be bright and able to succeed in the classroom despite distractions.

Social aggression appears to be related to other externalizing behaviors in middle childhood (Card et al., 2008), such as rule breaking and substance use. Remember that physical and social aggression are highly correlated; the average intercorrelation across many studies is .76 (Card et al., 2008).

Engaging in social aggression also seems to be related to internalizing problems. Children high on social aggression report more loneliness and depression than non-socially aggressive children (Crick & Grotpeter, 1995). Children high on social aggression are rated by teachers as higher on internalizing problems than their non-socially aggressive peers (Crick, 1997). Third graders high on social aggression as assessed by peer nominations tended to have more symptoms of anxious depression and withdrawn depression in fourth grade (Crick, Ostrov, & Werner, 2006). A comprehensive meta-analysis found that social aggression is uniquely related to internalizing problems (Card et al., 2008).

PHYSICAL AGGRESSION IN ADOLESCENCE

Overall, most youths continue to decline in the frequency with which they fight physically across adolescence (Dodge, Coie, et al., 2006). One study of rural adolescents' self-reports of physical aggression found that youths increase in physical aggression in adolescence from age 11 to 15, then decline from age 15 to 18 (Karriker-Jaffe, Foshee, Ennett, & Suchindran, 2008). However, a few highly aggressive individuals persist and maybe even increase in their aggression, and adolescence is when most serious youth violence begins (Dodge, Coie, et al., 2006; Dodge, Greenberg, Malone, & the Conduct Problems Prevention Research Group, 2008). Children who began aggressive and antisocial behavior early ("the early starter group") persist during adolescence, and these early starters may be joined by an adolescent-onset group who initiate antisocial conduct as a result of the influence of deviant peers and perhaps as a way to demonstrate pseudomaturity (Moffitt & Caspi, 2001).

Research that examines growth and change in physical aggression during adolescence finds somewhat mixed results for an adolescent-onset group for physical aggression. Because growth trajectories are empirically derived, they tend to vary across samples and contexts. An investigation of a large sample of boys from Montreal found little support for an adolescent-onset group (Brame, Nagin, & Tremblay, 2001). Adolescent physical-aggression trajectories were measured by self-reports, and four groups emerged: no aggression (64%), increasing aggression (16%), decreasing aggression (15%), and high aggression (5%). The high-aggression group increased between ages 13 and 16, then decreased thereafter. There was not a group that seemed to begin behaving aggressively in adolescence; the growth in aggression by the increasing group was slight. Although membership in the high-aggression trajectory in childhood (as assessed by teacher reports) predicted membership in the high-trajectory group in adolescence, the most common transition from childhood to adolescence was movement into the low-aggression group.

Other trajectory studies have found empirical support for an adolescent-onset group for physical aggression. A study with a mostly rural sample used latent growth mixture modeling to determine whether girls and boys followed different developmental trajectories for both familial and nonfamilial physical aggression in adolescence (Martino et al., 2008). For both genders, four trajectory groups emerged: no or low aggression (27% of boys and 48% of girls), desisting aggression (26% of boys and 18% of girls), adolescent aggression (28% of boys and 19% of girls), and persistent high aggression (19% of boys and 15% of girls). Although several other studies support the existence of an adolescent-onset group for antisocial behavior more broadly (Fergusson & Horwood, 2002; Lahey et al., 2006; see Moffitt et al., 2008, for a discussion), these studies do not examine aggression specifically.

Origins and Explanations

Most causal factors that contribute to high levels of physical aggression early in life continue to operate in adolescence. Early risk factors may predict and be mediated by the impact of later risk factors and may also contribute directly to growth in aggression via a dynamic cascade model (Dodge et al., 2008). Risk factors in this model include early adverse environments, early harsh parenting, poor preparedness for school, conduct problems, low school achievement, low parental monitoring, and affiliating with a deviant peer group. This model was tested with the control sample from a large prevention trial, and the children were followed from kindergarten through high school. The results clearly indicated that diverse factors working in concert predicted serious violence in adolescence, that risk factors are correlated and each domain affects the next in developmental sequence, that each subsequent risk factor mediates the effects of earlier risk factors on adolescent violence, and that each risk domain explains unique and incremental variance in adolescent violence (Dodge et al., 2008).

Developmental Consequences

Longitudinal evidence suggests that aversive behavior toward others in early childhood is the beginning of a developmental pathway that leads to physical fighting in middle childhood and violent crime in adolescence (Loeber & Hay, 1997). Most violent crime begins in adolescence (see Dodge, Coie, et al., 2006, for a helpful overview). Self-report data from the National Youth Survey (NYS) suggest that age 17 may be the peak of violent offenses; 19% of boys and 12% of girls report having committed at least one serious violent offense (Elliott & Huizinga, 1983). Base rates of violent offenses are higher for boys than girls, but evidence suggests that the developmental pathway is the same and that the mean age of onset for physical fighting is remarkably similar for boys ($M = 12.42$) and girls ($M = 12.60$; Gorman-Smith & Loeber, 2005). That some youths increase sharply in physical aggression during adolescence may be related to the fact that physical aggression becomes positively related to peer popularity (see Crick, Murray-Close, Marks, & Mohajeri-Nelson, 2008, for a review).

Children who fight physically are at risk for other negative outcomes during adolescence, including dropping out of school (Kupersmidt & Coie, 1990), covert delinquency and substance abuse (Harachi et al., 2006), and violence in romantic relationships (Capaldi & Crosby, 1997). Girls who fight are at heightened risk for adolescent motherhood (Miller-Johnson et al., 1999; Serbin et al., 1998; Underwood, Kupersmidt, & Coie, 1996), as well as gynecological problems, sexually transmitted diseases, obstetrical complications, close spacing of births, being insensitive and unresponsive parents, and having children prone to behavior problems (Serbin et al., 1998).

SOCIAL AGGRESSION IN ADOLESCENCE

Although many claim that social aggression is most frequent and intense during adolescence (Bjorkqvist et al., 1992; Crick et al., 1999; Underwood, 2003), few studies have examined growth and change in this developmental period. Ongoing longitudinal studies are assessing social aggression, along with physical aggression, so information may soon be available as to whether individuals follow different developmental trajectories for social aggression across adolescence. In early adolescence, even the high-social-aggression groups seem to be decreasing (Underwood et al., 2009; Vaillancourt et al., 2007), but trajectories jointly estimated by social and physical aggression suggest that there is a subgroup that is high and rising on both types of aggression through age 13 (Underwood et al., 2009).

Social aggression may take different forms in adolescence as autonomy increases, friendships become more intimate, and romantic relationships form. Gossip may become more extensive and personal as a means of exploring identity (Gottman & Mettetal, 1986), youths may use gossip to explore the moral boundaries of acceptable conduct (Fine, 1986), and gossip may be transmitted via text messaging or online communication. Youths may hurt one another by disrupting each others' emerging romances (Crick et al., 1999). As investigators begin to study social aggression in adolescence, it will be important to test whether new behaviors are used in the service of hurting others by disrupting relationships. One study with 11- to 15-year-olds in England asked youths to rate a large number of specific aggression behaviors on how often they hear or see them and on harmfulness (Coyne, Archer, & Eslea, 2006). On frequency, participants reported seeing and hearing the most verbal aggression, followed by social aggression and then physical aggression. Items rated as high in frequency included: "gossiping" (social), "make fun of someone so it makes them look stupid" (social), "calling mean names" (verbal), and "hitting or punching" (physical; p. 302). Interestingly, the second most frequent of the many behaviors examined was "giving a dirty look" (social). Items rated high on harmfulness included some that were low on frequency: "anonymous mean notes" (social), "breaking confidences" (social), "threaten to break off friendship" (social), and "make fun of clothes or personality to a person's face" (verbal).

Origins and Explanations

Little is known about how factors such as biology, temperament, and parenting might influence individual differences in adolescent social aggression. Adolescents' exposure to marital conflict may relate to their aggression with peers; one study of adjudicated youths in Canada found that girls who witnessed mothers' aggression toward partners were more aggressive with their friends and that boys who were more exposed to fathers' aggression were more aggressive with their friends (Moretti, Obsuth, Odgers, & Reebye, 2006). The scant evidence available suggests that peer factors may also contribute to social aggression. Highly socially aggressive youths are central in their social networks (Xie, Swift, Cairns, & Cairns, 2002), which likely enhances their power to manipulate and exclude others. Also, as girls move through adolescence, engaging in social aggression becomes positively related to peer popularity (Cillessen & Mayeux, 2004; Rose, Swenson, & Waller, 2004); growth in social aggression may be related to peer reinforcement. Young adolescents tend to affiliate with peers who are similar to them on physical fighting and social aggression, and affiliation with socially aggressive peers contributes to growth in social bullying above and beyond individuals' initial levels (Espelage et al., 2003).

Developmental Consequences

Whereas social aggression is linked to peer rejection in childhood, during adolescence social aggression becomes positively related to perceived popularity with peers (Cillessen & Mayeux, 2004; Prinstein & Cillessen, 2003; Rose et al., 2004; see Crick et al., 2008, for a discussion). Popular youths may need to malign and exclude others to achieve and protect popular status (Adler & Adler, 1995), or being popular may empower youths to harm others. Adolescents who engage in social aggression but are also high on prosocial behaviors and self-efficacy are most likely to be high on perceived popularity (Puckett, Aikins, & Cillessen, 2008), perhaps because social self-efficacy indicates adept deployment of social aggression and accompanying prosocial behaviors may make social aggression more palatable to peers.

Experts have proposed that for girls, engaging in social aggression may increase risk for three types of adjustment problems: problems to which girls and women are vulnerable (such as depression and eating disorders), syndromes with symptoms that resemble social aggression (such as borderline personality disorder), and externalizing problems (because social and physical aggression are often highly correlated; Crick & Zahn-Waxler, 2003). Further research is needed on all of these points, but it is important to note that the evidence to date is clear that gender does not moderate the relation between engaging in social aggression and maladjustment (Card et al., 2008).

Whether engaging in social aggression confers greater risk for disorders more frequent among girls and women remains unclear. Many studies suggest that engaging in social aggression predicts internalizing problems (Card et al, 2008), but most of these studies have been conducted with younger samples, and little evidence is available for adolescents. In a study with a sample of 9th through 12th graders, engaging in social aggression was not associated with depressive symptoms, though socially aggressive boys were higher on loneliness than non-socially aggressive boys (Prinstein, Boergers, & Vernberg, 2001). Only one published study has examined the association between engaging in social aggression and eating disorder symptoms; for a sample of college women, peer nominations for social aggression were related to self-reports of bulimia symptoms (Werner & Crick, 1999). Further research is needed to examine whether engaging in social aggression relates to eating disorder symptoms for younger adolescents of both genders. Although the behaviors involved in social aggression resemble symptoms of borderline personality features, again, more research is needed to understand this link. The same study with college students just described found that women high on social aggression reported more borderline personality features (Werner & Crick, 1999).

Evidence is mixed for the relation between engaging in social aggression in adolescence and other externalizing symptoms. On the one hand, high correlations between indirect and direct aggression (Card et al., 2008) and problem behavior theory (Jessor & Jessor, 1977) would suggest that social aggression might be part of a constellation of other antisocial behaviors, and some evidence supports this hypothesis. Engaging in social aggression has been shown to be associated with externalizing symptoms for high school students (Prinstein et al., 2001). Social aggression seems to be a salient characteristic of adjudicated girls. For a sample of detained girls, proactive social aggression was strongly and uniquely associated with callous-unemotional traits (Marsee & Frick, 2007). Antisocial girls in therapeutic foster care programs report frequently engaging in social aggression (71% reported perpetrating social aggression in a single 24-hour period; Chamberlain & Moore, 2002), and therapeutic foster care programs now seek to reduce social aggression (Leve, Chamberlain, & Reid, 2005). A Canadian study of adjudicated girls and boys found that self-reports of social aggression were correlated with having committed physical assault ($r = .47$; Moretti, Holland, & McKay, 2001).

On the other hand, one of the few studies that directly tested problem behavior theory with a large Canadian sample found that a latent problem behavior construct explained only 11% of the variance in social aggression (Willoughby, Chalmers, & Busseri, 2004). Self-reports of social aggression were highly correlated with direct aggression ($r = .60$) and moderately correlated with major ($r = .26$) and minor ($r = .31$) delinquency but more weakly associated with other problem behaviors such as substance use, sexual activity, and gambling (rs ranged from .15 to .22). Additional longitudinal studies with adolescents are needed to understand how social aggression relates to emerging antisocial behaviors for both genders.

PREVENTION AND INTERVENTION

Because persistent childhood aggression predicts negative outcomes, both concurrently and predictively, scholars and policymakers have prioritized the development of programs to reduce and prevent physical aggression. Effective approaches to reducing physical aggression include: stimulant medication (to help with attention problems often associated with aggressive behavior and perhaps to increase responsiveness to intervention; Frick, 2001), parent management training (to teach parents to refrain from coercive exchanges and to reinforce positive behavior; Patterson, DeBaryshe, & Ramsey, 1986), school-based programs such as the Good Behavior Game (Ialongo et al., 1999) and the PATHS curriculum (Providing Alternative THinking Strategies; Greenberg & Kusche, 1993), and social-cognitive skills training (such as the Coping Power Program; Lochman & Wells, 2004). A comprehensive intervention program combining the aforementioned strategies resulted in long-lasting reductions in aggression and antisocial behavior (e.g., the Fast Track program; Conduct Problems Prevention Research Group [CPPRG], 2004). For youths already in the justice system, a program called Multidimensional Treatment Foster Care (MTFC) reduces antisocial behavior by offering placement with foster parents trained to provide consistent monitoring and consequences for misbehavior, but also reinforcement for positive change and adult mentoring (Chamberlain, 2003).

Although all of these approaches have been shown to be effective, policymakers and the public have yet to embrace and invest in youth violence prevention, possibly because we cling to metaphors for youth violence that are not supported by evidence and that have failed to inspire creative intervention, such as the Superpredator metaphor (Dodge, 2008). In a groundbreaking paper, Dodge (2008) proposed new frames for the prevention of youth violence: preventive dentistry (in which prevention is practiced at multiple levels and corrective action taken when problems emerge), heart disease prevention (in which knowledge of distal risk factors guides prevention of more proximal causes), and literacy promotion (in which children are taught skills in regulating emotions and controlling behaviors as part of their regular education).

Although very few programs to prevent social aggression have been empirically tested, a pioneering study of a Social Aggression Prevention Program (SAPP) found that school-based group intervention with girls led to improvements in problem solving and a trend toward reduction in social aggression for those girls initially high in social aggression (Capella & Weinstein, 2006). In this prevention program, fifth-grade girls were randomly assigned to either the SAPP or a reading club. The SAPP consisted of discussion and role playing designed to increase awareness of social aggression, build empathy, develop positive leadership, and practice positive resolution of social conflicts, with an emphasis on the group's role in reinforcing or interrupting the behavior. This type of school-based approach offers great promise for reducing social aggression. It could guide interventionists in adding components to programs to reduce physical aggression and in enhancing therapeutic foster care programs that now seek to reduce social aggression, as well as other antisocial behavior (Leve et al., 2005).

PRESSING RESEARCH QUESTIONS

Research on physical aggression is rich with multi-method, multi-informant, prospective longitudinal investigations, as well as decades' worth of clever experimental and cross-sectional studies, but important questions remain. Current research priorities emphasize the role of biological factors such as genes and brain functioning as illuminated by new imaging techniques (Moffitt et al., 2008). However, although biology undoubtedly has a critical role, it will be important to remember that biological explanations are not ultimate answers, because biological variables interact with and are influenced by psychosocial factors (Caspi et al., 2002; Pollak, 2006). Integrating biological and psychosocial factors will require sophisticated transactional models to do justice to the complexity of the development of aggressive behavior.

More information is needed about how the processes by which aggressive behaviors unfold, in real and developmental time. We must resist the temptation to rely on questionnaires that assess aggressive behavior (or victimization) as if it is a personality trait. To understand the processes by which episodes of aggression take place, observational methods can illuminate social processes when possible and ecologically valid, and innovative methods can also reveal social processes that may happen outside of adult sight: semistructured interviews, diary methods, and time sampling using handheld computers or even smart phones. If we seek to understand how to prevent and reduce aggression, we need to carefully analyze the factors that support aggression escalating and what types of conditions make it stop—specifically, what peers or even victims, as well as adults, might be able to do to respond effectively.

Researchers and policymakers still sorely need more information about how physical and social aggression unfold across developmental time and how these behaviors relate to one another. Do children high on social aggression in preschool continue to malign and exclude peers as they move into elementary school? And what are the consequences of social aggression for academic and social adjustment at each developmental stage? Social and physical aggression are highly correlated in numerous studies (Card et al., 2008), but how do these behaviors relate to each other at the individual level or in terms of social processes? Does social aggression confer additional developmental risk over and above physical aggression?

Last, it is vitally important that we continue to consider gender seriously in investigating childhood aggression. Despite the fact that boys and men hit more than girls and women, girls who fight are important to study because they are at serious risk and because they transmit behavior problems to the next generation (Serbin et al., 1998). Gender differences in the frequency of engaging in social aggression may not be large enough to matter (Card et al., 2008), but gender may affect social aggression in ways we have yet to examine. Girls may enact social aggression more toward their friends than boys do, girls may feel more threatened when victimized by social aggression, and engaging in and being victimized by social aggression may have very different social and emotional consequences for girls and boys. Both girls and boys manipulate and fight. Understanding more about gender and aggression will force us to be sensitive to the struggles of all perpetrators and the plights of all victims and guide the development of maximally effective interventions for all aggressive youths.

ACKNOWLEDGMENTS

Preparation of this chapter was supported by Grant Nos. R01 MH63076, R01 HD060995, and K02 MH073616 from the National Institutes of Health.

SUGGESTED READINGS

Brendgen, M., Boivin, M., Vitaro, F., Bukowski, W. M., Dionne, G., Girard, A., et al. (2008). Linkages between children's and their friends' social and physical aggression: Evidence for a gene–environment interaction? *Child Development, 79,* 13–29.

Capella, E., & Weinstein, R. (2006). The prevention of social aggression among girls. *Social Development, 15,* 434–459.

Dodge, K. A. (2006). Translational science in action: Hostile attributional style and the development of aggressive behavior problems. *Development and Psychopathology, 18,* 791–814.

Dodge, K. A. (2008). Framing public policy and prevention of chronic violence in American youths. *American Psychologist, 63,* 573–590.

NICHD Early Child Care Research Network. (2004). Trajectories of physical aggression from toddlerhood to middle childhood. *Monographs of the Society for Research in Child Development, 69*(4), Serial No. 278.

REFERENCES

Adler, P. A., & Adler, P. (1995). Dynamics of inclusion and exclusion in preadolescent cliques. *Social Psychology Quarterly, 58*(3), 145–162.

Archer, J. (2004). Sex differences in aggression in real-world settings: A meta-analytic review. *Review of General Psychology, 8,* 291–322.

Archer, J., & Coyne, S. M. (2005). An integrated review of indirect, relational, and social aggression. *Personality and Social Psychology Review, 9,* 212–230.

Arnold, D. H., Hanrock, S., Ortiz, C., & Stowe, R. M. (1999). Direct observation of peer rejection acts and their temporal relation with aggressive acts. *Early Childhood Research Quarterly, 14,* 183–196.

Baumrind, D. (1989). Rearing competent children. In W. Damon (Ed.), *Child development today and tomorrow* (pp. 349–378). San Francisco: Jossey-Bass.

Bjorkqvist, K. (1994). Sex differences in physical, verbal, and indirect aggression: A review of recent research. *Sex Roles, 30,* 177–188.

Bjorkqvist, K., Lagerspetz, K., & Kaukiainen, A. (1992). Do girls manipulate and do boys fight? Developmental trends in regard to direct and indirect aggression. *Aggressive Behavior, 18,* 117–127.

Bjorkqvist, K., & Niemela, P. (1992). New trends in the study of female aggression. In K. Bjorkqvist & P. Niemela (Eds.), *Of mice and women: Aspects of female aggression* (pp. 3–16). San Diego, CA: Academic Press.

Bjorkqvist, K., Osterman, K., & Kaukiainen, A. (1992). The development of direct and indirect aggressive strategies in males and females. In K. Bjorkqvist & P. Niemela (Eds.), *Of mice and women: Aspects of female aggression* (pp. 51–64). San Diego, CA: Academic Press.

Bonica, C., Arnold, D. H., Fisher, P. H., Zeljo, A., & Yershova, K. (2003). Relational aggression, relational victimization, and language development in preschoolers. *Social Development, 12,* 551–562.

Brame, B., Nagin, D. S., & Tremblay, R. E. (2001). Developmental trajectories of physical aggression from school entry to late adolescence. *Journal of Child Psychology and Psychiatry, 42,* 503–512.

Brendgen, M., Boivin, M., Vitaro, F., Bukowski, W. M., Dionne, G., Girard, A., et al. (2008). Linkages between children's and their friends' social and physical aggression: Evidence for a gene–environment interaction? *Child Development, 79,* 13–29.

Brendgen, M., Dionne, G., Girard, A., Boivin, M., Vitaro, F., & Perusse, D. (2005). Examining genetic and environmental effects on social aggression: A study of six-year-old twins. *Child Development, 76,* 930–946.

Broidy, L. M., Nagin, D. S., Tremblay, R. E., Bates, J. E., Brame, B., Dodge, K. A., et al. (2003). Developmental trajectories of childhood disruptive behaviors and adolescent delinquency: A six-site, cross-national study. *Developmental Psychology, 39,* 222–245.

Brown, S. A., Arnold, D. H., Dobbs, J., & Doctoroff, G. L. (2007). Parenting predictors of relational aggression among Puerto Rican and European American school-age children. *Early Childhood Research Quarterly, 22,* 147–159.

Buchanan, C. M., Maccoby, E. E., & Dornbusch, S. M. (1991). Caught between parents: Adolescents' experience in divorced homes. *Child Development, 62,* 1008–1029.

Bushman, B. J., & Anderson, C. A. (2001). Media violence and the American public: Scientific facts versus media misinformation. *American Psychologist, 56,* 477–489.

Buss, A. H. (1961). *The psychology of aggression.* New York: Wiley.

Buss, A. H., & Plomin, R. (1984). *Temperament: Early developing personality traits.* Hillsdale, NJ: Erlbaum.

Cairns, R. B., & Cairns, B. D. (1994). *Lifelines and risks: Pathways of youth in our time.* New York: Cambridge University Press.

Cairns, R. B., Cairns, B. D., Neckerman, H. J., Gest, S., & Gariepy, J. (1988). Social networks and aggressive behavior: Peer support or peer rejection? *Developmental Psychology, 24,* 815–823.

Capaldi, D. M., & Crosby, L. (1997). Observed and reported psychological and physical aggression in young at-risk couples. *Social Development, 6,* 184–206.

Capella, E., & Weinstein, R. (2006). The prevention of social aggression among girls. *Social Development, 15,* 434–459.

Card, N. A., Stucky, B. D., Sawalani, G. M., & Little, T. D. (2008). Direct and indirect aggression during childhood and adolescence: A meta-analytic review of gender differences, intercorrelations, and relations to maladjustment. *Child Development, 79,* 1185–1229.

Caspi, A., McClay, J., Moffitt, T. E., Mil, J., Martin, J., Craig, I. W., et al. (2002). Role of genotype in the cycle of violence in maltreated children. *Science, 297,* 851–854.

Chamberlain, P. (2003). *Treating chronic juvenile offenders: Advances made through the Oregon Multidimensional Treatment Foster Care Model.* Washington, DC: American Psychological Association.

Chamberlain, P., & Moore, K. J. (2002). Chaos and trauma in the lives of adolescent females with antisocial behavior and delinquency. In R. Greenwald (Ed.), *Trauma and juvenile delinquency: Theory, research, and interventions* (pp. 79–108). Binghamton, NY: Haworth Press.

Cillessen, A. H. N., & Mayeux, L. (2004). From censure to reinforcement: Developmental changes in the association between aggression and social status. *Child Development, 75,* 147–163.

Coie, J. D., Belding, M., & Underwood, M. K. (1988). Aggression and peer rejection in childhood. In B. B. Lahey & A. Kazdin (Eds.), *Advances in clinical child psychology* (Vol. 11, pp. 125–158). New York: Plenum Press.

Coie, J. D., & Dodge, K. A. (1998). Aggression and antisocial behavior. In N. Eisenberg (Ed.), *Handbook of child psychology* (pp. 779–862). New York: Wiley.

Coie, J. D., & Krehbiel, G. (1984). Effects of academic tutoring on the social status of low achieving, socially rejected children. *Child Development, 55,* 1465–1478.

Coie, J. D., & Kupersmidt, J. B. (1983). A behavioral analysis of emerging social status in boys' groups. *Child Development, 54,* 1400–1416.

Comstock, G. (2008). A sociological perspective on television violence and aggression. *American Behavioral Scientist, 51,* 1184–1211.

Conduct Problems Prevention Research Group. (2004). The effects of the Fast Track program on serious problem outcomes at the end of elementary school. *Journal of Clinical Child and Adolescent Psychology, 33,* 650–661.

Coyne, S. M., & Archer, J. (2005). The relation between indirect and physical aggression on television and in real life. *Social Development, 14,* 324–338.

Coyne, S. M., Archer, J., & Eslea, M. (2004). Cruel intentions on television and in real life: Can viewing indirect aggression increase viewers' subsequent indirect aggression? *Journal of Experimental Child Psychology, 88,* 234–253.

Coyne, S. M., Archer, J., & Eslea, M. (2006). "We're not friends anymore! Unless … " The frequency and harmfulness of indirect, relational, and social aggression. *Aggressive Behavior, 32,* 294–307.

Coyne, S. M., & Whitehead, E. (2008). Indirect aggression in animated Disney films. *Journal of Communication, 58,* 382–395.

Crick, N. R. (1995). Relational aggression: The role of intent attributions, feelings of distress, and provocation type. *Development and Psychopathology, 7,* 313–322.

Crick, N. R. (1996). The role of overt aggression, relational aggression, and prosocial behavior in the prediction of children's future social adjustment. *Child Development, 67,* 2317–2327.

Crick, N. R. (1997). Engagement in gender normative versus gender nonnormative forms of aggression: Links to social-psychological adjustment. *Developmental Psychology, 33,* 610–617.

Crick, N. R., Bigbee, M. A., & Howes, C. (1996). Gender differences in children's normative beliefs about aggression: How do I hurt thee? Let me count the ways. *Child Development, 67,* 1003–1014.

Crick, N. R., Casas, J. F., & Mosher, M. (1997). Relational and overt aggression in preschool. *Developmental Psychology, 33*(4), 589–600.

Crick, N. R., & Grotpeter, J. K. (1995). Relational aggression, gender, and social-psychological adjustment. *Child Development, 66,* 710–722.

Crick, N. R., Grotpeter, J. K., & Bigbee, M. A. (2002). Relationally and physically aggressive children's intent attributions and feelings of distress for relational and instrumental provocations. *Child Development, 73,* 1134–1142.

Crick, N. R., Murray-Close, D., Marks, P. E. L., & Mohajeri-Nelson, N. (2008). Aggression and peer relationships in school-age children: Relational and physical aggression in group and dyadic contexts. In K. H. Rubin, W. M. Bukowski, & B. Laursen (Eds.), *Handbook of peer interactions, relationships, and groups* (pp. 287–321). New York: Guilford Press.

Crick, N. R., & Ostrov, J. M., & Kawabata, Y. (2007). Relational aggression and gender: An overview. In D. J. Flannery, A. T. Vazsonyi, & I. D. Waldman (Eds.), *Cambridge handbook of violent behavior and aggression* (pp. 245–259). New York: Cambridge University Press.

Crick, N. R., Ostrov, J. M., & Werner, N. E. (2006). A longitudinal study of relational aggression, physical aggression, and children's social-psychological adjustment. *Journal of Abnormal Child Psychology, 34,* 131–142.

Crick, N. R., Wellman, N. E., Casas, J. F., O'Brien, M. A., Nelson, D. A., Grotpeter, J. K., et al. (1999). Childhood aggression and gender: A new look at an old problem. In D. Bernstein, (Ed.), *Nebraska Symposium on Motivation* (pp. 75–140). Lincoln: University of Nebraska Press.

Crick, N. R., & Werner, N. E. (1999). Response decision processes in relational and overt aggression. *Child Development, 69,* 1630–1639.

Crick, N. R., & Zahn-Waxler, C. (2003). The development of psychopathology in females and males: Current progress and future challenges. *Development and Psychopathology, 15,* 719–742.

Cullerton-Sen, C., Cassidy, A. R., Murray-Close, D., Cicchetti, D., Crick, N. R., & Rogosch, F. A. (2008). Childhood maltreatment and the development of relational and physical aggression: The importance of a gender-informed approach. *Child Development, 79,* 1736–1751.

Cummings, E. M., Davies, P. T., & Campbell, S. B. (2000). *Developmental psychopathology and family process: Theory, research, and clinical implications.* New York: Guilford Press.

Delveaux, K. D., & Daniels, T. (2000). Children's social cognitions: Physically and relationally aggressive strategies and children's goals in peer conflict situations. *Merrill–Palmer Quarterly, 46,* 672–692.

Dettling, A. C., Gunnar, M. R., & Donzella, B. (1999). Cortisol levels of young children in full-day childcare centers: Relations with age and temperament. *Psychoneuroendocrinology, 24,* 519–536.

Dishion, T. J. (2000). Cross-setting consistency in early adolescent psychopathology: Deviant friendships and problem behavior sequelae. *Journal of Personality, 68,* 1109–1126.

Dodge, K. A. (2006). Translational science in action: Hostile attributional style and the development of aggressive behavior problems. *Development and Psychopathology, 18,* 791–814.

Dodge, K. A. (2008). Framing public policy and prevention of chronic violence in American youths. *American Psychologist, 63,* 573–590.

Dodge, K. A., Bates, J. E., & Pettit, G. S. (1990). Mechanisms in the cycle of violence. *Science, 250,* 1678–1683.

Dodge, K. A., & Coie, J. D. (1987). Social information processing factors in reactive and proactive aggression in children's peer groups. *Journal of Personality and Social Psychology, 53,* 1146–1158.

Dodge, K. A., Coie, J. D., & Lynam, D. (2006). Aggression and antisocial behavior in youth. In W. Damon (Series Ed.) & N. Eisenberg (Vol. Ed.), *Handbook of child psychology: Vol. 3. Social, emotional, and personality development* (pp. 719–788). Hoboken, NJ: Wiley.

Dodge, K. A., Dishion, T. J., & Lansford, J. E. (Eds.). (2006). *Deviant peer influences in programs for youth: Problems and solutions.* New York: Guilford Press.

Dodge, K. A., Greenberg, M. T., Malone, P. S., & the Conduct Problems Research Group. (2008). Testing an idealized dynamic cascade model of the development of serious violence in adolescence. *Child Development, 79,* 1907–1927.

Dodge, K. A., Pettit, G. S., Bates, J. E., & Valente, E. (1995). Social information-processing patterns partially mediate the effect of early physical abuse on later conduct problems. *Journal of Abnormal Psychology, 104,* 632–643.

Dodge, K. A., & Sherrill, M. R. (2006). Deviant peer group effects in youth mental health interventions. In K. A. Dodge, T. J. Dishion, & J. E. Lansford (Eds.), *Deviant peer influences in programs for youth: Problems and solutions.* New York: Guilford Press.

Elliott, D. S., & Huizinga, D. (1983). Social class and delinquent behavior. *Criminology, 21,* 149–177.

Ellis, W. E., & Zarbatany, L. (2007). Peer group status as a moderator of group influence on children's deviant, aggressive, and prosocial behavior. *Child Development, 78,* 1240–1254.

Espelage, D. L., Holt, M. K., & Henkel, R. R. (2003). Examination of peer-group contextual effects on aggression during early adolescence. *Child Development, 74,* 205–220.

Fabes, R. A., Shepard, S. A., Guthrie, I. K., & Martin, C. L. (1997). Roles of temperamental arousal and gender-segregated play in young children's social adjustment. *Developmental Psychology, 33,* 693–702.

Fagot, B. I., & Hagan, R. (1985). Aggression in toddlers: Responses to the assertive acts of boys and girls. *Sex Roles, 12,* 341–351.

Fagot, B. I., Leinbach, M. D., & Hagan, R. (1986). Gender labeling and the adoption of sex-typed behaviors. *Developmental Psychology, 22,* 440–443.

Farver, J. M. (1996). Aggressive behavior in preschoolers' social networks: Do birds of a feather flock together? *Early Childhood Research Quarterly, 11,* 333–350.

Fergusson, D. M., & Horwood, L. J. (2002). Male and female offending trajectories. *Development and Psychopathology, 14,* 159–177.

Feshbach, N. D. (1964). The function of aggression and the regulation of aggressive drive. *Psychological Review, 71,* 257–272.

Feshbach, N. (1969). Gender differences in children's modes of aggressive responses toward outsiders. *Merrill–Palmer Quarterly, 15,* 249–258.

Fine, G. A. (1986). The social organization of adolescent gossip. In J. Cook-Gumperz, W. Corsara, & J. Streek (Eds.), *Children's worlds and children's language* (pp. 405–423). Berlin: Mouton.

Frick, P. J. (2001). Effective interventions for children and adolescents with conduct disorder. *Canadian Journal of Psychiatry, 46,* 597–608.

Frodi, A., Macaulay, J., & Thome, P. (1977). Are women always less aggressive than men?: A review of the experimental literature. *Psychological Bulletin, 84,* 635–657.

Galen, B. R., & Underwood, M. K. (1997). A developmental investigation of social aggression among children. *Developmental Psychology, 33,* 589–600.

Giles, J. W., & Heyman, G. D. (2005). Young children's beliefs about the relationship between gender and aggressive behavior. *Child Development, 76,* 107–121.

Gorman-Smith, D., & Loeber, R. (2005). Are developmental pathways in disruptive behaviors the same for girls and boys? *Journal of Child and Family Studies, 14,* 15–27.

Gottman, J., & Mettetal, G. (1986). Speculations about social and affective development: Friendship and acquaintanceship through adolescence. In J. M. Gottman & J. G. Parker (Eds.), *Conversations with friends: Speculations on affective development* (pp. 192–237). New York: Cambridge University Press.

Greenberg, M. T., & Kusche, C. A. (1993). *Promoting social and emotional development in deaf children: The PATHS project.* Seattle: University of Washington Press.

Grotpeter, J. K., & Crick, N. R. (1996). Relational aggression, overt aggression, and friendship. *Child Development, 67,* 2328–2338.

Harachi, T. W., Fleming, C. B., White, H. R., Ensminger, M. E., Abbott, R. D., Catalano, R. F., et al. (2006). Aggressive behavior among girls and boys during middle childhood: Predictors and sequelae of trajectory group membership. *Aggressive Behavior, 32,* 279–293.

Harré, R., & Lamb, R. (1983). *The encyclopedic dictionary of psychology.* Oxford, UK: Blackwell.

Hart, C. H., DeWolf, D. M., & Burts, D. C. (1992). Linkages among preschoolers' playground behavior, outcome expectations, and parental disciplinary strategies. *Early Education and Development, 3,* 265–283.

Hart, C. H., Ladd, G. W., & Burleson, B. R. (1990). Children's expectations of the outcomes of social strategies: Relations with sociometric status and maternal disciplinary styles. *Child Development, 61,* 127–137.

Hart, C. H., Nelson, D. A., Robinson, C. C., Olsen, S. F., & McNeilly-Choque, M. K. (1998). Overt and relational aggression in Russian nursery-school-age children: Parenting style and marital linkages. *Developmental Psychology, 34,* 687–697.

Hudley, C. A., & Graham, S. (1993). An attributional intervention to reduce peer-directed aggression among African American boys. *Child Development, 64,* 124–138.

Huesmann, L. R. (1998). The role of social information processing and cognitive schemas in the acquisition and maintenance of habitual aggressive behavior. In R. Geen & E. Donnerstein (Eds.), *Human aggression: Theories, research, and implications for policy* (pp. 73–109). New York: Academic Press.

Huesmann, L. R., Moise-Titus, J., Podolski, C. L., & Eron, L. D. (2003). Longitudinal relations between children's exposure to TV violence and their aggressive and violent behavior in young adulthood: 1977–1992. *Developmental Psychology, 39,* 201–221.

Ialongo, N. S., Werthamer, L., Kellam, S. G., Brown, C. H., Wang, S., & Lin, Y. (1999). Proximal impact of two first-grade preventive interventions on the early risk behaviors for later substance abuse, depression, and antisocial behavior. *American Journal of Community Psychology, 27,* 599–641.

Jessor, R., & Jessor, S. L. (1977). *Problem behavior and psychosocial development: A longitudinal study of youth.* New York: Academic Press.

Karriker-Jaffe, K. J., Foshee, V. A., Ennett, S. T., & Suchindran, C. (2008). The development of aggression during adolescence: Sex differences in trajectories of physical and social aggression among youth in rural areas. *Journal of Abnormal Child Psychology, 36,* 1227–1336.

Kaukiainen, A., Bjorkqvist, K., Lagerspetz, K., Osterman, K., Salmivalli, C., Rothberg, S., et al. (1999). The relationships between social intelligence, empathy, and three types of aggression. *Aggressive Behavior, 25,* 81–89.

Kellam, S. G., Ling, X., Merisca, R., Brown, C. H., & Ialongo, N. (1998). The effect of the level of aggression in the first-grade classroom on the course and malleability of aggressive behavior into middle school. *Development and Psychopathology, 10,* 165–185.

Kerig, P. K., Brown, C., & Patenaude, R. (2001, April). Ties that bind: Coparenting, parent–child relations, and triangulation in post-divorce interpersonal conflicts. In M. El-Shiekh (Chair), *Marital conflict and child outcomes: Processes, risk variables, and protective factors.* Symposium presented at the biennial meeting of the Society for Research in Child Development, Minneapolis, MN.

Kindermann, T. A. (1993). Natural peer groups as contexts for individual development: The case of children's motivation in school. *Developmental Psychology, 29,* 970–977.

Kingston, L., & Prior, M. (1995). The development of patterns of stable, transient, and school-age onset of aggressive behavior in young children. *Journal of the American Academy of Child and Adolescent Psychiatry, 34,* 348–358.

Kokko, L., Tremblay, R. E., Lacourse, E., Nagin, D. S., & Vitaro, F. (2006). Trajectories of prosocial behavior and physical aggression in middle childhood: Links to adolescent school dropout and physical violence. *Journal of Research on Adolescence, 16,* 403–428.

Kupersmidt, J. B., & Coie, J. D. (1990). Preadolescent peer status, aggression, and school adjustment as predictors of externalizing problems in adolescence. *Child Development, 61,* 1350–1362.

Ladd, G. W. (1990). Having friends, keeping friends, making friends, and being liked by peers in the classroom: Predictors of children's early school adjustment? *Child Development, 61,* 1081–1100.

Ladd, G. W., & Burgess, K. B. (1999). Charting the relationship trajectories of aggressive, withdrawn, and aggressive/withdrawn children during early grade school. *Child Development, 70,* 910–929.

Ladd, G. W., & Price, J. M. (1987). Predicting children's social and school adjustment following the transition from preschool to kindergarten. *Child Development, 58,* 1168–1189.

Lahey, B. B., Van Hulle, C. A., Waldman, I. D., Rodgers, J. L., D'Onofrio, B. M., Pedlow, S., et al. (2006). Testing descriptive hypotheses regarding sex differences in the development of conduct problems and delinquency. *Journal of Abnormal Child Psychology, 34,* 737–755.

Lansford, J. E., Deater-Deckard, K., Dodge, K. A., Bates, J. E., & Pettit, G. S. (2004). Ethnic differences in the link between physical discipline and later adolescent externalizing behaviors. *Journal of Child Psychology and Psychiatry, 45,* 801–812.

Lengua, L. L., West, S. G., & Sandler, I. N. (1998). Temperament as a predictor of symptomatology in children: Addressing contamination of measures. *Child Development, 69,* 164–181.

Leve, L. D., Chamberlain, P., & Reid, J. B. (2005). Intervention outcomes for girls referred from juvenile justice: Effects on delinquency. *Journal of Consulting and Clinical Psychology, 73,* 1181–1185.

Lochman, J. E., & Wells, K. C. (2004). The coping power program for preadolescent aggressive boys and their parents: Outcome effects at the 1–year follow-up. *Journal of Consulting and Clinical Psychology, 72,* 571–578.

Loeber, R., & Hay, D. (1997). Key issues in the development of aggression and violence from childhood to early adulthood. *Annual Review of Psychology, 48,* 371–410.

Maccoby, E. E. (1998). *The two sexes: Growing up apart, coming together.* Cambridge, MA: Harvard University Press.

Maccoby, E. E., & Jacklin, C. N. (1974). *The psychology of gender differences.* Stanford, CA: Stanford University Press.

Marcus, N. E., Lindahl, K. M., & Malik, N. M. (2001). Interparental conflict, children's social cognitions, and child aggression: A test of a mediational model. *Journal of Family Psychology, 15,* 315–333.

Marsee, M. A., & Frick, P. J. (2007). Exploring the cognitive and emotional correlates to proactive and reactive aggression in a sample of detained girls. *Journal of Abnormal Child Psychology, 35,* 969–981.

Martin, C. L., & Fabes, R. A. (2001). The stability and consequences of young children's same-sex peer interactions. *Developmental Psychology, 37,* 431–446.

Martino, S. C., Ellickson, P. L., Klein, D. J., McCaffrey, D., & Edelen, M. O. (2008). Multiple trajectories of physical aggression among adolescent boys. *Aggressive Behavior, 34,* 61–75.

McNeilly-Choque, M. K., Hart, C. H., Robinson, C. C., Nelson, L. J., & Olsen, S. F. (1996). Overt and relational aggression on the playground: Correspondence among different informants. *Journal of Research in Childhood Education, 11,* 47–67.

Miller-Johnson, S., Winn, D., Coie, J. Maumary-Gremaud, A., Hyman, C., Terry, R., et al. (1999). Motherhood during the teen years: A developmental perspective on risk factors for childbearing. *Development and Psychopathology, 11,* 85–100.

Moffitt, T. E. (1993). "Life-course-persistent" and "adolescent-limited" antisocial behavior: A developmental taxonomy. *Psychological Review, 100,* 674–701.

Moffitt, T. E. (2005). The new look at behavioral genetics in developmental psychopathology: Gene–environment interplay in antisocial behaviors. *Psychological Bulletin, 131,* 533–554.

Moffitt, T. E., Arseneault, L., Jaffee, S. R., Kim-Cohen, J., Koenen, K. C., Odgers, C. L., et al. (2008). Research review: DSM-V conduct disorder: Research needs for an evidence base. *Journal of Child Psychology and Psychiatry, 49,* 3–33.

Moffitt, T. E., & Caspi, A. (2001). Childhood predictors differentiate life-course-persistent and adolescent-limited antisocial pathways among males and females. *Development and Psychopathology, 13,* 355–375

Moretti, M. M., Holland, R., & McKay, S. (2001). Self–other representations and relational and overt aggression in adolescent girls and boys. *Behavioral Sciences and the Law, 19,* 109–126.

Moretti, M. M., Obsuth, I., Odgers, C. L., & Reebye, P. (2006). Exposure to maternal versus paternal partner violence, PTSD, and aggression in adolescent girls and boys. *Aggressive Behavior, 32,* 385–395.

Murray-Close, D., & Crick, N. R. (2007). Gender differences in the association between cardiovascular reactivity and aggressive conduct. *International Journal of Psychophysiology, 65,* 103–113.

Murray-Close, D., Crick, N. R., & Galotti, K. M. (2006). Children's moral reasoning regarding physical and relational aggression. *Social Development, 15,* 345–372.

Murray-Close, D., Ostrov, J. M., & Crick, N. R. (2007). A short-term longitudinal study of growth in relational aggression during middle childhood: Associations with gender, friendship intimacy, and internalizing problems. *Development and Psychopathology, 19,* 187–203.

Nelson, D. A., Hart, C. H., Yang, C., Olsen, J. A., & Jin, S. (2006). Aversive parenting in China: Associations with child physical and relational aggression. *Child Development, 77,* 554–572.

NICHD Early Child Care Research Network. (2004). Trajectories of physical aggression from toddlerhood to middle childhood. *Monographs of the Society for Research in Child Development, 69*(4, Serial No. 278).

Osterman, K., Bjorkqvist, K., Lagerspetz, K. M. J., Kaukiainen, A., Landau, S. F., Fraczek, A., et al. (1998). Cross-cultural evidence of female indirect aggression. *Aggressive Behavior, 24,* 1–8.

Ostrov, J. M., & Crick, N. R. (2007). Forms and functions of aggression during early childhood: A short-term longitudinal study. *School Psychology Review, 36,* 22–43.

Paik, H., & Comstock, G. (1994). The effects of television violence on antisocial behavior: A meta-analysis. *Communication Research, 21,* 516–546.

Paquette, J. A., & Underwood, M. K. (1999). Young adolescents' experiences of peer victimization: Gender differences in accounts of social and physical aggression. *Merrill–Palmer Quarterly, 45,* 233–258.

Park, J. H., Essex, M. J., Zahn-Waxler, C., Armstrong, J. M., Klein, M. H., & Goldsmith, H. H. (2005). Relational and overt aggression in middle childhood: Early child and family risk factors. *Early Education and Development, 16,* 233–256.

Parke, R. D., Kim, M., Flyr, M., MacDowell, D. J., Simpkins, S. D., Killian, C. M., et al. (2001). Managing marital conflict: Links with children's peer relationships. In J. H. Grych & F. D. Fincham (Eds.), *Interparental conflict and child development* (pp. 291–314). New York: Cambridge University Press.

Patterson, G. R. (1982). *Coercive family process.* Eugene, OR: Castalia.

Patterson, G. R. (1986). Performance models for antisocial boys. *American Psychologist, 41,* 432–444.

Patterson, G. R., DeBaryshe, B. D., & Ramsey, E. (1989). A developmental perspective on antisocial behavior. *American Psychologist, 44,* 329–335.

Pollak, S. D. (2006). Early adversity and mechanisms of plasticity: Integrating affective neuroscience with developmental approaches to psychopathology. *Development and Psychopathology, 17,* 735–752.

Prinstein, M. J., Boergers, J., & Vernberg, E. M. (2001). Overt and relational aggression in adolescents: Social-psychological adjustment of aggressors and victims. *Journal of Child Clinical Psychology, 30,* 479–491.

Prinstein, M. J., & Cillessen, A. H. N. (2003). Forms and functions of adolescent peer aggression associated with high levels of peer status. *Merrill–Palmer Quarterly, 49,* 310–342.

Puckett, M. B., Aikins, J. W., & Cillessen, A. H. N. (2008). Moderators of the association between relational aggression and perceived popularity. *Aggressive Behavior, 34,* 563–576.

Raine, A. (2008). From genes to brain to antisocial behavior. *Current Directions in Psychological Sciences, 17,* 323–328.

Rodkin, P. C., Farmer, T. W., Pearl, R., & Van Acker, R. (2000). Heterogeneity of popular boys: Antisocial and prosocial configurations. *Developmental Psychology, 36,* 14–24.

Rose, A. J., Swenson, L. P., & Waller, E. M. (2004). Overt and relational aggression and perceived popularity: Developmental differences in current and prospective relations. *Developmental Psychology, 40,* 378–387.

Rosen, L. H., Underwood, M. K., Gentsch, J. K., Radhar, A., & Wharton, M. E. (2011). *Adult recollections of peer victimization during middle school: Forms and consequences.* Manuscript under review.

Rys, G. S., & Bear, G. G. (1997). Relational aggression and peer relations: Gender and developmental issues. *Merrill–Palmer Quarterly, 43,* 87–106.

Sandstrom, M. J. (2007). A link between mothers' disciplinary strategies and children's relational aggression. *British Journal of Developmental Psychology, 25,* 399–407.

Sears, R. R. (1961). Relation of early socialization experiences to aggression in middle childhood. *Journal of Abnormal Psychology, 63,* 466–492.

Serbin, L. A., Cooperman, J. M., Peters, P. L., Lehoux, P. M., Stack, D. M., & Schwartzmen, A. E. (1998). Intergenerational transfer of psychosocial risk in women with childhood histories of aggression, withdrawal, or aggression and withdrawal. *Developmental Psychology, 34,* 1246–1262.

Serbin, L. A., Moller, L. C., Gulko, J., Powlishta, K. K., & Colburne, K. A. (1994). The emergence of gender segregation in toddler playgroups. *New Directions in Child Development, 65,* 7–18.

Snyder, J. R. (1998). Marital conflict and child adjustment: What about gender? *Developmental Review, 18,* 390–420.

Snyder, J., Horsch, E., & Childs, J. (1997). Peer relationships of young children: Affiliative choices and the shaping of aggressive behavior. *Journal of Child Clinical Psychology, 26,* 145–156.

Stipek, D., & Miles, S. (2008). Effects of aggression on achievement: Does conflict with teachers make it worse? *Child Development, 79,* 1721–1735.

Stormshak, E. A., Bierman, K. L., Bruschi, C., Dodge, K. A., Coie, J. D., and the Conduct Problems Prevention Research Group. (1999). The relation between behavior problems and peer preference in different classroom contexts. *Child Development, 70,* 169–182.

Strassberg, Z., Dodge, K. A., Pettit, G. S., & Bates, J. E. (1994). Spanking in the home and children's subsequent aggression towards kindergarten peers. *Development and Psychopathology, 6,* 445–461.

Sullivan, H. S. (1953). *The interpersonal theory of psychiatry.* New York: Norton.

Talbott, E. (1997). Reflecting on antisocial girls and the study of their development: Researchers' view. *Exceptionality, 7,* 267–272.

Tremblay, R. E., Japel, C., Perusse, D., McDuff, P., Boivin, M., Zoccolillo, M., et al. (1999). The search for the age of "onset" of physical aggression: Rousseau and Bandura revisited. *Criminal Behavior and Mental Health, 9,* 8–23.

Underwood, M. K. (2003). *Social aggression among girls.* New York: Guilford Press.

Underwood, M. K., Beron, K. J., Gentsch, J. K., Galperin, M. B., & Risser, S. D. (2008). Interparental conflict resolution strategies, parenting styles, and children's social and physical aggression with peers. *International Journal of Behavioral Development, 32,* 549–562.

Underwood, M. K., Beron, K. J., & Rosen, L. (2009). Continuity and change in social and physical aggression from middle childhood through early adolescence. *Aggressive Behavior, 35,* 357–375.

Underwood, M. K., Beron, K. J., & Rosen, L. (2011). Joint trajectories for social and physical aggression as predictors of adolescent maladjustment: Internaliing symptoms, rule-breaking behaviors, and borderline and narcissistic personality features. *Development and Psychopathology, 23,* 659–678.

Underwood, M. K., & Coie, J. D. (2004). Future directions and priorities for prevention and intervention. In M. Putallaz and K. L. Bierman (Eds.), *Aggression, antisocial behavior, and violence among girls: A developmental perspective* (pp. 289–301). New York: Guilford Press.

Underwood, M. K., Galen, B. R., & Paquette, J. A. (2001). Hopes rather than fears, admirations rather than hostilities: A response to Archer and Bjorkqvist. *Social Development, 10,* 275–280.

Underwood, M. K., Kupersmidt, J. B., & Coie, J. D. (1996). Childhood peer sociometric status and aggression as predictors of adolescent childbearing. *Journal of Research on Adolescence, 6,* 201–223.

Vaillancourt, T., Brendgen, M., Boivin, M., & Tremblay, R. E. (2003). A longitudinal confirmatory factor analysis of indirect and physical aggression: Evidence of two factors over time? *Child Development, 74,* 1628–1638.

Vaillancourt, T., Miller, J. T., Fagbemi, J., Cote, S., & Tremblay, R. E. (2007). Trajectories and predictors of indirect aggression: Results from a nationally representative sample of Canadian children aged 2–10. *Aggressive Behavior, 33,* 314–326.

Werner, N. E., & Crick, N. R. (1999). Relational aggression and social-psychological adjustment in a college sample. *Journal of Abnormal Psychology, 108,* 615–623.

Werner, N. E., & Crick, N. R. (2004). Maladaptive peer relationships and the development of relational and physical aggression during middle childhood. *Social Development, 13,* 495–514.

Willoughby, T., Chalmers, H., & Busseri, M. A. (2004). Where is the syndrome? Examining co-occurrence among multiple problem behaviors in adolescence. *Journal of Consulting and Clinical Psychology, 72,* 1022–1037.

Wright, J. C., Giammarino, M., & Parad, H. W. (1986). Social status in small groups: Individual–group similarity and the social "misfit." *Journal of Personality and Social Psychology, 50,* 523–536.

Xie, H., Swift, D. J., Cairns, B. D., & Cairns, R. B. (2002). Aggressive behaviors in social interaction and developmental adaptation: A narrative analyses of interpersonal conflicts during early adolescence. *Social Development, 11*, 205–224.

Zahn-Waxler, C., & Polanichka, N. (2004). All things interpersonal: Socialization and female aggression. In M. Putallaz & K. L. Bierman (Eds.), *Aggression, antisocial behavior, and violence in girls: A developmental perspective* (pp. 48–68). New York: Guilford Press.

10

The Science
of Moral Development

Lawrence J. Walker
Jeremy A. Frimer

The title of this chapter may seem mundane, even forgettable, at first glance. But on reflection, the title may cause the reader some apprehension. We suspect such a reaction is sourced to two related paradoxes—each a seemingly nonkosher befuddlement of concepts—in the title itself. Ponder, then, these two questions: First, how can the descriptive method of psychological science—which can catalogue how matters *are*—inform the prescriptive domain of morality, which dictates how matters *ought to be*? And second, how can impersonal scientific observations examine moral phenomena that are personal, subjective experiences? We introduce this chapter by exploring these paradoxes, which will allow us to carve out a paradigmatic space for the science of morality. By describing the discipline's subject matter and what it can and cannot achieve, this exercise will also provide a framework for approaching the different content areas within this domain, which make up the subject matter of this chapter.

THE INTERPLAY OF SCIENCE AND MORALITY

Can Descriptive Psychology Inform Prescriptive Morality?

A first source of hesitation may arise from an unusual application of science: to the study of morality. Historically, morality has fallen outside the purview of science, more often addressed by religious figures, social commentators, philosophers, and societal leaders. Morality, after all, is inherently *prescriptive*; by contrast, the epistemic toolkit of science is explicitly *descriptive*. Contributing to a prescriptive discipline using a descriptive device may appear to be an impossible task, a mixing of categories. Drawing conclusions about what *ought to be* based on observations of an existing state of affairs is such a verboten deed that philosophers (Moore, 1903) have applied the pejorative label "the naturalistic fallacy." So, how can the descriptive method of science approach or inform moral prescriptions?

As is presupposed in the chapter's title, we believe that the coordination of science and morality is not only feasible but, in fact, worthwhile and productive. As a method for acquiring knowledge, science needs a subject matter, a set of claims to test empirically. The subject matter (e.g., reasoning vs. emotions) may be selected either by deliberately ascribing to a particular prescriptive philosophy or by more passively riding a zeitgeist. This adoption of a prescriptive theory, whether explicit or implicit, marks a critical turning point, which often favors certain methods and arguments over others. (These turning points are highlighted in each section of this chapter.) As will become apparent, some of the diversity within the psychological study of moral development can be primarily attributed to the differing paradigmatic assumptions underlying the enterprises. To help situate a scientific study, each enterprise needs to clearly acknowledge the prescriptive claims about morality underlying the empirical work. In this sense, psychological science is a "consumer" of moral philosophy.

The influence between moral psychology and philosophy, however, is not unidirectional. Science contributes to our understanding of prescriptions by testing descriptive assertions that are part of the foundation of prescriptive claims (Johnson, 1996). Often, prescriptive codes entail descriptive premises. For example, Kant's (1785/1964) categorical imperative prescribes a method for reasoning through moral conflicts, built on the assumption that abstract reasoning is an essential step in acting appropriately. Notice that the latter (namely, that the quality of one's reasoning influences behavior) is an empirical claim—one that has been challenged using scientific methods (Blasi, 1980; Haidt, 2001). In this way, psychological science can bolster or undermine the foundation of moral claims.

This opening discussion is meant to (1) draw attention to some anticipated concerns about the application of science to morality; (2) set a paradigmatic boundary around this field of study; and (3) foreshadow some of the ways that scientific work can interplay with morality. Exploring the second apparent paradox built into the application of science to morality will help pinpoint the kinds of topics studied in this field.

Can Impersonal Science Examine Personal Moral Phenomena?

To return to possible reactions to the title of this chapter, we now address the second paradox therein. Experiencing morality—be it a reasoned argument about right or wrong, a stab of guilt, or a sense of compassion for the hurting—is a personal, subjective affair; the phenomenon of morality is located inside the individual (the moral agent). By contrast, science, as the systematic study of natural phenomena, is impersonal, verifiably witnessed by multiple observers. How can scientists study phenomena that exist uniquely in the subjective experience of individuals? This problem is not unique to moral psychology (e.g., similar concerns are evident in the study of attitudes, the self-concept, and so on), but the solution within each discipline may be somewhat different.

The solution that scientists of morality have adopted is to conceive of moral beings not only as subjects (experiencing their world in moral terms) but also as objects (as having certain psychological mechanisms and structures that interact with their experience). Researchers study the latter—the psychological *functioning* of persons experiencing, forming, and reacting to their morality. This distinction hopefully helps to frame the subject matter of the discipline as being the psychological processes that are at play in individuals' moral experience.

The Subject Matter of Moral Development

Demystifying this second paradox is intended to locate the subject matter of the discipline. What, then, is this subjective psychological matter that makes up the moral experience? Early theories highlighted different components of the moral experience. Freud's (1927) psychoanalytic approach to morality focused on the development of the superego, acquired primarily through identification with the same-sex parent; moral functioning in his theory was limited to emotion regulation processes. This emphasis on affect marginalized moral judgment, which was viewed as being readily distorted by defense mechanisms. Skinner's (1938) behaviorist approach focused on the acquisition of overt behaviors, shaped and conditioned through environmental contingencies. Cognitive and affective processes were regarded as epiphenomenal and irrelevant; and eventually Skinner (1971) explicitly eschewed the notion of morality altogether. In essence, behaviorism argued against the idea of a science of moral development. Piaget's (1932/1977) cognitive-developmental approach focused on moral judgment, which was held to develop as a function of structural growth and cognitive disequilibrium. In this approach, moral behavior was essentially regarded as a by-product of moral cognition. Thus the early history of the field was characterized by a seemingly rigid "partitioning" of the moral domain, which obscured its complexity and the interdependent nature of its components.

The contemporary study of moral development is, at least superficially, more pluralistic in that each "school" acknowledges that moral functioning references not a single but several processes. This scaffold allows us to provide a brief outline of the evolution of the science of moral development by exploring particular topics in their historical context. Our initial attention in this chapter is on the development of moral reasoning, given the dominance of Kohlberg's (1969) cognitive-developmental model in the field for some time and the fact that much of the later work either built on his framework or was an explicit reaction to it. For example, the neo-Kohlbergian approach (advocated by Rest, Narvaez, Bebeau, & Thoma, 1999) entailed a significant conceptual and methodological extension of Kohlberg's approach, with a focus on moral schemas.

Some of the blunter challenges to Kohlberg's model, giving rise to substantial controversy, included Gilligan's (1982) positing of gender-related moral orientations, Turiel's (1983) notion of domain distinctions, and Haidt's (2001) emphasis on moral intuition and the relegation of deliberative reasoning. One of the problems, however, of the conceptual focus on moral cognition is that it tends to slight the moral competencies of young children, who are largely inarticulate on moral matters. Thus our attention shifts to early conscience development and the significance of various moral emotions (Eisenberg, Spinrad, & Sadovsky, 2006). Finally, the imperfect, indeed weak, relation that is typically evident between moral cognition and behavior leads to a discussion of aspects of moral motivation, including moral personality and identity, which intends to answer the question, "Why be moral, anyway?"

STAGES

A major impetus for the psychological study of moral development was World War II, with its horrors of global conflagration, over 60 million casualties, the Holocaust, and the releasing of nuclear weapons on civilian populations. In its aftermath, social scientists struggled to explain such pernicious behavior. Personality psychologists speculated about the functioning of the authoritarian personality (Adorno, Frenkel-Brunswik, Levinson, & Sanford, 1950); social psychologists focused on the contextual pressures that contribute to obedience to authorities (Milgram, 1974; Zimbardo, Banks, Haney, & Jaffe, 1973); and developmental psychologists pointed to deficiencies in processes of moral judgment (Kohlberg, 1969).

Kohlberg's Stage Model

Among the intellectual tasks that Kohlberg engaged in was explaining how most Germans could be complicit or even actively participate in the heinous projects of the Third Reich. Kohlberg's general approach was to differentiate three different types (or levels) of moral reasoning: personal, conventional, and principled. (Two stages compose each level, as discussed later.) The personal, preconventional level largely characterizes the thinking of children. Whereas the conventional level is the most common form of reasoning for adults, this orientation left the German masses grossly underequipped to adequately challenge the broader Nazi culture. The rarely acquired principled, postconventional level, by contrast, provides a basis for critically examining the deeds of authorities and moving against the same when good reasons so dictate.

Kohlberg's claim was not just that these three types of thought differ from one another but that principled reasoning is *better* than conventional reasoning, which is, in turn, *better* than preconventional reasoning. By "better," Kohlberg meant that the former is better able to solve moral problems, is more equilibrated, and is more philosophically defensible than the latter. This prescriptive claim aimed to defend against, even defeat, ethical relativism—the notion that morality can only be defined and scrutinized relative to a culture—and thus provided a sound basis for rejecting the likes of Nazism. Kohlberg's empirical project was to substantiate this prescriptive claim using scientific, descriptive methods—to "Commit the Naturalistic Fallacy and Get Away with It," as he brashly put it (Kohlberg, 1971). The core of Kohlberg's approach was to argue that if the ordering of the adequacy of these structures of reasoning is correct, then this order will be evident in the natural world, in individual human development. This postulation reframed the sequence into a developmental stage model of moral reasoning (see Colby & Kohlberg, 1987), one that was claimed to be cross-culturally applicable.

The first two stages make up the preconventional level. At Stage 1 (*heteronomy*), children understand the dictates of authorities and the physical consequences of actions as defining right and wrong. Stage 2 (*exchange*) reasoning focuses on serving one's own interests and so cooperative interaction is based on notions of simple exchange. The next two stages reflect the conventional level of moral reasoning and are typical of the thinking of older adolescents and adults. Stage 3 (*expectations*) entails conforming to expectations, having good motives, and keeping mutual relationships. The focus of Stage 4 (*social system and conscience*) is on maintenance of the social order and meeting the demands of conscience. Finally, Stages 5 and 6 compose the principled, postconventional level. Stage 5 (*prior rights and social contract*) is evidenced by a small minority of adults who reason in terms of nonrelative values and mutual standards that reflect a social contract. The theoretical end point of the model is Stage 6 (*universal ethical principles*), which entails self-chosen universal principles of justice that focus on equality of rights and respect for the dignity of human beings (Kohlberg, Boyd, & Levine, 1990). The "logic" of the stage order reflects the increasing complexity of social perspective that each entails: from self alone, to self and another, to the primary reference group, to broader society, and then beyond society.

Kohlberg's (1981, 1984) model quickly came to dominate the field of moral development because of its bold conceptual claims and significant practical implications. His approach reflected not only the psychological tradition of Piaget's (1932/1977) structural-developmental theory but also the Western philosophical tradition of the Enlightenment thinkers (such as Immanuel Kant, 1785/1964). More than any other scientist in the field of moral development, Kohlberg was aware of and explicit about the philosophical framing of his model. His 1981 book, *The Philosophy of Moral Development*, embraced a formalist, deontological moral philosophy that emphasized the centrality of reasoning in moral functioning and that specified universal principles of justice as the developmental end point. Furthermore, Kohlberg was clear about what he meant by moral development: progression through the moral reasoning stage sequence.

How did Kohlberg suggest that one measure these stages of moral reasoning? Kohlberg's Moral Judgment Interview (MJI) entails prompting a participant to reason through several challenging, hypothetical moral dilemmas, which were designed to "test the limits" of people's moral understandings. The most classic of these is the "Heinz dilemma," wherein Heinz, having exhausted all other alternatives, needs to decide whether to steal a pharmaceutical drug to save his wife's life. Responses are scored using a laborious but highly specific coding manual (Colby & Kohlberg, 1987).

Empirical Claims

With this background in mind, we can now examine the heart of Kohlberg's conceptual and scientific enterprise. His project entailed a series of empirical claims. First, he claimed that each stage of moral reasoning is psychologically real—not merely an ad hoc abstraction but indeed representing a holistic structure in the natural world. This assertion was extended into the scientific realm to claim that individuals are relatively consistent in their moral reasoning across different contexts, either "in" a stage or "in transition" between adjacent stages, but not straddling two nonadjacent stages (e.g., Stages 2 and 4). The extant evidence (Walker, 1988) indicates that people are typically found to be consistent in their stage of moral reasoning across varying contexts (e.g., in responding to hypothetical vs. real-life dilemmas); only under fairly intense situational pressure does this consistency begin to crack.

Next, Kohlberg claimed that these stage structures are not only real but are ordered relative to one another in a highly specific, namely invariant, way. Developmentally, this was translated to mean that the progress of acquisition of the stages is irreversibly forward, one stage at a time (no regressions and no stage skipping). The rate and eventual end point of development may vary, but not the order of the stages. Longitudinal evidence (Colby, Kohlberg, Gibbs, & Lieberman, 1983; Walker, Gustafson, & Frimer, 2007) has confirmed that people do develop through the stages in the order specified, with few violations of the sequence.

A third claim of Kohlberg's model holds that successive stages represent better equilibrated reasoning in that they hierarchically integrate the concepts of previous stages. That is, a later stage is both psychologically and ethically superior. Available evidence suggests that people do recognize the increasing moral adequacy of successive moral stages by favoring the highest stage within the range of their comprehension (Walker, de Vries, & Bichard, 1984). Thus, the validity of Kohlberg's model of moral reasoning development has received considerable empirical support and therein is his foremost contribution to the discipline.

Developmental Mechanism of Disequilibrium

An understanding of Kohlberg's stage model raises the question of how one progresses through the stages. What developmental processes underlie transitions? The core developmental mechanism in cognitive-developmental theory is disequilibrium, which is the subjective experience of conflict, puzzlement, or inadequacy (Kohlberg, 1984; Piaget, 1975/1985). Kohlberg saw disequilibrium as being of paramount developmental importance in spite of (perhaps because of) such associated discomfort. Disequilibrium is held to propel (or motivate) structural reorganization toward more equilibrated stages of thinking. Note that the structural-developmental mechanism for development differs sharply from the identification–internalization process proposed by the psychoanalytic approach and from the conditioning and observational learning process proposed by the behavioral approach.

Various research strategies have examined the viability of the construct of disequilibrium as a mechanism for moral reasoning development (see Walker, 2004, for a review). Perhaps the most illustrative of these has examined disequilibrium within the family context. Walker, Hennig, and Krettenauer (2000) found that contrasting parenting styles were differentially predictive of children's moral reasoning development. The parents of children who evidenced considerable moral growth were particularly child-centered in their techniques, scaffolding their child's development by eliciting the child's opinions, posing appropriate probing questions, and checking for understanding. This was typically accomplished in the context of emotional support and attentiveness, along with the challenging stimulation of more sophisticated reasoning. These techniques reflect a disequilibrating Socratic style that can be strongly effective in inducing rethinking. In contrast, the parents of children who evidenced minimal development seemed to undermine their children's processing by engaging in overwhelmingly opinionated and challenging interactions, being hostile and critical, and being ego defensive. This parenting style interferes with children's meaningful engagement with moral issues and diminishes their experience of disequilibrium that might foster more mature moral understandings.

The conceptual richness and empirical strength of Kohlberg's model and methodology allowed their domination of the field of moral psychology for almost a generation. As has been seen in this section, empirical support did accrue for the validity of the stage model and for the developmental mechanism it posited. But, not surprisingly, Kohlberg's model attracted a number of significant challenges that speak to its limitations. To anticipate what follows, Kohlberg's approach embodies an incomplete depiction of the functioning of a moral agent. This claim does not diminish the model's substantial contributions to our understanding of moral reasoning but rather places these contributions within a more comprehensive framework.

SCHEMAS

The viability of Kohlberg's enterprise eventually was stymied by his labor-intensive interview and subjective coding system. Conducting and coding interviews consumed an inordinate amount of resources, and so research on the model began to languish from lack of an efficient methodology.

Rest (1979) developed the Defining Issues Test (DIT), loosely based on Kohlberg's approach, as a multiple-choice alternative to Kohlberg's MJI. The accessibility and relative ease of use of the DIT quickly vaulted it to the position of measure-of-choice in the moral development field. On the DIT, participants respond to a series of hypothetical dilemmas (as on the MJI). However, unlike the MJI, in which participants actually reason aloud regarding the moral problems, on the DIT participants simply evaluate brief fragmentary examples of moral judgments (by rating and then ranking them). The recommended index of moral judgment development is not a stage score but rather the P score, which is an indicator of how highly an individual ranks postconventional items.

Neo-Kohlbergian Approach

Although the DIT approach initially surfed the rising tide of Kohlberg's moral stage model by providing a methodological alternative, over time it also introduced some significant conceptual reformulations, becoming known as the neo-Kohlbergian approach (Rest et al., 1999). In the neo-Kohlbergian approach, focus is on tacit moral understandings rather than on the articulation of moral reasons (as with the MJI). The premise is that people often know more than they can tell. In that sense, the DIT can be considered akin to a projective test because it presents brief questions or fragments of reasoning (not elaborated arguments) to which participants impute meaning as they respond to the test items. The DIT is construed as a device for activating moral schemas and for assessing these schemas in terms of relevance judgments.

The items on the DIT were initially intended as examples of reasoning at Kohlberg's moral stages, but the neo-Kohlbergian approach (Rest et al., 1999) now explicitly abandons those stages and instead proposes three developmental moral schemas: personal interest, maintaining norms, and postconventional. These schemas are understood as general knowledge structures that facilitate information processing. They differ from stages in that they are not defined in terms of underlying structural operations; rather, they are more concrete and entail more content.

Moral Schemas

The personal-interest schema references the personal stake that individuals have in the consequences of their actions and entails some of the themes in Kohlberg's Stages 2 and 3. The maintaining-norms schema aligns with Kohlberg's Stage 4 and references generally accepted norms and role structures for governing a society. The postconventional schema appeals to shared ideals that are impartial in their formulation and logically coherent in fostering consensus. Kohlberg was often criticized for aligning his psychological theory with a particular philosophical tradition that espoused formalist principles of justice and respect for persons. The neo-Kohlbergian model circumvents this criticism by not embracing principled morality or any other recognizable moral philosophy, but instead advocating a less philosophically pure "common morality" that is characterized in generic postconventional terms (merely reflecting judgments that tend to cluster and to be endorsed by relatively mature people).

Neo-Kohlbergians have long held antipathy to the strong stage model in the moral domain (Rest, 1979), arguing against defining development as progression through a sequence of "hard" stages of reasoning and instead conceptualizing development as "softer" changes involving shifting distributions of reasoning across schemas. The emphasis of the neo-Kohlbergian approach has been on the shift from conventional to postconventional moral understandings. The DIT is not intended to tap the moral schemas that are predominant in childhood, and its cognitive demands preclude its use with participants younger than adolescence. This emphasis pinpoints one of the major limitations of the model and the measure: It does not offer much insight into the moral functioning of children.

Construct Validity

Researchers within the neo-Kohlbergian framework, however, have amassed a considerable amount of evidence attesting to the construct validity of the DIT (Rest et al., 1999), and their program of research is illustrative in that regard. A sampling of these findings include: differences in moral judgment level between groups that vary in age, education, or expertise; progressive changes in level of moral judgment in longitudinal studies and in moral education interventions; relationships to political attitudes; prediction of moral behavior; evidence of internal structure (factor-analytic studies yield factors reflecting the three moral schemas); and discriminant validity (moral judgment is not merely a reflection of other variables such as verbal ability).

Although Rest and his colleagues introduced both conceptual and methodological innovations to the Kohlbergian framework (see Walker, 2002, for a review), they believe that the general approach remains generally useful and valid (hence the *neo-*Kohlbergian moniker). For example, the approaches share the emphasis on the personal construction of moral meanings in their understanding of moral epistemology. They explicitly share an emphasis on the cognitive aspects of moral functioning. Both approaches are unabashedly developmental, eschewing any definition of morality that aligns it with adherence to conventional norms and claiming that a principled or postconventional form of moral reasoning is more defensible from a philosophical perspective. Despite the considerable empirical success of the Kohlbergian and neo-Kohlbergian paradigms, the tandem encountered significant challenges for other reasons, which quickly heightened controversy in the field.

ORIENTATIONS

Gilligan (1982) may have provided the most direct challenge to dominant models in moral psychology with her well-publicized arguments regarding gender and morality, arguments made during the ascendency of feminism in America. Her contentions were twofold. First, Gilligan claimed that the moral thinking of women is qualitatively different ("In a Different Voice") from that of men; women's morality is characterized by an ethic of care, and men's by an ethic of justice. These moral orientations are held to reflect a fundamental difference in the way that women and men orient to life. Second, she claimed that influential theories of human development (including Kohlberg's) are biased against women's experiences. In her view, Kohlberg's approach misconstrues women's distinctive voice on morality and hence portrays women as being morally deficient.

Gendered Moral Orientations

Gilligan's primary proposal was that men and women typically have different moral orientations. A moral orientation is a conceptually distinctive framework for understanding and organizing one's morality. Men, she argued, typically have a justice orientation, based on their individualistic sense of self, identity derived from vocation, detached objectivity, and preference for abstract rules and principles. In contrast (and she does hold that these are fundamentally incompatible perspectives), women characteristically have a care orientation, based on their interdependent sense of self, identity derived from relationships, sensitivity not to hurt, concern for the well-being of self and others, and a focus on maintaining harmonious relationships.

Gilligan's claim of gender-related moral orientations raised questions of their developmental origins. Borrowing from neopsychoanalytic theory, Gilligan and Wiggins (1987) proposed that these orientations arise in young boys' and girls' relationships with parents; in particular, in their differential experiences of attachment and inequality. Gilligan surmised that girls are both attached to and identify with their mothers; and so their identities develop in the context of maintaining this relationship. Thus, for girls, the experience of attachment, of maintaining connections with others, is central to their self-definitions, whereas the experience of inequality is not as relevant. Their developmental outcome is an orientation toward care and the maintenance of relationships. In contrast, although boys are also initially attached to their mothers, they come to identify with their fathers; and so their identities develop as they detach from the mother and begin to relate to the father's power and status. Thus, for boys, the experience of inequality and the need for independence become central to their self-definitions. Their developmental outcome is an orientation toward justice and a separate sense of self.

Gilligan's theorizing attracted widespread attention, with scientific examination of her claims (a fuller discussion is provided by Walker, 2006). A fundamental issue concerns whether the characterization of individuals as having a specific moral orientation accurately captures how they actually function. In Gilligan's view, the notion of an orientation implies that people should be relatively consistent (across contexts and over time) in their reliance on that orientation. However, the available evidence does not support this claim (Walker & Frimer, 2009b). In a typical examination of this issue, participants were prompted to reason through two real-life moral problems, and their orientation on each was scored as either *justice* or *care* (Pratt, Golding, Hunter, & Sampson, 1988). Only 60% of their sample evidenced the same orientation on the two moral dilemmas, a level of consistency that does not differ from chance. Thus empirical examination has not supported the claim of consistency; most people use a mix of both types of reasoning, with no evident preference, undermining the naturalistic claim of moral orientations.

Setting aside the question of consistency in moral orientations, Gilligan's primary claim concerned gender differences, with men orienting to justice and women to care. This claim proved to be provocative and prompted considerable research on the issue, culminating in Jaffee and Hyde's (2000) review and meta-analysis of 113 studies. Overall, they found that gender differences were not evident in most studies (73% of the studies that assessed care reasoning and 72% of those that assessed justice reasoning). In short, there is no compelling evidence for the strong gender polarity in moral orientations claimed by Gilligan.

In follow-up analyses, Jaffee and Hyde (2000) compared studies using standard hypothetical dilemmas (including those designed to elicit either justice or care reasoning) with those using personally generated, real-life dilemmas. Gender differences were generally weak and not significant when participants were responding to standard dilemmas, whereas moderate effects were found when participants were reasoning through real-life dilemmas. Given that the real-life dilemmas were idiosyncratic, this latter pattern of moderate gender differences may be explained by a methodological artifact. That is, the occasional findings of gender differences on real-life dilemmas could merely be a function of the different moral problems that women and men tend to encounter and choose to relate, rather than a dispositional difference in moral orientation.

This hypothesis was corroborated by Walker, de Vries, and Trevethan's (1987) finding that, within different types of real-life dilemmas (namely, personal vs. impersonal), gender differences in moral orientations were not evident. The apparent gender differences in moral orientations with real-life dilemmas reflect a methodological artifact. En masse, the evidence reveals that people do not consistently focus on a single moral orientation but, instead, use reasoning that reflects the nature of the moral problem under consideration. Gilligan's claim of gender differences in moral orientations has thus far not fared well against scientific scrutiny.

Another of Gilligan's claims concerns the developmental origins of these orientations. Unfortunately, she did not present any supportive empirical evidence relevant to this issue, nor did she explain how the dimensions of inequality and attachment might be directly assessed in early parent–child relationships. One should not expect that such psychoanalytic theorizing would be readily amenable to empirical test. Also note Gilligan's implication that relationships with peers and with other adults are not particularly relevant to moral development. Turiel (2006) challenged that implication and the claim that these dimensions are strongly related to gender by noting that the experience of inequality is more salient for girls and women in patriarchal societies and that the experience of attachment is salient for boys in the context of groups, team sports, and gangs. The only study that is tangentially relevant to Gilligan's claims regarding developmental origins of the orientations was conducted by Lollis, Ross, and Leroux (1996). But, in observing parents' interactions with their preschoolers, they found no indication that girls receive more care-oriented reasoning or that boys receive more justice-oriented reasoning from either parent.

Conceptual issues regarding Gilligan's theory have also been raised. One recurring question concerns her prescriptive claim of what moral maturity entails. Is the care orientation ethically preferable? Are the two orientations equally valid but fundamentally incompatible? Is moral maturity represented by integration of the two orientations? Gilligan (1982) provides conflicting answers on this score. As was discussed at the outset of this chapter, specifying the developmental end point (and thus the prescriptive claim) is critical in evaluating any model of human development. Other conceptual problems with Gilligan's theory have been identified, including: its reinforcement of restrictive and traditional stereotypes about the sexes, its rigid dichotomization on the basis of gender, and its limited scope of moral responsibility (only within the sphere of familiar, personal relationships).

Gender Bias in Dominant Models

Regardless of the validity of Gilligan's claim of gendered moral orientations, we can consider her second major claim: that influential theories of human development—particularly Kohlberg's—are biased against females and their ethic of care. Gilligan (1982) alleged that Kohlberg's approach indicates a lower stage of moral reasoning for women than for men and that such evidence confirms the pervasive gender bias of Kohlberg's model.

As is becoming a pattern, Gilligan's claim of gender bias is at odds with the data. Walker (1984) conducted a meta-analysis of the 80 existing studies of gender differences in Kohlberg's model and found that gender was not a significant predictor of moral stage as Gilligan assumed; indeed, gender explained an infinitesimal portion (1/2000th) of the variability in moral reasoning development. Thoma (1986) similarly reviewed gender differences on the DIT and found a small effect *favoring females*; and, to put this effect into context, age and education were found to be 250 times more powerful in predicting level of moral judgment than was gender. Perish in the scientific gauntlet did Gilligan's allegation of gender bias; her claim has been "convincingly debunked" (Jaffee & Hyde, 2000, p. 707).

This section of the chapter has revealed that gender explains a negligible amount of the variability in moral reasoning development and that Gilligan is substantially incorrect in that regard. This, of course, does not speak to the possibility that gender might be an important variable in other aspects of moral functioning (such as moral emotions or moral character), and it does not negate the many other positive contributions that Gilligan has made to moral psychology in general—by drawing attention to the need to have better representative samples in psychological research; by raising awareness of the limited scope of theoretical perspectives in moral psychology; by expanding our conceptions of moral development with the broadening emphasis on care; and by introducing the methodology of eliciting self-generated real-life dilemmas which has yielded new insights about the moral lives of real people.

DOMAINS

All of the theoretical perspectives considered to this point in the chapter have centered on the development of moral intellect, with their prescriptive claims thus far sending inarticulate preschool children to the moral basement. But we can rightly ask whether anything foundational in moral development occurs early in the lifespan. This section and the next explore early indicators of moral sensibilities in the development of younger children.

Early Moral Awareness

Evidence is beginning to accumulate to indicate that the moral lives of young children are already rich. Wright and Bartsch (2008), for example, analyzed everyday conversations of children between 2 and 5 years of age, attempting to provide a window on their moral awareness. They documented that, even at the youngest ages, children readily engage in morally relevant conversations with adults. There was a clear tendency for these preschoolers to be active rather than passive in their moral conversations; that is, to introduce moral issues rather than merely respond to adult leads. This is not what the cognitive-developmental tradition would have predicted; in that framework, children are premorally self-focused.

Both Piaget (1932/1977) and Kohlberg (1969) described young children as heteronomous, as having unilateral respect for authorities who dictate what is right and wrong. However, studies of children's reasoning about authority (Laupa, Turiel, & Cowan, 1995) have revealed a more differentiated view. For example, Tisak (1986) found that children do draw boundaries around parents' jurisdiction based on the nature of the action involved: Almost all children accorded parents the authority to make a rule prohibiting stealing; fewer children gave this response when the rule involved family chores; and almost none allowed that parents should regulate friendships. Although these findings suggest that children respect parental authority at least in the moral domain, Damon (1977) found that even preschool children rejected the legitimacy of a parental injunction to steal from or to harm someone else, suggesting that children understand that moral rules are not subject to parental whims. Clearly, the moral universe of young children is not simply determined by the dictates of authority. Indeed, these findings indicate that children's view of authority varies with the domain of social knowledge.

Domains of Social Knowledge

In Kohlberg's framework, personal, conventional, and moral considerations are jumbled together in early life and only gradually become differentiated over the course of development. Turiel's (1983) conceptual challenge to this view claimed that personal, conventional, and moral knowledge constitute distinct conceptual domains, each of which (1) is understood even by young children, (2) entails its own unique sort of social experience, and (3) develops independently from the other domains.

Turiel's domain theory identifies three domains. The *moral* domain pertains to issues of justice, rights, and human welfare, and so entails prescriptive judgments about how people should behave toward each other. Prototypical moral transgressions would be inherently wrong actions, such as hitting or stealing. The *conventional* domain pertains to arbitrary but shared norms in behavior that serve to coordinate people's interactions. Prototypical social conventions would be types of attire or modes of address (e.g., "Yes, sir"). The *personal* domain pertains to matters of individual prerogative that apply primarily to the self and fall outside the purview of moral concern and social regulation. Prototypical personal issues would be choice of friends and personal appearance.

Research on this model indicates that even preschool children make distinctions across these domains, in accord with theoretical criteria (Smetana, 2006). Typically, the research paradigm involves presenting children with simple, hypothetical vignettes that are prototypical of each domain and then eliciting their judgments (and justifications). For moral transgressions (such as hitting or lying), children assert that the wrongness of this action is not dependent on the existence of a rule and that it would be wrong to alter this rule. These rule contingency and rule alterability criteria reflect the philosophical notion that moral rules are prescriptive. Children similarly assert that it would be wrong for another society not to have such a rule and that it would be wrong to engage in this action even if that society had no rule. These rule and act generalizability criteria reflect the notion that moral rules are universally applicable. Thus moral rules are viewed as independent of social regulation and generalizable across contexts.

In contrast, social conventions (such as forms of greeting or address) are rule-dependent and hold normative force only within the social system in which they were formed. Thus a conventional violation (e.g., referring to schoolteachers by their first names) is wrong only if there is an explicit prohibition, and these rules can readily vary across social contexts. Personal issues (such as the choice of friends) are judged by children to be under individual jurisdiction and not subject to either moral or conventional regulation.

How do such domain distinctions arise in children's social understanding? Domain theory holds that the emergence of these different conceptual systems can be explained by the qualitatively different forms of social interaction that children experience. Nucci and Weber (1995), for example, found in an observational study that mothers of preschoolers restricted children's actions in the moral and the conventional domains but negotiated personal matters and accorded children a fair amount of freedom. And although both children and adults respond to moral transgressions, children are less likely than adults to respond to conventional violations because of their arbitrary nature and social origins (Smetana, 2006).

Definition of the Moral Domain

The evidence from the domain approach is compelling in its demonstration that young children have more complex social understandings than was previously presumed—in particular, in distinguishing between unalterable moral imperatives, arbitrary social norms, and areas of personal jurisdiction. However, a couple of related issues surrounding the approach should be flagged. One concern focuses on its paradigmatic assumptions regarding the nature of the moral domain—defined narrowly as pertaining only to issues of justice, rights, and human welfare. This definition circumscribes the scope of the domain to be exclusively interpersonal and excludes intrapsychic functions (such as values and identity), even if these functions are responsible for motivating one to live out the "morally good life." A more complete account of development includes both the differentiation of morality from the personal and also the later integration of the two (Piaget, 1975/1985).

The other concern deals with the frequent reliance on simplistic prototypical vignettes to tap each domain, which yields evidence that these domains are more strongly demarcated than is either typical or appropriate in everyday life. Although social conventions may be arbitrary, that does not mean that they are void of moral significance. For example, gender roles are obvious social conventions (arbitrary, changeable, specific to contexts), but gender inequality certainly has moral implications (Okin, 1989). Similarly, substance abuse reflects the personal domain (as a matter of personal jurisdiction), but that activity is rife with moral implications for self and others. The domain approach has yet to accord sufficient attention to children's and adolescents' developing ability to handle multifaceted events in their social worlds and, in particular, to appreciate the moral implications of many personal choices and actions.

EMOTIONS

Young children evidence a moral sense not only in the form of social knowledge but also by way of emotional dispositions. Based on observations of toddlers' reactions to flawed objects, Kagan (1981) made an intriguing suggestion. He speculated that young children's interest in and distress over broken objects reflects an emerging sense of propriety—an awareness of standards and how things ought to be. This emerging sense would set the important psychological building blocks for aspects of conscience, including guilt, shame, and similar self-conscious emotions.

Self-Conscious Emotions

Kochanska, Casey, and Fukumoto (1995) unpacked this assertion to predict that differences in toddlers' sensitivity to flawed objects would predict their emotional reactions to their own transgressions. These researchers compared 2- and 3-year-olds' reactions to flawed and whole objects; in another context, they assessed the toddlers' behavior in response to contrived mishaps (in which the children were led to believe that they had caused damage to the experimenter's valued possession). Toddlers' reactivity to this whole–flawed quality of objects predicted their responses to their own apparent wrongdoing, as evidenced by distress during mishaps and subsequent apologetic comments and reparative attempts. These findings indicate that young children's ability to appreciate standards and their violations—to experience right and wrong—perhaps reflects an early-arriving "moral instinct" (Pinker, 2008).

Other-Oriented Emotions

Moral behavior can be motivated not only by "negative" self-conscious emotions, such as guilt and shame, but also by more "positive" other-oriented emotions, such as empathy and sympathy. When do children first experience empathy, and how does it develop from then on? Hoffman's (2000) stage theory posits that empathy emerges early and that infants are biologically predisposed to experience a primitive form, given the evidence that newborns cry selectively in response to other infants' cries. Moving from this initial stage of global empathic distress, toddlers develop to a stage of undifferentiated, egocentric empathy in which they often fail to distinguish their own and the other's internal states, and so their prosocial behaviors are sometimes misguided (e.g., a toddler might try to console another child by proffering his or her own security blanket). Later, in the preschool years, children typically reach a stage at which they evidence empathy for another's feelings based on simple perspective taking and an appreciation of a wider range of emotions. Then, by later childhood, development proceeds to a stage of empathy for others' general condition or plight beyond the immediate situation, based on broader social understandings. Note that, in Hoffman's model, emotion and cognition become increasingly interwoven as development proceeds.

This conceptualization of the moral capabilities of infants and toddlers challenges the cognitive-developmental caricature of the young child as "premoral" and overwhelmingly egocentric. Zahn-Waxler, Radke-Yarrow, Wagner, and Chapman (1992) provided empirical corroboration of the notion that empathy-related responding begins early in the lifespan, behavior that is not merely based on parental directives or coercive fear. They assessed infants' responses to others' distress in a sample of 1-year-olds followed longitudinally for a year. Mothers reported their children's responses to emotion events, including ones witnessed by the children (e.g., parents arguing), and the children's behaviors in response to simulated distress incidents (e.g., mother feigning choking). Findings indicated that both empathic concern and prosocial behaviors increase over this age range, suggesting that young children are not purely egocentric but are actively involved in the emotional lives of others.

How does empathy lead to prosocial behavior, and how can this process go awry? Eisenberg and colleagues (2006) propose an answer. They conceptualize empathy as being value-neutral, as an affective response similar to what the other is feeling. This empathic response can lead either to personal distress (a self-focused, aversive reaction to another's emotional state) or to sympathy (an emotional response involving feelings of concern for the other). Personal distress is likely to lead to egoistic reactions and reflects poor social competence, whereas sympathy more likely motivates prosocial behavior. Thus the ability to regulate emotional reactions may figure prominently in activating moral behavior.

Temperament and Socialization Influences

If early-appearing moral emotions have some biological or temperamental origin, then that raises the question of the corresponding role of socialization influences on children's conscience development. Kochanska's (1997) research nicely melds these two effects. Her goodness-of-fit model focuses on the interplay between the child's temperament and parental socialization in fostering the development of conscience and suggests that there may be different socialization processes that promote moral internalization in children with different temperaments. She suggests that, for temperamentally anxious children, deemphasizing power assertion and instead relying on psychological discipline that capitalizes on the child's internal discomfort will be most effective. In contrast, for temperamentally fearless children, discipline (either power assertive or psychological) will be ineffective because it induces minimal anxiety; rather, effective parenting should capitalize on the secure relationship between parent and child. Kochanska's study with 2- and 3-year olds initially assessed children's temperament and mother–child interactions and then, a year later, assessed conscience development (cheating on games and moral themes in projective stories). As hypothesized, inductive discipline predicted moral internalization for temperamentally fearful children, whereas a secure attachment to a responsive mother predicted moral internalization for temperamentally fearless children. In sum, these and other findings (Thompson, Meyer, & McGinley, 2006) indicate that the influence of early socialization experience may be mediated by the child's temperamental profile.

The now compelling data regarding young children's moral sensibilities prompt interest in the socialization influences that might foster these nascent understandings and emotions. Parent–child interactions, particularly in the context of disciplinary situations, are rife with moral implications and entail strong relational incentives for learning self-regulation. Grusec (2006) argues for the importance of the type of information parents present and how it is communicated and received. Accurate perception of the parent's message is achieved through attention getting, clarity, redundancy, and consistency, whereas acceptance of the message depends on a warm relationship and the child's belief that the value was self-generated rather than externally imposed.

Research on moral emotions has challenged the once-prevailing view that young children are essentially premoral—lacking the moral emotions and insights to regulate moral behavior. Instead, a more sharply focused image of toddlers and preschoolers is one of emerging moral sensitivities: awareness of standards as well as self-conscious and other-oriented moral emotions.

INTUITION

Until the turn of the millennium, approaches emphasizing conscious, deliberative, rational processes of moral decision making largely dominated the field of moral development (e.g., Gilligan, 1982; Kohlberg, 1984; Piaget, 1932/1977; Rest et al., 1999; Turiel, 1983). Recently, this zeitgeist faced a stiff challenge from theoretical perspectives claiming that moral judgments are more typically the result of quick, automatic intuitions and, as such, that these moral intuitions provide a more veridical description of moral functioning. This section surveys what we know and have yet to learn about these dual processes within the moral domain. Although most theories of moral reasoning thus far reviewed are clearly developmental in perspective (with research on participants across the lifespan), most theories of moral intuition lack a developmental perspective, and relevant research with children is currently missing.

Dual-Process Theories

Dual-process theories have been of interest to the more general study of cognition for some time (Sherry & Schacter, 1987; Shiffrin & Schneider, 1977), but only in the last decade have such models come to the fore in moral psychology. Dual-process theories posit a bifurcation of mental processing. The intuitive System 1 (as it is known) is a quick, automatic, associative, affectively imbued parallel processor that functions outside of conscious awareness. In contrast, the deliberative System 2 is a slow, effortful, rule-governed serial processor that functions within the individual's awareness. Each system may govern its own class of behavior (namely, System 1 governs nonverbal "body language" and System 2 governs verbal expression; Dovidio, Kawakami, & Gaertner, 2002). Their functional independence, however, only goes so far; the two processes interact in synchronic functioning and diachronically in the course of development (Lapsley & Hill, 2008; Wegner & Bargh, 1998).

Critical to our understanding of moral development is how each system contributes to everyday moral decision making. This is not a trite issue for the field, because Kohlberg (1981), for example, was adamant that the moral quality of behavior was set by the individual's conscious intention, effectively ruling out intuitive processes. For Kohlberg, what differentiates amoral actions (e.g., classically conditioned, biologically determined, or reflex-governed movements) from actions of the moral kind is a conscious control function that affords the individual a choice to act or not act and thus forms a basis for moral responsibility (Blasi, 2009; Turiel, 2006). This standing challenge to the role of moral intuition beckons a response: What brings intuition into the moral domain?

Affective Intuition Models

Social Intuitionist Model

Various models of moral intuition have been proposed (see Lapsley & Hill, 2008, for a recent overview), but, for the sake of highlighting issues, we make a dichotomous classification between those that front-load moral functioning with affective intuitions (bequeathed by evolution) and those that back-end the process with heuristic intuitions (emerging through experience). The front-load approach is illustrated by Haidt's (2001, 2008) social intuitionist model (SIM), which represents what is likely the most brazen challenge to Kohlberg's perspective on moral judgment. To Haidt, intuitions are primarily "gut feeling," affective evaluations, constitutive of evolutionarily based human nature and prior to moral judgment and reasoning. According to the SIM, these intuitions are the default system for governing our moral universe, with later evolving capacities for language and higher order reasoning subservient to it. Moral judgments, then, are typically the result of quick and automatic moral intuitions; and moral reasoning, if and when it is produced, typically only factors in later to justify (rationalize) the prior intuitive judgment and serve as a social means of impression management.

What brings Haidt's brand of intuition into the moral domain is not the quality that Kohlberg demanded (namely, agentic choice) but rather a stripped-down sense of morality based on the felt experience of rightness and wrongness arising from evolutionary adaptiveness. Within the SIM, the adequacy of a moral judgment cannot be evaluated based on a justifying reason, as reason does not play a causal role in the formation of the former; what makes one moral judgment better developed than another, and therefore what prescriptive claim is being advanced, remains unclear (Jacobson, 2008; Narvaez, 2008). For this reason, the SIM has little to say about moral development, and it is thin on developmental considerations.

Evidence proffered in support of the SIM (Haidt & Bjorklund, 2008a) includes the phenomenon of "moral dumbfounding"—people's sometime puzzled inability to justify a strongly held moral conviction. Haidt argues that, if reasons cannot be produced to justify a moral judgment, then it must have been, by default, created via intuition. The classic illustration of this phenomenon involves a vignette about sibling incest in which no apparent harm comes of the act. Virtually all participants contend that the incest is wrong, and they maintain this stance even when unable to provide a reason. Other evidence, supportive of the model, includes the finding that manipulating affective processes can affect subsequent moral judgments.

Challenges to the SIM have been many (Sinnott-Armstrong, 2008) and have prompted a drastic shrinking of the scope and applicability of Haidt's earlier claims. Narvaez (2008) took philosophical issue with Haidt's claim of the ubiquity of moral intuition by identifying commonplace aspects of moral deliberation for which affective intuitions are simply inadequate; for example, in assessing the moral quality of past decisions, setting personal goals and evaluating progress toward them, reconciling multiple considerations and competing values, and making evaluations of right and wrong. Haidt and Bjorklund (2008b), in response, acknowledge that the SIM does not apply when more consequential decisions about morally relevant actions involving self and others are being considered; rather, the SIM pertains only to evaluative judgments about the character or actions of others when relatively little is at stake (as in aesthetic judgments).

The Personal–Impersonal Dimension

The SIM affords intuitive processing inordinate sway in the formation of moral judgments. By comparison, the remainder of the accounts reviewed here distribute the load more evenly and in a more sophisticated way. Of these accounts, the smallest role afforded to reasoning is advanced in the perspective of Greene, Sommerville, Nystrom, Darley, and Cohen (2001). They divide moral experience along a personal–impersonal dimension and argue that personal situations (in which one is faced with directly inflicting harm on another person) activate an intuitive–emotional center in the brain; in contrast, impersonal experiences (in which harm may ensue but is not caused by direct action) are handled by more rational centers.

Tests of Greene's theory come in the context of hypothetical scenarios involving a trolley (Hauser, Cushman, Young, Jin, & Mikhail, 2007). The trolley is moving quickly along the tracks, out of control. Ahead, on the tracks, are five people who are about to be hit and killed by the careening trolley. Participants are asked whether or not they would undertake a specific action to save the five lives when doing so would cost the life of one innocent bystander.

Participants tend to respond differently depending on how the averting action is framed. In the trolley condition, activating a switch will cause the trolley to change tracks, hitting and killing a single innocent bystander. The death of this one person would be caused by a remote action; thus this condition represents an impersonal moral dilemma. Almost univocally, participants say that they would indeed pull the switch, sacrificing one life to save five. In contrast, the footbridge condition elicits a different response. In this condition, the averting action involves pushing a man (of considerable heft) off the footbridge onto the tracks, killing him but derailing the train and saving the other five lives. In a rational framework, the two dilemmas are indistinguishable—the calculus in intention and human life is equal. Nevertheless, participants tend to take a different stance on the second (personal) one, claiming that they would not push the man and therefore allow the five to die.

To test the relevance of the personal–impersonal distinction to moral functioning, Greene and colleagues (2001) had participants respond to the trolley and footbridge conditions while in an fMRI machine. They found that different areas of the brain were activated between the two conditions, with intuitive–emotional centers more active during the personal dilemma and more deliberative, working-memory centers more active during the impersonal dilemma. The implication of these results is that our moral universe may be divided into two different processes depending on the nature of the action. Greene and colleagues are clear that this is a descriptive claim, not a prescriptive one; that is, this is a theory of how judgments are formed, not a theory of how judgments ought to be formed. Whatever the better (or least bad) response to these dilemmas may be, Greene's and Haidt's theories have little to say about how to judge the moral validity of intuitions, what moral maturity would entail, and which developmental processes might lead to it.

Heuristic Intuition Models

Unlike Greene's and Haidt's front-load perspectives, in which affective intuitions emerge from some biological module, back-end theories focus on those moral intuitions that are in some way learned and informed by prior reasoning (Pizarro & Bloom, 2003). These theories, therefore, have the potential to contribute more to our understanding of the development of intuitive judgment and, at least, have the potential to implicate developmental processes.

Heuristics and Biases

One approach to moral intuition development advances the view that everyday moral functioning is often controlled by moral heuristics—shortcuts or rules of thumb—that may contribute to errors in judgment (Sunstein, 2005). These heuristics and biases, although viable in some specific contexts, can lead to substantial errors in moral decisions if generalized without deliberation. The imperative, therefore, is to apply these learned shortcuts only in the contexts in which they were formed and to engage deliberative reasoning otherwise.

Much of the empirical work regarding heuristics and biases has been conducted in domains that involve factual knowledge (Kahneman, 2003). Less apparent is how to assess heuristic errors in the moral domain, in which agreement on what constitutes an error is more elusive. Pizarro, Uhlmann, and Bloom's (2003) approach is illustrative in that regard. They asked participants to compare a pair of vignettes: a causally normal scenario (in which an ill-intentioned action causes negative consequences) versus a causally deviant scenario (in which the same ill intention is enacted but ineffectual, and instead something else intervenes, producing the same negative consequences). Participants were prompted to rely on intuition to evaluate each act. Implicitly defining intuitive judgments as being fundamentally irrational, Pizarro and colleagues classified any response other than an equal evaluation of the actions in the two vignettes as an intuitive one because it deviates from the normative standard of evaluating exclusively on the basis of intentions. What remains unclear is how participants interpreted the instruction on this task to respond intuitively; some may have taken it as an instruction to take an illogical position. In any case, a measure that instructs participants to deliberately be intuitive does some violence to the meaning of the construct.

Expertise

Distinguished from the heuristics-and-biases approach is the expertise tradition, which regards moral intuitions as a developmentally advanced form of cognition that has become efficient, accurate, and highly automatized. In this perspective, novices are more likely to be dumbfounded and to use unreliable moral heuristics; with practice, these same individuals can become experts. This is achieved by addressing moral issues intentionally and deliberatively, taking a rational approach. Repetition of this process trains the intuitive system to the point of becoming equal to the task of managing similar moral conflicts. In this conceptualization, automaticity in moral functioning does not necessarily imply that the judgment or behavior is unintentional or uncontrollable (think of skills such as riding a bicycle, playing video games, or interpreting political machinations). Controlled and reflective reasoning processes thus hold an influential role in the diachronic development of intuition and may perform important functions (such as overriding an intuition) in certain circumstances (see Wegner & Bargh, 1998).

Lapsley and Narvaez (2004) operationalize moral expertise as an individual-differences personality variable, defined by the ready accessibility of moral concepts and schemas, ones that have been consistently and frequently activated. Their research (Narvaez, Lapsley, Hagele, & Lasky, 2006) compared moral experts (those for whom moral schemas were readily accessible) with moral novices (those for whom other schemas were predominant) and found that moral expertise was predictive of better information processing when dealing with morally relevant material on a spontaneous trait-inference task and a lexical decision-making task. Thus the expertise framework proffers the back-end view that some intuitions are a product of explicit moral understandings that become intuitive and implicit over the course of development; however, research within this framework has yet to be undertaken with children.

Definition of Intuition

It should now be apparent that little agreement has yet arisen regarding the processes characterizing moral intuition, with a clear divergence between the front-load view of affective evaluations and the back-end view of heuristic cognitions. Obviously, the psychological definition of intuition is an important issue, but consensus has been elusive. Topolinski and Strack (2008) have proposed four defining aspects of intuitive functioning: (1) operating outside of conscious awareness, (2) entailing fast and efficient decision making, (3) activated automatically, and (4) affectively charged. None of the extant measures of moral intuition tap all of these aspects; indeed, deliberative responding to contrived scenarios (e.g., incestuous siblings, trolley problem, causally deviant stories) hardly seems to be an approach that strikes close to the mark. The challenge for the field is to frame intuitive and rational approaches in a way that provides a meaningful account of their mutual conflicts, complementarities, and developing interdependence. With few exceptions, developmental considerations have yet to be explored; for this reason, the field of intuition has only begun to emerge as a topic of moral development.

PERSONALITY

Our review of moral reasoning, emotion, and intuition has shed light on how individuals respond to conflict situations, but by studying morality primarily as responses to moral problems, the more proactive side of morality has been neglected. When asked to name a moral hero, most people think of someone who is proactively compassionate, not someone who is particularly adept at resisting temptation or resolving dilemmas (Walker, Pitts, Hennig, & Matsuba, 1995). To fill in our picture of the morally developed individual, the focus of this section is on the psychological aspects of more supererogatory functioning (good to do but not necessarily required). This approach mostly augments what we know from these other enterprises, but it also offers an important conceptual challenge.

Dualistic Conception of Human Nature

The initial impetus for interest in moral development can be credited to the efforts of Piaget and Kohlberg, who advocated deliberative judgment as the primary moral function. This stance reflected the formalist assumptions of Enlightenment-era philosophers who viewed human nature dualistically, pitting reason against the self's more primal desires. As previously reviewed, in this framework, moral cognition was exalted—viewed as both necessary to define the moral quality of situations and as adequate to motivate moral action. Meanwhile, personal desires were not merely benignly neglected but, rather, explicitly denigrated as potentially corrupting influences that the moral agent must somehow overcome (Kohlberg, 1981).

Two challenges have been mounted against this dualistic framing. The first is empirical: Level of moral reasoning does not have adequate predictive validity, typically explaining about 10% of the variability in moral action (Blasi, 1980; Walker, 2004) and thus implying that the singular emphasis on moral cognition may be missing something important in moral functioning. The second challenge is more conceptual: If, as the dualism suggests, "doing the good" means acting on what one believes to be the right course and somehow overcoming self-interest, then precisely what interest does the agent have in the action? If morality runs counter to one's self-interest, then why be moral in the first place? The answer advocated by scholars of moral personality stems from the Aristotelian tradition, which highlights the role of virtuous character.

Personality Functioning of Moral Exemplars

In everyday temptations, emotional pangs or the voice of reason may often be sufficient to steer one down the path of decency. But when we consider moral exemplars—individuals who consistently live by a lofty moral code, devoting their lives to doing right by others—these moral functions seem to have insufficient motivational thrust in themselves. Premising the study of the moral personality is a suspicion that, on some deeper motivational plane, the actions of these moral exemplars are subtly, and in some kind of enlightened sense, self-enhancing (Colby & Damon, 1992).

Researchers have approached this claim by studying moral exemplars, aiming to understand their functioning. Studying more banal populations would yield limited insights into these highly adaptive modes of moral functioning, especially if banal and heroic populations function in some qualitatively different way. This does not imply that exemplars are different kinds of people from the rest of us. Approaching the study of moral exemplars through a developmental lens inspires the possibility that these exemplars are simply more mature instances of ordinary people. The focus is, first, on identifying the ways in which their personalities are extraordinary and, second, on exploring how those personality functions may have developed (if they did).

Our interest here is on the motivational aspects of personality. One of the landmark studies of moral exemplarity is Colby and Damon's (1992) qualitative analysis of a small sample of social activists. They proposed four processes in moral personality development, including (1) a continuing desire and capacity to change; (2) a balancing of certainty about moral ideals with openness to new ideas; (3) a stance of positivity, love, humility, and an underlying faith; and (4) an identity that integrates personal and moral goals. Such findings are suggestive, as are those from similar exemplar research (Oliner, 2003), but the lack of psychometrically valid measures and appropriate comparison groups renders the interpretation of these findings fragile.

Follow-up studies have confirmed some of Colby and Damon's suspicions. Hart and Fegley (1995), for example, studied adolescent care exemplars, teenagers who had taken on exceptional volunteer service activities or family responsibilities. They were extensively interviewed regarding qualities and aspects of the self. In contrast to comparison adolescents, these care exemplars used more moral personality traits in their self-attributions, more strongly incorporated their ideal selves into their actual selves, and evidenced greater continuity in their self-understanding.

Walker and Frimer (2007, 2009a) assessed the functioning of two different types of moral exemplars (namely, caring vs. brave). These nationally recognized caring and brave exemplars were demographically matched to comparison participants drawn from the community. The study employed multiple measures (including several personality inventories and an extensive interview), tapping all three levels of personality description (McAdams, 1995): (1) dispositional traits (broad and decontextualized dimensions of personality), (2) characteristic adaptations (motivational and developmental aspects of personality that are more particular to contexts), and (3) integrative life narratives (the psychosocial construction of a personal identity).

One of the issues framing Walker and Frimer's (2007) research examined whether a foundational core, common to both the brave and caring exemplars, could be identified. Five personality variables were identified as foundational, with pronounced differences between exemplar and comparison groups: themes of agency and of communion, redemption sequences (the tendency to reframe transformative life events such that some benefit is discerned out of adversity), the identification of helpers in early life, and secure childhood attachments.

Integrated Identity

Although these findings may seem to be of the "motherhood and apple pie" variety, the finding that exemplars expressed strong themes of *both* agency and communion calls for pause. Agency captures self-enhancing, "yes I can" type themes (e.g., achievement, mastery); communion is depicted in solidarity with and in helping others. This finding challenges the dualism between self-interest and morality identified at the outset of this section: If doing the good requires suppressing one's own self-interest, then the dualism would predict that moral exemplars would be lower on agency, not higher, than comparisons. Instead, the self seems to be among the benefactors of the exemplars' actions, as represented by enhanced levels of agency.

This exemplar research has identified a range of personality variables that may be implicated in development toward moral maturity. Missing as yet is a developmental account of how these personality outcomes came about and how "creatures like us" (Flanagan, 1991) could become like them. One attempt to fill in the developmental story was seeded by Colby and Damon's (1992) impression that, rather than seeing the two in tension, moral exemplars tended to fuse their personal and moral goals. This notion that the self's interests and moral concerns are integrated in moral maturity provides an empirical inroad to the lofty notion of enlightened self-interest and, in doing so, adds to our understanding of the development of moral motivation. This speculative notion, however, has only recently been subjected to empirical test.

The traditional view (e.g., Schwartz's [1992] values paradigm) is that agency represents the self-enhancing aspects of motivation, whereas communion represents the other-enhancing aspects, and that these motivations are, by their respective natures, mutually interfering. Frimer and Walker (2009) have, however, recently proposed a *reconciliation model* of moral identity development. In their model, the individual development of each of these competing motivations necessarily proceeds in segregation throughout childhood and adolescence until their evolving importance but growing tension produces a disequilibrating crisis. This disequilibrium can be reduced either by abandoning one motivation or the other (resulting in either unmitigated agency or unmitigated communion) and thus stagnating in development or by more adaptively integrating agency and communion—a reconciliation between these two fundamental motives.

To operationalize and test the reconciliation model, Frimer and Walker (2009) had participants respond to a self-understanding interview; their responses were coded in terms of value orientations. Of particular interest were the agentic values of power and achievement and the communal values of benevolence and universalism. An integrated identity was operationalized as the tendency to weave together agentic and communal values in the same segment of the narrative. Participants (university student club leaders representing a variety of worldviews and interests) also completed several measures tapping prosocial behaviors. As predicted by the reconciliation model, the integration of agency and communion positively predicted moral behaviors. In a morally integrated identity, agency brings life to communion and communion imparts agency with a greater purpose. This notion of an integrated identity that reconciles the self and morality has greater potential to explain the developmental roots of moral motivation than those conceptual frameworks that regard them as fundamentally at loggerheads.

CONCLUSIONS AND FUTURE DIRECTIONS

As prefigured in its title, this chapter was framed by the seeming paradox of using science's descriptive, outsider observations to examine morality's prescriptive, inner experience. Our intent in highlighting this tension was to focus attention on the critical paradigmatic assumptions underlying psychological theories of moral development and to clarify the respective boundaries of, and relationships between, developmental science and moral philosophy. We claim that moral philosophy and psychological science can be mutually informative.

In this chapter we surveyed several different human functions (including reasoning, intuition, emotions, and personality) as they relate to the moral experience. As is now readily apparent, the domain is expansive and entails the dynamic interplay of various aspects of cognition, emotion, and behavioral expression. But among these bodies of conceptual and empirical work are entrenched differences of opinion about which psychological process drives an individual's moral life (e.g., empathy vs. reasoning vs. values). Ultimately, these various processes work together in the whole person, and so integrating insights from across schools of thought represents important work to be done (Reed, 2009)—but not just yet. Development, at both the level of the individual person and at the level of the scientific enterprise, involves an initial stage of differentiation, which both precedes and motivates a move toward integration (Werner, 1957). We believe that, with the possible exception of Kohlberg's theory, each of the approaches to moral development has yet to be properly clarified and scientifically substantiated. Therefore, we contend that differentiating each approach should continue until which time integration becomes a meaningful possibility.

Moral reasoning has long been regnant in the study of moral development, but its dominant role has recently been sharply challenged by claims regarding the significance of intuitive processes in moral functioning. This challenge prompts two critical issues for future work. One question is largely conceptual and concerns the moral validity of intuition: What brings automatic, intuitive processes into the moral domain given that morality is typically understood to require that the individual has an opportunity to choose a course of action (Turiel, 2006)?

A second research direction calls for a meaningful analysis of the functional relationship between deliberative and intuitive processes in moral cognition (both in a synchronic moment and, through time, diachronically). Something approaching a consensus appears to be forming that dual processes are operative, but their respective roles in governing different classes of behavior in any instance and how they influence each other in real time remain to be properly explored. Similarly, explication of the developmental nature of moral intuition has yet to make it to the scientific table. What is the typical developmental trajectory of the affective and heuristic aspects of moral intuition? How are later forms more adequate or profound than earlier forms? What are the developmental roots of these intuitive processes? And what are the cognitive and social mechanisms underlying developmental change? Consider in these regards the contrasting perspectives on intuition that were reviewed: affective intuitions that arise prior to judgment and reasoning versus heuristic intuitions that are one output of the honed exercise of moral reflection. Embedded within this conceptual enterprise is the empirical challenge of devising appropriate means by which to assess moral intuition and thus test theory. Addressing these questions will be no small task but will be of considerable practical import for socialization efforts in fostering moral growth.

As noted earlier, the privileged position long accorded moral rationality in the field consequently slighted the moral competencies of young children whose elocutionary skills are nascent. Evolving evidence, however, speaks to the moral sensitivities of young children, both in terms of differentiated understandings of social domains and the development of self- and other-oriented emotions. Developmental differentiation has been demonstrated in children making domain distinctions, appropriately treating different types of social questions using different rules. The value of the approach would be advanced by research that addresses the requisite second part of development—integration—perhaps evident in adolescents' and adults' developing ability to handle multifaceted events in their social worlds and, in particular, to appreciate the moral implications of many choices and actions.

To round out our suggestions for future directions, we consider the morally relevant aspects of personality and identity as a way to understand the motivation to be moral. The bald concern is that moral knowledge, in itself, does not seem sufficient to impel moral action, particularly when one's morality dictates that one should act against one's self-interest. Moral psychology ought to be constrained by psychologically feasible motivational mechanisms. Future research needs to clarify when and how personal and moral goals developmentally differentiate and then integrate, how these developmental states affect (and are affected by) situations and behavior, and what factors can facilitate or thwart such a process. Perhaps, then, we will be in a better space to answer the questions, "Why live the morally good life?" and "How can we make this outcome the norm, rather than the exception?"

SUGGESTED READINGS

Colby, A., & Damon, W. (1992). *Some do care: Contemporary lives of moral commitment.* New York: Free Press.

Gilligan, C. (1982). *In a different voice: Psychological theory and women's development.* Cambridge, MA: Harvard University Press.

Killen, M., & Smetana, J. G. (Eds.). (2006). *Handbook of moral development.* Mahwah, NJ: Erlbaum.

Kohlberg, L. (1984). *Essays on moral development: Vol. 2. The psychology of moral development.* San Francisco: Harper & Row.

Narvaez, D., & Lapsley, D. K. (Eds.). (2009). *Personality, identity and character: Explorations in moral psychology.* New York: Cambridge University Press.

Rest, J. R., Narvaez, D., Bebeau, M. J., & Thoma, S. J. (1999). *Postconventional moral thinking: A neo-Kohlbergian approach.* Mahwah, NJ: Erlbaum.

Sinnott-Armstrong, W. (Ed.). (2008). *Moral psychology: Vol. 2. The cognitive science of morality: Intuition and diversity.* Cambridge, MA: MIT Press.

Turiel, E. (2006). The development of morality. In W. Damon & R. M. Lerner (Series Eds.) & N. Eisenberg (Vol. Ed.), *Handbook of child psychology: Vol. 3. Social, emotional, and personality development* (6th ed., pp. 789–857). Hoboken, NJ: Wiley.

REFERENCES

Adorno, T. W., Frenkel-Brunswik, E., Levinson, D. J., & Sanford, R. N. (1950). *The authoritarian personality.* New York: Harper.

Blasi, A. (1980). Bridging moral cognition and moral action: A critical review of the literature. *Psychological Bulletin, 88,* 1–45.

Blasi, A. (2009). The moral functioning of mature adults and the possibility of fair moral reasoning. In D. Narvaez & D. K. Lapsley (Eds.), *Personality, identity, and character: Explorations in moral psychology* (pp. 396–440). New York: Cambridge University Press.

Colby, A., & Damon, W. (1992). *Some do care: Contemporary lives of moral commitment.* New York: Free Press.

Colby, A., & Kohlberg, L. (1987). *The measurement of moral judgment* (Vols. 1–2). New York: Cambridge University Press.

Colby, A., Kohlberg, L., Gibbs, J., & Lieberman, M. (1983). A longitudinal study of moral judgment. *Monographs of the Society for Research in Child Development, 48*(1–2, Serial No. 200).

Damon, W. (1977). *The social world of the child.* San Francisco: Jossey-Bass.

Dovidio, J. F., Kawakami, K., & Gaertner, S. L. (2002). Implicit and explicit prejudice and interracial interaction. *Journal of Personality and Social Psychology, 82,* 62–68.

Eisenberg, N., Spinrad, T. L., & Sadovsky, A. (2006). Empathy-related responding in children. In M. Killen & J. G. Smetana (Eds.), *Handbook of moral development* (pp. 517–549). Mahwah, NJ: Erlbaum.

Flanagan, O. (1991). *Varieties of moral personality: Ethics and psychological realism.* Cambridge, MA: Harvard University Press.

Freud, S. (1927). *The ego and the id* (J. Riviere, Trans.). London: Hogarth Press.

Frimer, J. A., & Walker, L. J. (2009). Reconciling the self and morality: An empirical model of moral centrality development. *Developmental Psychology, 45,* 1669–1681.

Gilligan, C. (1982). *In a different voice: Psychological theory and women's development.* Cambridge, MA: Harvard University Press.

Gilligan, C., & Wiggins, G. (1987). The origins of morality in early childhood relationships. In J. Kagan & S. Lamb (Eds.), *The emergence of morality in young children* (pp. 277–305). Chicago: University of Chicago Press.

Greene, J. D., Sommerville, R. B., Nystrom, L. E., Darley, J. M., & Cohen, J. D. (2001, September 14). An fMRI investigation of emotional engagement in moral judgment. *Science, 293,* 2105–2108.

Grusec, J. (2006). The development of moral behavior and conscience from a socialization perspective. In M. Killen & J. G. Smetana (Eds.), *Handbook of moral development* (pp. 243–265). Mahwah, NJ: Erlbaum.

Haidt, J. (2001). The emotional dog and its rational tail: A social intuitionist approach to moral judgment. *Psychological Review, 108,* 814–834.

Haidt, J. (2008). Morality. *Perspectives on Psychological Science, 3,* 65–72.

Haidt, J., & Bjorklund, F. (2008a). Social intuitionists answer six questions about moral psychology. In W. Sinnott-Armstrong (Ed.), *Moral psychology: Vol. 2. The cognitive science of morality: Intuition and diversity* (pp. 181–217). Cambridge, MA: MIT Press.

Haidt, J., & Bjorklund, F. (2008b). Social intuitionists reason, in conversation. In W. Sinnott-Armstrong (Ed.), *Moral psychology: Vol. 2. The cognitive science of morality: Intuition and diversity* (pp. 241–254). Cambridge, MA: MIT Press.

Hart, D., & Fegley, S. (1995). Prosocial behavior and caring in adolescence: Relations to self-understanding and social judgment. *Child Development, 66,* 1346–1359.

Hauser, M., Cushman, F., Young, L., Jin, R. K.-X., & Mikhail, J. (2007). A dissociation between moral judgments and justifications. *Mind and Language, 22,* 1–21.

Hoffman, M. L. (2000). *Empathy and moral development: Implications for caring and justice.* Cambridge, UK: Cambridge University Press.

Jacobson, D. (2008). Does social intuitionism flatter morality or challenge it? In W. Sinnott-Armstrong (Ed.), *Moral psychology: Vol. 2. The cognitive science of morality: Intuition and diversity* (pp. 219–232). Cambridge, MA: MIT Press.

Jaffee, S., & Hyde, J. S. (2000). Gender differences in moral orientation: A meta-analysis. *Psychological Bulletin, 126,* 703–726.

Johnson, M. L. (1996). How moral psychology changes moral theory. In L. May, M. Friedman, & A. Clark (Eds.), *Minds and morals: Essays on cognitive science and ethics* (pp. 45–68). Cambridge, MA: MIT Press.

Kagan, J. (1981). *The second year: The emergence of self-awareness.* Cambridge, MA: Harvard University Press.

Kahneman, D. (2003). A perspective on judgment and choice: Mapping bounded rationality. *American Psychologist, 58,* 697–720.

Kant, I. (1964). *Groundwork of the metaphysic of morals* (H. J. Paton, Trans.). New York: Harper & Row. (Original work published 1785)

Kochanska, G. (1997). Multiple pathways to conscience for children with different temperaments: From toddlerhood to age 5. *Developmental Psychology, 33,* 228–240.

Kochanska, G., Casey, R. J., & Fukumoto, A. (1995). Toddlers' sensitivity to standard violations. *Child Development, 66,* 643–656.

Kohlberg, L. (1969). Stage and sequence: The cognitive-developmental approach to socialization. In D. A. Goslin (Ed.), *Handbook of socialization theory and research* (pp. 347–480). Chicago: Rand McNally.

Kohlberg, L. (1971). From is to ought: How to commit the naturalistic fallacy and get away with it in the study of moral development. In T. Mischel (Ed.), *Cognitive development and epistemology* (pp. 151–235). New York: Academic Press.

Kohlberg, L. (1981). *Essays on moral development: Vol. 1. The philosophy of moral development.* San Francisco: Harper & Row.

Kohlberg, L. (1984). *Essays on moral development: Vol. 2. The psychology of moral development.* San Francisco: Harper & Row.

Kohlberg, L., Boyd, D. R., & Levine, C. (1990). The return of Stage 6: Its principle and moral point of view. In T. Wren (Ed.), *The moral domain: Essays in the ongoing discussion between philosophy and the social sciences* (pp. 151–181). Cambridge, MA: MIT Press.

Lapsley, D. K., & Hill, P. L. (2008). On dual processing and heuristic approaches to moral cognition. *Journal of Moral Education, 37,* 313–332.

Lapsley, D. K., & Narvaez, D. (2004). A social-cognitive approach to the moral personality. In D. K. Lapsley & D. Narvaez (Eds.), *Moral development, self, and identity* (pp. 189–212). Mahwah, NJ: Erlbaum.

Laupa, M., Turiel, E., & Cowan, P. A. (1995). Obedience to authority in children and adults. In M. Killen & D. Hart (Eds.), *Morality in everyday life: Developmental perspectives* (pp. 131–165). Cambridge, UK: Cambridge University Press.

Lollis, S., Ross, H., & Leroux, L. (1996). An observational study of parents' socialization of moral orientation during sibling conflicts. *Merrill–Palmer Quarterly, 42,* 475–494.

McAdams, D. P. (1995). What do we know when we know a person? *Journal of Personality, 63,* 365–396.

Milgram, S. (1974). *Obedience to authority.* New York: Harper & Row.

Moore, G. E. (1903). *Principia ethica.* Cambridge, UK: Cambridge University Press.

Narvaez, D. (2008). The social-intuitionist model: Some counter-intuitions. In W. Sinnott-Armstrong (Ed.), *Moral psychology: Vol. 2. The cognitive science of morality: Intuition and diversity* (pp. 233–240). Cambridge, MA: MIT Press.

Narvaez, D., Lapsley, D. K., Hagele, S., & Lasky, B. (2006). Moral chronicity and social information processing: Tests of a social cognitive approach to the moral personality. *Journal of Research in Personality, 40,* 966–985.

Nucci, L., & Weber, E. K. (1995). Social interaction in the home and the development of young children's conceptions of the personal. *Child Development, 66,* 1438–1452.

Okin, S. M. (1989). *Justice, gender, and the family.* New York: Basic Books.

Oliner, S. P. (2003). *Do unto others: Extraordinary acts of ordinary people.* Boulder, CO: Westview.

Piaget, J. (1977). *The moral judgment of the child* (M. Gabain, Trans.). Harmondsworth, UK: Penguin. (Original work published 1932)

Piaget, J. (1985). *The equilibration of cognitive structures: The central problem of intellectual devel-*

opment (T. Brown & K. J. Thampy, Trans.). Chicago: University of Chicago Press. (Original work published 1975)

Pinker, S. (2008, January 13). The moral instinct. *New York Times Magazine*, pp. 32–37, 52–58.

Pizarro, D. A., & Bloom, P. (2003). The intelligence of the moral intuitions: Comment on Haidt (2001). *Psychological Review, 110,* 193–196.

Pizarro, D. A., Uhlmann, E., & Bloom, P. (2003). Causal deviance and the attribution of moral responsibility. *Journal of Experimental Social Psychology, 39,* 653–660.

Pratt, M. W., Golding, G., Hunter, W., & Sampson, R. (1988). Sex differences in adult moral orientations. *Journal of Personality, 56,* 373–391.

Reed, D. C. (2009). A multi-level model of moral functioning revisited. *Journal of Moral Education, 38,* 299–313.

Rest, J. R. (1979). *Development in judging moral issues.* Minneapolis: University of Minnesota Press.

Rest, J. R., Narvaez, D., Bebeau, M. J., & Thoma, S. J. (1999). *Postconventional moral thinking: A neo-Kohlbergian approach.* Mahwah, NJ: Erlbaum.

Schwartz, S. H. (1992). Universals in the content and structure of values: Theoretical advances and empirical tests in 20 countries. *Advances in Experimental Social Psychology, 25,* 1–65.

Sherry, D. F., & Schacter, D. L. (1987). The evolution of multiple memory systems. *Psychological Review, 94,* 439–454.

Shiffrin, R. M., & Schneider, W. (1977). Controlled and automatic human information processing: II. Perceptual learning, automatic attending and a general theory. *Psychological Review, 84,* 127–190.

Sinnott-Armstrong, W. (Ed.). (2008). *Moral psychology: Vol. 2. The cognitive science of morality: Intuition and diversity.* Cambridge, MA: MIT Press.

Skinner, B. F. (1938). *The behavior of organisms.* New York: Appleton-Century-Crofts.

Skinner, B. F. (1971). *Beyond freedom and dignity.* New York: Knopf.

Smetana, J. G. (2006). Social-cognitive domain theory: Consistencies and variations in children's moral and social judgments. In M. Killen & J. G. Smetana (Eds.), *Handbook of moral development* (pp. 119–153). Mahwah, NJ: Erlbaum.

Sunstein, C. R. (2005). Moral heuristics. *Behavioral and Brain Sciences, 28,* 531–573.

Thoma, S. J. (1986). Estimating gender differences in the comprehension and preference of moral issues. *Developmental Review, 6,* 165–180.

Thompson, R. A., Meyer, S., & McGinley, M. (2006). Understanding values in relationships: The development of conscience. In M. Killen & J. G. Smetana (Eds.), *Handbook of moral development* (pp. 267–297). Mahwah, NJ: Erlbaum.

Tisak, M. S. (1986). Children's conceptions of parental authority. *Child Development, 57,* 166–176.

Topolinski, S., & Strack, F. (2008). Where there's a will—there's no intuition. The unintentional basis of semantic coherence judgments. *Journal of Memory and Language, 58,* 1032–1048.

Turiel, E. (1983). *The development of social knowledge: Morality and convention.* Cambridge, UK: Cambridge University Press.

Turiel, E. (2006). Thought, emotions, and social interactional processes in moral development. In M. Killen & J. G. Smetana (Eds.), *Handbook of moral development* (pp. 7–35). Mahwah, NJ: Erlbaum.

Walker, L. J. (1984). Sex differences in the development of moral reasoning: A critical review. *Child Development, 55,* 677–691.

Walker, L. J. (1988). The development of moral reasoning. *Annals of Child Development, 5,* 33–78.

Walker, L. J. (2002). The model and the measure: An appraisal of the Minnesota approach to moral development. *Journal of Moral Education, 31,* 353–367.

Walker, L. J. (2004). Gus in the gap: Bridging the judgment–action gap in moral functioning. In D. K. Lapsley & D. Narvaez (Eds.), *Moral development, self, and identity* (pp. 1–20). Mahwah, NJ: Erlbaum.

Walker, L. J. (2006). Gender and morality. In M. Killen & J. G. Smetana (Eds.), *Handbook of moral development* (pp. 93–115). Mahwah, NJ: Erlbaum.

Walker, L. J., de Vries, B., & Bichard, S. L. (1984). The hierarchical nature of stages of moral development. *Developmental Psychology, 20*, 960–966.

Walker, L. J., de Vries, B., & Trevethan, S. D. (1987). Moral stages and moral orientations in real-life and hypothetical dilemmas. *Child Development, 58*, 842–858.

Walker, L. J., & Frimer, J. A. (2007). Moral personality of brave and caring exemplars. *Journal of Personality and Social Psychology, 93*, 845–860.

Walker, L. J., & Frimer, J. A. (2009a). Moral personality exemplified. In D. Narvaez & D. K. Lapsley (Eds.), *Personality, identity and character: Explorations in moral psychology* (pp. 232–255). New York: Cambridge University Press.

Walker, L. J., & Frimer, J. A. (2009b). "The song remains the same": Rebuttal to Sherblom's re-envisioning of the legacy of the care challenge. *Journal of Moral Education, 38*, 53–68.

Walker, L. J., Gustafson, P., & Frimer, J. A. (2007). The application of Bayesian analysis to issues in developmental research. *International Journal of Behavioral Development, 31*, 366–373.

Walker, L. J., Hennig, K. H., & Krettenauer, T. (2000). Parent and peer contexts for children's moral reasoning development. *Child Development, 71*, 1033–1048.

Walker, L. J., Pitts, R. C., Hennig, K. H., & Matsuba, M. K. (1995). Reasoning about morality and real-life moral problems. In M. Killen & D. Hart (Eds.), *Morality in everyday life: Developmental perspectives* (pp. 371–407). Cambridge, UK: Cambridge University Press.

Wegner, D. M., & Bargh, J. A. (1998). Control and automaticity in social life. In D. T. Gilbert, S. T. Fiske, & G. Lindzey (Eds.), *Handbook of social psychology* (4th ed., Vol. 1, pp. 446–496). Boston: McGraw-Hill.

Werner, H. (1957). The concept of development from a comparative and organismic point of view. In D. B. Harris (Ed.), *The concept of development* (pp. 125–148). Minneapolis: University of Minnesota Press.

Wright, J. C., & Bartsch, K. (2008). Portraits of early moral sensibility in two children's everyday conversation. *Merrill–Palmer Quarterly, 54*, 56–85.

Zahn-Waxler, C., Radke-Yarrow, M., Wagner, E., & Chapman, M. (1992). Development of concern for others. *Developmental Psychology, 28*, 126–136.

Zimbardo, P. G., Banks, W. C., Haney, C., & Jaffe, D. (1973, April 8). The mind is a formidable jailer: A Pirandellian prison. *New York Times Magazine*, Section 6, pp. 38–46.

11

Prosocial Behavior

Joan E. Grusec
Amanda Sherman

As 12-year-old Craig Kielburger was flipping through the *Toronto Star* searching for comics, he was struck by the story of a South Asian boy who had been sold into slavery at age 4 and had spent 6 years chained to a carpet-weaving loom. The boy, Iqbal, captured the world's attention by speaking out for children's rights. Craig knew he had to help. He gathered together a small group of his classmates, and they began an organization whose goal was to free children from poverty and exploitation. Today Free the Children is the world's largest network of children helping children through education.

How do children learn to show concern and consideration for others? How does selfless behavior develop? How have humans evolved to assist others? To what extent is prosocial behavior influenced by genetic predispositions? And how do these predispositions interact with the experiences that children have, both at home and in the larger community, that might facilitate or be detrimental to a desire to reach out and share with others? These are important questions to be addressed in this chapter.

We begin the chapter with a discussion of characteristics of prosocial behavior that make it particularly challenging to study. We then move on to a discussion of the evolutionary, genetic, and experiential underpinnings of the behavior and how they interact.

CHALLENGES IN STUDYING PROSOCIAL BEHAVIOR

Interest in Prosocial and Antisocial Behavior Compared

We start this section with an observation about the level of attention researchers have paid to the topic of concern for others, or prosocial behavior, and how that compares

263

with the level of attention devoted to its opposite, antisocial behavior. A search of the PsycINFO database indicates that interest in the latter has consistently outstripped interest in the former: Researchers have been much more concerned with behavior that is disruptive to societal functioning than in behavior that promotes societal harmony and peace. For example, in the period from 2000 to 2010, there were 3,419 publications dealing with antisocial behavior, of which 901 dealt with children. In contrast, there were only 1,601 publications focused on prosocial behavior, with 531 of those addressed to questions about children. A similar pattern can be seen for earlier years. In 1990–1999, 2,007 publications were about antisocial behavior, with 532 having to do with children; in contrast, 1,010 publications were about prosocial behavior, with 388 focused on children. Why this differential interest? There seems no obvious answer, other than the fact that the commission of a hurtful act is apparently more salient and perhaps incomprehensible than the expression of concern for others, which is apparently less noticeable, although not necessarily more easily understood.

Complexity of Prosocial Behavior

It is also true that prosocial behavior in many ways is more complex than antisocial behavior and therefore offers more challenges to the investigator. Accordingly, it is easy to identify behaviors that are antisocial or harmful to others, but it is more difficult to identify those that are helpful. Long ago Kant (1788/1956) pointed this out in his discussion of perfect and imperfect duties, with the former involving actions of omission, such as not lying and not stealing, and the latter involving actions of commission, such as sharing and helping. Perfect duties require only that individuals not engage in a certain action, and so they can be performed at all times, whereas imperfect duties require a consideration or selectivity in the time, place, and object of behavior. The following quote illustrates the point quite nicely in its focus on the decisions that need to be made before an individual behaves in a prosocial way: "I should help or give to *deserving* individuals who are in X level of *need*, and are *dependent* on *me* for help, when I can *ascertain and perform* the necessary behavior and when the *cost* or *risk* to me does not exceed Y *amount* of my currently available resources" (Peterson, 1982, pg. 202).

Some of the decisions required before one can act prosocially include knowledge of how the recipient of the prosocial behavior is going to react. Although the intentions of the actor are positive, prosocial behavior can be experienced negatively by recipients (Fisher, Nadler, & Whitcher-Alagna, 1982). For example, being the object of consideration from others may elicit feelings of failure, inferiority, and dependency. Given that people want to feel independent and self-reliant, receiving assistance intimates that they are not and is therefore threatening. Older individuals, for example, who still see themselves as healthy and strong may not be pleased to be offered a seat on a subway or bus. Expressions of concern can become embarrassing for someone who has just tripped and fallen in public because they draw attention to the individual's clumsiness. Prosocial behavior can also lead to unwanted feelings of obligation, particularly if reciprocation is difficult or unpleasant. All these possibilities simply add to the confusion and challenge that surround this area of social functioning. Thus they make it difficult for agents of socialization such as parents and teachers to decide when prosocial behavior should be encouraged and when it should not. There is a great deal of learning that has to go on before an individual can be seen as truly efficient at the task of appropriate concern for others.

Ambivalence by agents of socialization about prosocial behavior has been observed in several studies. It is not always praised by parents or teachers (Caplan & Hay, 1989; Grusec, 1991), nor is it encouraged in young children (Rheingold, 1982). Undoubtedly, there are several reasons for this lack of enthusiasm. One has to do with the negative impact of prosocial behavior on recipients. Additionally, parents try to protect their children from engaging in too much self-sacrifice, a distinct possibility when individuals work to assist others, possibly at some or considerable expense to their own comfort. As well, some adults may feel that prosocial behavior should occur naturally, independent of adult approval. Mothers often discourage help from their children because of their children's lack of expertise and the fact that they often create more trouble than they save (Rheingold, 1982). It should be noted, however, that ambivalence about prosocial behavior is not universal: It is more likely to be seen in Western European cultures as opposed to non-Western cultures (e.g., Hindu Indian) in which social responsibility is more duty-based and seen to be as important as ensuring that justice is achieved (Miller & Bersoff, 1992).

Definitions of Prosocial Behavior

There are additional concerns that make the study of prosocial behavior challenging. One has to do with the nature of the actions that constitute it. Researchers have generally defined prosocial behavior as helping, sharing, showing consideration and concern, defending, and making restitution after deviation. However, these behaviors are somewhat arbitrary, as Greener and Crick (1999) noted in a study in which they asked 8- to 11-year-old children what boys and girls do when they want to be nice to people. The list of activities provided by the children was markedly different from those described by adult researchers. For the children, being nice meant using humor, being friends (such as by asking people about themselves), avoiding being mean, including people in the play group, ending a conflict, sharing or caring, hanging around with people, and trusting them by, for example, telling them secrets. The most frequent examples of being nice were being friends, inclusion in the group, and sharing and caring, with sharing and caring seen as more appropriate for peers of the opposite sex. Other groups might well give different exemplars of being nice or behaving prosocially. What this means for those who carry out, as well as those who read about, research on prosocial behavior is that they need to know how prosocial behavior has been operationalized: Not all forms of niceness, let alone conceptions of it, are identical, and conclusions about one might be very different from conclusions that could be drawn about another.

Meanings of Prosocial Behavior

Yet another source of confusion for the study of prosocial behavior is that the same behavior may have entirely different meanings for both the actor and the recipient and may be conducted for entirely different reasons. Suppose, for example, that someone notices a neighbor struggling to carry a large and awkward package into her house and goes to the neighbor's house to offer assistance. There are any number of possible reasons for that offer. It may be that the donor experiences empathically the discomfort being experienced by the neighbor, or experiences a sympathetic response, and therefore acts prosocially in order to alleviate the neighbor's distress. Indeed, this is an aspect of prosocial behavior that has been a central focus for theorists and researchers who study it. But prosocial behavior can also occur because the donor has a strongly internalized principle that others in difficulty should be assisted, because the donor is friendly and sees an opportunity to strike up a conversation, because the donor is about to ask the neighbor for permission to cut a branch from a tree overhanging the donor's garden and sees this as a good opportunity to establish an accommodating relationship, because the donor has grown up in a household where people routinely offer help when needed, and so on. Although the act is the same, the meaning and the learning experiences that went into the promotion of that act are vastly different.

EVOLUTIONARY, GENETIC, AND SOCIALIZATION ANALYSES

The Evolution of Prosocial Behavior

The focus of this chapter is on the conditions that lead to individual differences in prosocial behavior. Thus we discuss features of the child and of the child's environment that produce concern for others (or kindness). We digress briefly, however, to look at prosocial behavior from another perspective and to ask a somewhat different question, which has to do with why human beings, as well as members of other species, exhibit prosocial behavior at all. This question has been addressed by evolutionary theorists, generally in the context of discussions of altruism, that is, of behavior that aids or provides benefits to another at some cost to the altruist. (The difficulty in identifying whether a behavior is performed at some cost to the donor has led developmental psychologists to prefer the term *prosocial behavior*, which requires no such distinction between costly behavior and that which is not). Altruism, that aspect of prosocial behavior that requires self-sacrifice, does pose a problem from an evolutionary perspective that posits survival and reproduction as central explanatory mechanisms. Thus aggression is easy to understand: Its role in survival and reproduction is simple to infer. But self-sacrifice and possible threats to the altruist's survival are less easy to understand.

Hamilton (1964) provided a solution to the problem by suggesting that any behaviors that benefit others with whom genes are shared are likely to be favored by natural selection. A mother who sacrifices her life in the course of protecting her children, for example, is behaving in a highly adaptive manner because her children's genes, which are copies of her own, will be transmitted into the gene pool. In this way she is increasing her own genetic fitness over what it would have been if only she had survived. Hamilton's notion of kin selection, of course, does not address the issue of why prosocial behavior should exist between unrelated members of a group. That problem was solved by positing the concept of reciprocal altruism (Trivers, 1971). Trivers argued that survival and reproductive success are also more likely when help is received from non-kin, but here there has to be a mechanism ensuring that the exchange of help is equivalent so that the exchange of benefits and sacrifice balances out over time. Accordingly, early hominids appear to have developed a mechanism for the detection of cheating that makes them sensitive to those individuals who have failed to return favors and thus unlikely to continue helping them. An example of the operation of this mechanism is the finding that people are better at identifying pictures of individuals who have been described as not trustworthy than they are if those individuals are described with other adjectives (Mealey, Daood, & Krage, 1996).

Yet another set of explanations comes from multilevel selection theory (Wilson,

1997). This theory suggests that selection for altruism can occur at a group rather than an individual level. There are conditions in which it would be adaptive for all members of a group to be altruistic, regardless of whether or not their altruism was reciprocated. Thus groups in competition with other groups for resources would be at an advantage if, on average, their members were more altruistic. When groups are isolated or not in competition, then noncontingent altruism would, of course, be a disadvantage. Finally, costly-signaling theory (Grafen, 1990; Zahavi, 1977) attempts to account for actions that involve a great deal of self-sacrifice and that are unlikely to be reciprocated, as, for example, in the case of the wealthy philanthropist. It is argued that in these cases the behavior increases the attractiveness of the donor as a mate or increases the donor's level of dominance. Conspicuous and costly altruism thus signals that the actor has multiple resources that will aid survival. It can also provide insurance against future adversity when the donor no longer has resources and may be more likely to receive help from those who were previously assisted.

It is important to note that there is no conflict between evolutionary approaches and the more traditional ones taken by developmental and social psychologists (McAndrew, 2002). Social developmentalists are concerned with the immediate or proximal causes of prosocial behavior, whereas evolutionary theorists are interested in the origins and functions or distal causes of prosocial behavior. Each area is informative for the other, however. In the case of social developmental psychology, sensitivity to general proclivities of human beings that have evolved over time makes it easier to understand why some behaviors are particularly difficult to modify and others remarkably easy. In the former case, those who desire to modify a child's actions are working against strong tendencies whereas, in the latter, they are working in concert with evolved predispositions.

Evolutionary theory explains why all members of the human species have an inclination to behave in a prosocial way. There are, however, large individual differences among humans that, as we have noted, have been the chief object of attention by developmentalists. Different experiences account for some of these differences. Genetic variation also accounts for some of them, with the latter of particular interest to investigators in recent years. Thus there is now a growing body of evidence, using the methodology of behavior genetics, that speaks to the role of genes in the development of prosocial behavior. And even more recently researchers, using the methods of molecular genetics, have begun to identify specific genes involved in the expression of concern for others. We begin with a discussion of the role of genes and then turn to the role of experience. Most important is the fact that genes and environment interact, that is, the effects of a particular experience may be moderated by the individual's genetic features and the expression of an individual's genetic features may be moderated by a particular experience.

The Genetic Underpinnings of Prosocial Behavior

Quantitative Behavior Genetics and Prosocial Behavior

Quantitative behavior genetics studies rely on comparisons between sets of individuals who have different degrees of genetic overlap: These may be, for example, monozygotic and dyzygotic twins, parents and children, siblings and stepsiblings, or adopted and biological children, for whom, in all cases, the average degree of genetic overlap is clear. Most common are studies comparing monozygotic/identical and dyzygotic/

fraternal (same-sex) twins, with the former having all their genes in common and the latter, on average, having half their genes in common. Researchers compare the similarity between the two groups in the behavior of interest (in the present case, prosocial behavior). They assume that both kinds of twins, given their identical age and that they are growing up in the same household, share at least to an extent a common environment (which could include not only parental encouragement or discouragement of prosocial behavior but also similarity between twins as they respond reciprocally to each other's actions). Because of the shared environment, any differences between identical and fraternal twins must be mediated by their different genetic compositions, as well as by features of their environment that are not shared. Knowing the correlation between measures of prosocial behavior for monozygotic and dyzygotic twins allows calculation of the extent to which prosocial behavior reflects genetic differences, environmental differences (nonshared environment), and the shared environment.

CHILD STUDIES

Most behavior genetics studies, primarily using mothers' reports of their children's prosocial behavior, have found both genetic and shared environmental effects. However, heritability contributes less to prosocial behavior in toddlers and young children than does shared environment, with heritability coefficients generally ranging from 0% to 30–40% (Knafo & Plomin, 2006; Zahn-Waxler, Robinson, & Emde, 1992; Zahn-Waxler, Schiro, Robinson, Emde, & Schmitz, 2001). Recently, Knafo and Israel (2009) found no shared environmental effects on the prosocial behavior of Israeli 3-year-olds. They note that the studies that have found shared environmental effects have all been conducted in Western, Anglophone countries and that their finding may reflect a different preschool experience in Israel, which provides a more uniform environment for all children. This observation underlines the important fact that there is nothing absolute about calculations of heritability and shared and nonshared environments: The more uniform an environment, the more room there is for genes to be seen to affect the amount of prosocial behavior that individuals exhibit.

A reminder of the complexity of prosocial behavior appears in a study by Zahn-Waxler et al. (1992) in which the response of 14- to 36-month old twins to their mothers' feigned distress was assessed at several time points. Prosocial acts were coded as trying to help or comfort, showing concern, expressing personal distress at the distress of the mother, showing indifference, and trying to understand the mothers' distress. Indifference and attempts at understanding showed some shared environmental influences, but only at 20 and 24 months, with no evidence of shared environmental influences for the other acts. Genetic effects were found at most ages for help/comfort, concern, and attempts at understanding, but they varied from 10% to 42%. There was a genetic effect for indifference only at 14 and 36 months, and self-distress was accounted for mainly by nonshared environment.

Changes in the degree of genetic mediation occur with age. Knafo and Plomin (2006), for example, found that genetic effects increased in importance between 2 and 7 years (26–37% at age 2 to 51–72% at age 7) and that shared environment effects decreased, becoming negligible by 7 years. Part of the explanation for the increased importance of genetic effects is that cognitive skills such as the ability to take the perspective of others, which are genetically influenced, come into play in the child's developing prosocial behavior. Thus they add to the genetic underpinnings of the child's prosocial abilities. Shared environment plays a reduced role as the range of extrafamilial experiences increases and as children seek out environments that support their genetic predispositions. Also, as we shall see later in this chapter, many parenting influences interact with children's temperamental or prosocial predispositions and, given the way behavior genetics calculations are done, the variance accounted for by these interactions is included in the heritability component.

ADOLESCENT AND ADULT STUDIES

In a review of the literature, Knafo and Plomin (2006) concluded that the majority of studies demonstrate considerable genetic influence (sometimes more than 70%) and little shared environmental influence on prosocial behavior in adolescents and adults. This trend makes sense for the same reasons proposed earlier for increases in genetic influence as children age. However, differences in methodology may also account for some of the observed changes. Thus studies of young children have relied on reports by others or observations of prosocial behavior, whereas studies with adults have generally used self-report questionnaires. Because self-report questionnaires are susceptible to biased patterns of responding, as well as to social desirability biases, both of which may be heritable tendencies, the role of genetic influence may be exaggerated.

Molecular Genetics and Prosocial Behavior

Identification of the variety of specific genes involved in prosocial behavior is just beginning. These include polymorphisms (different forms of DNA sequences at a given point on a gene) of the dopamine D4 receptor gene, which have been associated with young women's reports of selflessness (Bachner-Melman et al., 2005), as well as with preschool twins' sharing with each other (DiLalla, Elam, & Smolen, 2009). The dopaminergic system has been shown to relate to conscientiousness (Dragan & Oniszczenko, 2007), a possible feature of prosocial behavior. Other polymorphisms are related to oxytocin and arginine vasopressin hormones that have been associated with a variety of social traits, such as affiliation and social bonding (Israel et al., 2008). Both polymorphisms in the oxytocin receptor gene, as well as the length of the promoter region of the gene that codes for the arginine vasopressin receptor, have been associated with donation of money to a stranger (Israel et al., 2009; Knafo et al., 2008). As well, Knafo et al. (2008) found that adults with long versions of the arginine vasopressin 1a receptor reported more prosocial behavior on a questionnaire. Clearly, many genes will be found to be involved in prosocial behavior (Chakrabarti et al., 2009, report 19 that are associated with young adults' self-reported empathy). Additionally to be expected are gene-by-gene interactions, gene-by-environment interactions, and differential timing of activation of genes associated with prosocial behavior.

Socialization of Prosocial Development

Genes cannot manifest themselves in the absence of experience, and it is to experience that we now turn. Much has been learned about the impact of family, peers, teachers, and the media on the socialization of concern for others, although there are confusing and inconsistent findings in the literature (Eisenberg, Fabes, & Spinrad, 2006). Recently, Grusec and Davidov (2010) have argued that some order can be brought to these inconsistencies by thinking in terms of domains of socialization. The argument is that a given agent of socialization can have different forms of relationships with children at different points in time and that successful socialization depends on the relationship, that is, on the domain in which the dyad is operating. Moreover, the particular child outcome will depend on the domain in which socialization takes place.

Grusec and Davidov (2010) have identified five domains. The first is the *protection* domain: The need for protection is activated when a child is anxious or distressed, and the appropriate action from the agent of socialization is protection from or alleviation of distress. With respect to prosocial behavior, events in the protection domain affect the child's empathic capacity, which, in turn, underlies concern for others. The second domain is *reciprocity*. In this case, socialization agent and child are partners in a relationship of equality in which they are motivated to exchange favors. Socialization agents who comply with the child's reasonable requests are more likely to have children who will in turn comply with their requests. In this domain, prosocial behavior is willingly given as part of a mutual exchange of favors. In the third, the *control* domain, the socialization agent has greater power than the child and is thereby able to exert that power in order to promote desired behavior. This can occur either through the use of rewards and punishment contingent on prosocial behavior or in a more subtle way that is less threatening to the child's sense of autonomy (e.g., through the use of minimal amounts of punishment in combination with reasoning). In the latter case children may come to attribute prosocial behavior to personal choice: This attribution results in prosocial behavior that is relatively resistant to change and that reflects principled behavior that is seen as inherently proper and in keeping with the individual's self-concept. In the case of control by reinforcement contingencies, prosocial behavior can occur in order to receive praise or reinforcement or to avoid punishment. The fourth domain, *guided learning*, involves teaching by the socialization agent of skills and knowledge that occurs within the child's zone of proximal development, that is, at a level that is matched to the child's level of understanding and mastery of the task being taught. Prosocial behavior in this domain occurs because, given the deep understanding that is facilitated by such teaching, its necessity and importance is clearly understood and accepted. Finally, prosocial behavior can also be socialized in the *group participation* domain. Socializing agents in this domain take advantage of the child's desire to be part of the social group and to act like other members of the group. Through rituals, routines, and habitual acts, children are exposed to examples of behaviors that are associated with the group. In this domain prosocial behavior is routine, expected, and unquestioned. When questioned, however, its practice is in danger of being rejected.

THE DEVELOPMENT OF PROSOCIAL BEHAVIOR

Using a domains perspective, we turn now to a description of how prosocial behavior develops through the combined forces of and interplay between genes and environment. We begin with infancy and early childhood, then move to middle childhood, and finally to adolescence. It should be noted that each domain of socialization is represented in each phase of development, given that the domains come into play at various points in the first two or three years of life and that they operate throughout the course of development. Accordingly, the child's need for protection occurs from the very beginning of life. Mutual reciprocity emerges very early in the life of infants (Adamson & Bakeman, 1991). Control becomes necessary in the second year of life, once children become mobile and their desire for mastery of the environment comes into play. Interactions involving guided learning emerge during the second year as language and the ability to understand and internalize complex explanations develops (Vygotsky, 1978). Finally, group participation becomes salient when adherence to the rules of group life and the desire for ritual become strong in the second to fourth years of life (Emde, Biringen, Clyman, & Oppenheim, 1991).

Infancy and Early Childhood

Features of Prosocial Behavior

Newborns cry in response to the cries of other infants, a rudimentary form of empathy that reflects personal distress, given that they do not yet have a sense of self versus other (Sagi & Hoffman, 1976). At 6 months they may respond to the cry of another baby by crying themselves, or else they may ignore the cry or simply look at the other child (Hay, Nash, & Pedersen, 1981). By the age of 12–14 months young children begin to show concern when others are distressed, including touching and verbally reassuring them (Zahn-Waxler et al., 1992). Sometimes the comforting behavior may be inappropriate, as when an object the child uses for self-soothing is offered to another. Nevertheless, the attempts to help, even if unskilled because of cognitive limitations, are evident. Indeed, prosocial behavior increases as cognitive abilities increase. These abilities include being able to take the perspective of the other, being able to make the distinction between self and other as evidenced by self-recognition in a mirror, and emotion knowledge (Zahn-Waxler et al, 1992; Garner, Jones, & Palmer, 1994). Young children also display inappropriate or insensitive responses to distress in others, such as laughing, aggression, or ignoring, and these responses decline with age (Radke-Yarrow, Zahn-Waxler, & Chapman, 1982). Rheingold (1982) has documented another form of prosocial behavior involving young children's desire to be helpful with household tasks such as folding laundry and sweeping. Mothers, as noted earlier, tend not to react positively to these desires given the inefficiency of the children's actions.

Socialization Processes

PROTECTION DOMAIN

The child's need for protection and care is present at the very beginning of life, and how caregivers respond to that need plays a large role in the development of empathy and prosocial behavior. Caregivers who are sensitively responsive to children's distress or anxiety foster children's ability to cope with their own distress, as well as that of others. Children's lack of confidence in protection impairs the development of important neurobiological systems associated with stress (Gunnar, 2000). In addition, lack of confidence means that the threatening features of stressful situations are not reduced by knowledge that they will or can be dealt with. The important role played by features of the child in this aspect of the socialization process is evident in the observation that what is stressful for one child is not for another, and what is comforting for one child is not for another. Thus child temperament and developmental status are important variables that influence what the child perceives to be sensitive and responsive caregiving (Buck, 1991).

Research indicates that children of appropriately sensitive mothers are better at regulating their own distress and negative emotions (e.g., Cassidy, 1994), as well as showing greater empathy for the distress of others and responding in a helpful way. The capacity to show empathy is facilitated by children's ability to regulate their own arousal in response to the distress of others and therefore remain focused on the problems of the other, rather than being overwhelmed by personal distress occasioned by the other's distress (Eisenberg, Wentzel, & Harris, 1998; Davidov & Grusec, 2006). Indeed, when children experience high levels of personal distress, the evidence indicates that they are more likely to try to escape from the situation than to do something to improve it (Eisenberg, Fabes, & Spinrad, 2006). It is significant that being able to appreciate the distress of others also reduces the incidence of antisocial behavior because the negative consequences of one's own actions for the welfare of others are more easily comprehended (Eisenberg et al., 1998; Hoffman, 1970).

As noted earlier, interactions do frequently occur between characteristics of the child that are genetically mediated (e.g., temperament) and parenting. Relevant to the domain of protection is a study by Valiente and colleagues (2004) of a sample of children between the ages of 55 and 97 months of age. They found that parents who usually expressed their negative emotions were more likely to have children who reported feeling sympathetic when others were distressed. This relation held, though, only in the case of children who were high in effortful control, that is, good at concentrating on and persisting at a task. Valiente et al. (2004) suggest that exposure to moderately high levels of negative emotion may promote sympathy when children are able to manage their emotions but not when such management is more difficult.

RECIPROCITY DOMAIN

Mutual positive and frequently playful exchanges between adult caregivers and children begin to occur early in infancy and form the basis for exchanges of favors or compliance between two partners who now have an egalitarian relationship (Adamson & Bakeman, 1991; Parpal & Maccoby, 1985). In the case of prosocial behavior, this means that requests from others for help and concern are more likely to be responded to in a willing and cooperative way. We note that, in this analysis, prosocial behavior is conceived as happening in response to a request rather than spontaneously, although the requests may not be particularly salient. For example, a partner with whom a reciprocal relationship has developed might only need to indicate a need for assistance rather than have to ask for it directly.

CONTROL DOMAIN

In this domain parents and other agents of socialization have more power and control over resources and so are in a position to exert their authority when they wish to encourage prosocial behavior. As noted earlier, there are two possibilities with respect to outcomes in this domain. One is that children's behavior is controlled by reinforcement contingencies and that children engage in acts such as helping others because they hope for reward of some kind (of either a social or material nature) or to avoid punishment. The other possibility is that a positive social behavior is internalized, that is, socialization experiences are of such a nature that they minimize the child's belief that behavior is externally motivated and maximize beliefs that it is driven by internal motives, that is, internalized (Grusec, 1983; Hoffman, 1970; Lepper, 1983). Behavior that is clearly externally motivated may be seen as less optimal because it relies on the presence of the reward agent, although Patterson and Fisher (2002) have argued that such behavior becomes habitual simply as a result of repetition. It is also the case that some more subtle forms of reward for helping, such as social approval, may be less likely to produce attributions to external sources of motivation (Smith, Gelfand, Hartmann, & Partlow, 1979).

It is in the domain of control that interactions between genes and parenting styles or between temperament and parenting styles have been most frequently reported. These interactions have been reported particularly in the case of antisocial behavior, as well as internalizing problems (Bates & Pettit, 2007). Nevertheless, a few have been found in which prosocial behavior is the outcome of interest. Cornell and Frick (2007), for example, report that children who were identified by their teachers as uninhibited, that is, who were described as sensation seeking (e.g., liking to jump off swings while they were still high off the ground) and fearless, were lower in empathy (assessed by mothers' responses to a questionnaire) than those who were inhibited. However, they also found that for uninhibited children consistent discipline and empathy were positively related, whereas for inhibited children consistent discipline and empathy were unrelated. Cornell and Frick (2007) suggest that children who are temperamentally inhibited may be protected against less optimal parenting.

In a recent study Knafo and Israel (2009) assessed interactions between a genetic polymorphism, the exon III repeat region of the DRD4 receptor, and parenting. In the case of this polymorphism, the presence of a DRD4 7-repeat allele has been associated with attention-deficit/hyperactivity disorder (ADHD) and novelty seeking (Faraone, Doyle, Mick, & Biederman, 2001). Knafo and Israel found that for 7-absent children there was no relation between parenting and prosocial behavior, whereas for 7-present children there was. In the latter case mothers who reported that they were warm and reasoned with their children rated their children as prosocial. Mothers who reported that they used punishment also had children who were observed to be more prosocial. Again, as in the Cornell and Frick study, inhibition seems to serve as a protective factor against less optimal parenting.

GUIDED LEARNING DOMAIN

As children's verbal skills improve, parents and teachers talk to them about social and emotional issues. In order for learning to take place, the talk must be within the child's zone of proximal development, that is, involve a task the child has not yet mastered but can with the aid of a more proficient agent of socialization (Vygotsky, 1978). Learning must be supported or scaffolded so that it is adjusted to the child's increasing level of understanding (Wood, Bruner, & Ross, 1976). Because this learning is so closely matched to the child's understanding, it allows considerable depth of comprehension and internalization of the relevant information (e.g., Gauvain, 2005). Preschoolers who display high levels of empathy and prosocial behavior have parents who frequently discuss the causes of their emotions (Denham, Bassett, & Wyatt, 2007). Moreover, toddlers whose mothers try to explain emotions when talking to them and who direct them to label emotions are more likely to attempt to understand the emotional states of others, as well as to express concern for others (Garner, 2003). Puntambekar and Hübscher (2005) note that when the teaching is matched closely to the child's abilities, teacher and child are especially likely to arrive at a shared understanding of the task.

GROUP PARTICIPATION DOMAIN

A notable feature of children's behavior that is seen most strongly between the ages of 2 and 4 years is an almost obsessive concern with the proper display of conventional routines (Evans et al., 1997; Emde et al., 1991). Children appear to believe that there is one certain way in which things are done, and they resist efforts to change established routines. If the routines include being helpful to others, then this desire to be like other members of the social group provides another way in which prosocial behavior can be facilitated. By creating routines and rituals for their children and by exposing them to examples of concern for others, caregivers encourage the adoption of such actions. Thus the parent–child relationship in this domain involves membership in a common social group that helps to foster a sense of self-identity that comes from belonging to that group. One area in which children learn through observation of prosocial behavior, although certainly not the only one, involves events associated with the caregiver's response to distress. Caregivers, in the course of reacting to children's negative emotions by either accepting, discouraging, or ignoring them, provide a potent model that forms a basis for how children learn to react to the negative emotions of others.

Middle Childhood

During middle childhood the socialization of prosocial behavior continues, and, given children's increased exposure to their influence, peers and teachers come to assume increasingly important roles as socializing agents. The way in which children react to distress in themselves and others nevertheless continues to be an area of concern for parents.

Protection Domain

The way parents help their children deal with negative emotions and the impact of this aid on prosocial behavior remains important through middle childhood. For example, Eisenberg, Fabes, and Murphy (1996) found that mothers who provided moderate encouragement of emotion expression had 8- to 11-year-old children who displayed both high quantities and high quality of comforting. The finding held for both boys and girls. For fathers, moderate and low levels of encouragement of emotion expression were related to high-quality comforting in girls; there was no effect for boys. Vinik, Almas, and Grusec (2011) found that mothers who were more knowledgeable about what their 10- to 12-year-old children found to be comforting when they were distressed (and who, presumably, were better able to help them deal with distress) had children who coped better and who were reported to be more prosocial by their teachers.

Reciprocity Domain

In a study of 11- to 13-year-old European American and African American children, Lindsey, Colwell, Frabutt, Chambers, and MacKinnon-Lewis (2008) found that shared positive affect between mother and child was associated with higher levels of prosocial behavior (as reported by the mothers). Shared negative affect predicted lower levels of prosocial behavior, although only for European American children.

Control Domain

In studies of prosocial behavior relevant to the control domain, socialization theorists have remained focused on the undermining effects of external motivation on children's acceptance of prosocial values and enactment of prosocial behavior. Previously we noted that social reinforcement has been demonstrated to have fewer negative effects on helping behavior than material reinforcement (Smith et al., 1979). Another form of subtle consequence has been studied by Grusec and her colleagues (Grusec, Kuczynski, Rushton, & Simutis, 1978; Grusec & Redler, 1980), who told 7- to 10-year-old children after they had shared winnings from a game that they must have shared because they were the kind of people who liked to help others. The children subsequently were more prosocial than those who were praised for sharing. These character attributions were not effective with 5-year-olds, perhaps a reflection of the fact that children do not think of themselves as having enduring dispositional characteristics until they are 7 or 8 years of age (Livesley & Bromley, 1973; Peevers & Secord, 1973).

Additional evidence for the problematic nature of rewards comes from a study with 7- to 11-year-olds (Fabes, Fultz, Eisenberg, May-Plumlee, & Christopher, 1989), in which children who were rewarded with a toy for being helpful became more helpful in the immediate situation. However, later helping was undermined when rewards were no longer available, although only for children whose mothers felt positive about the use of rewards in general. In addition, these mothers reported that their children were generally less prosocial than did mothers who felt less positive about the use of rewards.

Group Participation Domain

Models of prosocial behavior continue to be important in the developmental process. A number of experimental studies conducted in the 1970s and 1980s have shown that children match their behavior to that of adults who donate rewards to others during the middle childhood years (see Grusec, 1982, for a review). And in a meta-analysis of 34 studies of prosocial media exposure, including a number of studies of children in middle childhood, Mares and Woodard (2005) concluded that children who watch more prosocial content in the media behave significantly more prosocially.

Adolescence

Historically, the prosocial behavior of adolescents has been an understudied area relative to the prosocial behavior of younger children (Hoffman, 1980; Eisenberg, 1990; Fabes, Carlo, Kupanoff, & Laible, 1999). It is only in the past decade that research on adolescence has begun to move from a focus on negative topics—such as adolescent moodiness and hormones, parent–adolescent conflict and distance, and adolescent social deviance—to more positive topics, such as prosocial behavior (see Smetana, Campione-Barr, & Metzger, 2006; Steinberg & Morris, 2001).

Adolescence is a developmental period characterized by growing autonomy from the family and increased time spent in the company of peers (Larson, Richards, Moneta, Holmbeck, & Duckett, 1996). There is considerable evidence that groups of peers initiate and perpetuate cycles of prosocial exchanges (Bukowski & Sippola, 1996; Eisenberg & Fabes, 1998): This seems particularly so in the case of groups that are highly influential because, for example, they are trend setters, are physically attractive (in the case of girls), and engage in prestigious activities such as team sports (Ellis & Zarbatany, 2007). The negative impact of peers on prosocial behavior has also been documented. Thus a comparison of pairs of delinquent and nondelinquent male adolescent friends revealed that delinquent dyads reacted positively to rule-breaking topics and were less likely to reinforce prosocial discussions (Dishion, Spracklen, Andrews, & Patterson, 1996). Nevertheless, although peers are significant, the influence of mothers and fathers continues to be important (e.g., Carlo, Fabes, Laible, & Kupanoff, 1999).

In our discussion we again organize the relevant literature according to socialization domains. We then turn to a discussion of volunteerism, which is unique because it not only promotes prosocial behavior but is also itself a form of prosocial behavior.

Protection Domain

Parents continue to be a source of emotional support during adolescence. Accordingly, Barry, Padilla-Walker, Madsen, and Nelson (2008) assessed adolescents' self-disclosure to mothers (defined as "telling her everything," turning to mothers for emotional support with personal problems, and receipt of maternal aid in helping to solve problems) and linked it to internalization of values (defined as adolescent self-reports of internal as opposed to external motivation for positive social behavior). They found that self-disclosure predicted internalization of the three prosocial moral values of fairness, honesty, and kindness. Adolescents' internalized values were, in turn, positively related to their self-reported prosocial tendencies for behaviors that occurred in a private context but not those occurring when others were watching, suggesting that internally motivated behavior is likely to reveal itself in contexts in which there is no opportunity for social approval. Other research has found that adolescents who reported a secure attachment relationship with their parents, characterized by trust in the accessibility and responsiveness of both mothers and fathers, also reported that they would engage in a variety of prosocial behaviors (Laible, Carlo, & Roesch, 2004).

Reciprocity Domain

Recipients of positive behavior from others frequently experience gratitude, which, in turn, has been linked with prosocial behavior (McCullough, Kilpatrick, Emmons, & Larson, 2001; Tsang, 2006). Thus studies of gratitude could be seen to reflect events in the reciprocity domain. Froh, Yurkewicz, and Kashdan (2009) examined the influence of parenting on feelings of gratitude by asking young adolescents to estimate the extent to which they had felt grateful, thankful, and appreciative since the prior day and the degree to which they felt their families were supportive. The researchers found that boys who reported higher levels of family support also reported more feelings of gratitude. Girls, on the other hand, felt highly grateful regardless of level of family support, a finding in accord with past research that has found girls more likely to express gratitude than boys (Gordon, Musher-Eizenman, Holub, & Dalrymple, 2004). The implication of these sex differences and of the role of gratitude in the development of prosocial behavior remains to be examined.

Adolescents' participation in organized sports can also be linked to events in the reciprocity domain. Thus, in a study of adolescents' perceptions of the emotional climate of their sporting environment, those who considered their teammates and coaches to be trusting of one another, respectful, and fair reported engaging in more prosocial behaviors in their everyday lives (Rutten, Stams, Biesta, Schuengel, Dirks, & Hoeksma, 2007). In a study of youths attending a summer sports program, those who felt valued by their team members and who recognized their team environments as receptive, accepting, and supportive reported greater confidence in their abilities to regulate their positive emotions and empathize with others. This confidence in turn predicted their performance of prosocial behaviors (Gano-Overway, Newton, Magyar, Fry, Kim, & Guivernau, 2009). One conclusion, then, is that contexts that promote mutuality and shared positive climates indirectly affect adolescents' development of kindness toward others by helping them to recognize and value their team members' needs and feelings; this skill is then generalized to others outside the sporting context in order to promote adolescents' general prosocial orientations. No doubt some of the characteristics of involvement in organized sports also contribute to behavior in other domains, as we describe below.

Control Domain

In the control domain, studies are consistent with research with younger children finding that praise, when compared with material rewards, is associated with greater incorporation of prosocial moral values and expressions of prosocial behavior. In one study, for example, mothers were asked what parenting practices they used with their adolescents to promote prosocial behaviors (Carlo, McGinley, Hayes, Batenhorst, & Wilkinson, 2007). Associations between social reinforcement (i.e., praise) and adolescents' self-reported prosocial behaviors in several different hypothetical contexts (giving aid in times of extreme crisis or emergency, responding to others' requests for help, responding to observed emotional distress, and anonymous giving) were found. These associations were indirect, with the adolescents' self-reported empathic concern and perspective-taking ability mediating the relation between maternal social reinforcement and adolescents' prosocial behavior. In contrast, mothers' use of material rewards was not significantly related to adolescents' empathic concern and perspective-taking ability, although it was directly related to public helping.

We note that social reinforcement has its problems, however. Thus Roth (2008) compared the effects of autonomy-supportive parenting (taking the child's perspective, providing meaningful rationales, granting choices, and allowing criticism and independent thinking) with those of conditional regard or social reinforcement, that is, providing affection and approval for prosocial behavior. Adolescents reported on their parents' past use of these techniques, with those whose parents were autonomy-supportive more likely to display internalized prosocial motives, feeling that they had a sense of choice over their actions. These adolescents also reported practicing prosocial behaviors that were based on others' needs and desires (e.g., "When I'm helping another person, it is important for me to know how he or she would like to be helped"), rather than motivated by the approval or appreciation of others (e.g., "When I am helping another person, it is important for me to know that he or she appreciates me for doing so"). In contrast, adolescents who reported having parents who exercised high levels of conditional regard were more likely to report that their prosocial behaviors were motivated by gaining the appreciation or approval of others. These adolescents also said that they had feelings of internal compulsion to perform prosocial behaviors, which is commonly referred to as introjection (a weak form of internalization). Although these adolescents took in the prosocial values of their parents, they did not accept them as their own. Instead, their prosocial behavior was motivated by the need to enhance their own self-esteem. We conclude, then, that social reinforcement may lead to some form of incorporation of values but not to truly internalized standards of behavior.

Guided Learning Domain

Youths' participation in team sports is a context in which teaching and encouragement of such prosocial skills as cooperation and consideration of others occurs. Accordingly, adolescents who participate in organized sports have been found to exhibit more self-reported prosocial behaviors (e.g., comforting, helping, sharing) relative to those who do not (Linver, Roth, & Brooks-Gunn, 2009). Longitudinal research has also compared adolescents of low-income families who participated in extracurricular team sports with matched adolescents who were involved in religious activities, clubs and youth groups, programs at recreation or community centers, and private lessons. Of the five activities, the researchers reported that involvement in team sports during middle childhood was most consistently related to positive psychosocial outcomes in adolescence, including parent-reported prosocial behavior. Children who spent time at clubs, youth groups, and religious activities, however, also had relatively high levels of psychosocial functioning and prosocial behavior (Ripke, Huston, & Casey, 2006). It is true that team sports encourage cooperation and consideration of others, but clubs, youth groups, and religious activities also appear to allow for interactions with peers that involve working together toward a common goal, which is important for the development of prosocial behavior in the guided learning domain.

Group Participation Domain

One way in which children are trained to be socially responsible is through the assignment of household duties. Thus many parents believe that sharing household work is an important route to concern for others (Goodnow, 1988), although the evidence is mixed. In one study that attempted to unravel some of the confusion around the topic, Grusec, Goodnow, and Cohen (1997), working with Australian and Canadian families, investigated the kind of household work children were assigned and the way in which it was assigned. They found that routine work done for others, such as setting the table for dinner or taking out the garbage, was associated with spontaneous concern for others (indexed by mothers who kept journal accounts of their children's prosocial actions). Routine work done for oneself, such as keeping one's room clean, as well as work for oneself or for others that was done in response to a request, showed no such relation. In fact, there was some evidence of a negative relation between both routine and requested work that involved caring for the self and spontaneous concern for others. Grusec et al. (1997) concluded that everyday routines involving specific kinds of household chores provide an excellent opportunity for children to learn about societal expectations and to practice meeting them. Interestingly, it takes time for these routines to be adopted, with results apparent for older children (12–14 years) but not younger (9–11 years).

Volunteerism: A Special Case

In spite of a relative scarcity of research on prosocial behavior in adolescence, one area has received considerable attention: adolescents' participation in volunteer community service activities. Volunteerism is a central topic of study because it is not only an activity that promotes and fosters prosocial development, but it is also a prosocial behavior in its own right. Volunteer work is also much more commonly practiced in adolescence than at younger ages and usually occurs over some sustained period of time.

What do we know about the socialization of volunteerism? First, it can occur within the group participation domain. Research has shown that volunteering adolescents were more likely to have parents who were also involved in community service activities (Keith, Nelson, Schlabach, & Thompson, 1990). Other research has found that adolescents whose parents were highly involved in their school activities throughout high school (e.g., discussing school activities, asking what the adolescent was studying, and PTA participation) had a 30% greater likelihood of volunteering for community service 2 years after high school graduation than adolescents of disengaged parents (Zaff, Moore, Papillo, & Williams, 2003). These parents not only provide an example of community service through their own involvement in their adolescents' schools but also likely manage their adolescents' exposure to other prosocial models (i.e., good teachers and responsible peer groups). Aside from providing opportunities for observational learning, many parents also operate in the guided learning domain. These parents choose to talk to their adolescents directly about initiating community service and in doing so communicate to them the benefits and importance of donating one's time to serve others (Yates & Youniss, 1996). Moreover, adolescents may learn social responsibility from educational television programming. One study found that regularly watching television programs with informative content was predictive of adolescents' weekly time spent participating in community service extracurricular activities. Although the link between educational television and volunteerism is not immediately apparent, the researchers speculated that viewing informative content may cultivate an interest in the broader community environment (Anderson, Huston, Schmitt, Linebarger, & Wright, 2001).

Recent longitudinal studies have allowed causal inferences about the relation between volunteerism and prosocial behavior. Accordingly, Fredricks and Eccles (2006) have reported that youths' participation in volunteer service or civil rights activities in grade 11 predicted their charitable, social service, and political involvement 1 year after graduation from high school. Voluntarily helping an organization or individual may reinforce adolescents' developing self-concepts about their own prosocial orientations. Another study found that youths' involvement in community helping activities at age 17 predicted higher scores 2 years later on an index of the significance of moral values to the adolescent. Over this period of time the adolescents increased their emphasis on the importance of holding prosocial moral values, such as trustworthiness, honesty, kindness, caring, fairness, integrity, and being a good citizen (Pratt, Hunsberger, Pancer, & Alisat, 2003).

Empirical evidence for the effectiveness of mandatory school-based community service programs on the enhancement of adolescents' civic interest or engagement has been largely inconsistent (Newmann & Rutter, 1983; Melchior, 1998; Yates & Youniss, 1996). Problems arise from the comparison of volunteer activities that are not similar, from large variation in structure between programs, from disparity in requirements for time commitment, and from lack of random assignment of research participants by investigators. Metz and Youniss (2005), using a design that corrected for these methodological inconsistencies, examined two cohorts of high school students; one was required to complete 40 hours of curricular community service, whereas the second did not participate in any community service activities. The researchers also measured all of the students' views on community service participation at baseline. At the end of grade 12, the researchers asked only the students who had been initially disinclined to volunteer for their views on civil service engagement. The disinclined students from the two cohorts were significantly different in their views; only the students who were required to volunteer said that they would increase their community involvement in the years ahead after graduation. These findings suggest that even when adolescents are required to engage in community service (sometimes grudgingly), the involvement still has positive effects on their prosocial development.

CULTURAL DIFFERENCES IN PROSOCIAL BEHAVIOR

Most of the research and theory discussed to this point has been conducted in a Western cultural context. Studies of prosocial behavior in other cultures, of course, are imperative to a more comprehensive understanding of how concern for others develops. Many years ago Whiting and Whiting (1975) reported that children in Kenya, Mexico, and the Philippines were more likely to offer help or support than children in Okinawa, India, and the United States. Whiting and Whiting attributed these differences to the fact that the first group of children was more likely to be assigned responsibility for the care of younger children. Given that mothers in these countries were more likely to be contributing to the family economy, they needed to delegate some of their workload, and, accordingly, they set the conditions for greater participation in prosocial activities.

Cultures also differentially value different forms of prosocial behavior. In the case of so-called individualist cultures (primarily North American and Western European), self-assertion, self-expression, and self-actualization are valued, whereas in collectivist cultures (most of the rest of the world) the emphasis is on propriety, fitting in, and harmonious family relationships (Markus & Kitayama, 1991). Not surprisingly, unsolicited or spontaneous prosocial behavior is viewed more positively in individualist cultures, incidentally a bias seen in the predisposition of Western researchers to see internalized moral values as the best socialization outcome. In contrast, reciprocal or solicited prosocial behavior is more highly valued among those with a more collectivist orientation (Miller & Bersoff, 1992), a reflection of the emphasis on interdependence and compliance with social roles as opposed to autonomy and feelings of self-generation. This differential emphasis is also seen in a report by Kemmelmeier, Jambor, and Letner (2006). They found that volunteerism and charitable giving across the United States was higher in those states that were rated as higher on individualism. If volunteerism and charitable giving reflect concern for strangers and the more abstract valuation of the community, then one should expect to find helping directed toward family members as a feature of prosocial behavior for those scoring higher on collectivism.

Finally, we note an example of how opposing values may inhibit displays of prosocial behavior. The example comes from the observation that, in cultures in which deference to authority is a prominent value, individuals may be reluctant to offer assistance to older individuals because it could cause the latter to lose face (Trommsdorf, Friedlmeier, & Mayer, 2007).

CONCLUSION

In this chapter we have tried to show how the complex interplay between evolutionary principles, genetic predispositions, and social and cultural experiences contributes to the development of prosocial behavior. We have also tried to emphasize how interrelated these various approaches are: It is impossible to understand the emergence of any social behavior without an appreciation of the intimate interconnectedness of our evolutionary history, our genetic makeup, our socialization experiences, and the impact of the values of the culture in which we live on those socialization experiences. We have also tried to emphasize the problems involved in the study of prosocial behavior, not only in terms of the multiple meanings that have been assigned to the concept but also of the multiple domains in which its socialization takes place. Finally, we note that a focus on what makes people reach out to assist others is at least as important as a focus on what keeps them from doing harm to others.

RESEARCH QUESTIONS REMAINING

This review of the literature on prosocial development makes clear that there is still much to be learned about how children learn to become responsive to the needs of others. One direction this learning may take is toward the current major interest in the biological aspects of social development, with a focus on genetic, hormonal, and neurological changes that accompany the developmental process. This interest will be manifested in increasing knowledge of prosocial behavior and its constituent parts, particularly as the approaches of neuroscience become integrated with those of social and cultural psychology.

Another question needing to be addressed is the role of fathers in the socialization process. Also, we need to know more about events in middle childhood and adolescence and how particular changes in physical, cognitive, and emotional functioning in that time period lead to changes in concern for others. The domain analysis presented here suggests that the goal of concern for others can be achieved in a variety of ways. The question here is whether the nature of that concern for others depends on the way in which it was socialized. Are children whose parents nurture their empathic capacity in the protection domain particularly caring only for others who are clearly experiencing distress? Does the expression of prosocial behavior that develops in the domain of mutual reciprocity require the clear possibility that it can be reciprocated? What form of socialization produces a deeply principled concern for others that is impervious to external pressure?

A final and important direction for developmental researchers involves the need for more longitudinal studies that thereby enable some inference of causality. These studies are costly both in terms of time and resources. But they, along with intervention studies and experimental investigations, will be the only way we can really answer the question that is the focus of this chapter: How do we produce caring individuals in a world that is too often spoiled by selfishness and greed?

SUGGESTED READINGS

Eisenberg, N., Fabes, R. A., & Spinrad, T. L. (2006). Prosocial development. In N. Eisenberg (Vol. Ed.), *Handbook of child psychology: Vol. 3. Social, emotional, and personality development* (pp. 646–718). Hoboken, NJ: Wiley.

Gregory, A. M., Light-Häusermann, J. H., Rijsdijk, F., & Eley, T. C. (2009). Behavioral genetic analyses of prosocial behavior in adolescents. *Developmental Science, 12*, 165–174.

Knafo, A., Zahn-Waxler, C., Van Hulle, C., Robinson, J., & Rhee, S. H. (2008). The developmental origins of a disposition toward empathy: Genetic and environmental contributions. *Emotion, 8,* 737–752.

Malti, T., Gummerum, M., Keller, M., & Buchmann, M. (2009). Children's moral motivation, sympathy, and prosocial behavior. *Child Development, 80,* 442–460.

Shirtcliff, E. A., Vitacco, M. J., Graf, A. R., Gostisha, A. J., Merz, J. L., & Zahn-Waxler, C. (2009). Neurobiology of empathy and callousness: Implications for the development of antisocial behavior. *Behavioral Sciences and the Law, 27,* 137–171.

REFERENCES

Adamson, L. B., & Bakeman, R. (1991). The development of shared attention during infancy. In R. Vasta (Ed.), *Annals of child development* (Vol. 8, pp. 1–41). London: Kingsley.

Anderson, D. R., Huston, A. C., Schmitt, K. L., Linebarger, D. L., & Wright, J. C. (2001). Extracurricular activities. *Monographs of the Society for Research in Child Development, 66*(1), 90–99.

Bachner-Melman, R., Zohar, A. H., Bacon-Shnoor, N., Yoel, E., Nemanov, L., Gritsenko, I., & et al. (2005). Link between vasopressin receptor AVPR1A promoter region microsatellites and measures of social behavior in humans. *Journal of Individual Differences, 26,* 2–10.

Barry, C. M., Padilla-Walker, L. M., Madsen, S. D., & Nelson, L. J. (2008). The impact of maternal relationship quality on emerging adults' prosocial tendencies: Indirect effects via regulation of prosocial values. *Journal of Youth and Adolescence, 37,* 581–591.

Bates, J. E., & Pettit, G. S. (2007). Temperament, parenting, and socialization. In J. E. Grusec & P. D. Hastings (Eds.), *Handbook of socialization* (pp. 153–177). New York: Guilford Press.

Buck, R. (1991). Temperament, social skills, and the communication of emotions: A developmental-interactionist view. In D. G. Gilbert & J. J. Connolly (Eds.), *Personality, social skills, and psychopathology: An individual differences approach* (pp. 85–105). New York: Wiley.

Bukowski, W. M., & Sippola, L. K. (1996). Friendship and morality. In W. M. Bukowski & A. F. Newcomb (Eds.), *The company they keep: Friendship in childhood and adolescence* (pp. 238–261). Cambridge, UK: Cambridge University Press.

Caplan, M. Z., & Hay, D. (1989). Preschoolers' responses to peers' distress and beliefs about bystander intervention. *Journal of Child Psychology and Psychiatry, 30,* 231–242.

Carlo, G., Fabes, R. A., Laible, D., & Kupanoff, K. (1999). Early adolescence and prosocial moral behavior: II. The role of social and contextual influences. *Journal of Early Adolescence, 19*(2), 133–147.

Carlo, G., McGinley, M., Hayes, R., Batenhorst, C., & Wilkinson, J. (2007). Parenting styles or practices?: Parenting, sympathy, and prosocial behaviors among adolescents. *Journal of Genetic Psychology, 168,* 147–176.

Cassidy, J. (1994). Emotion regulation: Influences of attachment relationships. *Monographs of the Society for Research in Child Development, 59,* 228–283.

Chakrabarti, B., Dudbridge, F., Kent, L., Wheelwright, S., Hill-Cawthorne, G., Allison, C., et al. (2009). Genes related to sex steroids, neural growth, and social-emotional behavior are associated with autistic traits, empathy, and Asperger syndrome. *Autism Research, 2,* 157–177.

Cornell, A. H., & Frick, P. J. (2007). The moderating effects of parenting styles in the association between behavioral inhibition and parent-reported guilt and empathy in preschool children. *Journal of Clinical Child and Adolescent Psychology, 36,* 305–318.

Davidov, M., & Grusec, J. E. (2006). Untangling the links of parental responsiveness to distress and warmth to child outcomes. *Child Development, 77,* 44–58.

Denham, S. A., Bassett, H. H., & Wyatt, T. (2007). The socialization of emotional competence. In J. E. Grusec & P. D. Hastings (Eds.), *Handbook of socialization* (pp. 614–637). New York: Guilford Press.

DiLalla, L. F., Elam, K. K., & Smolen, A. (2009). Genetic and gene–environment interaction effects on preschoolers' social behaviors. *Developmental Psychobiology, 51*(6), 451–464.

Dishion, T. J., Spracklen, K. M., Andrews, D. M., & Patterson, G. R. (1996). Deviancy training in male adolescent friendships. *Behavior Therapy, 27,* 373–390.

Dragan, W. L., & Oniszczenko, W. (2007). An association between dopamine D4 receptor and transporter gene polymorphisms and personality traits, assessed using NEO-FFI in a Polish female population. *Personality and Individual Differences, 43,* 531–540.

Eisenberg, N. (1990). Prosocial development in early and mid-adolescence. In R. Montemayor, G. R. Adams, & T. P. Gullotta (Eds.), *From childhood to adolescence: A transitional period?* (Vol. 2, pp. 240–269). Newbury Park, CA: Sage.

Eisenberg, N., & Fabes, R. A. (1998). Prosocial development. In W. Damon (Series Ed.) & N. Eisenberg (Vol. Ed.), *Handbook of child psychology: Vol. 3. Social, emotional, and personality development* (5th ed., pp. 701–778). New York: Wiley.

Eisenberg, N., Fabes, R., & Murphy, B. C. (2006). Parents' reactions to children's negative emotions: Relations to children' social competence and comforting. *Child Development, 67,* 2227–2247.

Eisenberg, N., Fabes, R. A., & Spinrad, T. L. (2006). Prosocial development. In N. Eisenberg (Vol. Ed.), *Handbook of child psychology: Vol. 3. Social, emotional, and personality development* (pp. 646–718). Hoboken, NJ: Wiley.

Eisenberg, N., Wentzel, M., & Harris, J. D. (1998). The role of emotionality and regulation in empathy-related responding. *School Psychology Review, 27,* 506–521.

Ellis, W. E., & Zarbatany, L. (2007). Peer group status as a moderator of group influence on children's deviant, aggressive, and prosocial behavior. *Child Development, 78*(4), 1240–1254.

Emde, R. N., Biringen, Z., Clyman, R. B., & Oppenheim, D. (1991). The moral self of infancy: Affective core and procedural knowledge. *Developmental Review, 11,* 251–270.

Evans, D. W., Leckman, J. F., Carter, A., Reznick, J. S., Henshaw, C., King, R. A., et al. (1997). Ritual, habit, and perfectionism: The prevalence and development of compulsive-like behavior in normal young children. *Child Development, 68,* 58–68.

Fabes, R. A., Carlo, G., Kupanoff, K., & Laible, D. (1999). Early adolescence and prosocial/moral behavior: I. The role of individual processes. *Journal of Early Adolescence, 19*(1), 5–16.

Fabes, R. A., Fultz, J., Eisenberg, N., May-Plumlee, T., & Christopher, F. S. (1989). Effects of rewards on children's prosocial motivation: A socialization study. *Developmental Psychology, 25,* 509–515.

Faraone, S. V., Doyle, A. E., Mick, E., & Biederman, J. (2001). Meta-analysis of the association between the 7-repeat allele of the dopamine D_4 receptor gene and attention-deficit/hyperactivity disorder. *American Journal of Psychiatry, 158,* 1052–1057.

Fisher, J. D., Nadler, A., & Whitcher-Alagna, S. (1982). Recipient reactions to aid. *Psychological Bulletiin, 91,* 27–54.

Fredricks, J., & Eccles, J. (2006). Is extracurricular participation associated with beneficial outcomes?: Concurrent and longitudinal relations. *Developmental Psychology, 42*(4), 698–713.

Froh, J. J., Yurkewicz, C., & Kashdan, T. B. (2009). Gratitude and subjective well-being in early adolescence: Examining gender differences. *Journal of Adolescence, 32*(3), 633–650.

Gano-Overway, L. A., Newton, M., Magyar, T. M., Fry, M. D., Kim, M., & Guivernau, M. R. (2009). Influence of caring youth sport contexts on efficacy-related beliefs and social behaviors. *Developmental Psychology, 45*(2), 329–340.

Garner, P. W. (2003). Child and family correlates of toddlers' emotional and behavioral responses to a mishap. *Infant Mental Health Journal, 24,* 580–592.

Garner, P. W., Jones, D. C., & Palmer, D. J. (1994). Social cognitive correlates of preschool children's sibling caregiving behavior. *Developmental Psychology, 30,* 905–911.

Gauvain, M. (2005). Scaffolding in socialization. *New Ideas in Psychology, 23,* 129–139.

Goodnow, J. J. (1988). Children's household work: Its nature and functions. *Psychological Bulletin, 103,* 5–26.

Gordon, A. K., Musher-Eizenman, D. R., Holub, S. C., & Dalrymple, J. (2004). What are children thankful for?: An archival analysis of gratitude before and after the attacks of September 11. *Applied Developmental Psychology, 25,* 541–553.

Grafen, A. (1990). Biological signals as handicaps. *Journal of Theoretical Biology, 144,* 517–546.

Greener, G., & Crick, N. R. (1999). Normative beliefs about prosocial behavior in middle childhood: What does it mean to be nice? *Social Development, 8,* 349–363.

Grusec, J. E. (1982). The socialization of altruism. In N. Eisenberg (Ed.), *The development of prosocial behavior* (pp. 139–166). New York: Academic Press.

Grusec, J. E. (1983). The internalization of altruistic dispositions: A cognitive analysis. In E. T. Higgins, D.N. Ruble, & W. W. Hartup (Eds.), *Social cognition and social development* (pp. 275–293). New York: Cambridge University Press.

Grusec, J. E. (1991). Socializing concern for others in the home. *Developmental Psychology, 27,* 338–342.

Grusec, J. E., & Davidov, M. (2010). Integrating different perspectives on socialization theory and research: A domain-specific approach. *Child Development, 81,* 687–709.

Grusec, J. E., Goodnow, J. J., & Cohen, L. (1997). Household work and the development of children's concern for others. *Developmental Psychology, 32,* 999–1007.

Grusec, J. E., Kuczynski, L., Rushton, J. P., & Simutis, Z. M. (1978). Modeling, direct instruction, and attributions: Effects on altruism. *Developmental Psychology, 14,* 51–57.

Grusec, J. E., & Redler, E. (1980). Attribution, reinforcement, and altruism: A developmental analysis. *Developmental Psychology, 16,* 525–534.

Gunnar, M. R. (2000). Early adversity and the development of stress reactivity and regulation. In C. A. Nelson (Ed.), *The Minnesota Symposia on Child Psychology: Vol. 31. The effects of early adversity on neurobehavioral development* (pp. 163–200). Mahwah, NJ: Erlbaum.

Hamilton, W. D. (1964). Genetical evolution of social behavior. *Journal of Theoretical Biology, 7,* 1–52.

Hay, D. F., Nash, A., & Pedersen, J. (1981). Responses of six-month-olds to the distress of their peers. *Child Development, 52,* 1071–1075.

Hoffman, M. L. (1970). Moral development. In P.H. Mussen (Ed.), *Carmichael's manual of child psychology* (Vol. 2, pp. 261–360). New York: Wiley.

Hoffman, M. L. (1980). Moral development in adolescence. In J. Adelson (Ed.), *Handbook of adolescent psychology* (pp. 295–343). New York: Wiley.

Israel, S., Lerer, E., Shalev, I., Uzefovsky, F., Reibold, M., Bachner-Melman, R., et al. (2008). Molecular genetic studies of the arginine vasopressin 1a receptor (AVPR1a) and the oxytocin receptor (OXTR) in human behavior: From autism to altruism with some notes in between. *Progress in Brain Research, 170,* 435–449.

Israel, S., Lerer, E., Shalev, I., Uzefovsky, F., Riebold, M., Laiba, E., et al. (2009). The oxytocin receptor (*OXTR*) contributes to prosocial fund allocations in the dictator game and the social value orientations task. *PLoS One, 4*(5), e5535.

Kant, I. (1956). *Critique of practical reason.* New York: Macmillan. (Original work published 1788)

Keith, J. G., Nelson, C. S., Schlabach, J. H., & Thompson, C. J. (1990). The relationship between parental employment and three measures of early adolescent responsibility: Family related, personal, and social. *Journal of Early Adolescence, 10,* 399–415.

Kemmelmeier, M., Jambor, E. E., & Letner, J. (2006). Individualism and good works: Cultural variations in giving and receiving across the United States. *Journal of Cross-Cultural Psychology, 37,* 327–344.

Knafo, A., & Israel, S. (2009). Genetic and environmental influences on prosocial behavior. In M. Mikulincer & P. R. Shaver (Eds.), *Prosocial motives, emotions, and behavior* (pp. 149–167). Washington, DC: American Psychological Association.

Knafo, A., Israel, S., Darvasi, A., Bachner-Melman, R., Uzefovsky, F., Cohen, L., et al. (2008). Individual differences in allocation of funds in the dictator game and postmortem hippocampal mRNA levels are correlated with length of the arginine vasopressin 1a receptor (AVPR1a) RS3 promoter-region repeat. *Genes, Brain, and Behavior, 7,* 266–275.

Knafo, A., & Plomin, R. (2006). Prosocial behavior from early to middle childhood: Genetic and environmental influences. *Developmental Psychology, 42,* 771–786.

Laible, D. J., Carlo, G., & Roesch, S. C. (2004). Pathways to self-esteem in late adolescence: The role of parent and peer attachment, empathy, and social behaviours. *Journal of Adolescence, 27,* 703–716.

Larson, R. W., Richards, M. H., Moneta, G., Holmbeck, G., & Duckett, E. (1996). Changes in adolescents' daily interactions with their families from ages 10–18: Disengagement and transformation. *Developmental Psychology, 32,* 744–754.

Lepper, M. (1983). Social control processes, attributions of motivation, and the internalization of social values. In E. T. Higgins, D. N. Ruble, & W. W. Hartup (Eds.), *Social cognition and social development: A sociocultural perspective* (pp. 294–330). New York: Cambridge University Press.

Lindsey, E. W., Colwell, M. J., Frabutt, J. M., Chambers, J. C., & MacKinnon-Lewis, C. (2008). Mother–child dyadic synchrony in European American and African American families during early adolescence: Relations with self-esteem and prosocial behavior. *Merrill–Palmer Quarterly, 54,* 289–315.

Linver, M. R., Roth, J. L., & Brooks-Gunn, J. (2009). Patterns of adolescents' participation in organized activities: Are sports best when combined with other activities? *Developmental Psychology, 45*(2), 354–367.

Livesley, W. J., & Bromley, D. B. (1973). *Person perception in childhood and adolescence.* Oxford, UK: Wiley.

Mares, M., & Woodard, E. (2005). Positive effects of television on children's social interactions: A meta-analysis. *Media Psychology, 7,* 301–322.

Markus, H. R., & Kitayama, S. (1991). Culture and the self: Implications for cognition, emotion, and motivation. *Psychological Review, 98,* 224–253.

McAndrew, F. T. (2002). New evolutionary perspectives on altruism: Multilevel-selection and costly-signaling theories. *Current Directions in Psychological Science, 11,* 79–82.

McCullough, M. E., Kilpatrick, S. D., Emmons, R. A., & Larson, D. B. (2001). Is gratitude a moral affect? *Psychological Bulletin, 127,* 249–266.

Mealey, L., Daood, C., & Krage, M. (1996). Enhanced memory for faces of cheaters. *Evolution and Human Behavior, 17,* 119–128.

Melchior, A. (1998). *Final report: National evaluation of Learn and Serve America and community-based programs.* Waltham, MA: Brandeis University, Center for Human Resources.

Metz, E. C., & Youniss, J. (2005). Longitudinal gains in civic development through school-based required service. *Political Psychology, 26*(3), 413–437.

Miller, J. G. E., & Bersoff, D. M. (1992). Culture and moral judgment: How are conflicts between justice and interpersonal responsibilities resolved? *Journal of Personality and Social Psychology, 62,* 541–554.

Newmann, F., & Rutter, R. (1983). *The effects of high school community service programs on students' social development: Final report.* Madison: University of Wisconsin Center for Educational Research.

Parpal, M., & Maccoby, E. E. (1985). Maternal responsiveness and subsequent child compliance. *Child Development, 56,* 1326–1334.

Patterson, G. R., & Fisher, P. A. (2002). Recent developments in our understanding of parenting, bidirectional effects, causal models, and the search for parsimony. In M. H. Bornstein (Ed.) *Handbook of parenting* (Vol. 3, pp. 59–88). Mahwah, NJ: Erlbaum.

Peevers, B. H., & Secord, P. E. (1973). Developmental changes in attribution of descriptive concepts to persons. *Journal of Personality and Social Psychology, 27,* 120–128.

Peterson, L. (1982). Altruism and the development of internal control: An integrative model. *Merrill–Palmer Quarterly, 28,* 197–222.

Pratt, M., Hunsberger, B., Pancer, S. M., & Alisat, S. (2003). A longitudinal analysis of personal values socialization: Correlates of a moral self-ideal in late adolescence. *Social Development, 12*(4), 563–585.

Puntambekar, S., & Hübscher, R. (2005). Tools for scaffolding students in a complex learning environment: What have we gained and what have we missed? *Educational Psychologist, 40,* 1–12.

Radke-Yarrow, M., Zahn-Waxler, C., & Chapman, M. (1982). Children's prosocial dispositions and behavior. In E. M. Hetherington (Ed.), *Handbook of child psychology: Vol 4. Socialization, personality and social development* (pp. 469–546). New York: Harper & Row.

Rheingold, H. (1982). Little children's participation in the work of adults: A nascent prosocial behavior. *Child Development, 53,* 114–125.

Ripke, M., Huston, A., & Casey, D. M. (2006). Low-income children's activity participation as a predictor of psychosocial and academic outcomes in middle childhood and adolescence. In A. Huston & M. Ripke (Eds.), *Developmental contexts in middle childhood: Bridges to adolescence and adulthood* (pp. 260–282). New York: Cambridge University Press.

Roth, G. (2008). Perceived parental conditional regard and autonomy support as predictors of young adults' self-versus-other-oriented prosocial tendencies. *Journal of Personality, 76*(3), 513–534.

Rutten, E., Stams, G., Biesta, G., Schuengel, C., Dirks, E., & Hoeksma, J. (2007). The contribution of organized youth sport to antisocial and prosocial behavior in adolescent athletes. *Journal of Youth and Adolescence, 36*(3), 255–264.

Sagi, A., & Hoffman, M. L. (1976). Empathic distress in the newborn. *Developmental Psychology, 12,* 175–176.

Smetana, J., Campione-Barr, N., & Metzger, A. (2006). Adolescent development in interpersonal and societal contexts. *Annual Review of Psychology, 57*(1), 255–284.

Smith, C. L., Gelfand, D. M., Hartmann, D. P., & Partlow, M. E. (1979). Children's causal attributions regarding helping. *Child Development, 50,* 203–210.

Steinberg, L., & Morris, A. S. (2001). Adolescent development. *Annual Review of Psychology, 52,* 83–110.

Trivers, R. (1971). The evolution of reciprocal altruism. *Quarterly Review of Biology, 46,* 35–57.

Trommsdorff, G., Friedlmeier, W., & Mayer, B. (2007). Sympathy, distress, and prosocial behaviour of preschool children in four cultures. *International Journal of Behavioural Development, 31,* 284–293.

Tsang, J. (2006). Gratitude and prosocial behavior: An experimental test of gratitude. *Cognition and Emotion, 20,* 138–148.

Valiente, C., Eisenberg, N., Fabes, R. A., Shepard, S. A., Cumberland, A., & Losova, S. H. (2004). Prediction of children's empathy-related responding from their effortful control and parents' expressivity. *Developmental Psychology, 40,* 911–926.

Vinik, J., Almas, A. N., & Grusec, J. E. (2011). Mother's knowledge of what distresses and what comforts their children predicts children's coping, empathy, and prosocial behavior. *Parenting: Science and Practice, 11,* 56–71.

Vygotsky, L. S. (1978). *Mind in society: The development of higher psychological processes.* Cambridge, MA: Harvard University Press.

Whiting, B. B., & Whiting, J. W. M. (1975). *Children of six cultures: A psycho-cultural analysis.* Cambridge, MA: Harvard University Press.

Wilson, D. S. (1997). Incorporating group selection into the adaptionist program: A case study involving human decision making. In J. A. Simpson & D. T. Kenrick (Eds.), *Evolutionary social psychology* (pp. 345–386). Hillsdale, NJ: Erlbaum.

Wood, D. J., Bruner, J. S., & Ross, G. (1976). The role of tutoring in problem solving. *Journal of Child Psychology and Psychiatry, 17,* 89–100.

Yates, M., & Youniss, J. (1996). A developmental perspective on community service in adolescence. *Social Development, 5,* 85–111.

Zaff, J., Moore, K., Papillo, A., & Williams, S. (2003). Implications of extracurricular activity participation during adolescence on positive outcomes. *Journal of Adolescent Research, 18*(6), 599–630.

Zahavi, A. (1977). Reliability in communication systems and the evolution of altruism. In B. Stonehouse & C.M. Perrins (Eds.), *Evolutionary ecology* (pp. 253–259). London: Macmillan Press.

Zahn-Waxler, C., Robinson, J. L., & Emde, R. N. (1992). The development of empathy in twins. *Developmental Psychology, 28,* 1038–1047.

Zahn-Waxler, C., Schiro, K., Robinson, J. L., Emde, R. N., & Schmitz, S. (2001). Empathy and prosocial patterns in young MZ and DZ twins. In R. N. Emde & J. K. Hewitt (Eds.), *Infancy to early childhood: Genetic and environmental influences on developmental change* (pp. 141–162). New York: Oxford University Press.

Part IV

Contexts for
Social Development

12

Gender

Campbell Leaper
Rebecca S. Bigler

Gender shapes human lives in large and small ways. Whether a person is female or male influences her or his clothing, hobbies, social interactions, occupations, and incomes. To consider the pervasiveness of gender in our daily lives, imagine what it would be like if a person tried to live outside of the categories "male" and "female." That is the premise of Lois Gould's (1978) fictional children's story about a child named X who was raised by its parents without revealing its gender to others. In the story, X encounters resistance from peers, teachers, and other parents who want to treat X as a girl or a boy. In the story's happy ending, the other children begin to emulate X once they realize that X is having twice as much fun as they are. That is, without being constrained by traditional gender categories, X has the flexibility to pursue a greater range of play activities.

The idea of not revealing one's gender to other people may seem like something that could only happen in a children's story. However, a Swedish couple is not revealing the gender of their 2½-year-old child named Pop. According to the mother, "We want Pop to grow up more freely and avoid being forced into a specific gender mould at the outset" (Dowling, 2010, p. 3). In addition, Shane Whalley is a real-life adult example of someone who avoids being defined by the binary gender categories of "female" or "male." Shane is the education coordinator of the Gender and Sexuality Center at the University of Texas and uses gender-neutral terms of address (e.g., "ze" instead of "he" or "she" and "hir" instead of "his" or "her"). Living outside of society's gender categories has created challenges for Shane in gendered public spaces, such as bathrooms and locker rooms.

The fictional story of X, as well as the real cases of Pop and Shane Whalley, bring into stark relief society's reliance on gender to define and constrain human experience.

In the present chapter, we review some of the ways in which this occurs in children's lives. We describe children's gender development during three age periods: infancy and early childhood (approximately birth–5 years), middle childhood (approximately 6–12 years), and adolescence (approximately 13–18 years). Because children construct their own beliefs about gender and use these beliefs to guide their behavior, we focus on the role of children's cognitions, affect, and behavior in shaping their gender development. At the same time, because children are born into a world in which gender has significant meaning, we highlight the ways in which other people's gender-stereotyped expectations and behaviors differentially affect girls' and boys' beliefs, goals, and behaviors. However, because gender affects virtually every facet of individuals' lives, we are unable to review every important aspect of gender development. We concentrate on subjects most closely linked to social development and hope that readers will be inspired to read more broadly on other related topics.

SETTING THE STAGE

Gender Roles and Inequality in Society

There are two universal truths about gender that are important to note. First, gender is an important social category in every culture. Societies in which gender is largely meaningless exist only in the world of science fiction (e.g., Ursula Le Guin's [1969] *The Left Hand of Darkness*). Nonetheless, the use of gender categories varies across cultures. In most contemporary cultures, gender is defined as two groups: males and females. Individuals who are born outside of those categories (e.g., individuals with characteristics of males and females at birth) are routinely fitted into one category or the other via some combination of pharmaceuticals, surgery, and social treatment. Some cultures, however, have included more than two gender categories. For example, some Native American cultures had a third gender category for individuals who did not fit into either "female" or "male" categories (see Lang, 1998). Nonetheless, gender remains important to society, even when there are more than two gender categories.

The second universal truth is that the status of gender groups is unequal in all cultures. In every culture that has been examined, men enjoy higher levels of status than women. However, the degree of difference in status between the two genders varies across cultures and over historical time. The World Economic Forum (2007) assigned 128 countries scores based on information concerning relative differences in women's and men's (1) economic participation and opportunity, (2) educational attainment, (3) political empowerment, and (4) health and survival. This report ranked Sweden, Norway, Finland, Iceland, and New Zealand as the most egalitarian. The United States ranked 35th, trailing behind countries such as Croatia, Bulgaria, Costa Rica, Namibia, and Estonia. In sum, all research on gender has taken place within contexts in which gender is viewed as a meaningful attribute and in which men enjoy greater power and status than do women.

Understanding Gender Similarities and Differences

Across the history of gender research, scholars have focused on identifying potential differences between females (as a group) and males (as a group). The research typically has addressed two questions: (1) Are there reliable differences between the genders? (2) How large are any differences between the genders?

Are There Reliable Differences between the Genders?

Many researchers have measured some particular characteristic (e.g., height, verbal ability, depression, aggression) among males and females with the goal of determining whether the two groups were different. Researchers must use statistical tests to determine whether a difference exists. A statistically significant difference between the genders is one that is reliable. That is, the statistical test rules out fluctuation that is random with at least 95% confidence (if .05 probability is the criterion for statistical significance). It is important to understand, however, that a statistically reliable effect does not necessarily indicate a large group difference. With large samples, statistically significant gender differences can be detected that are negligible in magnitude and thus can be practically meaningless. For example, although firstborn children score reliably higher on IQ tests than later-born children, the difference in IQ performance is so small that it carries no practical significance in society. That is, employers do not preferably hire firstborns, teachers do not stereotypes first-borns as smarter than later-borns.

How Large Are Any Differences between the Genders?

In addition to examing *whether* differences exist, researchers consider the *size* of any observed gender difference. To do so, researchers consider the distribution of scores for males and females on some measure. Even when there is a statistically reliable difference on some attribute or behavior, there is typically much overlap between girls and boys and much variability within each gender (Hyde, 2005). More than 85% of overlap in scores between girls and boys reflects an average gender difference of negligible size. Meaningful differences, when they are found, may be small (67–85% overlap), moderate (53–66% overlap), or large (less than 53% overlap) in magnitude (Cohen, 1988). When several studies have tested for gender differences in the same behavior, researchers can use a technique known as *meta-analysis*, whereby the average effect size and statistical significance across studies is computed.

Another important point is that the magnitude of average gender difference for many behaviors is not fixed but varies—sometimes dramatically—across (1) countries, (2) contexts, and (3) historical time (Best & Thomas, 2004; Wood & Eagly, 2002). For example, the difference between male and female world-class running performances steadily diminished across the twentieth century (Whipp & Ward, 1992). Thus it is important to exercise caution in drawing conclusions about gender differences from single contexts or time points.

Finally, it is worth noting that, because most behaviors are determined by multiple factors, a statistically reliable predictor may actually account for a very small percentage of the variation. Meaningful effects can be small, moderate, or large when they, respectively, account for at least 1%, 6%, or 14% (or more) of the variation. Thus, even when a factor such as gender has been show to account for 15% of the variation (a large effect), 85% of the variation across individuals is explained by other factors.

Theoretical Frameworks

Theoretical frameworks are vital to interpreting data about gender differences. That is, researchers' explanations of *why* males and females differ depend on their theoretical orientation. Furthermore, such frameworks guide researchers' designs of new empirical studies. We next review several major theories of gender role development. They include models that variously emphasize societal factors (social role theory), cognitive factors (cognitive-developmental theory, gender schema theory), and a combination of cognitive and interpersonal factors (social cognitive theory, developmental intergroup theory). The theories are not mutually exclusive and overlap somewhat. To limit the scope of the chapter, we focus on social and cognitive explanations, although it is important to acknowledge that biological factors are also related to gender development (see Blakemore, Berenbaum, & Liben, 2009; Hines, 2004).

Social Role Theory

Social role theory—as advanced by Eagly and her colleagues (Eagly, 1987; Wood & Eagly, 2002)—focuses on the influence of institutionalized roles in imposing opportunities or constraints on people's behavior. When family and occupational roles are allocated on the basis of gender, women and men (as well as girls and boys) are expected to engage in different behaviors (i.e., roles). These expectations shape the kinds of opportunities that are available to individuals during development. For example, the role of caregiver is nearly universally imposed more strongly on women than men. Consistent with cultural expectations, women take care of children and elderly parents more often then men and work in caretaking jobs (e.g., day care, nursing) more often than men. Also, in childhood, girls experience frequent opportunities and obligations to practice nurturance through doll play and babysitting.

When gender is used to organize social roles in society, people tend to expect women's and men's traits and actions to correspond to their typical roles (Eagly, 1987). Men's traditional roles as economic providers emphasize self-assertive and task-oriented behaviors, whereas women's traditional roles as caregivers stress affiliative and expressive behaviors. Thus, in both childhood and adulthood, there tend to be average gender differences in people's self-perceived assertive and affiliative traits (Bassen & Lamb, 2006; Boldizar, 1991). In addition, children and adults tend to hold gender stereotypes attributing affiliative traits to females and assertive traits to males (Best & Thomas, 2004; Liben & Bigler, 2002; Serbin, Powlishta, & Gulko, 1993). These divisions are also reflected in small average gender differences in assertive and affiliative behavior among children (Leaper & Smith, 2004) and adults (Leaper, Anderson, & Sanders, 1998; Leaper & Ayres, 2007).

Cognitive-Developmental Theory

Cognitive-developmental theorists focus on the changes that occur in children's thinking about gender across development (see Martin, Ruble, & Szkrybalo, 2002). According to Kohlberg (1966), the processes begin with categorizing other people's gender (gender labeling) around 2 years of age and labeling one's own gender (gender identity) around 3 years. These abilities are followed by the understanding that gender (1) remains stable over time (gender stability) and (2) is consistent across situations despite changes in appearance (gender consistency), an understanding that usually emerges by around 6 years of age. According to cognitive-developmental theories, children's changing understandings of gender affects their gender-related behavior. So, for example, a young boy who believes that he can grow up to be a mommy (i.e., who lacks gender stability) may happily practice breast-feeding a baby doll. In contrast, a child who fully understands the permanence of gender may be much more motivated to adhere to gender-typed norms (see Martin et al., 2002). Additional cognitive skills have been hypothesized to affect gender role development, including the acquisition of multiple classification skill (Bigler & Liben, 1992), social perspective-taking abilities (Brown & Bigler, 2005), and understanding gender roles as social conventions (Carter & Patterson, 1982; Katz & Ksansnak, 1994).

Gender Schema Theory

Gender schema theory reflects an information-processing approach to the study of gender development (Bem, 1981; Liben & Signorella, 1980; Martin & Halverson, 1981). According to this theory, children formulate personal theories of what it means to be a girl or a boy known as *gender schemas*. They use these gender concepts to guide information processing and to regulate behavior. Thus, children categorize objects and events as either for females or for males. They subsequently approach and value what is considered for their own gender, and they ignore and devalue what is associated with the other gender. Also, children's gender schemas affect information encoding and retrieval in two ways. First, children are more likely to remember information about their own than about the other gender (Signorella, Bigler, & Liben, 1993). Second, children are more likely to recall gender-stereotypic than gender-counterstereotypic information (e.g., Martin & Halverson, 1981). Indeed, children have sometimes been found to change counter-stereotypic information so that it becomes *stereotypic* in memory. For example, after being shown a picture of a male *cooking* at a stove, a boy later recalled that he had seen a man *fixing* a stove (Liben & Signorella, 1980).

Gender schemas are multidimensional in three ways (Signorella, 1999). First, children establish schemas for the self (i.e., identity and personal preferences) and schemas for others (i.e., stereotyped knowledge and attitudes). Self-schemas and attitudes about others are not strongly related. To illustrate, a girl may endorse the view that "both men and women can be firefighters" (a belief concerning others) and simultaneously state that she personally is uninterested in becoming a firefighter (a belief concerning the self). Second, gender schemas are applied to different domains, including traits, activities, and roles. Among domains, children and adults appear to have less gender-typed views of traits than of activities and roles. Finally, gender schemas contain both cognitive and affective components. The *cognitive component* refers to knowledge and beliefs that children form of themselves and others (e.g., gender identity, gender stereotypes), whereas the *affective component* refers to evaluative judgments (i.e., positive or negative) about gender (e.g., gender-typed values and preferences).

Social Cognitive Theory

Bandura's (1986) social cognitive theory has proven useful in psychology for understanding people's behavior in a wide range of domains. Bussey and Bandura (1999) used social cognitive theory to explain the process of gender role development. They proposed that gender learning occurs in three ways. First, children learn about gender through *observation* of male and female models (e.g., parents, teachers, peers, TV characters). Second, children learn from *enactive experience*; that is, they learn about gender norms and expectations from the reactions of others to their own or to other people's behavior (e.g., encouragement or disapproval for playing with particular toys).

Finally, children learn about gender via *direct teaching* (e.g., a parent tells a child that a particular behavior is only for girls or boys, as in "Boys don't cry!").

Social cognitive theory is perhaps most notable for outlining how these three forms of learning are internalized so that children's gender development is *self-guided*. That is, the child becomes self-motivated to conform to the gender norms of her or his society. First, Bussey and Bandura (1999) argued that social sanctions imposed by adults and peers are internalized as personal standards and become self-sanctions. So, for example, a boy who has been teased by his peers for wearing a pink shirt will become self-motivated to avoid all pink items and may even join his peers in teasing others for their nonconformity to gender norms. Second, Bussey and Bandura (1999) argued that self-evaluations have an important motivational influence on behavior. When individuals experience positive self-evaluations for their behavior, they gain a sense of personal agency, known as *self-efficacy*. Self-efficacy is strongly tied to the motivation to repeat a behavior. Thus, for example, when a boy receives positive feedback for playing football, he will come to value and feel competent at football. As a consequence, he will be self-motivated to play football in the future. Conversely, when children receive negative sanctions for cross-gender-typed activities, it becomes less likely that they will practice and develop self-efficacy in these areas.

Developmental Intergroup Theory

Bigler and Liben (2007) advanced a theory grounded in both cognitive-developmental theory (reviewed previously) and intergroup theory. According to intergroup theory, people derive esteem from their group memberships, and thus they are motivated to maintain and to enhance their social identities. Related processes include ingroup favoritism (favoring characteristics associated with the ingroup) and assimilation to ingroup norms (see Harris, 1995; Leaper, 2000b; Tajfel & Turner, 1979). Thus, once people belong to a group, they tend to view it more positively than other groups. This can lead to stereotyping and negatively evaluating members of other groups.

Developmental intergroup theory addresses how children's cognitive abilities interact with environmental conditions to produce gender stereotyping and prejudice. For example, young children's tendency to focus on perceptually salient characteristics (e.g., Piaget, 1970) is conducive to stereotyping. Also, children's (and adults') tendency to essentialize groups—that is, to see group members as sharing important, innate, unobservable traits and tendencies (e.g., Gelman, 2003)— facilitates gender stereotyping and prejudice.

In addition, developmental intergroup theory takes into account the conditions that make some human characteristics (e.g., gender) but not others (e.g., handedness) the basis of stereotyping and prejudice. First, children are especially likely to stereotype on the basis of groups that are *perceptually discriminable* (i.e., groups that can be visually detected). Gender is a highly salient perceptual category, in part because of social conventions concerning gender differences in hairstyle, clothing, and makeup. Second, children are especially likely to stereotype groups that are *labeled explicitly*. Gender is regularly marked in people's speech through the use of gendered pronouns ("he" or "she") and generics (e.g., "Girls like dolls"; e.g., Gelman, Taylor, & Nguyen, 2004; Hyde, 1984; Leaper & Bigler, 2004). Finally, children are especially likely to stereotype groups that are physically separate or segregated. As discussed later, girls and boys typically play apart from one another.

GENDER DEVELOPMENT IN INFANCY AND EARLY CHILDHOOD

Developmental Patterns

Children's Gender-Related Thinking

Children develop their first understandings of gender between birth and age 2 years (see Martin et al., 2002, for a review). Children are capable of distinguishing men's from women's faces as they approach 1 year of age, although only when such faces contain gender-related cues (females with makeup and long hair). Verbal signs of a gender concept appear around 1½ to 2 years of age when children begin to use gender to label other people (i.e., gender labeling). By age 3, children typically demonstrate knowledge of their own gender (i.e., gender identity). Once children see themselves as belonging to their gender group, gender becomes a social identity. Between 3 and 6 years of age, children develop an understanding of gender constancy (reviewed earlier). During this age period, children also begin to form stereotypes about physical features (e.g., girls wear dresses), activities (e.g., boys play with trucks), traits (e.g., boys get into fights), and occupational roles (e.g., women are nurses). Beginning as early as 18 months of age, children's gender schemas shape their interest and memory for gender-related events (see Martin et al., 2002).

Gender-Typed Behavior

During their first year, girls and boys are generally very similar in behavior. Average gender differences in behavior become more apparent in the second year of life (see Blakemore et al., 2009; Leaper & Friedman, 2007, for reviews). Girls tend to acquire language at a faster rate than do boys (Gleason & Ely, 2002). In addition, boys are generally more physically active than are girls, whereas girls generally demonstrate more self-control and less impulsivity than do boys (Else-Quest, Hyde, Goldsmith, & Van Halle, 2006).

Gender-typed play preferences emerge by around 2 years (see Blakemore et al., 2009; Leaper & Friedman, 2007, for reviews). On average, boys favor construction toys and active forms of play, whereas girls tend to prefer dolls. As children begin to engage in pretend play, average gender differences are also seen in the "scripts" of such play. Girls are more apt to emphasize domestic themes (e.g., playing house), whereas boys are apt to emphasize action-adventure and aggressive themes (e.g., playing super-heroes). Also, rough-and-tumble play is more common among boys than girls during early childhood. Although there are average gender differences in play behavior, not all girls and boys are alike. Furthermore, girls are more likely than boys to demonstrate flexibility in their play choices and to engage in both feminine- and masculine-stereotyped activities.

Researchers have found that average gender differences in styles of social interaction begin to emerge between 2 and 5 years of age. In general, boys are more likely than girls to use power-assertive behaviors such as directives and physical aggression. In contrast, girls are more likely than boys to use affiliative and collaborative behaviors, such as building positively on other speakers' actions or statements. Girls are also more likely than boys to use strategies to deescalate conflicts when they occur (see Leaper & Smith, 2004; Maccoby, 1998; Rose & Rudolph, 2006, for reviews).

One of the most important aspects of gender development during early childhood is an increasing preference for same-gender peers (see Leaper, 1994; Maccoby, 1998). By around 3 years of age, children commonly favor same-gender peers for play. This tendency for gender segregation increases in strength during the course of the preschool years and remains stable until adolescence.

Cognitive and Motivational Influences

A combination of cognitive and motivational factors contributes to young children's gender development. As addressed later, gender schemas and socialization pressures are strongly implicated in the development of many forms of gender-typed behavior. However, average gender differences in maturation and temperament may be partly responsible for some behavioral differences. Most notably, behavioral compatibility rather than ingroup identity may guide children's initial preferences for same-gender peers. Thus boys who like active and rough play may be drawn to play with one another, whereas many girls may find this kind of play aversive and thereby avoid playing with boys (Moller & Serbin, 1996; Pellegrini, Long, Roseth, Bohn, & Van Ryzin, 2007). In support of the behavioral compatibility explanation, physically active girls often approach boys for play during early childhood (Pellegrini et al., 2007). However, most girls who like physical activity eventually affiliate with other girls rather than with boys (Pellegrini et al., 2007). Thus children's social identities as girls or boys ultimately take precedence over behavioral compatibility in guiding peer contacts. Consistent with this premise, Martin, Fabes, Evans, and Wyman (1999) observed that between 3 and 6 years of age, children increasingly anticipated more peer approval for selecting same-gender play partners.

Much of gender development is a process of self-socialization guided by children's gender schemas and personal standards. As children's gender stereotyping increases during the preschool years, their preferences for gender-typed play and same-gender peers also increase (e.g., Martin & Little, 1990). The link between gender stereotyping and gender-typed preferences is probably the result of causal processes that run in *both* directions. That is, children's gender stereotypes lead them to make certain play choices, such as selecting an unfamiliar toy because it was labeled as for their gender (Martin, Eisenbud, & Rose, 1995); however, children's play experiences can simultaneously lead them to develop gender stereotypes such as observing that girls, but not boys, are playing with dolls.

Environmental Influences

Parents

ROLE MODELING

Although women and men participate in the U.S. workforce at approximately equal rates, mothers and fathers often conform to gender-stereotypic roles in the home (see Leaper, 2002, for a review). For example, women are more likely than men to be responsible for child care and housework. Increased gender equality in family roles, however, is associated with a reduced likelihood of children's gender stereotyping (see Best & Thomas, 2004, for a review). Interestingly, parental sharing of household duties is associated with reduced gender stereotyping even among children of lesbian parents (Fulcher, Suftin, & Patterson, 2008).

Parents may also model gender-typed styles of communication. According to a meta-analysis (Leaper et al., 1998), there are small average differences between mothers and fathers. Mothers were more talkative than were fathers when interacting with their infant or toddler children (but not with older children). Also, mothers were more likely than fathers to use affiliative speech (e.g., supportive comments), and fathers were more likely than mothers to use assertive speech (e.g., directives). These average gender differences in parents' language style parallel those seen in children (see Leaper & Smith, 2004); however, it is unclear whether parental modeling contributes to gender differences in children's communication.

DIFFERENTIAL TREATMENT

Parents regularly perceive and treat daughters and sons differently, a process that starts with newborns and continues through adulthood. One of the most consistent ways in which parents tend to treat girls and boys differently is through the encouragement of gender-typed play. In a meta-analysis considering various parenting behaviors, Lytton and Romney (1991) identified the encouragement of gender-typed play activities as the most reliable means by which parents treat sons and daughters differently. Of course, parents vary in how strongly they encourage gender-typed (and discourage cross-gender-typed) play. Parents' genders and attitudes are two known moderators. First, fathers are more likely than mothers to promote gender-typed activities in their children (Lytton & Romney, 1991). Perhaps for this reason, boys are often attentive to their fathers' reactions to gender-typed and cross-gender-typed play (Raag & Rackliff, 1998). Second, parents with traditional gender attitudes are more likely than egalitarian parents to reinforce their children's gender-typed play (Fagot, Leinbach, & O'Boyle, 1992). (Of course, these factors are themselves related; fathers are more likely than mothers to hold traditional gender attitudes.) Nonetheless, many parents who hold gender-egalitarian beliefs unwittingly act in gender-stereotyped ways with their children (e.g., Friedman, Leaper, & Bigler, 2007; Weitzman, Birns, & Friend, 1985).

Parents may explicitly or implicitly endorse gender stereotypes when talking with their children. Explicit endorsement of stereotypes might occur in the form of prescriptive statements such as "boys don't cry" or "dolls are for girls, not boys." In contrast, implicit endorsement of stereotypes occurs when parents highlight gender in relation to some behavior ("those *girls* are feeding the ducks" instead of "those *children* are feeding the ducks") or through the use of essentialist statements whereby a broad generalization is made about males or females ("boys play football"). Gelman et al. (2004) found that these forms of gender labeling were common among a sample of middle-class American mothers who held gender-egalitarian beliefs. Similarly, in a study of mothers reading to their preschool children, Friedman, Leaper, and Bigler (2007) found that implicit stereotyping was four times more likely than explicit stereotyping. Whether a mother had a son or a daughter was, however, predictive of their behavior. Mothers of daughters highlighted *counterstereotypical* content about female story characters more often than did mothers of sons. Mothers of sons highlighted *stereotypical* content about male story characters more often than did mothers of daughters.

A CAVEAT REGARDING PARENTS' DIFFERENTIAL TREATMENT

Although it is apparent that many parents treat boys and girls differently, the *reason* for their behavior is not clear. It is possible that parents' gender-stereotypic beliefs and expectations lead them to act differently with daughters and sons (*parent-driven effect*). It is also possible, however, that girls and boys may act differently themselves and thereby *elicit* different reactions from parents (*child-driven effect*). So, for example, parents may buy dolls for daughters (but not sons) based on their personal belief that girls (but not boys) should practice nurturance. Or parents may buy dolls for daughters (but not sons) because girls (but not boys) *request* that their parents purchase such items. Most researchers now believe that both parent- and child-driven effects operate during development. That is, parents' gendered expectations guide their behavior toward sons and daughters and, simultaneously, children's own gender-related dispositions affect their behavior toward their parents.

Peers

As young children spend more time with peers, they have the opportunity to observe other boys' and girls' behavior. That is, peers become role models for gender-typed behavior. Peers also become enforcers of conformity through their use of approval and disapproval (e.g., Fagot, 1977). The potential impact of peers on young children's gender typing was demonstrated in Martin and Fabes's (2001) longitudinal study that followed preschool children from fall to spring. They found that the amount of time that children spent with same-gender peers was positively related to later increases in gender-typed behavior. In other words, those children who played with same-gender peers most often became more gender-typed over time.

Because girls' and boys' peer groups differ in structure (e.g., group size) and content (e.g., play activities), gendered social norms and personal standards tend to emerge. Some writers have even described males and females as living in different "gender cultures" (Maccoby, 1998; Maltz & Borker, 1982; Thorne & Luria, 1986). Indeed, children's gender-typed play activities can create different opportunities for practicing particular behaviors (Goodwin, 2001; Huston, 1985; Leaper, 2000a). During masculine-stereotyped play activities, children are apt to practice self-assertive behaviors (e.g., competition). In contrast, during feminine-stereotyped play activities, they are apt to practice a combination of affiliative and self-assertive behaviors (e.g., nurturance and mutual collaboration). These different play activities both reflect and foster different social norms regarding the expression of self-assertion and affiliation.

There is an important difference between girls' and boys' ingroup socialization. Males typically are afforded greater status and power in society than are females. Group status has some important consequences for behavior (Harris, 1995; Leaper, 1994). First, members of high-status groups are usually more invested in maintaining group boundaries than are members of low-status groups (e.g., Bigler, Brown, & Markell, 2001). Consistent with the greater status and power traditionally accorded to males in society, boys are more likely than girls to endorse gender stereotypes (e.g., Rowley, Kurtz-Costes, Mistry, & Feagans, 2007) and to initiate and maintain role and group boundaries (e.g., Sroufe, Bennett, Englund, Urban, & Shulman, 1993). Thus gender-typing pressures tend to be more rigid for boys than for girls. Second, the characteristics associated with high-status groups are typically valued more than those of low-status groups. Hence, masculine-stereotyped attributes (e.g., bravery, toughness) tend to be valued more than feminine-stereotyped attributes (e.g., kindness, emotionality), especially in highly male-dominated cultures (Hofstede, 2000). Although cross-gender-typed behavior can sometimes enhance a girl's status (e.g., "tomboys" are often well liked), it typically diminishes a boy's status ("sissies" are seldom well liked). Accordingly, cross-gender-typed behavior tends to be more common among girls than boys.

Media

Gender-stereotyped messages are commonly transmitted in television programs, commercials, video games, child-oriented web pages, and other electronic media (e.g., Cherney & London, 2006; Leaper, Breed, Hoffman, & Perlman, 2002; Thompson & Zerbinos, 1995). For example, TV commercials for children's toys regularly underscore the message that action-adventure and construction toys are for boys, whereas doll play and fashion accessories are for girls (Signorielli, 2001). Several studies have documented that TV commercials and programs contribute to children's developing beliefs about gender-normative roles and behavior. According to Oppliger's (2007) meta-analysis, significant average effect sizes that were small but meaningful were seen in both experimental and nonexperimental studies.

Another potentially influential source for learning stereotypes is the literature that parents read to their young children. One form of bias is the underrepresentation of female characters. Although the ratio has become more equitable over the years, males are still more common in titles and pictures (Gooden & Gooden, 2001). In addition, storybooks tend to portray characters (verbally and pictorially) in terms of gender-stereotyped personality traits and activities (Diekman & Murnen, 2004), including many books touted as "nonsexist." It is important to note, though, that media potentially can be used to counteract stereotypes (e.g., see Mares & Woodard, 2005). Studies have, for example, examined the effectiveness of egalitarian books and videos to reduce children's gender stereotyping (see Liben & Bigler, 1987). The effects of such interventions appear to quite small because (1) such egalitarian messages are swamped in number by the available gender-stereotyped messages and (2) children tend to forget and distort counterstereotypic information at high rates.

GENDER DEVELOPMENT IN MIDDLE CHILDHOOD

Developmental Patterns

Gender-Related Thinking

Middle childhood spans approximately 6–12 years of age. By 6 years, children understand that gender is a consistent and stable entity (i.e., gender constancy). They also begin to recognize that gender roles are based on social conventions. This allows for somewhat increased flexibility in gender typing (e.g., Carter & Patterson, 1982). However, most children continue to adhere to gender-typed norms because they have internalized gender-typed values or they want to maintain peer approval.

As part of the gender-typing process, girls and boys tend to develop different self-concepts regarding assertion and affiliation (Boldizar, 1991; Rose & Rudolph, 2006). On average, boys are more likely to stress assertive over affiliative goals in their relationships. Also, boys are more likely to have positive self-concepts of their assertive traits (e.g., being independent or competitive) than their affiliative traits (e.g., being understanding or supportive). In contrast, girls are more likely than boys to value affiliative goals (or a combination of affiliative and assertive goals) and to have positive self-concepts regarding affiliative traits (or both affiliative and assertive traits). Impor-

tantly, these gender-typed interpersonal goals reflect and perpetuate gender inequalities in power and status because assertive goals and behaviors (e.g., independence,
competition) are more empowering than affiliative goals and behaviors (e.g., nurturance, expressivity). Furthermore, enacting these differences in activities and roles mir-
rors the gendered division of labor in adulthood (Wood & Eagly, 2002).

Gender-Typed Behavior

During middle childhood, children affiliate in primarily same-gender peer networks.
Children who violate this convention risk peer rejection (Sroufe et al., 1993). Within
their gender-segregated peer groups, children are most likely to participate in gender-
typed play activities. However, there is usually more flexibility in activity choices
among girls than boys. For example, it is now common for girls in the United States
and other Western societies to participate in organized sports, but it is still rare for
boys to engage in doll play (Cherney & London, 2006). Although children generally
affiliate with same-gender peers, cross-gender contact is tolerated in some contexts.
Cooperative cross-gender interactions often occur in children's homes and neighborhoods, where companion choices may be limited, and in public settings when children
can attribute the contact to an external cause, such as a teacher assigning students to
groups (Strough & Covatto, 2002; Thorne & Luria, 1986).

Average gender differences in other behaviors are seen in middle childhood. Boys
continue to be higher than girls in activity level, and the magnitude of this difference
widens with age (Eaton & Enns, 1986). Self-assertive and antisocial forms of behavior
are more likely among boys than girls. For example, higher average rates of directive
communication are seen among boys than girls (Leaper & Smith, 2004). Also, boys
are more likely than girls to be physically and verbally aggressive (Archer, 2004). In
contrast, girls tend to demonstrate greater self-control than do boys (Else-Quest et al.,
2006). Also, prosocial behaviors, including empathy (Eisenberg & Fabes, 1998), self-
disclosure (Rose & Rudolph, 2006), and affiliative communication (Leaper & Smith,
2004), are more common among girls than boys. These average differences in behavior
are all small in size and most common in the context of peer group interactions when
conformity pressures often are felt.

Cognitive-Motivational Influences

Average gender differences in interpersonal goals and values may underlie some gender
differences in social behavior. In a review of the literature, Rose and Rudolph (2006)
reported that boys were more likely than girls to value self-assertive over affiliative
goals. Therefore, boys may be more apt to appraise conflicts as competitions requiring the use of power-assertive strategies to enhance their status (Miller, Danaher, &
Forbes, 1986). Concern with establishing dominance and appearing tough may interfere with many boys' willingness to open up to friends (Leaper & Anderson, 1997;
Levant, 2005). This trend may also contribute to higher rates of physical and verbal
aggression among boys (Rose & Asher, 1999). Furthermore, as described earlier, self-
assertive and aggressive themes are common in boys' gender-typed play (e.g., "playing
war," competitive sports).

In their review, Rose and Rudolph (2006) noted that girls, in contrast to boys,
were more likely in studies to favor affiliative goals (or the coordination of affiliative
and assertive goals). For instance, Strough and Berg (2000) found that girls used more

affiliative speech than did boys because they valued affiliative goals to a greater extent than did boys; however, those boys who endorsed affiliative goals were also likely to use affiliative speech. Girls' emphasis on affiliative goals is also seen in their gender-typed play (e.g., "playing house," nurturing baby dolls).

Environmental Influences

Parents

ROLE MODELING

One might expect parents to exert a strong influence on their children's gender stereotypes and beliefs. Evidence suggests, however, that parents have only a small influence on their school-age children's gender schemas. In their meta-analysis, Tenenbaum and Leaper (2002) found no association between parents' and preschool-age children's gender schemas and a significant but weak average correlation between parents' and school-age children's gender-related beliefs. One reason that the correlation between parents' and children's gender schemas is so small may be that parents' beliefs and actions are often inconsistent (Leaper & Bigler, 2004). That is, parents may espouse egalitarian beliefs but act in gender-typed ways. Parents may need to "talk the talk" *and* "walk the walk" to produce egalitarian children. Consistent with this notion, a study reported that 10-year-old children were more likely to endorse egalitarian attitudes about family roles when their fathers were highly involved in child care (Deutsch, Servis, & Payne, 2001).

DIFFERENTIAL TREATMENT

Parents' (especially fathers') encouragement of gender-typed activities continues into middle childhood (Lytton & Romney, 1991). At the same time, children are experiencing gender-conformity pressures from peers and other social agents; therefore, they often prefer gender-typed activities. The path of least resistance for many parents is to support their children's ongoing gender-typed interests rather than to encourage a complementary set of nontraditional activities.

Different patterns of communication may also occur in parent–daughter and parent–son interactions during childhood. In their meta-analysis, Leaper et al. (1998) found that mothers tended to use more affiliative speech (supportive comments) and more self-assertive speech (directive comments) with daughters than with sons. Through a higher use of affiliative speech with daughters, mothers may reinforce greater closeness; conversely, through a lower rate of directive speech with sons, mothers may foster more autonomy. These speech patterns may also be related to gender differences in activity preferences. Many feminine-stereotyped toys (e.g., dolls, food sets) elicit affiliative speech, whereas many masculine-stereotyped toys (e.g., construction toys, action figures) elicit assertive speech (e.g., Caldera, Huston, & O'Brien, 1989; Leaper, 2000a). Thus, to the extent that girls and boys play with different activities, they are apt to practice different styles of talk.

Whereas parents tend to be more accepting of cross-gender-typed play in daughters than sons, they may be less tolerant of physical aggression in daughters than in sons. Although studies indicate that parents disapprove of physical aggression similarly in daughters and in sons during the preschool years, parents may be more lenient about aggression with sons than with daughters in middle childhood (Martin & Ross,

2005). Indeed, boys are less likely than girls to anticipate parental disapproval for physical aggression (Perry, Perry, & Weiss, 1989).

Media

Gender-typed images in the media continue to inform and strengthen boys' and girls' gender-typed beliefs and preferences during middle childhood. As seen during early childhood, television programs and advertisements shape children's toy requests (e.g., Robinson, Saphir, Kraemer, Varady, & Haydel, 2001). In addition, boys are more likely than girls to spend time watching violent TV programming and playing violent video games (Cherney & London, 2006). Importantly, experimental studies clearly indicate a causal link between exposure and subsequent behavior; that is, exposure to violent media (television and video games) can increase the likelihood of aggressive behavior in some children (see Ferguson, 2007; Paik & Comstock, 1994).

Language

Gender labeling is built into most languages. In English and many other languages, singular animate pronouns force a distinction between male ("he") and female ("she"), and gender-marked terms continue to be used to label occupations (e.g., mailman, actress, cowboy; see Henley, 1989; Hyde, 1984; Liben, Bigler, & Krogh, 2002). Research suggests that merely labeling gender may cause increases in the psychological salience of gender and the likelihood that children will infer that men and women differ in their personal attributes (Gelman, 2003). Indeed, Bigler (1995) reported that when teachers used gender terms to address their classes (e.g., "Good morning, boys and girls"), early elementary school students developed more gender-stereotypic attitudes.

An implicit form of gender bias occurs when the masculine linguistic form (e.g., "he" or "chairman") is used to apply to both genders. (By way of contrast, imagine if we used "chairwoman" to refer to both men and women.) Psychologically masculine linguistic forms do not function in a truly neutral manner. Researchers find that children and adults tend to imagine male characters when they hear or read sentences using masculine nouns or pronouns as generics (Henley, 1989; Hyde, 1984). Moreover, this linguistic practice implicitly conveys that males have higher status in society than do females. As a consequence, many organizations have developed policies against the use of the generic "he" and gender-specific occupational titles (e.g., the American Psychological Association's *Publication Manual*).

Peers

During middle childhood, children continue to look to their same-gender peers to infer what is considered appropriate for their gender (Bussey & Bandura, 1999). Besides wanting to fulfill the job descriptions of their social identities as girls and boys, children also want to gain approval and avoid disapproval from peers. Peers generally disapprove of cross-gender-typed behavior (Martin, 1989). Over time, children typically internalize the norms of their same-gender peer groups as personal beliefs, standards, and values that regulate their behavior (Bussey & Bandura, 1999).

The power of peer norms on children's behavior is further illustrated in studies finding that some gender differences in social behavior are more likely in same-gender than mixed-gender interaction. For example, Leaper and Smith's (2004) meta-analysis found an average difference favoring boys in the use of assertive speech—but the average difference only occurred among studies examining same-gender interactions; there was no average difference in mixed-gender interactions. Thus boys' self-presentation concerns with appearing assertive may be more salient when interacting with other boys than with girls. Communication style also depends on activity type. Leaper and Smith (2004) reported that the average gender difference in affiliative speech was greater in unstructured than in structured settings. In unstructured settings, girls and boys tend to select different play activities that call for different communication styles (see Goodwin, 2001; Huston, 1985; Leaper, 2000a). Conversely, when girls and boys are encouraged to participate in similar activities, they get the opportunity to practice similar behaviors.

One of the possible long-term consequences of gender-typed play is that girls experience more opportunities to develop intimacy-related skills, such as self-disclosure and listener support (see Leaper & Anderson, 1997). For example, when girls play house together, two or three girls construct a collaborative storyline (e.g., playing house). This kind of play helps to prepare girls for establishing intimate relationships based on affection and responsiveness. In contrast, boys' gender-typed play activities (e.g., construction toys and sport games) teach them how to relate to one another through shared tasks or competition. Intimacy for many boys is further undermined by the values associated with traditional masculinity, such as status orientation, emotional restraint, and homophobia (Levant, 2005). These values are often perpetuated in boys' macho sport culture (Messner, 1998; Zarbatany, McDougall, & Hymel, 2000). Conversely, when boys experience activities that promote affiliation and expressivity, intimate friendships are more likely (Zarbatany et al., 2000; see also Bukowski, Buhrmester, & Underwood, Chapter 7, this volume).

GENDER DEVELOPMENT IN ADOLESCENCE

Developmental Patterns

Gender-Related Thinking

Cognitive, social, and physical changes during adolescence can affect individuals' views and motives regarding gender. First, according to some theoretical models, adolescence is a period in which gender-role transcendence (also known as *androgyny*) is possible. This occurs when individuals incorporate both traditionally masculine and traditionally feminine attributes and goals into their self-concepts (e.g., Robinson & Green, 1981). Bem (1993) also referred to these individuals as gender aschematic because traditional notions of gender do not guide their self-concepts. Greater flexibility in gender-role self-concepts is more likely among girls than boys (e.g., Huston, 1985; Katz & Ksansnak, 1994). According to some researchers, gender-role flexibility allows children to develop a wider range of competencies. For example, one study found that adolescents with more flexible self-concepts scored significantly higher than other adolescents in perceived academic competence, perceived friendship intimacy, and self-worth (Rose & Montemayor, 1994).

There are other domains of self-concept in which girls tend to show more vulnerability than do boys. Recent meta-analyses document average gender differences in self-esteem, depression, and body image during adolescence. Kling, Hyde, Showers, and Buswell's (1999) meta-analysis indicated a small average gender difference in self-esteem favoring boys during adolescence; however, the difference was negligible during childhood and adulthood. In addition, Twenge and Nolen-Hoeksema (2002) indicated that a small average difference in depression—with girls higher than boys—emerges between late childhood and adolescence. Finally, Feingold and Mazzella (1998) indicated a moderate average difference in body image favoring boys among studies of adolescents; their analyses additionally revealed that the magnitude of gender difference has been significantly increasing over the last few decades.

Adolescence is also a period of change in gender attitudes. Cross-gender friendship and heterosexual dating increase during adolescence. As a consequence, Glick and Hilt (2000) proposed that benevolent sexist attitudes (i.e., the view that women need men's protection) often emerge. Although hostile sexist attitudes may continue (e.g., disparaging girls' abilities in sports or science), they may combine with benevolent sexist views that are reinforced through traditional adolescent dating scripts. For example, adolescents typically expect males to initiate and pay for dates. Partly because many girls internalize sexist ideology themselves, they may not recognize when they are victims of such sexism (see Leaper & Brown, 2008).

Gender-Typed Behavior

Although cross-gender contacts increase, peer affiliations remain primarily with members of the same gender during adolescence (Poulin & Pedersen, 2007). Within their same-gender friendships, signs of intimacy are more likely among girls than boys. For example, self-disclosure tends to be more common among girls than boys (Rose & Rudolph, 2006). Boys appear to turn to their female friends or dating partners (rather than their same-gender friends) to disclose personal thoughts and feelings (Kuttler, La Greca, & Prinstein, 1999; Poulin & Pedersen, 2007). Girls are also more likely than boys to view their friends as sources of social support (e.g., Frydenberg & Lewis, 1993). One reason may be that, on average, girls and boys respond to emotional disclosures differently. Studies have found that girls are more likely than boys to use supportive listening statements in adolescence and emerging adulthood (Burleson, 1982; Leaper, Carson, Baker, Holliday, & Myers, 1995). It is important to note, however, that gender differences in same-gender friendships are small and thus (1) many girls and boys have similar patterns of friendship and (2) there are large variations within each gender in friendship qualities—especially among boys (Camarena, Sarigiani, & Petersen, 1990; McDougall & Hymel, 2007; McNelles & Connolly, 1999; Radmacher & Azmitia, 2006).

With the onset of puberty, sexual interest and dating relationships increase. Among heterosexual youth, dating often begins in the context of mixed-gender groups (Connolly, Craig, Goldberg, & Pepler, 2004). Lesbian, gay, and bisexual youths typically have fewer dating relationships with same-gender partners due either to limited opportunities or to the social stigma in the school or the community (Diamond, Savin-Williams, & Dubé, 1999). For many sexual-minority youths, sexual identity and expression may not emerge until early adulthood.

Sexual harassment is a form of aggression that most adolescents experience or instigate (American Association of University Women [AAUW], 2001; Goldstein, Malanchuk, Davis-Kean, & Eccles, 2007; Leaper & Brown, 2008; McMaster, Connolly, Pepler, & Craig, 2002). Verbal sexual harassment includes making demeaning, homophobic, or unwanted comments with sexual themes. These comments might be made directly to the person or indirectly, through negative gossip. In addition, sexual harassment can involve physical aggression through unwanted touching or sexual coercion. Comparable rates of sexual harassment have been indicated for girls and boys in the United States (AAUW, 2001) and Canada (McMaster et al., 2002). However, boys were more likely than girls to experience some forms of sexual harassment (e.g., homophobic comments), whereas girls were more likely than boys to report other kinds of harassment (e.g., unwanted touching). Both girls and boys were more likely to identify cross-gender than same-gender peers as perpetrators of sexual harassment; however, boys were more likely than girls to experience same-gender sexual harassment. Furthermore, sexual-minority youths were especially at risk for sexual harassment (Williams, Connolly, Pepler, & Craig, 2005).

Romantic relationships are another arena in which aggressive behavior can occur. Studies in the United States suggest that this happens in approximately one-fourth of adolescent dating relationships, with the rates varying across different communities (Hickman, Jaycox, & Aronoff, 2004; O'Leary, Slep, Avery-Leaf, & Cascardi, 2008). Although both girls and boys may initiate aggressive behavior in dating relationships, it is more likely in boys than in girls (Wolitzky-Taylor et al., 2008). Many girls come to expect demeaning behaviors as normal in heterosexual relationships (Witkowska & Gådin, 2005), and adolescent girls who experience dating abuse may be at risk for dysfunctional and abusive relationships in adulthood (see Larkin & Popaleni, 1994).

Cognitive–Motivational Influences

An important new cognitive ability that emerges in adolescents is to think about the causes and consequences of gender stereotyping and prejudice. That is, adolescents can metacognitively reflect on their own and others' gender roles. As a consequence, they may be increasingly capable of recognizing gender prejudice and discrimination—including institutionalized forms of sexism. There is relatively little research on youths' perceptions of gender discrimination. Brown and Bigler (2005) proposed that a number of age-related cognitive skills affect the ability to perceive gender discrimination, including having an understanding of the meaning of stereotypes, an ability to make social comparisons, and an ability to make moral judgments about fairness and equity. For example, whereas children often justify gender discrimination based on social conventions (Killen & Stangor, 2001), adolescents may be less likely to rationalize such behavior as they gain greater awareness. In addition, Brown and Bigler (2005) postulated a set of individual and situational moderators that affect the likelihood of recognizing discrimination. For example, girls are more likely to recognize gender discrimination if they hold gender-egalitarian attitudes (Brown & Bigler, 2004; Leaper & Brown, 2008).

Average gender differences in affiliative and assertive goals continue into adolescence (Bassen & Lamb, 2006; Rose & Rudolph, 2006), with girls more likely to value affiliative goals (or a combination of affiliation and assertion) and boys more likely to value power-assertive goals. Gender-typed girls' affiliative goals can help motivate them toward intimacy in relationships. In contrast, traditional boys' power-assertive goals (e.g., concerns with dominance and appearing tough) can interfere with their willingness to open up to friends (Leaper & Anderson, 1997; Levant, 2005; Tolman, Spencer, Harmon, Rosen-Reynosa, & Striepe, 2004). Furthermore, traditional values among boys are usually associated with homophobic attitudes that impair their willingness to express vulnerable feelings or affection with same-gender friends (Levant,

2005). When boys shun intimacy with one another, they miss opportunities to practice the social skills associated with being a supportive listener in close relationships. Thus a difference in preference may develop into a difference in ability (see Leaper et al., 1995; MacGeorge, Gillihan, Samter, & Clark, 2003).

Environmental Influences

Parents

Research suggests that parents can affect gender-related variations in adolescents' developing self-concepts. Parents, for example, appear to influence adolescents' concerns about body image. McCabe and Ricciardelli (2005) found that boys were particularly attentive to fathers' messages about their weight and muscularity, whereas girls were especially sensitive to mothers' messages about their weight.

In addition, parents may contribute to gender-related variations in adolescents' intimacy. Many parents foster relatively more emotional autonomy in sons and more closeness in daughters (e.g., Ryan & Lynch, 1989). These patterns may be especially strong in Latin American and Asian heritage families (Chao & Tseng, 2002; Fuligni, Tseng, & Lam, 1999; Harwood, Leyendecker, Carlson, Asencio, & Miller, 2002). Some studies suggest that daughters show better social-emotional outcomes when their parents encourage autonomy; conversely, sons show better such outcomes when parents encourage intimacy (Grotevant & Cooper, 1985; Kenny, Lomax, Brabeck, & Fife, 1998; Leaper et al., 1989).

Media

In adolescence, boys are more likely than girls to play violent video games and to watch violent movies and television programs. These habits are associated with an increased likelihood of aggressive behavior (Ferguson, 2007; Paik & Comstock, 1994). Media consumption also shapes adolescents' developing self-concepts about their bodies. The pervasive bombardment of advertisements emphasizing sexualized and idealized images of female beauty are inescapable (American Psychological Association Task Force on the Sexualization of Girls, 2007). Frequent exposure to this sort of media is associated with body image disturbances in adolescent girls in several studies (Grabe, Ward, & Hyde, 2008). In addition, a highly muscular ideal of male appearance is regularly depicted in video games and modeled by professional athletes. Exposure to these media is negatively related to adolescent boys' body image across several studies (Barlett, Vowels, & Saucier, 2008).

Peers

Peers continue to have a strong impact on gender development during adolescence. First, peers can exaggerate adolescents' concerns regarding body image (Jones & Crawford, 2006; McCabe & Ricciardelli, 2005). Jones and Crawford (2006) documented such effects among girls and boys. Girls commonly discussed appearance-related topics (e.g., dieting) with one another, and overweight girls often experienced appearance-related teasing. Boys discussed muscle building and were more likely to be teased if they were either overweight or underweight. Teasing about physical appearance often occurs through sexual harassment. Studies find that repeated experience with sexual harassment is associated with lowered self-esteem, increased depression, and negative body image (Goldstein et al., 2007; Gruber & Fineran, 2008; Lindberg, Grabe, & Hyde, 2007). These negative effects may be stronger for girls and sexual minorities (Gruber & Fineran, 2008; Timmerman, 2005).

Gender-typed peer norms are additionally related to average gender differences in friendship intimacy and aggression. Among boys, traditional notions of masculinity emphasize emotional restraint, nonrelational attitudes toward sex, homophobia, and dominance (Levant, 2005). These values are antithetical to disclosing personal feelings or showing affection with same-gender friends. Many boys use homophobic and misogynist insults with one another as social sanctions to enforce these norms (Murnen & Smolak, 2000). The macho sports culture in most high schools tends to reinforce traditional notions of masculinity (including misogyny and homophobia) that limit the potential for intimacy in friendship and romantic relationships (Messner, 1998; Zarbatany et al., 2000). These social norms can create a context that makes physical aggression more acceptable for boys than for girls in peer relations and romantic relationships (Conroy, Silva, Newcomer, Walker, & Johnson, 2001).

Traditional social norms among girls emphasize the sharing of feelings as a means of attaining emotional closeness. Girls are more likely than boys to offer emotional support in response to disclosures (as reviewed earlier). Although self-disclosure is generally associated with psychological adjustment, excessive disclosure can be debilitating. When friends keep dwelling on an upsetting incident, it is known as corumination. Rose, Carlson, and Waller (2007) found that corumination was more common among girls than boys; also, corumination predicted increases in depression and anxiety in girls.

Although girls are less likely than boys to use direct aggression during adolescence, girls are equally as likely as boys to use indirect aggression (Card, Stucky, Sawalani, & Little, 2008). Whereas girls' use of physical aggression would likely be strongly reproached, the use of indirect strategies, such as social exclusion or negative gossip, is generally acceptable (see Underwood, 2003). Negative gossip about a third party can even be a way for girls to gain a sense of solidarity with one another (Leaper & Holliday, 1995; see also Underwood, Chapter 9, this volume).

DIRECTIONS FOR FUTURE RESEARCH

Although much has been learned about the role of gender in shaping social development, much is still left to learn, and new questions arise as gender roles in the United States and elsewhere evolve. One direction for future research and theory is to gain a better appreciation of how cultural and social-structural factors affect children's gender development. For example, as we have noted, men are more powerful than women in all countries. When do children become aware of this fact? And what are the consequences of such knowledge? One recent study reported that the majority of early elementary-school-age children were aware that all of the U.S. presidents have been male (Bigler, Arthur, Hughes, & Patterson, 2008). Approximately one-third of the children in the study argued that men held this high status position because they were more deserving of the role than women. However, another one-third attributed women's exclusion to gender discrimination. Future work is needed to explicate the process by which children detect gender discrepancies and explain them. Such work is especially needed in countries that show large discrepancies in the power and status afforded to males and females. It is our hope that such research will facilitate the development and implementation of social, educational, and legal policies that promote the optimal development of all children.

SUGGESTED READINGS

Bigler, R. S., & Liben, L. S. (2007). Developmental intergroup theory: Explaining and reducing children's social stereotyping and prejudice. *Current Directions in Psychological Science, 16*, 162–166.

Blakemore, J. E. O., Berenbaum, S. A., & Liben, L. S. (2009). *Gender development*. New York: Taylor & Francis.

Bussey, K., & Bandura, A. (1999). Social cognitive theory of gender development and differentiation. *Psychological Review, 106*, 676–713.

Hyde, J. S. (2005). The gender similarities hypothesis. *American Psychologist, 60*, 581–592.

Leaper, C. (2000). The social construction and socialization of gender. In P. H. Miller & E. K. Scholnick (Eds.), *Towards a feminist developmental psychology* (pp. 127–152). New York: Routledge Press.

Martin, C. L., Ruble, D. N., & Szkrybalo, J. (2002). Cognitive theories of early gender development. *Psychological Bulletin, 128*, 903–933.

Wood, W., & Eagly, A. H. (2002). A cross-cultural analysis of the behavior of women and men: Implications for the origins of sex differences. *Psychological Bulletin, 128*, 699–727.

REFERENCES

American Association of University Women. (2001). *Hostile hallways: Bullying, teasing, and sexual harassment in school*. Washington, DC: Author.

American Psychological Association Task Force on the Sexualization of Girls. (2007). *Report of the APA Task Force on the Sexualization of Girls*. Washington, DC: American Psychological Association. Retrieved from *www.apa.org/pi/wpo/sexualization.htm*.

Archer, J. (2004). Sex differences in aggression in real-world settings: A meta-analytic review. *Review of General Psychology, 8*, 291–322.

Bandura, A. (1986). *Social foundations of thought and action: A social cognitive theory*. Englewood Cliffs, NJ: Prentice-Hall.

Barlett, C. P., Vowels, C. L., & Saucier, D. A. (2008). Meta-analyses of the effects of media images on men's body-image concerns. *Journal of Social and Clinical Psychology, 27*, 279–310.

Bassen, C. R., & Lamb, M. E. (2006). Gender differences in adolescents' self-concepts of assertion and affiliation. *European Journal of Developmental Psychology, 3*, 71–94.

Bem, S. L. (1981). Gender schema theory: A cognitive account of sex typing. *Psychological Review, 88*, 354–364.

Bem, S. L. (1993). *The lenses of gender*. New Haven, CT: Yale University Press.

Best, D. L., & Thomas, J. J. (2004). Cultural diversity and cross-cultural perspectives. In A. H. Eagly, A. E. Beall, & R. J. Sternberg (Eds.), *The psychology of gender* (2nd ed., pp. 296–327). New York: Guilford Press.

Bigler, R. S. (1995). The role of classification skill in moderating environmental influences on children's gender stereotyping: A study of the functional use of gender in the classroom. *Child Development, 66*, 1072–1087.

Bigler, R. S., Arthur, A. E., Hughes, J. M., & Patterson, M. M. (2008). The politics of race and gender: Children's perceptions of discrimination and the U.S. presidency. *Analyses of Social Issues and Public Policy, 8*, 83–112.

Bigler, R. S., Brown, C. S., & Markell, M. (2001). When groups are not created equal: Effects of group status on the formation of inter-group attitudes in children. *Child Development, 72*(4), 1151–1162.

Bigler, R. S., & Liben, L. S. (1992). Cognitive mechanisms in children's gender stereotyping: Theoretical and educational implications of a cognitive-based intervention. *Child Development, 63*, 1351–1363.

Bigler, R. S., & Liben, L. S. (2007). Developmental intergroup theory: Explaining and reducing children's social stereotyping and prejudice. *Current Directions in Psychological Science, 16*, 162–166.

Blakemore, J. E. O., Berenbaum, S. A., & Liben, L. S. (2009). *Gender development.* New York: Taylor & Francis.

Boldizar, J. P. (1991). Assessing sex typing and androgyny in children: The Children's Sex Role Inventory. *Developmental Psychology, 27*, 505–515.

Brown, C. S., & Bigler, R. S. (2004). Children's perceptions of gender discrimination. *Developmental Psychology, 40*, 714–726.

Brown, C. S., & Bigler, R. S. (2005). Children's perceptions of discrimination: A developmental model. *Child Development, 76*, 533–553.

Burleson, B. R. (1982). The development of comforting communication skills in childhood and adolescence. *Child Development, 53*, 1578–1588.

Bussey, K., & Bandura, A. (1999). Social cognitive theory of gender development and differentiation. *Psychological Review, 106*, 676–713.

Caldera, Y. M., Huston, A. C., & O'Brien, M. (1989). Social interactions and play patterns of parents and toddlers with feminine, masculine, and neutral toys. *Child Development, 60*, 70–76.

Camarena, P. M., Sarigiani, P. A., & Petersen, A. C. (1990). Gender-specific pathways to intimacy in early adolescence. *Journal of Youth and Adolescence, 19*, 19–32.

Card, N. A., Stucky, B. D., Sawalani, G. M., & Little, T. D. (2008). Direct and indirect aggression during childhood and adolescence: A meta-analytic review of gender differences, intercorrelations, and relations to maladjustment. *Child Development, 79*, 1185–1229.

Carter, D. B., & Patterson, C. J. (1982). Sex roles as social conventions: The development of children's conceptions of sex-role stereotypes. *Developmental Psychology, 18*, 812–824.

Chao, R., & Tseng, V. (2002). Parenting of Asians. In M. H. Bornstein (Ed.), *Handbook of parenting: Vol. 4, Social conditions and applied parenting* (2nd ed., pp. 59–93). Mahwah, NJ: Erlbaum.

Cherney, I. D., & London, K. (2006). Gender-linked differences in the toys, television shows, computer games, and outdoor activities of 5– to 13–year-old children. *Sex Roles, 54*, 717–726.

Cohen, J. (1988). *Statistical power analysis for the behavioral sciences* (2nd ed.). Hillsdale, NJ: Erlbaum.

Connolly, J., Craig, W., Goldberg, A., & Pepler, D. (2004). Mixed-gender groups, dating, and romantic relationships in early adolescence. *Journal of Research on Adolescence, 14*, 185–207.

Conroy, D. E., Silva, J. M., Newcomer, R. R., Walker, B. W., & Johnson, M. S. (2001). Personal and participatory socializers of the perceived legitimacy of aggressive behavior in sport. *Aggressive Behavior, 27*, 405–418.

Deutsch, F. M., Servis, L. J., & Payne, J. D. (2001). Paternal participation in child care and its effects on children's self-esteem and attitudes toward gendered roles. *Journal of Family Issues, 22*, 1000–1024.

Diamond, L. M., Savin-Williams, R. C., & Dubé, E. M. (1999). Sex, dating, passionate friendships, and romance: Intimate peer relations among lesbian, gay, and bisexual adolescents. In W. Furman, B.B. Brown, & C. Feiring (Eds.), *The development of romantic relationships in adolescence* (pp. 175–210). New York: Cambridge University Press.

Diekman, A. B., & Murnen, S. K. (2004). Learning to be little women and little men: The inequitable gender equality of nonsexist children's literature. *Sex Roles, 50*, 373–385.

Dowling, T. (2010, June 23). The Swedish parents who are keeping their baby's gender a secret. *Guardian*, G2, p. 3.

Eagly, A. H. (1987). *Sex differences in social behavior: A social-role interpretation.* Hillsdale, NJ: Erlbaum.

Eaton, W. O., & Enns, L. R. (1986). Sex differences in motor activity level. *Psychological Bulletin, 100*, 19–28.

Eisenberg, N., & Fabes, R. A. (1998). Prosocial development. In W. Damon (Series Ed.) & N. Eisenberg (Vol. Ed.), *Handbook of child psychology: Vol. 3. Social, emotional, and personality development* (5th ed., pp. 701–778). New York: Wiley.

Else-Quest, N., Hyde, J., Goldsmith, H., & Van Hulle, C. (2006). Gender differences in temperament: A meta-analysis. *Psychological Bulletin, 132*, 33–72.

Fagot, B. I. (1977). Consequences of moderate cross-gender behavior in preschool children. *Child Development, 48*, 902–907

Fagot, B. I., Leinbach, M. D., & O'Boyle, C. (1992). Gender labeling, gender stereotyping, and parenting behaviors. *Developmental Psychology, 28*(2), 225–230.

Feingold, A., & Mazzella, R. (1998). Gender differences in body image are increasing. *Psychological Science, 9*, 190–195.

Ferguson, C. J. (2007). Evidence for publication bias in video game violence effects literature: A meta-analytic review. *Aggression and Violent Behavior, 12*, 470–482.

Friedman, C. K., Leaper, C., & Bigler, R. S. (2007). Do mothers' gender-related attitudes or comments predict young children's gender beliefs? *Parenting: Science and Practice, 7*, 357–366.

Frydenberg, E., & Lewis, R. (1993). Boys play sports and girls turn to others: Age, gender and ethnicity as determinants of coping. *Journal of Adolescence, 16*, 253–266.

Fulcher, M., Suftin, E. L., & Patterson, C. J. (2008). Individual differences in gender development: Associations with parental sexual orientation, attitudes, and division of labor. *Sex Roles, 58*, 330–341.

Fuligni, A. J., Tseng, V., & Lam, M. (1999). Attitudes toward family obligations among American adolescents with Asian, Latin American, and European backgrounds. *Child Development, 70*, 1030–1044.

Gelman, S. A. (2003). *The essential child: Origins of essentialism in everyday thought.* New York: Oxford University Press.

Gelman, S. A., Taylor, M. G., & Nguyen, S. P. (2004). Mother–child conversations about gender. *Monographs of the Society for Research in Children Development, 69*(1), vii–127.

Gleason, J. B., & Ely, R. (2002). Gender differences in language development. In A. M. De Lisi & R. De Lisi (Eds.), *Biology, society, and behavior: The development of sex differences in cognition* (pp. 127–154). Westport, CT: Ablex.

Glick, P., & Hilt, L. (2000). Combative children to ambivalent adults: The development of gender prejudice. In T. Eckes & H. N. Trautner (Eds.), *The developmental social psychology of gender* (pp. 243–272). Mahwah, NJ: Erlbaum.

Goldstein, S. E., Malanchuk, O., Davis-Kean, P. E., & Eccles, J. S. (2007). Risk factors of sexual harassment by peers: A longitudinal investigation of African American and European American adolescents. *Journal of Research on Adolescence, 17*, 285–300.

Gooden, A. M., & Gooden, M. A. (2001). Gender representation in notable children's picture books: 1995–1999. *Sex Roles, 45*, 89–101.

Goodwin, M. H. (2001). Organizing participation in cross-sex jump rope: Situating gender differences within longitudinal studies of activities. *Research on Language and Social Interaction, 34*, 75–106.

Gould, L. (1978). *X: A fabulous child's story.* New York: Daughters.

Grabe, S., Ward, L. M., & Hyde, J. S. (2008). The role of the media in body image concerns among women: A meta-analysis of experimental and correlational studies. *Psychological Bulletin, 134*, 460–476.

Grotevant, H. D., & Cooper, C. R. (1985). Patterns of interaction in family relationships and the development of identity exploration in adolescence. *Child Development, 56*, 415–428

Gruber, J. E., & Fineran, S. (2008). Comparing the impact of bullying and sexual harassment victimization on the mental and physical health of adolescents. *Sex Roles, 59*, 1–13.

Harris, J. R. (1995). Where is the child's environment?: A group socialization theory of development. *Psychological Review, 102*, 458–489.

Harwood, R., Leyendecker, B., Carlson, V., Asencio, M., & Miller, A. (2002). Parenting among Latino families in the U.S. In M. Bornstein (Ed.), *Handbook of parenting: Vol. 4: Social conditions and applied parenting* (2nd ed., pp. 21–46). Mahwah, NJ: Erlbaum.

Henley, N. M. (1989). Molehill or mountain?: What we know and don't know about sex bias in language. In M. Crawford & M. Gentry (Eds.), *Gender and thought: Psychological perspectives* (pp. 59–78). New York: Springer-Verlag.

Hickman, L. J., Jaycox, L. H., & Aronoff, J. (2004). Dating violence among adolescents: Prevalence, gender distribution, and prevention program effectiveness. *Trauma, Violence, and Abuse, 5,* 123–142.

Hines, M. (2004). *Brain gender.* New York: Oxford University Press.

Hofstede, G. (2000). Masculine and feminine cultures. *Encyclopedia of Psychology, 5,* 115–118.

Huston, A. C. (1985). The development of sex typing: Themes from recent research. *Developmental Review, 5,* 1–17.

Hyde, J. S. (1984). Children's understanding of sexist language. *Developmental Psychology, 20,* 697–706.

Hyde, J. S. (2005). The gender similarities hypothesis. *American Psychologist, 60,* 581–592.

Jones, D. C., & Crawford, J. K. (2006). The peer appearance culture during childhood: Gender and body mass variation. *Journal of Youth and Adolescence, 35,* 257–269.

Katz, P. A., & Ksansnak, K. R. (1994). Developmental aspects of gender role flexibility and traditionality in middle childhood and adolescence. *Developmental Psychology, 30,* 272–282.

Kenny, M. E., Lomax, R., Brabeck, M., & Fife, J. (1998). Longitudinal pathways linking adolescent reports of maternal and paternal attachments to psychological well-being. *Journal of Early Adolescence, 18,* 221–243.

Killen, M., & Stangor, C. (2001). Children's social reasoning about inclusion and exclusion in gender and race peer group contexts. *Child Development, 72,* 174–186.

Kling, K. C., Hyde, J. S., Showers, C. J., & Buswell, B. N. (1999). Gender differences in self-esteem: A meta-analysis. *Psychological Bulletin, 125,* 470–500.

Kohlberg, L. A. (1966). A cognitive-developmental analysis of children's sex role concepts and attitudes. In E. E. Maccoby (Ed.), *The development of sex differences* (pp. 82–173). Stanford, CA: Stanford University Press.

Kuttler, A. F., La Greca, A. M., & Prinstein, M. J. (1999). Friendship qualities and social-emotional functioning of adolescents with close, cross-sex friendships. *Journal of Research on Adolescence, 9,* 339–366.

Lang, S. (1998). *Men as women, women as men: Changing gender in Native American cultures.* Austin: University of Texas Press.

Larkin, J., & Popaleni, K. (1994). Heterosexual courtship violence and sexual harassment: The private and public control of young women. *Feminism and Psychology, 4,* 213–227.

Leaper, C. (1994). Exploring the consequences of gender segregation on social relationships. In W. Damon (Series Ed.) & C. Leaper (Issue Ed.), Childhood gender segregation. (*New Directions for Child Development*, No. 62, pp. 797–811). San Francisco: Jossey-Bass.

Leaper, C. (2000a). Gender, affiliation, assertion, and the interactive context of parent–child play. *Developmental Psychology, 36,* 381–393.

Leaper, C. (2000b). The social construction and socialization of gender. In P. H. Miller & E. K. Scholnick (Eds.), *Towards a feminist developmental psychology* (pp. 127–152). New York: Routledge Press.

Leaper, C. (2002). Parenting girls and boys. In M. H. Bornstein, *Handbook of parenting: Children and parenting* (2nd ed., Vol. 1, pp. 189–225). Mahwah, NJ: Erlbaum.

Leaper, C., & Anderson, K. J. (1997). Gender development and heterosexual romantic relationships during adolescence. In W. Damon (Series Ed.) & S. Shulman & W. A. Collins (Issue Eds.), *Romantic relationships in adolescence: Developmental perspectives* (*New Directions for Child Development*, No. 78, pp. 85–103). San Francisco: Jossey-Bass.

Leaper, C., Anderson, K. J., & Sanders, P. (1998). Moderators of gender effects on parents' talk to their children: A meta-analysis. *Developmental Psychology, 34,* 3–27.

Leaper, C., & Ayres, M. M. (2007). A meta-analytic review of gender variation in adults' language use: Talkativeness, affiliative speech, and assertive speech. *Personality and Social Psychology Review, 11,* 328–363.

Leaper, C., & Bigler, R. S. (2004). Gendered language and sexist thought. *Monographs of the Society for Research in Child Development, 69*(1), 128–142.

Leaper, C., Breed, L., Hoffman, L., & Perlman, C. A. (2002). Variations in the gender-stereotyped content of children's television cartoons across genres. *Journal of Applied Social Psychology, 32,* 1653–1662.

Leaper, C., & Brown, C. S. (2008). Perceived experiences with sexism among adolescent girls. *Child Development, 79,* 685–704.

Leaper, C., Carson, M., Baker, C., Holliday, H., & Myers, S. B. (1995). Self-disclosure and listener verbal support in same-gender and cross-gender friends' conversations. *Sex Roles, 33,* 387–404.

Leaper, C., & Friedman, C. K. (2007). The socialization of gender. In J. E. Grusec, & P. D. Hastings (Eds.), *Handbook of socialization: Theory and research* (pp. 561–587). New York: Guilford Press.

Leaper, C., Hauser, S. T., Kremen, A., Powers, S. I., Jacobson, A. M., Noam, G. G., et al. (1989). Adolescent–parent interactions in relation to adolescents' gender and ego development pathway: A longitudinal study. *Journal of Early Adolescence, 9,* 335–361.

Leaper, C., & Holliday, H. (1995). Gossip in same-gender and cross-gender friends' conversations. *Personal Relationships, 2,* 237–246.

Leaper, C., & Smith, T. E. (2004). A meta-analytic review of gender variations in children's language use: Talkativeness, affiliative speech, and assertive speech. *Developmental Psychology, 40,* 993–1027.

Le Guin, U. K. (1969). *The left hand of darkness.* New York: Harper & Row.

Levant, R. F. (2005). The crises of boyhood. In G. E. Good & G. R. Brooks (Eds.), *The new handbook of psychotherapy and counseling with men: A comprehensive guide to settings, problems, and treatment approaches* (2nd ed., pp. 161–171). San Francisco, CA: Jossey-Bass.

Liben, L. S., & Bigler, R. S. (1987). Reformulating children's gender schemata. In. L. S. Liben & M. L. Signorella (Eds.), *Children's gender schemata (New Directions for Child Development, No. 38,* pp. 89–105). San Francisco: Jossey-Bass.

Liben, L. S., & Bigler, R. S. (2002). The developmental course of gender differentiation: Conceptualizing, measuring, and evaluating constructs and pathways. *Monographs of the Society for Research in Child Development, 67*(2), 1–183.

Liben, L. S., Bigler, R. S., & Krogh, H. R. (2002). Pink and blue collar jobs: Children's judgments of job status and job aspirations in relation to sex of worker. *Journal of Experimental Child Psychology, 79,* 346–363.

Liben, L. S., & Signorella, M. L. (1980). Gender-related schemata and constructive memory in children. *Child Development, 51,* 11–18.

Lindberg, S. M., Grabe, S., & Hyde, J. S. (2007). Gender, pubertal development, and peer sexual harassment predict objectified body consciousness in early adolescence. *Journal of Research on Adolescence, 17,* 723–742.

Lytton, H., & Romney, D. M. (1991). Parents' differential socialization of boys and girls: A meta-analysis. *Psychological Bulletin, 109,* 267–296.

Maccoby, E. E. (1998). *The two sexes: Growing up apart, coming together.* Cambridge, MA: Belknap Press/Harvard University Press.

MacGeorge, E. L., Gillihan, S. J., Samter, W., & Clark, R. A. (2003). Skill deficit or differential motivation? Accounting for sex differences in the provision of emotional support. *Communication Research, 30,* 272–303.

Maltz, D. N., & Borker, R. (1982). A cultural approach to male–female miscommunication. In J. J. Gumperz (Ed.), *Language and social identity* (pp. 195–216). Cambridge, UK: Cambridge University Press.

Mares, M. L., & Woodard, E. (2005). Positive effects of television on children's social interactions: A meta-analysis. *Media Psychology, 7,* 301–322.

Martin, C. L. (1989). Children's use of gender-related information in making social judgments. *Developmental Psychology, 25,* 80–88.

Martin, C. L., Eisenbud, L., & Rose, H. (1995). Children's gender-based reasoning about toys. *Child Development, 66,* 1453–1471.

Martin, C. L., & Fabes, R. A. (2001). The stability and consequences of young children's same-sex peer interactions. *Developmental Psychology, 37,* 431–446.

Martin, C. L., Fabes, R. A., Evans, S. M., & Wyman, H. (1999). Social cognition on the playground: Children's beliefs about playing with girls versus boys and their relation to sex-segregated play. *Journal of Social and Personal Relationships, 16,* 751–771.

Martin, C. L., & Halverson, C. F. (1981). A schematic processing model of sex typing and stereotyping in children. *Child Development, 52,* 1119–1134.

Martin, C. L., & Little, J. K. (1990). The relation of gender understanding to children's sex-typed preferences and gender stereotypes. *Child Development, 61,* 1427–1439.

Martin, C. L., & Ross, H. S. (2005). Sibling aggression: Sex differences and parents' reactions. *International Journal of Behavioral Development, 29,* 129–138.

Martin, C. L., Ruble, D. N., & Szkrybalo, J. (2002). Cognitive theories of early gender development. *Psychological Bulletin, 128,* 903–933.

McCabe, M. P., & Ricciardelli, L. A. (2005). A prospective study of pressures from parents, peers, and the media on extreme weight change behaviors among adolescent boys and girls. *Behaviour Research and Therapy, 43,* 653–668.

McDougall, P., & Hymel, S. (2007). Same-gender versus cross-gender friendship conceptions: Similar or different. *Merrill-Palmer Quarterly, 53,* 347–380.

McMaster, L. E., Connolly, J., Pepler, D., & Craig, W. M. (2002). Peer to peer sexual harassment in early adolescence: A developmental perspective. *Development and Psychopathology, 14,* 91–105.

McNelles, L. R., & Connolly, J. A. (1999). Intimacy between adolescent friends: Age and gender differences in intimate affect and intimate behaviors. *Journal of Research on Adolescence, 9,* 143–159.

Messner, M. A. (1998). Boyhood, organized sports, and the construction of masculinities. In M.A. Messner (Ed.), *Men's lives* (pp. 109–121). Boston: Allyn & Bacon.

Miller, P. M., Danaher, D. L., & Forbes, D. (1986). Sex-related strategies for coping with interpersonal conflict in children aged five and seven. *Developmental Psychology, 22,* 543–548.

Moller, L. C., & Serbin, L. A. (1996). Antecedents of toddler gender segregation: Cognitive consonance, gender-typed toy preferences and behavioral compatibility. *Sex Roles, 35,* 445–460.

Murnen, S. K., & Smolak, L. (2000). The experience of sexual harassment among grade-school students: Early socialization of female subordination? *Sex Roles, 43,* 1–17.

O'Leary, K. D., Slep, A. M. S., Avery-Leaf, S., & Cascardi, M. (2008). Gender differences in dating aggression among multiethnic high school students. *Journal of Adolescent Health, 42,* 473–479.

Oppliger, P. A. (2007). Effects of gender stereotyping on socialization. In R. W. Preiss, B. M. Gayle, N. Burrell, M. Allen, & J. Bryant (Eds.), *Mass media effects research: Advances through meta-analysis* (pp. 199–214). Mahwah, NJ: Erlbaum.

Paik, H., & Comstock, G. (1994). The effects of television violence on antisocial behavior: A meta-analysis. *Communication Research, 21,* 516–546.

Pellegrini, A. D., Long, J. D., Roseth, C., Bohn, K., & Van Ryzin, M. (2007). A short-term longitudinal study of preschool children's sex segregation: The role of physical activity, sex, and time. *Journal of Comparative Psychology, 121,* 282–289.

Perry, D. G., Perry, L. C., & Weiss, R. J. (1989). Sex differences in the consequences that children anticipate for aggression. *Developmental Psychology, 25,* 312–319.

Piaget, J. (1970). Piaget's theory. In P. H. Mussen (Ed.), *Carmichael's manual of child psychology* (pp. 703–732). New York: Wiley.

Poulin, F., & Pedersen, S. (2007). Developmental changes in gender composition of friendship networks in adolescent girls and boys. *Developmental Psychology, 43,* 1484–1496.

Raag, T., & Rackliff, C. L. (1998). Preschoolers' awareness of social expectations of gender: Relationships to toy choices. *Sex Roles, 38,* 685–700.

Radmacher, K., & Azmitia, M. (2006). Are there gendered pathways to intimacy in early adolescents' and emerging adults' friendships? *Journal of Adolescent Research, 21,* 415–448.

Robinson, B. E., & Green, M. G. (1981). Beyond androgyny: The emergence of sex-role transcendence as a theoretical construct. *Developmental Review, 1,* 247–265.

Robinson, T. N., Saphir, M. N., Kraemer, H. C., Varady, A., & Haydel, K. F. (2001). Effects of reducing television viewing on children's requests for toys: A randomized controlled trial. *Journal of Developmental and Behavioral Pediatrics, 22,* 179–184.

Rose, A. J., & Asher, S. R. (1999). Children's goals and strategies in response to conflicts within a friendship. *Developmental Psychology, 35,* 69–79.

Rose, A. J., Carlson, W., & Waller, E. M. (2007). Prospective associations of corumination with friendship and emotional adjustment: Considering the socioemotional trade-offs of corumination. *Developmental Psychology, 43,* 1019–1031.

Rose, A. J., & Montemayor, R. (1994). The relationship between gender role orientation and perceived self-competency in male and female adolescents. *Sex Roles, 31,* 579–595.

Rose, A. J., & Rudolph, K. D. (2006). A review of sex differences in peer relationship processes: Potential tradeoffs for the emotional and behavioral development of girls and boys. *Psychological Bulletin, 132,* 98–131.

Rowley, S. J., Kutz-Costes, B., Mistry, R., & Feagans, L. (2007). Social status and a predictor of race and gender stereotypes in late childhood and early adolescence. *Social Development, 16,* 150–168.

Ryan, R. M., & Lynch, J. H. (1989). Emotional autonomy versus detachment: Revisiting the vicissitudes of adolescence and young adulthood. *Child Development, 60,* 340–356.

Serbin, L. A., Powlishta, K. K., & Gulko, J. (1993). The development of sex typing in middle childhood. *Monographs of the Society for Research in Child Development, 58*(2), 1–75.

Signorella, M. L. (1999). Multidimensionality of gender schemas: Implications for the development of gender-related characteristics. In W. B. Swann, Jr., & J. H. Langlois (Eds.), *Sexism and stereotypes in modern society: The gender science of J. T. Spence* (pp. 107–126). Washington, DC: American Psychological Association.

Signorella, M. L., Bigler, R. S., & Liben, L. S. (1993). Developmental differences in children's gender schemata about others: A meta-analytic review. *Developmental Review, 13,* 147–183

Signorielli, N. (2001). Television's gender-role images and contribution to stereotyping: Past, present and future. In D. G. Singer & J. L. Singer (Eds.), *Handbook of children and the media* (pp. 341–358). Thousand Oaks, CA: Sage.

Sroufe, L. A., Bennett, C., Englund, M., Urban, J., & Shulman, S. (1993). The significance of gender boundaries in preadolescence: Contemporary correlates and antecedents of boundary violation and maintenance. *Child Development, 64,* 455–466.

Strough, J., & Berg, C. A. (2000). Goals as a mediator of gender differences in high-affiliation dyadic conversations. *Developmental Psychology, 36,* 117–125.

Strough, J., & Covatto, A. M. (2002). Context and age differences in same- and other-gender peer preferences. *Social Development, 11,* 346–361.

Tajfel, H., & Turner, J. (1979). An integrative theory of intergroup conflict. In W. G. Austin & S. Worchel (Eds.), *The social psychology of intergroup relations* (pp. 94–109). Monterey, CA: Brooks-Cole.

Tenenbaum, H. R., & Leaper, C. (2002). Are parents' gender schemas related to their children's gender-related cognitions? A meta-analysis. *Developmental Psychology, 38,* 615–630.

Thompson, T. L., & Zerbinos, E. (1995). Gender roles in animated cartoons: Has the picture changed in 20 years. *Sex Roles, 32,* 651–673.

Thorne, B., & Luria, Z. (1986). Sexuality and gender in children's daily worlds. *Social Problems, 33,* 176–190.

Timmerman, G. (2005). A comparison between girls' and boys' experiences of unwanted sexual behaviour in secondary schools. *Educational Research, 47,* 291–306.

Tolman, D. L., Spencer, R., Harmon, T., Rosen-Reynoso, M., & Striepe, M. (2004). Getting close, staying cool: Early adolescent boys' experiences with romantic relationships. In N. Way & J. Y. Chu (Eds.), *Adolescent boys: Exploring diverse cultures of boyhood* (pp. 235–255). New York: New York University Press.

Twenge, J. M., & Nolen-Hoeksema, S. (2002). Age, gender, race, socio-economic status, and birth cohort differences on the Children's Depression Inventory: A meta-analysis. *Journal of Abnormal Psychology, 111,* 578–588.

Underwood, M. K. (2003). *Social aggression among girls.* New York: Guilford Press.

Weitzman, N., Birns, B., & Friend, R. (1985). Traditional and nontraditional mothers' communication with their daughters and sons. *Child Development, 56,* 894–898.

Whipp, B. J., & Ward, S. A. (1992). Will women soon outrun men? *Nature, 355,* 25.

Williams, T., Connolly, J., Pepler, D., & Craig, W. (2005). Peer victimization, social support, and psychosocial adjustment of sexual minority adolescents. *Journal of Youth and Adolescence, 34,* 471–482.

Witkowska, E., & Gådin, K. G. (2005). Have you been sexually harassed in school? What female high school students regard as harassment. *International Journal of Adolescent Medicine and Health, 17*, 391–406.

Wolitzky-Taylor, K. B., Ruggiero, K. J., Danielson, C. K., Resnick, H. S., Hanson, R. F., Smith, D. W., et al. (2008). Prevalence and correlates of dating violence in a national sample of adolescents. *Journal of the American Academy of Child and Adolescent Psychiatry, 47*, 755–762.

Wood, W., & Eagly, A. H. (2002). A cross-cultural analysis of the behavior of women and men: Implications for the origins of sex differences. *Psychological Bulletin, 128*, 699–727.

World Economic Forum. (2007). *The global gender gap report 2007.* Geneva, Switzerland: Author. Available at *www.weforum.org/pdf/gendergap/report2007.pdf*

Zarbatany, L., McDougall, P., & Hymel, S. (2000). Title gender-differentiated experience in the peer culture: Links to intimacy in preadolescence. *Social Development, 9*, 62–79.

13

Race, Ethnicity, and Social Class

Nancy E. Hill
Dawn P. Witherspoon

Children's social development is shaped by a complex milieu of economic, cultural, and historical factors (Bronfenbrenner & Morris, 2006; Conger, Conger, & Elder, 1997; Lerner, 2006; McLoyd, 1990). For ethnic minorities and low-income families, social development is shaped by social stratification due to racism and classism, resulting in disadvantage and foreclosed opportunities (Garcia Coll et al., 1996; Wilson, 2009). In contrast, Euro-American and wealthier families often experience advantages because social stratification processes work in their favor (Conley, 1999; Lareau, 2003). Among the demographic indicators, race, ethnicity, and socioeconomic status (SES) are the most widely used for comparing developmental outcomes and trajectories (Hill, 2006). Such categorizations have become increasingly salient as federal and local policies require schools to assess and work toward closing gaps in achievement; as prevention and intervention scientists, practitioners, and policymakers grapple with ethnic and economic disparities in juvenile delinquencies and incarceration; and as scientists, practitioners, and policymakers use race and SES as markers of risk and advantage. The increased importance of race, ethnicity, and SES coexists with the increased diversity among the U.S. population.

The American school population is becoming increasingly diverse. In the early 2000s, almost 40% of all students enrolled in public schools in the United States were from ethnic minority groups (National Center for Education Statistics [NCES], 2003), with an average of 63% ethnic minorities in large and midsize cities, 36% in suburban areas, and 21% in rural areas (NCES, 2003), with increasing diversity expected. Further, gaps between the wealthiest and poorest families have increased in the last third of the 20th century and the first decade of the 21st century. Because of the powerful influences of social stratification based on race, ethnicity, and SES in the United States (Garcia Coll et al., 1996; Wilson, 2009), coupled with increasing diversity, we can no longer ignore these constructs. It is imperative to consider race, ethnicity, and economics to more fully understand children's social development.

In this chapter, we outline the distinct and overlapping conceptualizations of race and ethnicity; examine the direct and indirect roles of SES, race, and ethnicity for children's development; and highlight the ways in which SES, race, and ethnicity are intertwined as they shape social development. First, because the terms *race*, *ethnicity*, *SES*, *poverty*, and *middle class* are common terms in the secular, policy, and scientific literature, they have both implicit and explicit meanings and connotations. To more accurately understand the impact of race, ethnicity, and SES for children's social development, we carefully define the scope of these terms. Second, the evidence supporting current theories of the effects of race, ethnicity, and SES on social development are critically reviewed and evaluated. These theories include social capital and identity, as well as theories outlining indirect effects through neighborhood composition and selection, family socialization patterns, and intergenerational transference of advantage and disadvantage. Third, we outline the synergies created at the nexus of race, ethnicity, and SES that influence social development, along with the ways in which these constructs have been confounded in society and in research designs to mask the true unique and interactive effects of each construct.

Confounds in prior research, at times, have misdirected programs and policies by focusing on race and invoking cultural-deficit explanations when economic or structural explanations are more appropriate and meaningful (Hill, 2006; Krieger, Williams, & Moss, 1997). Based on the unique and synergistic influences of race, ethnicity, and SES, we outline future directions for theory and research to prepare the field to direct and navigate the changing political and scientific landscape as it pertains to three constructs that have a vexing history and a politically charged present and future.

CONCEPTUALIZATIONS, DISTINCTIONS, AND ISSUES: RACE, ETHNICITY, AND SOCIOECONOMIC STATUS

Although some suggest that race and ethnicity are interchangeable (e.g., Phinney, 1996) or that the term *race* was abandoned in favor of its less politically charged counterpart *ethnicity* (Sollors, 1996), maintaining conceptual distinctions is necessary in order to understand how race and ethnicity are uniquely associated with and influence children's development (Hill, 2006; Hill, Murry, & Anderson, 2005). Further, even as the social sciences move away from biological explanations of race, the fields of genetics and medicine provide evidence of the role of biologically defined (apart from socially defined) race in human development (Stevens et al., 1992). In addition, biologically driven phenotypic characteristics elicit experiences, including racial profiling and discrimination that influence social development apart from culture or ethnicity (Harrison & Thomas, 2009). This requires the careful consideration of race, ethnicity, and SES.

What Is Race?

Conceptualizations of race range from strictly biological to strictly social constructions. Racial grouping is based on presumed genetic, biological, or physical similarities (Graham, Taylor, & Ho, 2009). For some, "race" is used as a proxy for impoverished background and results in meaningless categories and inaccurate information (Helms, Jernigan, & Mascher, 2005). Yet, because the emphasis on categorizing youth continues, racial grouping is used despite its ambiguous meaning. Amid controversy, biological definitions and social constructions of race remain. Indeed, the U.S. federal government, for the purposes of research (e.g., National Institutes of Health) and of the census, counts all categories except Hispanics (White, African American, Asian American, Pacific Islander, Native American) as being races. Hispanic is defined as an ethnicity. This creates the assumption that Hispanics can be of many races, which is true. In contrast, Whites, African Americans, Asian Americans, and others are assumed not to have ethnic backgrounds beyond their race, which is largely untrue.

Biological Constructions of Race

Since the 19th century, races have been viewed as subgroups of humans who display phenotypic (e.g., skin color, hair texture, eye shape) commonalities that are based on ancestral origin and genes (Smedley & Smedley, 2005). Although biological explanations for racial differences are controversial and often considered to be either outdated or the result of inadequate assessments of SES or other contextual factors (Krieger et al., 1997; Oakes & Rossi, 2003), social scientists have renewed their interest in the controversial exploration of genetics and race (Anderson & Nickerson, 2005). Genetically, humans are 99.9% identical, and researchers find that American conceptualizations of different racial groupings of individuals are not genetically distinct populations (Bonham, Warshauer-Baker, & Collins, 2005). However, variations in DNA can be used to categorize individuals as Africans, Caucasians, Pacific Islanders, East Asians, and Native Americans *only if* certain sampling criteria are met (e.g., the individuals' ancestors all come from one geographical area; Risch, Burchard, Ziv, & Tang, 2002; Rosenberg et al., 2002). Yet, many scholars find that biologically defined race is not a valid conceptualization (Smedley & Smedley, 2005), especially for understanding social development, and that race can be understood only through its interpretation by society—that is, its social construction.

Social Constructions of Race

A social construction is "the reality created internally by the person's perceptions of his or her world" (Liu, 2001, p. 149). This is often the central tenet of discussions of race, ethnicity, and SES on social development—it is a reality that is fashioned or developed by families, community, and society. In this vein, racial effects are a "socially constructed lay theory" that has psychological consequences and focuses on boundaries between people (Quintana, 1998, 2008; Quintana & McKown, 2008; Sollors, 1996). Race reflects differential power as much as any biological category; even young children are aware of it and begin to internalize it (Hirschfeld, 2008; Quintana, 2008). Because most social scientists do not directly assess race biologically, the vast majority of research can be interpreted through the lens of social construction.

What Is Ethnicity?

Although some propose that the term *ethnicity* should replace *race* because social scientists do not typically assess biological aspects of race, others suggest that race and ethnicity should be distinct (Hill, 2006; Hill et al., 2005). Ethnicity, as a construct distinct from race, was introduced to contest the belief in inherent biological differences between racial groups and to create focus on the cultural aspects of ethnicity and race (Zagefka, 2009). However, similar to the conceptualizations of race, there have been various definitions of *ethnicity* and *ethnic groups* (Cartrite, 2003). Ethnicity can be defined as the groups of people who identity themselves as interconnected because of shared history, common language, nationality, or ancestry (Smedley & Smedley, 2005). Here, the focus is on understanding the mechanisms or processes (e.g., culture) within a particular ethnic group that lead to group identity and that may manifest themselves in ways specific to that group and thereby have identifiable consequences (i.e., outcomes) for that group. Most often ethnicity is conceptualized as one's country of origin, with the assumption that it reflects a common culture. Studying ethnically based mechanisms and processes elucidates the heterogeneity within racial or ethnic groups (Phinney, 1996). Despite these distinctions, many researchers conflate race and ethnicity.

Distinguishing Race and Ethnicity

Because of the multiple definitions and the politically charged nature of the term *race*, many researchers use *race* and *ethnicity* interchangeably (Phinney, 1989, 1996). However, there are heuristic differences between race and ethnicity (Hill, 2006). Further, within a race, there may be multiple ethnicities. For example, within the African American racial group, there may be Caribbean and African ethnic groups, in addition to those who have a long history living in the United States. The converse is also true: Among ethnic groups, there are multiple races (e.g., Black Cubans). When researchers provide little conceptual distinction between race and ethnicity, we lose this heterogeneity and assume that between-group variability (e.g., Latino and African American) is greater than within-group variability. Moreover, this results in comparing racial groups (e.g., Blacks) with ethnic groups (e.g., Mexican Americans) and drawing cultural conclusions when groups vary significantly on within-group cultural heterogeneity. However, if we distinguish race and ethnicity as separate entities, we can identify the unique and interactive effects of each. Finally, understanding the extent to which social development is affected by the social constructions or evaluations of one's racial group or by ethnically or culturally based belief systems has a significant impact on developing programs and policies to support youth and families. Equally complex and often confounded with race and ethnicity is socioeconomic status.

Defining Social Class and Socioeconomic Status

Although links between social and economic standing and health have been well documented even in ancient times (Wilson, 2009), interest in SES among social scientists, especially among researchers and practitioners interested in children's development, peaked in the late 1960s and 1970s in the aftermath of the infamous Moynihan Report, which outlined disparities in developmental outcomes across SES and race. This report coincided with the initiation of then President Lyndon Johnson's War on Poverty and with the documentation of increasing income inequality (Sifers, Puddy, Warren, & Roberts, 2002). Because SES is strongly related to a wide range of physical and mental health, behavioral, social, and other developmental outcomes, there is increased interest in defining and assessing it. SES and its effects on developmental outcomes are conceptualized at the individual and at the community or society levels.

SES reflects the distributions of resources, power, and influence within a society and a person's or family's relative standing among others in society with regard to such resources, power, prestige, and influence (APA Task Force on Socioeconomic Status, 2007). At the societal level, indicators such as the extent of socioeconomic inequality between the wealthiest and poorest families, median income and/or education levels, and percent unemployment within a community are related to a wide variety of developmental outcomes for children and families (Hoff, Laursen, & Tardiff, 2002). For understanding mental health and developmental outcomes at the individual or family level, the most powerful indicators of SES are family income levels, parental education level, and occupational status or prestige (Jones & McMillan, 2001). To understand why and how SES relates to children's social development, we consider theories that explain the origins and processes that maintain social stratification in industrialized countries.

Interest in economic levels and their impact on health began in the late 1800s with a focus on occupational tools and occupational injury and morbidity (Ward, 1883). In the late 19th century, social scientists became interested in the social or environmental correlates (i.e., socio-) or known class (i.e., economic) variations in infant health and mortality, resulting in an interest in the intersection of "social" and "economic" positions and the creation of the concept and term *socioeconomic status* (SES; Oakes & Rossi, 2003). Although most individuals have implicit working definitions of SES, there is little agreement about what comprises the construct. The American Psychological Association (APA) Task Force on Socioeconomic Status (2007) described SES as the relative standing of an individual or group in terms of their income, education, and occupation. Despite increased interest in understanding the effects of SES on children's development, there is little conceptual or theoretical foundation to guide its measurement (Smith & Graham, 1995).

The fields of sociology and economics provide several theories about the origins of social stratification and the processes that promote and replicate it in society (Crompton, 1993; Marx, 1967). Although not as influential as they once were, Marxist theories on the "warring" and "clashing" classes suggest that industrialized societies contain two opposing classes that each relate to the production of goods: the "capitalists," who control industrial production and labor, and the "workers" or "laborers" (Kohn, 1969; Luster, Rhoades, & Haas, 1989). Through their control of production, "capitalists" have greater control over and access to resources, which provides them with more power, prestige, and social stature. In contrast, "laborers" are often under the control of capitalists, are at the mercy of company policies, and have little control or power—hence the rise of organized labor unions. Some theorists suggest that the separation of these classes, the internalization of the conflict between the classes, and the differing skills, levels of control, hierarchy, and authority associated with success for each class resulted in varying parental socialization patterns and goals (Kohn, 1969; Lareau, 2003), which reproduce class position from one generation to the next.

A second group of theories suggest that no society is truly classless and that social stratification is both desirable and necessary in order to function as a society (cf. Dahrendorf, 1969; Davis, 1942; Davis & Moore, 1945). The goal of a society is to distribute members into necessary social and occupational positions and motivate them to do the tasks of that position. If all positions and duties are equally appealing to individuals and equally important to the functioning of society and require similar levels of ability or talent, it matters very little who takes on which positions. Because this is hardly ever true, Davis (1942; Davis & Moore, 1945) identifies three types of rewards that are used to motivate people into needed societal positions and thereby create class positions: (1) financial resources; (2) leisure or entertainment; and (3) rewards that contribute to self-respect and ego enhancement (e.g., prestige). Such rewards are built into positions. Davis and Moore (1945) concluded that "Social inequity is thus an unconsciously evolved device by which societies insure that the most important positions are consciously filled by the most qualified persons" (p. 243). Those positions with the largest rewards are those that have the greatest importance to society and require the most training and talent. Correspondingly, the reward of the position must be commensurate with the sacrifice made to obtain the training. Unequal economic returns can be used to control entrance into positions and to motivate others to complete the required training for positions. For example, positions with low desirability but that are highly needed can be filled by increasing financial reward (i.e., comparatively high rate of pay relative to training required). In contrast, for other positions, such as physicians, increasing the prestige and influence associated with the position, along with financial rewards, can motivate a select number of people to complete the arduous training for a needed position.

Similarly, market-based theories of stratification implicate the supply and demand of talents, skills, and abilities in conferring rewards (Davis & Moore, 1945). These theories emphasize the scarcity of the abilities or training associated with the position. As described in Smith and Graham (1995), to increase and maintain public health, both physicians and garbage collectors are needed. However, the perceived scarcity of talent and the difficulty of training associated with the role of the physician increase the market value and therefore the prestige and rewards associated with being a physician.

Certain characteristics distinguish social stratification across societies, including the size of the disparities between the richest and the poorest in society, the degree of openness or opportunity, and the sense of class identity (e.g., labor unions create solidarity among the manufacturing class); yet stratification in and of itself is not harmful to society nor to classes of individuals within society (Davis & Moore, 1945). It is when social stratification and differential social position are coupled with disadvantage, perceived lack of value, deprivation, and downward classism that they have pernicious outcomes for children and youth. This includes the extent to which class mobility is managed by the oppression of particular groups. Here, race and class intersect and result in differential outcomes for individuals (Hill, 2006; Oakes & Rossi, 2003; Sollors, 1996).

Prior to addressing the intersections of race, ethnicity, and SES, it is important to carefully consider the measurement of SES, the assumptions underlying its measurement, and the utility of these measurements to understand how SES shapes children's social development. Despite widely known theories of the origins and purposes of social stratification and its association with a wide variety of developmental outcomes, the measurement of SES has largely been uninformed by theory and reflects expedience rather than theoretically based tools (Frable, 1997).

Measuring Socioeconomic Status

Often, the main purposes of assessing SES for social science research are to describe research participants and to use SES variables as statistical controls to better examine the associations among other variables of interest (Oakes & Rossi, 2003). An underlying assumption of assessments of SES is that it is continuous and linear, meaning that levels of impact between two points on the SES continuum are roughly equal regardless of where they fall along the full range of SES. That is, a $5,000 increase in income will have the same impact for families making $30,000 a year as it will for those making $200,000 a year. In contrast, assessments that are class- or status-based have as their underlying assumption that there is greater homogeneity within and greater heterogeneity between classes and that specific classes can be consistently defined. In addition, one must consider the level at which SES functions (i.e., the level of analysis)—individual, family, neighborhood, region, or society. For most social development outcomes, it is often the SES level of the primary caretaker or family that matters most, as it dictates a family's resources and standard of living. However, neighborhood- or societal-level SES becomes salient when community resources, hazards, and risks and their impact on social development are of interest (e.g., the impact of violence exposure on children's mental health). Next, we outline and evaluate the ways in which SES is measured in the social sciences.

Income, Including Poverty

Income, including the amount of money available to a family from all sources, is among the most widely used assessments, because it provides an indication of the standard of living and the extent to which material needs can be purchased (Entwisle & Astone, 1994; Krieger et al., 1997). Although it is key for understanding the familial economic resources, income is often the most difficult indicator to assess, because people consider it private and sensitive information (Entwisle & Astone, 1994; Krieger et al., 1997). In addition, income may not convey accurate information about spending power (Duncan, 1988), especially compared with an income-to-needs assessment. Further, income is only modestly correlated with education (APA Socioeconomic Task Force, 2007). However, because income fluctuates more than other SES indicators, it may be more useful for predicting changes in children's development (Duncan, 1996) and for understanding the impact of trajectories and changes in SES over time.

Related to income is the use of poverty as an indicator of SES. For the United States, poverty level is based on subsistence food levels for biological survival. In the United States, the method for calculating the poverty level was developed in 1964 and is based on the dollar value for the U.S. Department of Agriculture's economy food plan (Fisher, 1992). This dollar value is considered minimally necessary for biological survival in short-term emergency situations. This calculation was not intended to define poverty for the United States more generally, but to provide a snapshot of intense poverty in the United States, and it does not reflect current changes in expenses. Attempts to revise the calculation of the poverty line within the United States to a level that more accurately reflects an inability to meet one's needs have been met with resistance. Despite its problematic assessment, it is often used in research, because it defines families' eligibility for programs and resources that families and children need.

Among indicators of SES, income is one of the most common. However, because income is difficult to obtain, does not always reflect purchasing power, and does not reflect other aspects of SES such as social capital, prestige, and power, some argue that parental education level is a better marker of SES, especially for understanding its impact on children's social and academic development (Hoff et al., 2002; Krieger et al., 1997).

Education Level

Education level is one of the most widely used indicators of SES (Hoff et al., 2002). Higher parental education levels are associated with fewer behavioral problems, higher academic performance, and greater engagement in school (Blacklund, Sorlie, & Johnson, 1999). Part of its appeal is its ease of measurement. Further, education level is applicable to unemployed individuals (especially stay-at-home parents) and, therefore, is often a better indicator of the effects of socioeconomic influences on child development that are not due to financial resources.

Education level is also a marker of persistence (APA Task Force, 2007), especially between those who complete degrees and those who attend but do not graduate. Further, education level is a marker of individuals' exposure to broader social networks. Although some research on the relation between parental education level and children's developmental outcomes uses number of years completed, considerable evidence shows that the effects of education are discontinuous and that the points at which degrees are conferred have the most significant effect on outcomes (Hoff et al., 2002; Jones & McMillan, 2001), suggesting that the benefit of education is largely due to credentialing rather than the knowledge and skills learned.

Despite preferences for using education level, there are some disadvantages. First, education level has a smaller range and variability. The vast majority of Americans complete either high school or college, with very few people completing less than an eighth-grade education or receiving doctoral degrees. This reduced variability makes it a less sensitive indicator of SES differences in children's outcomes. Further, as the proportion of the population that graduates from high school increases, the lack of variability at the lower end of the education range diminishes, making it difficult to see the impact of education at lower SES levels (Krieger et al., 1997). Although some argue that education level influences children's development because it reflects parents' ability to provide cognitively stimulating home environments, others suggest that the credentials, knowledge, and skills that are translated into occupations and opportunities are the key to understanding the influence of parental education on children's social development. There is considerable research that focuses on the role of occupations and employment status as they influence parental beliefs and goals for their children, parenting practices, and ultimately children's development (Jin, Shah, & Svoboda, 1995).

Employment Status, Occupations, and Occupational Prestige

At its most basic level, assessments of occupation include employment status—whether parents work full or part time—and desire to work. Working can be beneficial, especially for those who are unemployed, are looking for work, and are financial providers for their families; unemployment is associated with greater mental and physical health problems (Fuller et al., 2002; Galambos & Lerner, 1991). However, early research suggested that maternal employment was associated with less secure mother–infant attachments and increased behavioral problems (Belsky & Eggebeen, 1991). More recent work is less conclusive and is often dependent on the extent to which mothers are the primary financial providers and the degree to which mothers view working as a part of their maternal role. For example, an evaluation of the New Hope Project, an employment intervention program, found that maternal employment increased children's positive behavior and decreased problem behavior, especially among boys, in part because of improvements in parenting (Epps & Huston, 2007).

In understanding the relation between occupational prestige/status and social development, assessments of the context of the work environment, control, time demands, schedules, flexibility, prestige (i.e., social capital), and hierarchical structure matter most (Kohn, 1969; Luster et al., 1989). Occupations at the higher end of the SES continuum feature greater intellectual challenges, greater use and affirmation of personal skills, and more opportunities to control working conditions (Marmot, Bosma, Hemingway, Brunner, & Stansfeld, 1997). In contrast, lower-SES occupations provide less control, autonomy, and flexibility, while being more hazardous and tedious. Further, nonstandard and inflexible hours have been associated with decreased marital stability and family cohesion (Presser, 2003) and a negative impact on cognitive and behavioral development for children and adolescents (Strazdin, Clements, Korda, Broom, D'Souza, 2004; Strazdin, Korda, Lim, Broom, & D'Souza, 2006). However, the negative effects of nonstandard work hours are not uniform. When nonstandard work schedules permit parents to manage their schedules to spend more time with children (e.g., one parent working nights and another days) and when such schedules increase the family income, there are positive effects for children's social development (Barnett & Gareis, 2007).

In addition to examining employment status, others have used the social standing or prestige of occupations as a marker of SES (Davis, 1942; Davis & Moore, 1945). Occupational prestige reflects the social influence and networks that benefit individuals through their occupations—distinct from the economic rewards of the position. Contemporary occupational prestige scales rank each occupation listed in the census according to typical educational requirements or average education level for the position and the average income of those holding that occupation; a prestige score ranges from roughly 0 to 100 (Featherman & Hauser, 1976, 1978; Nakao & Treas, 1994).

Although some argue that the conflation of education and income into a single indicator of occupational prestige muddles the potentially unique influences of each on development (Conley, 1999), assessments of occupational prestige reflect the social capital and social networks that are available to parents, which they can utilize to support their parenting practices and their children's development. One key benefit of education level, occupational prestige, and income is the ability to provide the resources needed to absorb the impact of sudden, unexpected income and occupational losses. The accumulation of these resources reflects wealth.

Wealth

Wealth is the accumulation of assets (e.g., investments, home and car ownership) and is positively associated with mental health and other outcomes for children and adults (Kingston & Smith, 1997). The key process by which wealth affects children's development is the provision of a cushion in times of job or income loss and through intergenerational transfers of wealth (Hacker, 1992). However, wealth is a key source of SES inequality and of ethnic disparities in SES. Many ethnic minority populations are experiencing decreasing gaps in education and occupational levels, but the gaps in wealth remain large (MacArthur Foundation, 2000).

Subjective Assessments

As important as any objective indicator of SES, people's own feelings about their socioeconomic standing and their perceptions about their ability to meet their economic needs can have a tremendous effect on their mental health and well-being (APA Task Force, 2007). Because individual assessments are not objective, many social and public policy scientists overlook subjective accounts of SES. It is common for people in the United States to identify as being "middle class," although income, education level, occupational prestige, wealth, and other indicators would suggest differently (Liu, 2001). Further, few people can pinpoint an exact definition of "middle class."

The MacArthur Foundation has developed theories and measures to assess subjective SES (Adler, Epel, Castellazzo, & Ickovics, 2000; Singh-Manoux, Adler, & Marmot, 2003). These assessments were related to physical and mental health outcomes even after objective SES indicators were controlled (MacArthur Foundation, 2000). The difference between responses of subjective economic standing and social standing may be especially useful for low-SES communities, in which standing in the community is less driven by economics and education and more by roles in community groups (Oakes & Rossi, 2003).

Evaluation of Assessments

Assessments of SES are not interchangeable. Each reflects a particular view, belief, or theory about the nature of SES and its relation to outcomes. Identifying the underlying theory as to why SES should affect the outcome of interest or why it should be statistically controlled in order to better understand the relations among other variables is central to selecting the appropriate measure (Boston, 1991). Identifying and understanding the psychological markers that represent the boundaries between socioeconomic classes and the relations between defined class or statuses and one's sense of "class consciousness" are also key to understanding how SES relates to outcomes and to selecting the appropriate assessments (Grundy & Holt, 2001).

Further, it is generally recommended that multiple assessments of SES be gathered so that the unique and interactive effects of each can be examined (APA Task Force, 2007; Entwisle & Astone, 1994; Hauser, 1994). Others argue specifically for the importance of combining both objective and subjective indicators of SES to understanding the relations between SES and developmental outcomes, especially as it is often the stress of not being able to meet one's economic needs, rather than low-SES status, that matters most (Oakes & Rossi, 2003; Turner & Oakes, 1986).

HOW RACE, ETHNICITY, AND SOCIOECONOMIC STATUS COMBINE TO AFFECT SOCIAL DEVELOPMENT

SES and socioeconomic resources are not equally distributed across racial and ethnic groups. As already noted, there are significant disparities in income and education level across racial and ethnic groups. Based on 2008 U.S. Census data of households,

African American income was 66% of that of Whites, 52% of that of Asian Americans, and 90% of that of Hispanics. Based on per capita income data, Hispanic households' per capita income is 90% of African Americans', 55% of Whites, and 52% of Asian Americans' household per capita income levels (Kao & Thompson, 2003). Further, there are significant gaps in wealth across ethnicity (Conley, 1999), and gaps in wealth are even greater when home ownership and home equity are not included in the calculations. The reason is largely that ethnic minorities were barred from property ownership for much of U.S. history and, even when minorities (especially African Americans) were able to purchase homes, they were barred from purchasing homes in neighborhoods in which housing values appreciated considerably (Shapiro, 2004). In educational attainment, Asian Americans have the lowest levels of high school dropout and the highest average educational attainment, followed by Euro-Americans, African Americans, Hispanics, and Native Americans (Mather, 2007). Although most of those who live in poverty are Euro-Americans, a greater proportion of the African American and Latino populations are impoverished.

As has been well established, the interrelations among indicators of SES vary across ethnicity (Hacker, 1992). The "payoff" of educational attainment is lower for African Americans and Latinos compared with Euro-Americans and Asian Americans (Charles, 2003; Wilson, 1987). Each year of education is associated with lower income increases for ethnic minorities than for Euro-Americans. Some suggest that these differences in payoff for education result in diminished engagement and attachment to school for African Americans and Latinos (Ogbu, 1981). However, others find that valuing education is an integral part of African American culture (Cross, 2011).

In research with immigrant populations, understanding and distinguishing SES and ethnic effects on family and social development are even more complex. Indicators of SES such as education level and occupation may have different meanings for and influences on immigrant families. Immigrants who come to the United States for political reasons may earn much less and work in lower-level positions than their educational and/or typical occupational levels in their countries of origin would suggest (APA Task Force, 2007), making it difficult to obtain a full sense of the economic standing of new immigrants. Further, education levels may hold various meanings across countries, especially if education level is measured in years rather than based on credentials.

Much of the research in the social sciences confounds race and ethnicity in ways that have undermined our ability to distinguish race, ethnic, and SES effects on parenting, family dynamics, and children's development (Garcia Coll et al., 1996; Hill, 2006; Krieger et al., 1997). Most research on ethnic minority children and families, especially African Americans and Latinos, is based on those from lower SES backgrounds. Further, comparative research on Euro-Americans and ethnic minorities often includes samples that vary systematically on SES. When drawing conclusions from these comparative studies, it is impossible to determine whether SES or ethnicity accounts for the differences (Hill, 2006). Indeed, one argument for more sensitive measures of SES is that without good socioeconomic information, disparities are often interpreted through a lens of racial differences in genetic endowment or behavioral choices rather than considering how the processes of racial discrimination and the structural constraints of social stratification create niches that limit potential and undermine developmental outcomes (Arnett, 1995; Hill, 2011). Few studies have examined socioeconomic variations *within* ethnic minority groups, making it difficult to disentangle effects due to ethnicity and race from those due to SES, and therefore we know very little about socioeconomic variations in family dynamics, parenting, and developmental outcomes among ethnic minorities (Hill, 2006).

RACE, ETHNICITY, SOCIOECONOMIC STATUS AS THEY AFFECT SOCIAL DEVELOPMENT

Children's social development is broadly defined as the competencies children gain that serve them as they engage interpersonally, internalize their society's and their culture's values, and benefit their mental and behavioral health. Socialization includes the establishment of limits or impulse control; preparation for roles within society, including citizenship, occupational roles, gender roles, and family roles; and the process of internalizing the values, morals, and sources of meaning defined by one's culture. Broad ecological and cultural theories highlight how the economic, racial, and ethnic context shapes children's development at multiple levels (Chao, 2000; Garcia Coll et al., 1996).

Singularly and in combination, race, ethnicity, and SES inform the socialization of children more directly through their influence on parenting beliefs and practices and less directly through their influence on family activities, peer groups, ingroup marriage, and residential segregation. Despite few studies that have systematically examined the unique and interactive effects of SES, race, and ethnicity for children's development, theories reflect four levels of influence: (1) macro processes, including cultural and structural processes of social stratification that change and create developmental contexts; (2) neighborhood and community factors as mediators of social class/ethnicity and children's outcomes; (3) socioeconomically, racially, and culturally informed family-level beliefs and practices, which, in turn, affect children's development; and (4) individual factors, including identity (i.e., ethnic and socioeconomic identities), perceived opportunity structures, and behavioral norms and attributions. Each of these is discussed in turn.

Level 1: Macro Processes: Structural, Cultural, and Stratification

Macro processes reflect a set of behaviors and attitudes that define and distinguish racial, ethnic, and economic groups. For example, the ideology that is most associated with those in the "middle class" includes an endorsement of the American Dream of class mobility and equal opportunities to achieve success (Liu, 2001). When this belief is endorsed, group status differences are accepted and tolerated because of perceived differential effort (Takaki, 1993). The scientific and popular press has documented the increased challenges to upward mobility for the current generation compared with prior generations. Today, it is harder for children to "do better" than their parents on indicators of SES than in prior generations. Some call these phenomena the "mobility myth"—increasing challenges to upward mobility and achieving the American Dream.

One of the chief macro-level processes is the relative wealth and poverty rates within society. Part of the reason that disparities in wealth and poverty are associated with children's development is their influence on power and access to resources—social capital (Bourdieu, 1973). Economic, racial, and ethnic segregation, coupled with the fact that funding sources for community schools are tied to property values and community resources, has resulted in a multi-tiered system of educational and other resources for children and families. This differential quality and access limits lower-

SES children's ability to be upwardly mobile socioeconomically. In their influential model for studying minority children, Garcia Coll and colleagues (1996) highlighted how factors associated with social stratification influence the environments in which children live. Families' social positions define and constrain children's access to the very resources that will permit them to reach their potential and that are characteristic of an open-mobility society. Such differential experiences and availability of educational and other resources across socioeconomic levels perpetuates class reproduction and creates a hardened class structure, because children and families are segregated institutionally by their economic and racial contexts (Fine & Burns, 2003; Lareau, 2003). This creates synergies of advantage—families with greater economic resources, even within the same community, are able to take advantage of private schools and other resources that provide differential access to opportunities and social networks. The advantage of greater access to such resources accumulates over time.

U.S. Cultural Beliefs about Upward Mobility

Pervasive in the American cultural lore is an endorsement of the Protestant work ethic and beliefs in meritocracy. Those from higher socioeconomic backgrounds and privileged ethnic groups (i.e., Euro-American) are more likely to attribute success to their own efforts and talents than are ethnic minorities and those from lower SES backgrounds (Argyle, 1994; Heaton, 1987). Further, those from privileged economic and ethnic backgrounds often have little understanding of the nature and pervasiveness of the accumulative advantages they enjoy that account, in part, for their success (Cozzarelli, Wilkinson, & Tagler, 2001; Furnham, 2003). In contrast, those from ethnic minority and low-income backgrounds are more likely to identify structural causes for success and failure (Cozzarelli et al., 2001; Furnham, 2003). As a result of the American endorsement of meritocracy, especially among privileged classes, the American public has a lower tolerance for supporting safety nets for the poor and underprivileged (e.g., universal health insurance, universal preschool, and even defining poverty in ways that capture the real experiences of poverty, rather than being based on biological survival, as noted above). Such safety nets have significant and positive impacts on children's development (Brooks-Gunn & Duncan, 1997).

Discrimination, Racism, and Oppression

The deep-rooted endorsement of meritocracy among those from privileged ethnic and SES backgrounds often results in discrimination, prejudice, and racism against others and is a mechanism through which SES, race, and ethnicity influence child and adolescent social development (Prillentensky, 1997). Discrimination is defined as negative attitudes and behaviors toward someone because of their group membership (Brown, 2008). Racism is comprised of both stereotypes (negative beliefs) and prejudice (attitudes) that manifests itself in discriminatory behaviors (Cooper, McLoyd, Wood, & Hardaway, 2008; McKown, 2004). Social class and classism are similar in their construction as race and racism. Race is not meaningful without racism, and differences in class levels do not result in differential outcomes without class-based discrimination and differential access to resources.

Although discrimination can be ambiguous or explicit, subtle or overt (Brown, 2008), most discriminatory acts are covert and ambiguous. Individuals perceive discrimination typically when it is "situationally unambiguous" (Brown, 2008, p. 139), or highly likely. As young people age, their perceptions of discrimination change. Older adolescents perceive more discrimination than younger adolescents (Greene, Way, & Pahl, 2006). This pattern is particularly true for African American adolescents (McKown, 2004; Rosenbloom & Way, 2004), who perceive at least one discriminatory act per year (Seaton, Caldwell, Sellers, & Jackson, 2008). One manifestation of discrimination is institutional racism (Cooper et al., 2008). Although youth experience few individual discriminatory acts, they may be aware of institutionalized racism that limits access to resources and education and strips many ethnic minorities of economic empowerment (Cooper et al., 2008; Harrison-Hale, McLoyd, & Smedley, 2004).

Distal and macro-level factors, including social address variables such as race, ethnicity, gender, and social class, reflect social position and stratification influences that are "at the core rather than at the periphery" (Garcia Coll et al., 1996, p. 1892) of development and may stymie *normal* development due to their overlapping and additive natures and because they result in segregation at the residential (e.g., neighborhood), economic, and social-psychological levels.

Level 2: Neighborhood and Community Processes

Neighborhoods are the primary location for social interactions (DuBois, 1903/1990) and access to educational and extracurricular resources as well as to recreation and high-quality, moderately priced food (Evans, 2004). Long-standing policies associated with real estate, mortgage lending, and housing—such as redlining—resulted in ethnically, racially, and economically segregated neighborhoods (Charles, 2003) that decreased ethnic minority families' economic status, access to resources, and ability to create wealth, especially for African Americans (Conley, 1999; McAdoo, 2002). Neighborhood segregation based on race and ethnicity is a key mechanism through which racial and ethnic inequality are perpetuated (Charles, 2003; Leventhal & Brooks-Gunn, 2000; Sampson, 2001). Inner cities of the United States were transformed between the 1970s and 1990s as a result of the changes in the American economy and the outmigration of jobs. This change resulted in the concentration of disadvantage for African Americans (Wilson, 2003). Individuals living in the communities of concentrated poverty experienced greater constraints in social capital due to limited employment opportunities, increased poverty, and social isolation (Wilson, 1987, 1993). This social and economic isolation increases racial and social class homogeneity, places these neighborhood residents on the margins of society and resources, and exposes them (especially African Americans) to environmental toxins and hazards (McGinnis, Williams-Russo, & Knickman, 2002).

Neighborhood Characteristics That Perpetuate Social Stratification

A family's residential location dictates the quality and availability of resources by determining the proximity to good jobs and schools, safety, and the quality of social networks (Wilson, 1987). Numerous systematic structural characteristics vary between neighborhoods. Neighborhood theories such as social disorganization (Shaw & McKay, 1942), concentration of poverty effects (Wilson, 1987), collective socialization (Jencks & Mayer, 1990), and collective efficacy (Sampson, Raudenbush, & Earls, 1997) highlight the ways neighborhoods' structural characteristics (including race, ethnicity, and SES) influence children's social development, in part through their impact on social capital.

Social disorganization theory (Shaw & McKay, 1942), one of the most widely cited theories, asserts that neighborhood structural factors (e.g., residential instability, poverty, ethnic heterogeneity, and single-parent households) thwart the likelihood that individuals will develop strong community ties and common norms (i.e., social control and collective socialization). Wilson (1987) expanded this theory to include the effects of systemic changes in the American economy that resulted in the accumulation of disadvantage (e.g., decreases in social resources and increases in social isolation). Aspects of the social structure that deplete residents' opportunities and life chances include joblessness, deteriorated social networks, and resource-poor institutions—intervening variables that explain neighborhood structural effects on youth outcomes (Wacquant & Wilson, 1993).

Differential social networks and access to resources often result in the reinforcement of social-class groups and the reproduction of class across generations (Moss, 2002; Saegert, Warren, & Thompson, 2001). Affluent neighborhoods have more human and social capital and greater efficacy to demand better schools and resources to support parenting and children's development. In contrast, areas of concentrated poverty have underfunded and lower quality schools. Therefore, children in these neighborhoods, especially ethnic minority children, receive lower quality educational instruction and attend fewer years of school; and, because of differential quality, the same level of education does not confer the same benefits (e.g., skill development, knowledge, and social capital) as it does in high-SES and Euro-American neighborhoods (Hacker, 1992; Massey, 1990; Shapiro, 2004; Wilson, 2009).

Five models explain the mediating processes that link neighborhood characteristics to youth outcomes (Jencks & Mayer, 1990). Based on the *institutional resource model*, resources such as schools, recreation centers, and neighborhood organizations increase accessibility of stimulating environments, which in turn enhances children's social development. The *relative deprivation model* posits that individuals evaluate their own situations relative to others, suggesting that even those residing in neighborhoods with greater overall resources can be affected by feelings of poverty based on the evaluation of their social standing compared with others. Similarly, the *competition model* suggests that residents compete for scarce resources, and the *contagion/epidemic model* asserts that problem behavior is modeled. Last, *collective socialization models* suggest that socially organized neighborhoods promote supervision and monitoring of youth and provide role models for younger residents, which in turn affect parenting behaviors. Each of these models has been utilized to explain neighborhood effects on youth's developmental outcomes.

Neighborhood Characteristics That Affect Familial Support and Response

Families raise children and define appropriate and effective parenting strategies in response to and in conjunction with their neighborhood context. A key mechanism of family support that is affected by neighborhood characteristics is collective socialization. Collective socialization is the willingness of adults to monitor and supervise youth who are not their own and to intervene when children misbehave, coupled with a consensus about acceptable conduct. This mechanism produces social control—the communication of implicit agreement on standards of behavior from multiple sources (Coulton, Korbin, Su, & Chow, 1995). Both collective socialization and social control develop in contexts in which neighbors know one another and trust that adults in the neighborhood will act in the best interests of children's development and diminish in the presence of disadvantage (Sampson, Morenoff, & Gannon-Rowley, 2002). Beliefs about raising children are formed not only by neighborhood context but also, and especially, by one's ethnic and economic backgrounds (i.e., Level 3; see next section).

Level 3: Family-Level Beliefs and Practices

Race, ethnicity, and SES shape beliefs and practices at the family level, and these in turn influence children's development (Hill, 2009; Hoff et al., 2002; McLoyd, 1990). Comparative research shows that, across SES levels, parents from higher SES backgrounds are more encouraging of egalitarian relationships and are less punitive than are parents from lower SES backgrounds, whereas lower SES mothers are more controlling and restrictive (Hoff et al., 2002; Pinderhughes, Dodge, Bates, Pettit, & Zelli, 2000). However, other research shows that more no-nonsense parenting strategies are appropriate in navigating the often high-risk neighborhoods in which many low-income families reside (Furstenberg et al., 1993). Further, goals, values, and types of parenting strategies vary based on racial and ethnic background (Garcia Coll et al., 1996; Hill, 2006, 2009). Ethnic minority parents, including African Americans, Asian Americans, and Latinos, and parents from lower SES backgrounds are often found to be more authoritarian, to use more discipline, and to assert greater authority (Brody & Flor, 1998; Chao, 1994; Garcia Coll, Meyer, & Brillon, 1995; Hill et al., 2005).

Even when similarities in parenting practices are found, often ethnic variations in values and beliefs underlie these practices (Hill, 2006, 2009). For example, Euro-American parents, especially middle-class parents, often endorse individualism, individual achievement, competition, and material well-being to a greater extent than do other groups (Julian, McKenry, & McKelvey, 1994; Lareau, 2003). African American parents often value interdependence, security, collective goals and common interests, and perseverance in the context of adversity (Billingsley, 1974; Hill et al., 2005). Most Asian American families, especially those from East Asian cultures such as Chinese, Japanese, and Korean cultures, tend to emphasize social harmony, social relationships, and moral virtues. Moreover, East Asian cultures emphasize filial piety, age stratification, and the veneration of age (Chao, 1994, 1995). As with Asian American and African American families, Latino parents place a primacy on social relationships and the dynamics of social interactions (Marin & Marin, 1991; Simoni & Perez, 1995). Several cultural values shape social relationships for Latinos, especially with those outside the family. Further, there is some agreement that Latinos tend to value familism, machismo, respeto, and interdependence (e.g., Hill, 2009). For each of these ethnic groups, endorsement of these values is associated with parenting strategies (Hill, 2006, 2009).

The premise of a linear relation between SES and adaptive parenting has been challenged (Lareau, 2003; Luthar, 2003), highlighting the ecological fit of particular parenting practices. Numerous attempts have been proposed to explain racial, ethnic, and SES variations in children's development and outcomes and parenting practices, some focusing on the defining role of a developmental niche. Parenting practices and family dynamics, and ultimately children's development, reflect several processes: (1) adaptations to social stratification processes (Garcia Coll et al., 1996); (2) the cohering of parenting practices based on the values and beliefs that are driven by the racial, ethnic, and economic niche in which families find themselves (Lareau, 2003); and (3) proactive parenting to promote attachments to one's ethnic group (Hughes et al., 2008).

Family Dynamics Shaped by Social Stratification

Some ethnic differences in mean levels of parenting practices may be due to research designs that confound ethnicity with lower SES. For example, even though being African American was associated with the use of harsher discipline, this relation was mediated by stress (Pinderhughes et al., 2000). That is, rather than assuming that harsher parenting is endemic to African American culture, we need to recognize that the increased stress potentially associated with racial discrimination, perceptions of reduced opportunities, and lower SES may result in harsher parenting practices (McLoyd, 1998). Further, Pinderhughes et al. (2000) found that ethnicity accounted for only 2% of the variance in discipline, but SES accounted for 26%. SES variations in parenting may be more meaningful than ethnic variations. (See Holden, Vittrup, & Rosen, Chapter 6, this volume.)

Similarly, it may be that lower SES serves to overwhelm and undermine parenting and increase parental mental health problems (Conger et al., 1997; McLoyd, 1998; Shonkoff & Phillips, 2000). The stressors associated with residing in an impoverished, high-risk neighborhood with insufficient economic resources foster harsh, inconsistent, and less warm parenting practices (Conger et al., 1997; Hill & Herman-Stahl, 2002; McLoyd, 1998). Similarly, unemployment, unstable employment, and financial strain are associated with increases in maternal emotional distress, depression, and punitive and harsh parenting (Elder, Eccles, Ardelt, & Lord, 1995). However, the deleterious effect of poverty and stress that undermines parenting is only part of the story. In addition to research emphasizing a linear relation between social stratification and parenting, there is evidence that indicators of social stratification function interactively to create a unique niche for development.

Family Dynamics Shaped by Cultural Niche

Parents' niches, especially job conditions and expectations, shape their parenting beliefs and practices (Kohn, 1969). One goal of parenting is to prepare youth for economic self-sufficiency, and as parents attempt to instill values that will serve their children well on the job market, many look to their own jobs as models of success. Some argue that parenting practices informed by one's job may serve to reproduce one's socio-economic position (Hoff et al., 2002; Kohn, 1969; Lareau, 2003). For example, the communication styles, expectations for control and autonomy, and reward structures experienced by parents at work are similar to those they utilize with their children (Crouter & McHale, 1993; Kohn, 1969; Luster et al., 1989). Further, low-prestige jobs with low autonomy, routine tasks, and little opportunity for complex work diminish parents' cognitive skills, whereas high-prestige positions promote initiative, creative problem solving, critical-thinking skills, and decision-making abilities. Parents bring these experiences to their parenting (Duncan & Magnuson, 2003).

Sociologist Annette Lareau demonstrated this intergenerational perpetuation of social class through her careful study of parenting practices among working and middle-class families (Lareau, 2003). She documented two types of parenting typologies that cohere to potentially reproduce social stratification. The first is called *concerted cultivation* and characterizes middle-class parents. Such parents proactively organize children's curricular and extracurricular activities, use extensive reasoning and negotiations with children that permit children to contest parental decisions, intervene with institutions, and advocate for their children. From these parenting patterns, children develop a sense of entitlement and a comfort level in engaging with adults—skills that will serve them well later in life. In contrast, the working class families engaged in the *accomplishment of natural growth*, which operates from the premise that children's development unfolds naturally with love and care. These parents believe that children are best served by understanding how to deal with authority, by understanding hierarchy and by learning to be self-sufficient through self-organized activities. Such parents provide ample space and opportunity for children to grow and develop, and they emphasize the importance of family by spending leisure time with cousins and extended family. These parents use directives and rarely permit children to question or challenge the parent. In contrast to the middle-class families, these children do not develop a sense of entitlement—they develop a sense of constraint, dependence, and powerlessness (Lareau, 2003). However, unlike their middle-class counterparts, they do learn how to manage their own time.

It might be tempting to criticize working-class parents for not parenting in ways that promote entitlement and the development of confidence in interacting with adults, but other research comparing wealthy and working-class families identified some of the hidden costs of the parenting practices that push children to succeed (Luthar, 2003). Under pressure to achieve, some children feel that their parents' love is conditional—based on their success at school and in extracurricular activities. Compared with children from lower-SES homes, children of wealthy families reported higher levels of depression, self-medicating drug and alcohol abuse, loneliness, and insecurity (Luthar, 2003). Indeed, rather than competing and not succeeding in extracurricular activities, some children feign sickness and injury to remove themselves from the pressures to be the best. Because the identification of these parenting strategies and the potential costs and benefits of such parenting strategies across SES is relatively recent, only longitudinal research that is yet to be done can determine the long-term implications of today's parenting practices, including concerted cultivation.

Most parents are genuinely concerned about the well-being of their children and want to do what is best for them. There are differences in belief systems about how best to reach parenting goals (Luster et al., 1983). Parenting beliefs and practices and the implicit expectations that they promote influence the ways in which children perceive their economic and cultural environment. Therefore, just as children replicate the cultural values of their parents and develop healthy ethnic identities, children often perpetuate the SES identity of their parents (Lareau, 2003; Wilson, 2009). Similarly, parenting practices proactively serve to protect and promote children's attachment and understanding of their ethnic and cultural background.

Family Dynamics to Promote Attachment to Cultural Niche (Ethnic Socialization)

Ethnic socialization is an important goal for parents of ethnic minority youth. Ethnic socialization was the most salient child-rearing goal among African American parents and the least salient among White parents (Hughes et al., 2008). Ethnic and cultural socialization is equally important for Asian and Mexican Americans (Huynh & Fuligni, 2008). The purposes of such socialization include wanting children to acquire knowledge about their ethnic/cultural groups that they can incorporate into their sense of self and preparing ethnic minority children to cope with discriminatory treatment and resisting negative stereotypes. In general there are four types of socialization (Hughes et al., 2006, 2008): (1) *cultural socialization*, which emphasizes cultural knowledge, histories, and values; (2) *preparation for bias*, which includes discussions about stereotypes, prejudice, and discrimination; (3) *egalitarianism*, which focuses on the value of diversity and equal treatment for groups; and (4) *promotion of mistrust*, which creates wariness of other groups and is the least endorsed ethnic socialization message (Hughes & Chen, 1999). However, Chinese American youth received more messages about mistrust than did Mexican or Euro-Americans (Huynh & Fuligni, 2008). In general, ethnic socialization practices buffer the negative effects of racial discrimination and prejudice (Garcia Coll et al., 1996) on youth outcomes (Quintana et al., 2006; Rivas-Drake, Hughes, & Way, 2009; Rodriguez, Umaña-Taylor, Smith, & Johnson, 2009).

Across ethnic groups, African American parents reported preparation for bias as a parenting goal most frequently, followed by Latino and White parents (Hughes et al., 2008). African American parents believed that preparation-for-bias messages were most important. Preparation for bias included conversations about discrimination and how to cope with it and were either proactive (i.e., initiated by the parent) or reactive (i.e., in response to a specific event). Egalitarianism was the second most frequently reported type of ethnic socialization among all ethnic groups, except for Chinese American parents and adolescents, who reported it the least. Parents communicate egalitarian messages by showing openness yet resistance to race as an appropriate category, discussing their strong egalitarian principles, stopping and correcting bias in their children, or exposing youth to individuals from diverse backgrounds.

The amount and content of racial and ethnic socialization messages also vary by SES and neighborhood context (i.e., racial heterogeneity and social disorganization). Middle-class parents report higher levels of cultural socialization than their lower-SES counterparts (Caughy, O'Campo, Randolph, & Nickerson, 2002). In neighborhoods with high levels of ethnic diversity, boys received more messages about how to cope with discrimination and cultural socialization messages than did their female counterparts. However, girls in predominantly African American neighborhoods reported more cultural socialization messages when they had a racism experience (Caughy, Nettles, O'Campo, & Lohrfink, 2006). Part of the ways in which culturally and economically informed parenting practices result in the replication of social stratification and the development of strong, healthy ethnic minority youth is through its ultimate impact on children's personality, mental health, and identity. (See also Weisner, Chapter 15, this volume.)

Level 4: Individual Processes

Race, ethnicity, and SES affect children's social development directly and indirectly through many of the processes outlined already in this chapter. In this final section, we describe ways in which race, ethnicity, and SES get "under the skin" of youth and shape who they become. Race, ethnicity, and SES affect children's and adolescents' behaviors, dispositions, and belief systems and their identity development.

Behaviors, Dispositions, and Belief Systems

If socioeconomic status and social class form ecological and developmental niches for youth, then it can be expected that people will act according to the norms of their niches, which will maintain and perpetuate their class positions (Liu, 2001). SES is associated with several dispositions and belief systems. Lower-SES environments are associated with diminished cognitive functioning, including problem-solving skills and memory (Hoff et al., 2002; Rabbitt, Donlan, Watson, McInnes, & Bent, 1995). Further, lower-SES environments and experiences of discrimination and oppression influence aspects of the personality. Because of greater exposure to violence and aggression and fewer successes in advocacy, people from lower-SES backgrounds tend to make more negative attributions to ambiguous situations (Barefoot et al., 1991; Cunradi, Caetano, Clark, & Schafer, 2000; Wilson, Kirtland, Ainsworth, & Addy, 2004). When racism and classism are internalized, they can result in feelings of frustration and stress (Liu, Soleck, Hopps, Dunston, & Pickett, 2004). Further, prolonged anger, frustration, and stress associated with discrimination and oppression are related to mental and physical health problems (Koskenvuo et al., 1988; Shekele, Vernon, & Ostfeld, 1991). These findings suggest that negative social environments are associated with a negative reactivity style and, in turn, affect social and emotional well-being.

Experiences within one's developmental niche, whether it is defined economically, racially, or ethnically, create knowledge about inequalities, opportunity structures, and stratification that are incorporated into a person's identity and worldview (Liu, 2001). Children's awareness of opportunity structures, stratification, and the differential prestige of occupations shapes their aspirations (Luzzo, 1996). Ethnic minority children are aware of racial and ethnic differences and discrimination, even before they understand their identity (Cross, Parham, & Helms, 1998). Children as young as 6 make attributions of discrimination, and by early adolescence, youth have a clearer understanding of discrimination as it relates to context and self (Brown & Bigler, 2005). Discrimination has detrimental impacts on academic achievement and increases the likelihood of engaging in delinquent behavior by reducing self-esteem and increasing anxiety and depression (Chavous, Rivas-Drake, Smalls, Griffin, & Cogburn, 2008; Seaton, 2009). Racial identity (Sellers, Copeland-Linder, Martin, & Lewis, 2006) and racial socialization (Harris-Britt, Valrie, Kurtz-Costes, & Rowley, 2007; Neblett, Philip, Cogburn, & Sellers, 2006; Rivas-Drake et al., 2009) buffer the effects of discrimination on well-being. All of these experiences shape who children become and how they define themselves.

Identity Development: Ethnic, Racial, and Socioeconomic Worldviews

Group identity is defined as the "part of an individual's self-concept which derives from knowledge of his membership in a social group (or groups) together with the value and emotional significance attached to that membership" (Tajfel, 1981, p. 225). Within this rubric, one's identity is determined by individual status within one's group (ingroup) and by the assessment of others (outgroup). Key to understanding identity are saliency, the extent to which the identity is meaningful; consciousness, the degree to which the individual is aware or conscious of his or her identity; attitudes of significant others (e.g., parents, peers); and one's own attitudes (Liu, 2001; Sellers, Rowley, Chavous, Shelton, & Smith, 1997). For those who want to fit in with their reference groups, each of these components is linked to and influences individuals' behaviors and lifestyles (Liu, 2001). Although there is considerable research on ethnic and racial identity, Liu (2001) argues that much of the research on SES has focused on the individuals' experiences (e.g., class discrimination, opportunities) rather than on cognitive processes associated with one's socioeconomic position. There is little research on SES identity and how it develops and affects behavior—that is, "how people make meaning in and sense of their particular occupation, education, or income rather than how these indices situate them within an objective economic hierarchy" (Liu, 2001, p. 152).

There are several well-developed and empirically grounded theories of ethnic/racial identity development. Although it is beyond the scope of this chapter to review the tenets of each of these theories, their foundations, commonalities, and some uniquenesses are discussed. First is Phinney's (1989) Ethnic Identity Development Model, which presumes to be applicable to all ethnic groups. Among the theories of identity development, the strength of Phinney's theory is its developmental focus and its basis in Erikson's (1968) work. Proposed stages approximate Marcia's (1966) stages of identity development. The four proposed stages have been validated, and individuals either remain stable or move to higher statuses over time (Phinney, 1989; Seaton, Schottham, & Sellers, 2006; see also Rosen & Patterson, Chapter 4, this volume).

The remaining theories are based on Black–White racial identity or Black–African American identity development. Among the extant theories, three are most widely cited and utilized: Cross's Nigrescence Model (Cross & Cross, 2008; Cross, Parham, & Helms, 1991; Cross et al., 1998), Sellers and colleagues' Multidimensional Model of Racial Identity (MMRI; Sellers et al., 1997; Sellers et al., 1998), and the Phenomenological Variant of Ecological Systems Theory (PVEST; Spencer, 1995; Spencer, Dupree, & Hartman, 1997). Each of these models expands and highlights essential features of the identity formation experience and the ways in which identity predicts individuals' social outcomes. Racial awareness (i.e., knowledge of differences between racial groups) is a precursor to racial identity formation. Preschoolers are aware of salient phenotypic characteristics of individuals (e.g., skin color, hair texture; Tatum, 1997). Racial identity develops in the context of neighborhoods, schools, families, and peer relationships and is a multidimensional construct (Stevenson, 1998).

Based in Cross's theory of Nigrescence, racial identity development is catalyzed by an event (encounter) that makes one's racial identity salient—often a discriminatory experience (Cross, 1991). This event sets in motion a series of explorations (immersion) and integrations in additional stages that lead to internalization. The final internalized identity remains relatively stable throughout one's life. Whereas the theory is developmental to the extent that it outlines the unfolding of identity development, it does not link the theory to a particular developmental stage of the individual. Others have integrated it into a developmental framework by outlining how the stages of racial identity manifest themselves at different developmental stages of life (late adolescence/early adulthood, midlife, late adulthood; Parham, 1989). More recently, a lifespan conceptualization of the evolution of Black identity has been incorporated into the original theory that includes the integration and salience of multiple identities and the role of contexts such as peer groups, schools, and neighborhoods (Cross & Cross, 2008; Cross & Fhagen-Smith, 2001).

A second theory fuses the social and racial identity literatures and focuses on attitudes and cognitions associated with the significance and meaning of race as they affect one's self-concept (MMRI; Sellers et al., 1997, 1998). Among its assumptions is that people have multiple identities that are hierarchically arranged and that the salience or hierarchy of any part of the identity is context dependent. Implicitly, the MMRI focuses on individual differences within each dimension at a given point in time rather than on a developmental sequence of transitions from one stage of identity formation to the next (Sellers et al., 1998). Further, the MMRI accounts for both one's own judgment and the evaluation of one's own racial group and identity (i.e., private regard) and the impact of what one believes *others* think of his or her racial group (i.e., public regard). Unique to the MMRI is the multifaceted way in which one's identity is defined, which better reflects the heterogeneous experiences and identity structures of diverse African Americans. These ideologies include nationalist (e.g., emphasizing the unique experience of Blackness, separateness and group solidarity), oppressed minority (e.g., emphasizing the common experiences of oppression and discrimination among minorities), assimilationist (e.g., emphasizing similarities between African American and American society and culture), and humanist (e.g., emphasizing commonalities among all humans). It is not assumed that the individual's orientation or worldview is a singular African American or Black identity.

In the PVEST, identity is defined as "the view minority youth take of themselves with respect to their micro-, meso-, and macro-level environments" (Spencer, Harpalani, & Dell'Angelo, 2002, p. 262). The PVEST takes a broader view of the role of the environment in shaping identity. Identity formation may be influenced by negative stereotypes, lack of positive role models, and the absence of culturally relevant instruction (Spencer & Markstrom-Adams, 1990), which may lead to diminished exploration of different identities and increased conformity (e.g., perpetuation of stereotypes). Identity formation is framed by focusing on resilience and normal development in high-risk contexts and is made up of five components that lie along a continuum from positive, protective, and supportive to negative, risk, and challenging (Spencer, 1995; Spencer et al., 1997). Therefore, PVEST examines social stratification factors related to risk and stress, as well as individual differences in perceptions of risk, stress, and coping mechanisms to explore and explain the mediating processes linked to resilience and vulnerability. Among theories of racial and ethnic identity development, the PVEST is one of the few that accounts for the intersection of racial identity and SES. However, others are beginning to account for an identity based on SES.

Socioeconomic identity development functions in similar ways to ethnic and racial identity. SES is considered an organizing factor that cannot be reduced to particular indicators. This SES-driven organizing factor creates a developmental niche for children and families (DeNavas-Walt, Proctor, & Smith, 2009). As individuals interact with people from similar economic backgrounds, they are socialized into particular belief systems and behavioral styles of the group (in this case, SES group; Kelly & Evans, 1995). Through mutual reinforcement, individuals come to see themselves as prototypical of that SES group. Thus, as individuals are upwardly mobile, they must also cultivate the language and behavioral styles of the higher class group to fit into and be accepted as a member of that economic group (Liu, 2001). Early conceptualizations of an SES-based identity, which included a "cultural" space (culture of poverty), have been criticized for "blaming the victim" for his or her differing outcomes rather than outlining the societal structures that perpetuate intergenerational poverty or wealth. Recent research focuses on socialization and contextual factors that shape behavioral and belief patterns that reflect a socioeconomic identity (Lareau, 2003; Liu, 2001; Luthar, 2003; Wilson, 2009). Further research that outlines the factors that shape a socioeconomic identity and the facets of the identity itself is sorely needed. In addition, research and theory that link ethnic, racial, and cultural identities to socioeconomic identities are virtually absent. Because of the confounding of racial and ethnic minority status with low SES in many studies, we are unable to differentiate the processes associated with an ethnic or cultural identity from adaptations to cope with SES stratification.

FUTURE DIRECTIONS

Whereas much of the research on the effects of social stratification in the United States has examined each construct separately or, at best, attempts to control one while examining another, it is important for the field to more fully examine the intersection of these constructs. For example, to adequately grasp racial and ethnic factors, the field needs to examine race and ethnicity simultaneously among African Americans and Latinos, ethnicity among Whites, and the range of SES within ethnic minority populations. In many studies, race and SES are confounded with a focus on urban, poor African American youth (Hill, 2006). The literature must expand to examine racially, ethnically, and socioeconomically diverse samples from heterogeneous neighborhoods to fully explore the nuanced relationships between individual attributes and neighborhood characteristics. In examining the full range of SES, Massey (2001) suggests that researchers examine neighborhoods along a continuum of poverty and affluence to capture both the normative developmental processes relating neighborhoods to youth social development and the risk trajectories and pathologies associated with neighborhood effects. Further, the PVEST model offers a useful theoretical framework for individuals who wish to explore the complex relations between social stratification variables such as race, ethnicity, and SES within various contexts.

Most theories of normative development do not include diverse samples, and only later are attempts made to be racially, ethnically, and economically inclusive. Given the increasing diversity of the U.S. population, to be relevant from a scientific, representative, and practical stance, these constructs of social stratification must become more central to research on children's social development.

SUGGESTED READINGS

Garcia Coll, C. T., Maberty, G., Jenkins, R., McAdoo, H. P., Crnic, K., Wasik, B., et al. (1996). An integrative model for the study of developmental competencies in minority children. *Child Development, 67,* 1891–1914.

Hill, N. E. (2006). Disentangling ethnicity, socioeconomic status, and parenting: Interactions, influences, and meaning. *Vulnerable Children and Youth Studies, 1*(1), 114–124.

Hoff, E., Laursen, B., & Tardiff, T. (2002). Socioeconomic status and parenting. In M. H. Bornstein (Ed.), *Handbook of parenting* (Vol. 2, pp. 231–252). Mahwah, NJ: Erlbaum.

Lareau, A. (2003). *Unequal childhoods: Class, race and family life.* Berkeley: University of California.

Quintana, S. M., & McKown, C. (2008). Introduction: Race, racism, and the developing child. In S. M. Quintana & C. McKown (Eds.), *Handbook of race, racism, and the developing child* (pp. 1–15). Hoboken, NJ: Wiley.

REFERENCES

Adler, N. E., Epel, E. S., Castellazzo, G., & Ickovics, J. R. (2000). Relationship of subjective and objective social status with psychological and physiological functioning: Preliminary data in healthy white women. *Health Psychology, 19*(6), 586–592.

American Psychological Association Task Force on Socioeconomic Status. (2007). *Report of the APA Task Force on Socioeconomic Status.* Washington DC: American Psychological Association.

Anderson, N. B., & Nickerson, K. J. (2005). Genes, race, and psychology in the genome era: An introduction. *American Psychologist, 60*(1), 5–8.

Argyle, M. (1994). *The psychology of class.* New York: Routledge.

Arnett, J. J. (1995). Broad and narrow socialization: The family in the context of a cultural theory. *Journal of Marriage and the Family, 57,* 617–628.

Barefoot, J. C., Peterson, B. L., Dahlstrom, W. G., Siegler, I. C., Anderson, N. B., & Williams, R. B., Jr. (1991). Hostility patterns and health implications: Correlates of Cook–Medley hostility scale in a national survey. *Health Psychology, 10,* 18–24.

Barnett, R. C., & Gareis, K. C. (2007). Shift work, parenting behaviors, and children's socioemotional well-being: A within-family study. *Journal of Family Issues, 28,* 727–748.

Belsky, J., & Eggebeen, D. (1991). Early and extensive maternal employment and young children's socioemotional development: Children of the National Longitudinal Survey of Youth. *Journal of Marriage and the Family, 53*(4), 1083–1098.

Billingsley, A. (1974). *Black families and the struggle for survival: Teaching our children to walk tall.* New York: Simon & Schuster.

Blacklund, E., Sorlie, P. D., & Johnson, N. J. (1999). A comparison of the relationships of education and nicotine with mortality: The National Longitudinal Mortality Study. *Social Science and Medicine, 49,* 1373–1384.

Bonham, V. L., Warshauer-Baker, E., & Collins, F. S. (2005). Race and ethnicity in the genome era: The complexity of the constructs. *American Psychologist, 60*(1), 9–15.

Boston, T. (1991). Race, class, and political economy: Reflections on an unfinished agenda. In A. Zegeye, L. Harris, & J. Maxted (Eds.), *Exploitation and exclusion: Race and class in contemporary U.S. society* (pp. 142–157). New York: Hans Zell.

Bourdieu, P. (1973). Cultural reproduction and social reproduction. In R. Brown (Ed.), *Knowledge, education, and cultural change* (pp. 56–68). London: Tavistock.

Brody, G. H., & Flor, D. L. (1998). Maternal resources, parenting practices, and child competence in rural, single-parent African American families. *Child Development, 69,* 803–816.

Bronfenbrenner, U., & Morris, P. A. (2006). The bioecological model of human development. In R. M. Lerner (Ed.), *Handbook of child psychology: Vol. 1. Theoretical models of human development* (6th ed., pp. 793–828). Hoboken, NJ: Wiley.

Brooks-Gunn, J., & Duncan, G. J. (1997). The effects of poverty on children. *The Future of Children, 7*(2), 55–71.

Brown, B. S., & Bigler, R. S. (2005). Children's perceptions of discrimination: A developmental model. *Child Development, 76*(3), 533–553.

Brown, C. S. (2008). Children's perceptions of racial and ethnic discrimination: Differences across children and contexts. In S. M. Quintana & C. McKown (Eds.), *Handbook of race, racism, and the developing child* (pp. 133–153). Hoboken, NJ: Wiley.

Cartrite, B. (2003). *Reclaiming their shadow: Ethnopolitical mobilization in consolidated democracies.* Boulder: University of Colorado.

Caughy, M. O. B., Nettles, S. M., O'Campo, P. J., & Lohrfink, K. F. (2006). Neighborhood matters: Racial socialization of African American children. *Child Development, 77*(5), 1220–1236.

Caughy, M. O. B., O'Campo, P. J., Randolph, S. M., & Nickerson, K. (2002). The influence of racial socialization practices on the cognitive and behavioral competence of African American preschoolers. *Child Development, 73*(5), 1611–1625.

Chao, R. K. (1994). Beyond parental control and authoritarian parenting style: Understanding Chinese parenting through the cultural notion of training. *Child Development, 65,* 1111–1119.

Chao, R. K. (1995). Chinese and European-American cultural models of the self reflected in mothers' child-rearing beliefs. *Ethos, 23,* 328–354.

Chao, R. K. (2000). Cultural explanations for the role of parenting in the school success of Asian American children. In R. W. Taylor & M. C. Wang (Eds.), *Resilience across contexts: Family, work, culture, and community* (pp. 333–363). Mahwah, NJ: Erlbaum.

Charles, C. Z. (2003). The dynamics of racial residential segregation. *Annual Review of Sociology, 29,* 167–207.

Chavous, T. M., Rivas-Drake, D., Smalls, C., Griffin, T., & Cogburn, C. (2008). Gender matters, too: The influences of school racial discrimination and racial identity on academic engagement outcomes among African American adolescents. *Developmental Psychology, 44*(3), 637–654.

Conger, R. D., Conger, K. J., & Elder, G. H. (1997). Family and economic hardship and adolescent adjustment: Mediating and moderating processes. In G. J. Duncan & J. Brooks-Gunn (Eds.), *Consequences of growing up poor* (pp. 288–310). New York: Russell Sage Foundation.

Conley, D. (1999). *Being black and living in the red: Race, wealth, and social policy in America.* Berkeley: University of California Press.

Cooper, S. M., McLoyd, V. C., Wood, D., & Hardaway, C. R. (2008). Racial discrimination and the mental health of African American adolescents. In S. M. Quintana & C. McKown (Eds.), *Handbook of race, racism, and the developing child* (pp. 278–312). Hoboken, NJ: Wiley.

Coulton, C. J., Korbin, J. E., Su, M., & Chow, J. (1995). Community level factors and child maltreatment rates. *Child Development, 66*(5), 1262–1276.

Cozzarelli, C., Wilkinson, A. V., & Tagler, M. J. (2001). Attitudes toward the poor and attributions for poverty. *Journal of Social Issues, 57,* 207–228.

Crompton, R. (1993). *Class and stratification: An introduction to current debates.* Cambridge, UK: Polity Press.

Cross, W. E. (1991). *Shades of black: Diversity in African American identity.* Philadelphia: Temple University Press.

Cross, W. E. (2011). The historical relationship between black identity and black achievement motivation. In N. E. Hill, T. L. Mann, & H. E. Fitzgerald (Eds.), *African American children's mental health: Development and context* (pp. 1–27). Santa Barbara, CA: ABC-CLIO Books.

Cross, W. E., & Cross, T. B. (2008). Theory, research, and models. In S. M. Quintana & C. McKown (Eds.), *Handbook of race, racism, and the developing child* (pp. 154–181). Hoboken, NJ: Wiley.

Cross, W. E., & Fhagen-Smith, P. (2001). Patterns of African American identity development: A life span perspective. In C. L. Wijeyesinghe & B. W. Jackson (Eds.), *New perspectives on racial identity development: A theoretical and practical anthology* (pp. 243–270). New York: New York University Press.

Cross, W. E., Parham, T. A., & Helms, J. E. (1991). The stages of black identity development: Nigrescence models. In R. L. Jones (Ed.), *Black psychology* (3rd ed., pp. 319–338). Berkeley, CA: Cobb & Henry.

Cross, W. E., Parham, T. A., & Helms, J. E. (1998). Nigrescence revisited: Theory and research. In R. L. Jones (Ed.), *African American identity development* (pp. 3–71). Hampton, VA: Cobb & Henry.

Crouter, A. C., & McHale, S. M. (1993). Temporal rhythms in family life: Seasonal variation in the relation between parental work and family processes. *Developmental Psychology, 29*(2), 198–205.

Cunradi, C. B., Caetano, R., Clark, C., & Schafer, J. (2000). Neighborhood poverty as a predictor of intimate partner violence among white, black, and Hispanic couples in the United States: A multilevel analysis. *Annals of Epidemiology, 10,* 297–308.

Dahrendorf, R. (1969). On the origins of inequality among men. In A. Beteile (Ed.), *Social inequality: Selected readings* (pp. 16–44). New York and Harmondsworth, UK: Penguin Books.

Davis, K. (1942). A conceptual analysis of stratification. *American Sociological Review, 7,* 309–321.

Davis, K., & Moore, W. E. (1945). Some principles of stratification. *American Sociological Review, 10*(2), 242–249.

DeNavas-Walt, C., Proctor, B. D., & Smith, J. C. (2009). *Income, poverty, and health insurance coverage in the United States, 2008* (No. P60-236). Washington, DC: U.S. Census Bureau.

DuBois, W. E. B. (1990). *The souls of black folk: Essays and sketches.* New York: Vintage. (Original work published 1903)

Duncan, G. J. (1988). The volatility of family income over the life course. In P. B. Baltes, D. L. Featherman, & R. M. Lerner (Eds.), *Lifespan development and behavior* (pp. 317–358). Hillsdale, NJ: Erlbaum.

Duncan, G. J. (1996). Income dynamics and health. *International Journal of Health Services, 26,* 419–444.

Duncan, G. J., & Magnuson, K. A. (2003). Off with Hollingshead: Socioeconomic resources, parenting, and child development. In M. H. Bornstein & R. H. Bradley (Eds.), *Socioeconomic status, parenting, and child development* (pp. 83–106). Mahwah, NJ: Erlbaum.

Elder, G. H., Eccles, J. S., Ardelt, M., & Lord, S. (1995). Inner-city parents under economic pressure: Perspective on the strategies of parenting. *Journal of Marriage and the Family, 57*(3), 771–784.

Entwisle, D., & Astone, N. M. (1994). Some practical guides for measuring youth's race/ethnicity and socioeconomic status. *Child Development, 65,* 1521–1540.

Epps, S. R., & Huston, A. C. (2007). Effects of a poverty intervention policy demonstration on parenting and child behavior: A test of the direction of effects. *Social Science Quarterly, 88,* 344–365.

Erikson, E. H. (1968). *Identity, youth, and crisis.* New York: Norton.

Evans, G. W. (2004). The environment of childhood poverty. *American Psychologist, 59,* 77–92.

Featherman, D. L., & Hauser, R. M. (1976). Prestige or socioeconomic scales in the study of occupational achievement? *Sociological Methods and Research, 4*(4), 403–422.

Featherman, D. L., & Hauser, R. M. (1978). *Opportunity and change.* New York: Academic Press.

Fine, M., & Burns, A. (2003). Class notes: Toward a critical psychology of class and schooling. *Journal of Social Issues, 59,* 841–860.

Fisher, G. M. (1992). The development and history of the poverty thresholds. *Social Security Bulletin, 55*(1), 43–46.

Frable, D. E. S. (1997). Gender, racial, ethnic, sexual, and class identities. *Annual Review of Psychology, 48,* 139–162.

Fuller, B., Caspary, G., Kagan, S. L., Gauthier, C., Huang, D. S.-C., Carroll, J., et al. (2002). Does maternal employment influence poor children's social development? *Early Childhood Quarterly, 17*(4), 470–497.

Furnham, A. (2003). Poverty and wealth. In S. C. Carr & T. S. Sloan (Eds.), *Poverty and psychology: From global perspective to local practice* (pp. 163–183). New York: Kluwer.

Furstenberg, F. F., Belzer, A., Davis, C., Levine, J. A., Morrow, K., & Washington, M. (1993). How families manage risk and opportunity in dangerous neighborhoods. In W. J. Wilson (Ed.), *Sociology and the public agenda* (pp. 231–258). Newbury Park, CA: Sage.

Galambos, N. L., & Lerner, J. (Eds.). (1991). *Employed mothers and their children.* New York: Garland.

Garcia Coll, C. T., Maberty, G., Jenkins, R., McAdoo, H. P., Crnic, K., Wasik, B., et al. (1996). An integrative model for the study of developmental competencies in minority children. *Child Development, 67,* 1891–1914.

Garcia Coll, C. T., Meyer, E., & Brillon, L. (1995). Ethnic and minority parenting. In M. H. Bornstein (Ed.), *Handbook of parenting: Vol. 2. Biology and ecology of parenting* (pp. 189–210). Mahwah, NJ: Erlbaum.

Graham, S., Taylor, A. Z., & Ho, A. Y. (2009). Race and ethnicity in peer relations research. In K. H. Rubin, W. M. Bukowski, & B. Laursen (Eds.), *Handbook of peer interactions, relationships, and groups* (pp. 394–413). New York: Guilford Press.

Greene, M. L., Way, N., & Pahl, K. (2006). Trajectories of perceived adult and peer discrimination among Black, Latino, and Asian American adolescents: Patterns and psychological correlates. *Developmental Psychology, 42*(2), 218–236.

Grundy, E., & Holt, G. (2001). The socioeconomic status of older adults: How should we measure it in studies of health inequalities? *Journal of Epidemiological Community Health, 55,* 895–904.

Hacker, A. (1992). *Two nations: Black and white, separate, hostile, unequal.* New York: Scribner.

Harris-Britt, A., Valrie, C., Kurtz-Costes, B., & Rowley, S. J. (2007). Perceived racial discrimination and self-esteem in African American youth: Racial socialization as a protective factor. *Journal of Research on Adolescence, 17*(4), 669–682.

Harrison, M. S., & Thomas, K. M. (2009). The hidden prejudice in selection: A research investigation on skin color bias. *Journal of Applied Social Psychology, 39*(1), 134–168.

Harrison-Hale, A. O., McLoyd, V. C., & Smedley, B. (2004). Race and ethnic status: Risk and protective processes among African American families. In K. I. Maton, C. J. Schellenbach, B. J. Leadbeater, & A. L. Solarz (Eds.), *Investing in children, youth, families, and communities: Strengths-based research and policy* (pp. 269–283). Washington, DC: American Psychological Association.

Hauser, R. M. (1994). Measuring socioeconomic status in studies of child development. *Child Development, 65,* 1541–1545.

Heaton, T. B. (1987). Objective status and class consciousness. *Social Science Quarterly 68*, 611–620.

Helms, J. E., Jernigan, M., & Mascher, J. (2005). The meaning of race in psychology and how to change it: A methodological perspective. *American Psychologist, 60*(1), 27–36.

Hill, N. E. (2006). Disentangling ethnicity, socioeconomic status, and parenting: Interactions, influences, and meaning. *Vulnerable Children and Youth Studies, 1*(1), 114–124.

Hill, N. E. (2009). Culturally based world views, family processes, and family school interactions. In S. L. Christenson & A. Reschly (Eds.), *The handbook on school–family partnerships for promoting student competence* (pp. 101–127). New York: Routledge.

Hill, N. E. (2011). Undermining partnerships between African-American families and schools: Legacies of discrimination and inequalities. In N. E. Hill, T. L. Mann, & H. E. Fitzgerald (Eds.), *African American Children's mental health: Development and context* (Vol. 1, pp. 199–230). Santa Barbara, CA: Praeger.

Hill, N. E., & Herman-Stahl, M. A. (2002). Neighborhood safety and social involvement: Associations with parenting behaviors and depressive symptoms among African American and Euro-American mothers. *Journal of Family Psychology, 16*(2), 209–219.

Hill, N. E., Murry, V. M., & Anderson, V. D. (2005). Sociocultural contexts of African American Families. In V. C. McLoyd, N. E. Hill, & K. A. Dodge (Eds.), *African American family life: Ecological and cultural diversity* (pp. 21–44). New York: Guilford Press.

Hirschfeld, L. A. (2008). Children's developing conceptions of race. In S. M. Quintana & C. McKown (Eds.), *Handbook of race, racism, and the developing child* (pp. 37–54). Hoboken, NJ: Wiley.

Hoff, E., Laursen, B., & Tardiff, T. (2002). Socioeconomic status and parenting. In M. H. Bornstein (Ed.), *Handbook of parenting* (Vol. 2, pp. 231–252). Mahwah, NJ: Erlbaum.

Hughes, D., & Chen, L. (1999). The nature of parents' race-related communications to children: A developmental perspective. In L. Balter & C. S. Tamis-LeMonda (Eds.), *Child psychology: A handbook of contemporary issues* (pp. 467–490). Philadelphia: Psychology Press.

Hughes, D., Rivas, D., Foust, M., Hagelskamp, C., Gersick, S., & Way, N. (2008). How to catch a moonbeam: A mixed-methods approach to understanding ethnic socialization processes in ethnically diverse families. In S. M. Quintana & C. McKown (Eds.), *Handbook of race, racism, and the developing child* (pp. 226–277). Hoboken, NJ: Wiley.

Hughes, D., Rodriguez, J., Smith, E. P., Johnson, D., Stevenson, H. C., & Spicer, P. (2006). Parents' ethnic socialization: A review of research and directions for future study. *Developmental Psychology, 42*(5), 747–770.

Huynh, V., & Fuligni, A. J. (2008). Ethnic socialization and the academic adjustment of adolescents from Mexican, Chinese, and European backgrounds. *Developmental Psychology, 44*(4), 1202–1208.

Jencks, C., & Mayer, S. (1990). The social consequences of growing up in a poor neighborhood. In L. E. Lynn & M. F. H. McGeary (Eds.), *Inner-city poverty in the United States* (pp. 111–186). Washington, DC: National Academy Press.

Jin, R. L., Shah, C. P., & Svoboda, T. J. (1995). The impact of unemployment on health: A review of the evidence. *Canadian Medical Association Journal, 153*, 529–540.

Jones, F. L., & McMillan, J. (2001). Scoring occupational categories for social research: A review of current practice with Australian examples. *Work, Employment, and Society, 15*(3), 539–563.

Julian, T. W., McKenry, P. C., & McKelvey, M. W. (1994). Cultural variations in parenting: Perceptions of Caucasian, African-American, Hispanic, and Asian American parents. *Family Relations, 43*, 30–37.

Kao, G., & Thompson, J. S. (2003). Racial and ethnic stratification in educational achievement and attainment. *Annual Review of Sociology, 29*, 417–442.

Kelly, J., & Evans, M. D. R. (1995). Class and class conflict in six Western nations. *American Sociological Review, 60*, 157–178.

Kingston, R. S., & Smith, J. P. (1997). Socioeconomic status and racial and ethnic differences in functional status associated with chronic diseases. *American Journal of Public Health, 87*, 805–810.

Kohn, M. L. (1969). *Class and conformity: A study of values.* Homewood, IL: Dorsey.

Koskenvuo, M., Kaprio, J., Rose, R. J., Sesaniemi, A., Sarna, S., & Heikkila, K. (1988). Hostility as a risk factor in mortality and ischemic disease in men. *Psychosomatic Medicine, 50*(4), 330–340.

Krieger, N., Williams, D. R., & Moss, N. E. (1997). Measuring social class in public health research: Concepts, methodologies, and guidelines. *Annual Review of Public Health, 18*, 341–378.

Lareau, A. (2003). *Unequal childhoods: Class, race and family life.* Berkeley: University of California.

Lerner, R. M. (2006). Developmental science, developmental systems, and contemporary theories of human development. In R. M. Lerner (Ed.), *Handbook of child psychology: Vol. 1. Theoretical models of human development* (6th ed., pp. 1–17). Hoboken, NJ: Wiley.

Leventhal, T., & Brooks-Gunn, J. (2000). The neighborhoods they live in: The effects of neighborhood residence on child and adolescent outcomes. *Psychological Bulletin, 126*, 309–337.

Liu, W. M. (2001). Expanding our understanding of multiculturalism: Developing a social class worldview model. In D. B. Pope-Davis & H. L. K. Coleman (Eds.), *The intersection of race, class, and gender in multicultural counseling* (pp. 127–170). Thousand Oaks, CA: Sage.

Liu, W. M., Soleck, G., Hopps, J., Dunston, K., & Pickett, T. (2004). A new framework to understand social class in counseling: The social class worldview and modern classism theory. *Multicultural Counseling and Development, 32*, 95–122.

Luster, T., Rhoades, K., & Haas, B. (1989). The relation between parenting values and parenting behavior: A test of the Kohn hypothesis. *Journal of Marriage and the Family, 51*, 139–147.

Luthar, S. S. (2003). The culture of affluence: Psychological costs of material wealth. *Child Development, 74*, 1581–1593.

Luzzo, D. A. (1996). Exploring the relationship between the perception of occupational barriers and career development. *Journal of Career Development, 22*(4), 239–248.

MacArthur Foundation. (2000). The MacArthur Scale of Subjective Social Status. Retrieved August 2009 from *www.macses.ucsf.edu/research/psychosocial/notebook/subjective.html.*

Marcia, J. E. (1966). Development and validation of ego identity status. *Journal of Personality and Social Psychology, 3*, 551–558.

Marin, G., & Marin, B. V. (1991). *Research with Hispanic populations.* Newbury Park, CA: Sage.

Marmot, M. G., Bosma, H., Hemingway, H., Brunner, E., & Stansfeld, S. (1997). Contribution of job control and other risk factors to social variations in coronary heart disease incidence. *Lancet, 350*, 235–239.

Marx, K. (1967). *Capital: A critique of political economy* (Vol. 1). New York: International.

Massey, D. S. (1990). American apartheid: Segregation and the making of the underclass. *American Journal of Sociology, 96*, 329–357.

Massey, D. S. (2001). Residential segregation and neighborhood conditions in U.S. metropolitan areas. In N. J. Smelser, W. J. Wilson, & F. Mitchell (Eds.), *America becoming: Racial trends and their consequences* (Vol. 1, pp. 391–434). Washington, DC: National Academy Press.

Mather, M. (2007). U.S. racial/ethnic and regional poverty rates converge, but kids are still left behind. Retrieved, May 14, 2010, from *www.prb.org/Articles/2007/USRacialEthnicAndRegionalPoverty.aspx.*

McAdoo, H. P. (Ed.). (2002). *Black children: Social, educational, and parental environments* (2nd ed.). Thousand Oaks, CA: Sage.

McGinnis, M., Williams-Russo, P., & Knickman, J. (2002). The case for more active policy attention to health promotion. *Health Affairs, 2*, 78–93.

McKown, C. (2004). Age and ethnic variation in children's thinking about the nature of racism. *Journal of Applied Developmental Psychology, 25*(5), 597–617.

McLoyd, V. C. (1990). The impact of economic hardship on black families and children: Psychological distress, parenting, and socioemotional development. *Child Development, 61*, 311–346.

McLoyd, V. C. (1998). Socioeconomic disadvantage and child development. *American Psychologist, 53*, 185–204.

Moss, N. (2002). Gender equity and socioeconomic inequality: A framework for the patterning of women's health. *Social Science and Medicine, 45*, 649–661.

Nakao, K., & Treas, J. (1994). Updating occupational prestige and socioeconomic scores: How the new measures measure up. *Sociological Methodology, 24*, 1–72.

National Center for Education Statistics. (2003). *Overview of public elementary and secondary schools and districts: School year 2001–2002.* Retrieved July 12, 2005, from *www.nces.ed.gov/pubs2003/overview03/table_11.asp.*

Neblett, E., Philip, C., Cogburn, C., & Sellers, R. M. (2006). African American adolescents' discrimination experiences and academic achievement: Racial socialization as a cultural compensatory and protective factor. *Journal of Black Psychology, 32*(2), 199–218.

Oakes, J. M., & Rossi, P. H. (2003). The measurement of SES in health research: Current practice and steps toward a new approach. *Social Science and Medicine, 56*, 769–784.

Ogbu, J. (1981). Origins of human competence: A cultural ecological perspective. *Child Development, 52*, 413–429.

Parham, T. A. (1989). Cycles of psychological nigrescence. *The Counseling Psychologist, 17*(2), 187–226.

Phinney, J. S. (1989). Stages of ethnic identity development in minority group adolescents. *Journal of Early Adolescence, 9*, 39–49.

Phinney, J. S. (1996). When we talk about American ethnic groups, what do we mean? *American Psychologist, 51*(9), 918–927.

Pinderhughes, E. E., Dodge, K. A., Bates, J. A., Pettit, G. S., & Zelli, A. (2000). Discipline responses: Influence of parents' socioeconomic status, ethnicity, and beliefs about parenting, stress, and cognitive–emotional processes. *Journal of Family Psychology, 14*(3), 380–400.

Presser, H. B. (2003). *Working in a 24/7 economy: Challenges for American families.* New York: Russell Sage Foundation.

Prillentensky, I. (1997). Values, assumptions, and practices: Assessing the moral implications of psychological discourse and action. *American Psychologist, 52*, 517–535.

Quintana, S. M. (1998). Children's developmental understanding of ethnicity and race. *Applied and Preventive Psychology, 7*, 27–45.

Quintana, S. M. (2008). Racial perspective-taking ability: Developmental, theoretical, and empirical trends. In S. M. Quintana & C. McKown (Eds.), *Handbook of race, racism, and the developing child* (pp. 16–36). Hoboken, NJ: Wiley.

Quintana, S. M., Aboud, F. E., Chao, R. K., Contreras-Grau, J., Cross, W. E., Hudley, C., et al. (2006). Race, ethnicity, and culture in child development: Contemporary research and future directions. *Child Development, 77*(5), 1129–1141.

Quintana, S. M., & McKown, C. (2008). Introduction: Race, racism, and the developing child. In S. M. Quintana & C. McKown (Eds.), *Handbook of race, racism, and the developing child* (pp. 1–15). Hoboken, NJ: Wiley.

Rabbitt, P., Donlan, C., Watson, P., McInnes, L., & Bent, N. (1995). Unique and interactive effects of depression, age, socioeconomic advantage, and gender on cognitive performance of normal healthy older people. *Psychology and Aging, 10*, 307–313.

Risch, N., Burchard, E., Ziv, E., & Tang, H. (2002). Categorization of humans in biomedical research: Genes, race and disease. *Genome Biology, 3*(7). Available at *genomebiology.com/2002/3/comment/2007.*

Rivas-Drake, D., Hughes, D., & Way, N. (2009). Public ethnic regard and perceived socioeconomic stratification: Associations with well-being among Dominican and black American youth. *Journal of Early Adolescence, 29*(1), 122–141.

Rodriguez, J., Umana-Taylor, A., Smith, E. P., & Johnson, D. J. (2009). Cultural processes in parenting and youth outcomes: Examining a model of racial–ethnic socialization and identity in diverse populations. *Cultural Diversity and Ethnic Minority Psychology, 15*(2), 106–111.

Rosenberg, N. A., Pritchard, J. K., Weber, J. L., Cann, H. M., Kidd, K. K., Zhivotovsky, L. A., et al. (2002). Genetic structure of human populations. *Science, 298*(5602), 2381–2385.

Rosenbloom, S. R., & Way, N. (2004). Experiences of discrimination among African American, Asian American, and Latino adolescents in an urban high school. *Youth and Society, 35*(4), 420–451.

Saegert, S., Warren, M. R., & Thompson, J. (2001). *Social capital in poor communities.* New York: Russell Sage Foundation.

Sampson, R. J. (2001). How do communities undergird or undermine human development?: What are the relevant contexts and what mechanisms are at work? In A. Booth & A. Crouter (Eds.), *Does it take a village?: Community effects on children, adolescents, and families* (pp. 3–30). Mahwah, NJ: Erlbaum.

Sampson, R. J., Morenoff, J. D., & Gannon-Rowley, T. (2002). Assessing "neighborhood effects":

Social processes and new directions in research. *Annual Review of Sociology, 28*(1), 443–478.

Sampson, R. J., Raudenbush, S. W., & Earls, F. (1997). Neighborhoods and violent crime: A multilevel study of collective efficacy. *Science, 277*(5328), 918–924.

Seaton, E. K. (2009). Perceived racial discrimination and racial identity profiles among African American adolescents. *Cultural Diversity and Ethnic Minority Psychology, 15*(2), 137–144.

Seaton, E. K., Caldwell, C. H., Sellers, R. M., & Jackson, J. S. (2008). The prevalence of perceived discrimination among African American and Caribbean black youth. *Developmental Psychology, 44*(5), 1288–1297.

Seaton, E. K., Scottham, K. M., & Sellers, R. M. (2006). The status model of racial identity development in African American adolescents: Evidence of structure, trajectories, and well-being. *Child Development, 77*(5), 1416–1426.

Sellers, R. M., Copeland-Linder, N., Martin, P., & Lewis, R. (2006). Racial identity matters: The relationships between racial discrimination and psychological functioning in African American adolescents. *Journal of Research on Adolescence, 16*(2), 187–216.

Sellers, R. M., Rowley, S. A. J., Chavous, T. M., Shelton, J. N., & Smith, M. A. (1997). Multidimensional Inventory of Black Identity: A preliminary investigation of reliability and construct validity. *Journal of Personality and Social Psychology, 73*(4), 805–815.

Sellers, R. M., Shelton, J. N., Cooke, D. Y., Chavous, T. M., Rowley, S. J., & Smith, M. A. (1998). A multidimensional model of racial identity: Assumptions, findings, and future directions. In R. L. Jones (Ed.), *African American identity development* (pp. 275–302). Hampton, VA: Cobb & Henry.

Shapiro, T. (2004). *The hidden costs of being African American: How wealth perpetuates inequality.* New York: Oxford University Press.

Shaw, C. R., & McKay, H. D. (1942). *Juvenile delinquency and urban areas: A study of rates of delinquents in relation to differential characteristics of local communities in American cities.* Chicago: University of Chicago Press.

Shekele, R. B., Vernon, S. W., & Ostfeld, A. M. (1991). Personality and coronary heart disease. *Psychosomatic Medicine, 53*, 179–184.

Shonkoff, J. P., & Phillips, D. A. (Eds.). (2000). *From neurons to neighborhoods: The science of early childhood of education.* Washington, DC: National Academies Press.

Sifers, S. K., Puddy, R. W., Warren, J. S., & Roberts, M. C. (2002). Reporting demographics, methodology and ethical procedures in journals of pediatric and child psychology. *Journal of Pediatric Psychology, 27*(1), 19–25.

Simoni, J. M., & Perez, L. (1995). Latinos and mutual support groups: A case for considering culture. *American Journal of Orthopsychiatry, 65*(3), 440–445.

Singh-Manoux, A., Adler, N. E., & Marmot, M. G. (2003). Subjective social status: Its determinants and its association with measures of ill-health in the Whitehall II study. *Social Science and Medicine, 56*(6), 1321–1333.

Smedley, A., & Smedley, B. (2005). Race as biology is fiction, racism as a social problem is real: Anthropological and historical perspectives on the social construction of race. *American Psychologist, 60*(1), 16–26.

Smith, T. E., & Graham, P. B. (1995). Socioeconomic stratification in family research. *Journal of Marriage and the Family, 57*(4), 930–940.

Sollors, W. (1996). Foreword: Theories of American ethnicity. In W. Sollors (Ed.), *Theories of ethnicity: A classical reader* (pp. x–xliv). New York: New York University Press.

Spencer, M. B. (1995). Old issues and new theorizing about African American youth: A phenomenological variant of ecological systems theory. In R. L. Taylor (Ed.), *African-American youth: Their social and economic status in the United States* (pp. 37–69). Westport, CT: Praeger.

Spencer, M. B., Dupree, D., & Hartman, T. (1997). A phenomenological variant of ecological systems theory (PVEST): A self-organization perspective in context. *Development and Psychopathology, 9*, 817–833.

Spencer, M. B., Harpalani, V., & Dell'Angelo, T. (2002). Structural racism and community health: A theory-driven model for identity intervention. In W. R. Allen, M. B. Spencer, & C. O'Connor (Eds.), *African American education: Race, community, inequality and achievement, A tribute to Edgar G. Epps* (pp. 259–282). Oxford, UK: Elsevier Science.

Spencer, M. B., & Markstrom-Adams, C. (1990). Identity processes among racial and ethnic minorities in American. *Child Development, 61*(2), 290–310.

Stevens, J., Keil, J. E., Rust, P. F., Tyroler, H. A., Davids, C. E., & Gazes, P. C. (1992). Body mass index and body girths as predictors of mortality in black and white women. *Archives of Internal Medicine, 152*(6), 1257–1262.

Stevenson, H. C. (1998). The confluence of the "both–and" in black racial identity theory: Response to Stokes, Murray, Chavez, and Peacock. In R. L. Jones (Ed.), *African American identity* (pp. 151–157). Hampton, VA: Cobb & Henry.

Strazdin, L., Clements, M. S., Korda, R. J., Broom, D. H., & D'Souza, R. M. (2006). Unsocialized work? Nonstandard work schedules, family relationship, and children's wellbeing. *Journal of Marriage and the Family, 68*, 394–410.

Strazdin, L., Korda, R. J., Lim, L. L-Y., Broom, D. H., & D'Souza, R. M. (2004). Around-the-clock: Parent work schedule and children's well-being in a 24-h economy. *Social Science and Medicine, 59*, 1517–1527.

Tajfel, H. (1981). *Human groups and social categories.* Cambridge, UK: Cambridge University Press.

Takaki, R. (1993). *A different mirror: A history of multicultural America.* Boston: Little, Brown.

Turner, J. C., & Oakes, P. J. (1986). The significance of the social identity concept for social psychology with reference to individualism, interactionism and social influence. *British Journal of Social Psychology, 25*, 237–252.

Tatum, B. D. (1997). *"Why are all the Black kids sitting together in the cafeteria?" and other conversations about race.* New York: Basic Books.

Wacquant, L. J. D., & Wilson, W. J. (1993). The cost of racial and class exclusion in the inner city. In W. J. Wilson (Ed.), *The ghetto underclass: Social science perspectives* (pp. 25–42). Newbury Park: Sage.

Ward, L. F. (1883). *Dynamic sociology or applied social science as based upon statistical sociology and less complex sciences.* New York: Appleton.

Wilson, D. K., Kirtland, K. A., Ainsworth, B. E., & Addy, C. L. (2004). Socioeconomic status and perceptions of access and safety for physical activity. *Annals of Behavioral Medicine, 29*, 20–28.

Wilson, W. J. (1987). *The truly disadvantaged: The inner city, the underclass, and public policy.* Chicago: University of Chicago Press.

Wilson, W. J. (1993). The underclass: Issues, perspectives, and public policy. In W. J. Wilson (Ed.), *The ghetto underclass: Social science perspectives* (pp. 1–24). Newbury Park, CA: Sage.

Wilson, W. J. (2003). Race, class, and urban poverty: A rejoiner. *Ethnic and Racial Studies, 26*(6), 1096–1114.

Wilson, W. J. (2009). *More than just race: Being black and poor in the inner city.* New York: Norton.

Zagefka, H. (2009). The concept of ethnicity in social psychological research: Definitional issues. *International Journal of Intercultural Relations, 33*(3), 228–241.

14

Child Care and Schools

Margaret Tresch Owen
Kristen L. Bub

Maria has had the same teacher since she began infant care 4 months
ago. Maria, her teacher Sarah, and her parents have a comfortable set of
rhythms. They know what to expect from each other. Most importantly,
Maria flows with the rhythm of each caregiving day and the predictable
back and forth of interaction (e.g., cooing, caregiving, responding, playing)
with both her parents and Sarah. With all of her loving caregivers, Maria
visibly brightens and responds to their talk and touch.
—RAIKES AND EDWARDS (2009, p. 1)

Adam, the first-grade teacher, bends over a set of connecting blocks with
Kwame. Tears are welling in Kwame's eyes, reflecting the frustration he
feels trying to solve a math problem. Adam reassures Kwame that math
can be hard work and proceeds to "think out loud" with him about how to
solve the problem, regrouping the connecting blocks.
—GALLAGHER AND MAYER (2008, p. 80)

According to the National Scientific Council on the Developing Child (2004),
"Relationships are the 'active ingredients' of the environment's influence on healthy
human development" (p. 1). From this viewpoint, this chapter reviews the research on
the child care and school contexts of children's lives and how they influence children's
development by (1) defining characteristics of caregiver–child and teacher–child interactions that characterize growth-promoting relationships in these contexts, (2) reviewing findings on the effects of child care and school and what they tell us about how
these contexts relate to children's development through relationship experiences with
caregivers, teachers, and peers, and (3) examining the links between home and child
care and home and school via caregiver–parent and teacher–parent relationships.

347

The transition to school was once considered a monumental change in children's lives, as they went from spending the majority of their days at home, typically with their mothers and siblings, to spending many hours at school with their teacher and classmates. Although starting school still represents a new phase in the lives of children and their families, most children today have considerable amounts of out-of-home and away-from-parents experiences before they "leave for school." In 2006, the U.S. Bureau of the Census estimated that 11.3 million children (79%) in the United States younger than 5 years experienced some form of child care. Child care is defined as any form of regular, nonmaternal care, including informal arrangements with relatives, care by a nanny in the child's home, care with a small group of unrelated children in the child-care provider's home, and center-based care, including day care centers, preschool, and early childhood programs. Given the time children spend in school and the large proportion they spend in child care, children's child-care and school experiences constitute important contexts of influence in their lives.

One of the most consistent findings in the developmental literature pertains to the effects of child-care quality on child outcomes (Lamb, 1998). Quality refers to the provision of nurturance and stimulation, which have received much study. We know far less about the specific qualities that support positive development in elementary school, although researchers have posited a variety of explanations, including the quality of the classroom climate and the quality of the teacher–child relationship (Hamre & Pianta, 2005).

Relationship qualities and transactions between caregivers and children, between teachers and children, and between children and their peers are considered proximal features of experience as contrasted with distal features, such as structural characteristics including caregiver-to-child or teacher-to-child ratios, class size and the number of peers, and education and training of caregivers and teachers. Today, researchers interested in the nature of children's experiences attend more to proximal or process-quality features of caregiver–child and teacher–child interactions than they have in the past, although both structural and process features have been found to matter for children's development. Process qualities, which focus on emotional support and content of instruction in caregiver–child and teacher–child interactions, have been shown to relate to a wide array of positive child outcomes across many notable studies of child care, including the Bermuda Study (Phillips, McCartney, & Scarr, 1987), the Chicago Study (Clarke-Stewart, Gruber, & Fitzgerald, 1994), the Child Care and Family Study (Kontos, Howes, Shinn, & Galinsky, 1995), the Cost, Quality, and Outcomes Study (Peisner-Feinberg & Burchinal, 1997), and the National Institute of Child Health and Human Development (NICHD) Study of Early Child Care and Youth Development (SECCYD; NICHD Early Child Care Research Network, 2003b); and school studies, including the National Education Longitudinal Study (Mayer, Mullens, & Moore, 2000), the Early Childhood Longitudinal Study—Kindergarten cohort (Rathbun & West, 2004), and the NICHD SECCYD (NICHD ECCRN, 2005).

In the sections ahead, we first present the general components of an ecological model of development, utilized broadly in most of the recent research on the effects of child-care and school contexts. We describe in this section the issue of selection factors and other features of the family that should be controlled for in studies of the effects of child care and school on children's development, as well as issues in the measurement of quality. Within the child-care-context section we address the effects of child care on parent–child relationships and the effects of relationships in child care on child developmental outcomes, including both caregiver–child and peer relationships.

We also discuss the relationship between parent and child-care provider. Within the school-context section, we address the effects of the teacher–child relationship, the parent–teacher relationship, and peer relationships in school on child developmental outcomes, concluding with a discussion of variations in these relationships as a function of child, family, and teacher characteristics.

AN ECOLOGICAL MODEL

The child-care and school literatures have matured, particularly since an ecological-developmental model has become widely adopted to address the influences of child-care and school contexts. Bronfenbrenner's (1979) ecological model highlights the role of the social context in shaping the development of children and emphasizes the multiple sources of environmental influences and the interconnection of relationships within and across environmental contexts. Such models recognize that families make choices about child care that are influenced by their economic resources and constraints, attitudes and beliefs about child rearing and child care, and child characteristics.

Like early child care research, early school research failed to incorporate an ecological perspective. Although many advances have been made, schools are often still considered the primary factor responsible for student outcomes. Indeed, policymakers have used the results of studies demonstrating that quality matters to argue that schools alone are responsible for student well-being and achievement and that they can protect children from environmental factors that place them at risk for poor outcomes. Yet numerous studies report that in comparison with the home environment, schools have little effect on developmental outcomes in general and on achievement in particular (e.g., Coleman, 1966). Thus researchers have argued that a more holistic approach, such as an ecological approach that considers the multiple individual and environmental factors associated with development, would allow for the identification of specific environments that foster children's positive outcomes, especially among "at-risk" children (Sameroff, Seifer, Barocas, Zax, & Greenspan, 1987).

Selection Factors and the Study of Child Care and School Effects

With the exception of experimental studies of model programs implemented to intervene with children at risk due to poverty, studies of the effects of child-care and school contexts are conducted in naturalistic settings that do not randomly assign children to different types and qualities of experience. This means that studies of child-care and school influences must carefully consider family selection factors when thinking about whether these experiences are related to child outcomes (Burchinal & Nelson, 2000; Duncan & Gibson-Davis, 2006). Studies examining the effects of early child care should disentangle the effects of care from differences among families who make different choices about the amount, as well as the type and quality, of child care used. For example, children from families with more income and higher parental education generally experience higher quality child care (Lamb, 1998; NICHD ECCRN, 1997a). If children in higher quality child care are better prepared to achieve well in school, is it due to their child-care experience or to advantages they experience at home? Similarly, the quality of the school a child attends may be influenced by family characteristics. For example, parents may choose a longer commute to work in order to purchase or rent a home in a particular school district that is thought to be of high quality. Poorer quality schools tend to be found in poorer neighborhoods, and parents' choices or lack of choice about where they reside will factor into attributions we can make about school effects (Foster & McLanahan, 1996). Family decisions about child care and schools may also be influenced by characteristics of the child. For example, girls tend to be in higher quality child care than boys (NICHD ECCRN, 1996), and children with poorer academic skills tend to be in higher quality classrooms, marked by high levels of teacher sensitivity, than children with better academic skills (Murnane, Willett, Bub, & McCartney, 2006). Child temperament can also play a role. Do children who are more difficult to care for receive poorer quality child care or develop more conflicted relationships with their caregivers and teachers? Child characteristics may directly influence the quality of caregiver–child and teacher–child interactions the child experiences.

From an ecological-developmental perspective it is recognized that effects of child care and school are nested within experiences that derive from many sources. Thus analyses of the effects of child care or school qualities that do not take into account family and child characteristics will result in potential misattributions or biased estimates of associations.

Measuring Qualities of Caregiver–Child and Teacher–Child Relationships That Matter

The measure of child-care quality developed for the SECCYD, the Observational Record of the Caregiving Environment (ORCE; NICHD ECCRN, 1996, 2000), was based on the assumption that care experiences can differ for individual children within the same classroom or setting. A setting-wide measure that captures the availability of age-appropriate materials or teacher-led learning activities is more typical in studies of child care (e.g., The Early Childhood Environment Rating Scale; Harms & Clifford, 1980). Measures of child-care quality that are individualized for the child can more accurately capture the quality of the child's experiences, compared with measures that are taken at the level of the classroom or home setting (Burchinal & Nelson, 2000), but such measures are influenced by individual child characteristics, making it more difficult to discern effects attributable to child care per se. For example, a child with greater language skills is more likely to initiate verbal contact with a caregiver and to elicit stimulation from teachers than a child who has poorer language skills. Measures that assess classroom quality in the school setting have also focused on classroom-wide features rather than on the experiences of individual children. The Classroom Assessment Scoring System (CLASS; La Paro & Pianta, 2003) is a modified version of the ORCE developed to assess individual children's experience in three critical domains: classroom emotional support, classroom organization, and classroom instructional support. Each domain addresses effective interactions between students and teachers that are known to contribute to students' school success.

CHILD CARE

A large literature on the effects of child care reveals both positive and negative associations with children's outcomes (see Lamb & Ahnert, 2006). Overall, the findings indicate positive effects of good quality care, as measured by both structural features and caregiver–child interactions, for cognitive and social outcomes; both positive and negative effects of center-based care; and negative effects linking greater quantity of care with child problem behaviors. It is important to note that the effects are generally modest and that parenting qualities typically have stronger and more consistent effects on child outcomes, even for children who experience large quantities of child care (NICHD ECCRN, 2006). In this section we describe the effects of child care on children's relationships with their mothers and discuss findings pertaining to positive and negative effects of caregiver relationships and peer relationships in child care. In addition, research on the relationship between child-care providers and parents are reviewed.

Child–Care Experiences and the Parent–Child Relationship

Given the importance attributed to maternal care in cultural ideals and psychological theories (McCartney & Phillips, 1988) and the employment of the majority of mothers with very young children, there has been widespread concern and controversy about effects of nonmaternal child care for young children, especially when begun during infancy (e.g., Ahnert, Pinquart, & Lamb, 2006; Belsky, 1986). One argument put forth has been that because of the need for parents to have sufficient time with their children to be able to engage in sensitive, stimulating care and to form close and warm relationships (Belsky, 1999; Jaeger & Weinraub, 1990; Sroufe, 1988), extensive child care could lead to developmental difficulties.

Such arguments and conclusions regarding developmental risk from child care were first made by Belsky (1986) based on a review of results linking extensive nonmaternal child care with a higher probability of insecure infant–mother attachment, coupled with linkages between more hours of child care and child behavior problems. This was followed by additional studies that found increased proportions of insecure infant–mother attachments among children with extensive nonparental care compared with children with limited child-care experience (Belsky & Rovine, 1988; Clarke-Stewart, 1989).

Deficiencies in the prevalent research from this time, however, precluded definitive conclusions. Studies' deficiencies included (1) the lack of an ecological approach incorporating characteristics of families associated with child-care usage, (2) lack of study of parenting influences on attachment, and (3) no measures of other features of child-care experience other than its quantity, namely, the quality of care, age of entry, and continuity of care experience. Another voiced criticism was that differences between attachments of children experiencing extensive child care and those without nonmaternal care might have been inflated because meta-analyses were generally based on published studies and did not include unpublished studies that were less likely to have found significant associations with child care (Roggman, Langlois, Hubbs-Tait, & Rieser-Danner, 1994). This controversy and the need to address questions about the effects of early child care within an ecological framework that measured children's experiences both in child care and in the home was largely the impetus for the government-initiated NICHD SECCYD, the largest, most extensive longitudinal study conducted in the United States on the effects of child care. The SECCYD recruited a large and diverse sample of 1,364 children and their families shortly after the children's births and included extensive measurement of child-care, family, and school experiences, together with a wide array of child outcomes. To date, the study has followed the children through age 15.

Child Care and Parenting Sensitivity

The more hours children spend in child care, the less time parents spend with their children (Flouri & Buchanan, 2003; Goldberg, Greenberger, & Nagel, 1996); but the hypothesized link to diminished parental sensitivity has not been confirmed. Analyses of maternal time-use data indicate that mothers of infants who spent more than 30 hours a week in child care spent 32% less time with their infants than mothers of infants not in child care, but they were not less sensitive in their interactions with their infants (Booth, Clarke-Stewart, Vandell, McCartney, & Owen, 2002). Other reports from the SECCYD have shown that more hours of child care are associated with less sensitive and engaged mother–child interactions, after controlling for multiple family, maternal, and child factors related to child-care features and maternal sensitivity (NICHD ECCRN, 1999; 2003b), but only for Caucasian children; for nonwhite children, more hours of care were associated with more sensitive parenting. Maternal depressive symptoms and income also moderated associations between child-care quantity and mother–child interaction (NICHD ECCRN, 1999). Thus, time in child care appears to hold somewhat different relationships with mother–child interactions, depending on certain characteristics of the mother and child.

Higher quality child-care experience, however, was consistently associated with slightly more sensitive and engaged mother–child interactions from early infancy through first grade in longitudinal analyses that accounted for variations related to multiple features of child-care and family and child characteristics (NICHD ECCRN, 2003b). What processes might link the quality of child care with sensitive, engaged mother–child interactions? The findings could stem from unmeasured selection factors, in that more sensitive mothers may choose child-care arrangements with similarly more engaged and stimulating child-care providers (i.e. higher quality). Alternatively, higher quality interactions between caregiver and child may serve as a model of more sensitive care for the mother and help to enhance her own positive interactions with her child—an effect of relationships on relationships. It may also be the case that children with greater competencies stemming from higher quality relationships in child care are easier interactive partners, engage more positively with their parents, and evoke more sensitive parenting (NICHD ECCRN, 1999).

Child Care and Infant–Mother Attachment

The SECCYD has been considered the most thorough investigation to date of the effects of child care on infant–mother attachment, despite limitations that include a sample that is not nationally representative, its size, and the possibility that the poorest quality child-care arrangements were likely not sampled, particularly at the youngest ages. Contrary to the meta-analytic findings based on earlier studies that examined effects of child care without adequately controlling for family selection effects or child-care quality, the SECCYD found that the amount, age of entry, quality, and stability of child care were unrelated to the security of infant–mother attachments, except when mothers provided less sensitive care to their children (NICHD ECCRN, 1997b). For infants whose mothers provided less sensitive parenting, extended experience with child care, lower quality child care, and more changes in child-care arrangements were each associated with an increased likelihood of developing insecure attachments with their mothers. Moreover, the strongest predictor of attachment security, regardless of children's experiences with child care, was the sensitivity of a mother's caregiving with her infant (namely positive regard for her infant, responsiveness, and lack of intrusiveness or hostility), suggesting that it is the quality of mother–child interactions rather than maternal absence or child-care experiences per se that determine the quality of attachment. Attachment security with the mother at age 3 was similarly compromised with greater amounts of child care for children with less sensitive mothers, but not for children who experienced sensitive parenting with their mothers (NICHD ECCRN, 2001; see also Roisman & Groh, Chapter 5, this volume).

Results from a large longitudinal study, conducted in Israel and paralleling the SECCYD in study design, have qualified the conclusions drawn from the SECCYD on child care and attachment. It should be noted that child care in Israel is provided by the state, and its quality is less confounded with socioeconomic status than is care in the United States. Children's experiences with very low-quality center care with large caregiver–child ratios were associated with an increased rate of insecure infant–mother attachment, regardless of the sensitivity of the mothers' care of their infants (Aviezer & Sagi-Schwartz, 2008). Children from the Israeli sample who received child care in family care settings or who received kibbutz home sleeping—both care types that likely supported closer caregiving relationships than did the poor-quality centers—were more likely to be securely attached to their mothers. However, similar to findings from the SECCYD, children with both less sensitive mothers and low-quality child care were most at risk for insecure attachments to their mothers. Thus the findings from Israel augment those reported by the SECCYD. The Israeli findings indicate that the quality of caregiver–child interactions in child care matter for children's attachment relationships with their mothers. The two studies together also suggest that secure child–mother attachments are not compromised by child care when caregiving in the care arrangement is of sufficient quality, although a threshold for "sufficient" has not been established.

Quality of the Child's Attachment to Caregivers in Child Care

The quality of the caregiver–child relationship in child care can also be described in terms of attachment security. From Ainsworth's (1967) early observations of the development of attachment relationships, it has been noted that children develop attachment relationships with those who become familiar to them and provide them with care. Given the time that children spend with child-care providers at very young ages, it makes sense that caregivers can serve as nonparental attachment figures for the child. The sensitivity of child-care providers' interactions with children in their care predicts the security of child–caregiver attachment in various types of child-care settings (Howes & Smith, 1995). Meta-analyses indicate that in child-care centers, secure child–caregiver attachments are predicted by warmth and sensitive caregiving that monitors the individual child's needs and the needs of the larger group (Ahnert et al., 2006). Compelling evidence for causal relationships between the quality of care and attachment security with care providers comes from an increase in the prevalence of secure attachments to caregivers following changes in Florida child-care state licensing policy that required fewer children per caregiver; there was also evidence of more complex play with peers and objects, greater adaptive language proficiency, and fewer problem behaviors of anxiety and hyperactivity (Howes et al., 1996).

Is a secure attachment to the child-care provider beneficial for the child's development? There are relatively few studies that address associations of attachment security with child-care providers and child outcomes (see review by Howes & Spieker, 2008), but several are suggestive of its importance and the processes involved. Longitudinal studies from Israel and the United States suggest that social competence with peers in early childhood is better predicted by the security of attachment to the child-care provider than by attachment to parents (Howes, Matheson, & Hamilton, 1994; Oppenheim, Sagi, & Lamb, 1988), perhaps reflecting the importance of caregiver support in the child-care context for developing interpersonal skills with peers in that context. In addition, early attachment security with child-care providers was found to predict the quality of teacher–child relationships in school better than early attachment security with mothers (Howes, Hamilton, & Phillipsen, 1998). Other studies, however, have found that attachment security scores based on a network of relationships with mother, father, and caregiver best predicted peer behavior in toddlerhood (Howes, Rodning, Galluzzo, & Myers, 1988) and general social competence (van IJzendoorn, Sagi, & Lambermon, 1992).

Given that children form attachments with their caregivers in child care, what is the effect of the many changes in caregiving relationships that typically occur in children's child-care arrangements across early childhood? For example, over 36% of children in the SECCYD experienced changes in primary child-care providers in their first year (NICHD ECCRN, 1997b). Howes and Hamilton (1993) found that 44% of children from ages 1 to 4 experienced three to four changes in caregivers, and only 12% experienced only a single change. Changes are due to center care practices of age segregation in classrooms, necessitating moves to new classrooms; parents starting and stopping care arrangements; changes in parents' work schedules and jobs; and high rates of caregiver turnover (an average 43%) in child-care centers (Whitebook, Howes, & Phillips, 1998). Changes in care matter. Howes and Hamilton (1993) found that children with more changes in caregivers had more difficulties with peer relations, but children whose relationships with their caregivers changed in a positive direction had more positive relationships with their peers and were less withdrawn and aggressive (Howes & Hamilton, 1993). Changes in caregivers also occur for many children whose parents cobble together multiple arrangements to cover their child-care needs. Children who experienced increasing numbers of care arrangements across the week had associated increases in behavior problems and decreases in prosocial behavior (Morrissey, 2009). These effects were more evident among girls and when the children were younger.

Child Care and Externalizing Behavior Problems: Processes of Influence from the Perspective of Relationships with Caregivers and Peers

Negative effects of child care have been found in associations between more hours of early child care and externalizing problems, such as assertive, disobedient, and aggressive behaviors (Bates et al., 1994; Loeb, Bridges, Bassok, Fuller, & Rumberger, 2007; Magnuson, Meyers, Ruhm, & Waldfogel, 2004). In the SECCYD this association was found at 24 months (NICHD ECCRN, 1998) and at 54 months and in kindergarten (NICHD ECCRN, 2003a). A recent reanalysis of the SECCYD data using longitudinal modeling of associations between child-care experiences and externalizing behavior replicated the earlier cross-sectional findings, with associations found at 24 and 54 months but not at 36 months (McCartney et al., 2010). This study was able to provide greater understanding of this negative effect of child-care experience from the perspective of relationships in child care. Child-care hours were more strongly related to externalizing behavior when children were in lower quality child care and when children spent a greater proportion of time with a group of peers that was larger in size than recommended by experts.

These findings suggest that the processes involved in negative associations between the amount of child care and externalizing problems include the children's quality of relationships with their caregivers and peers in those settings. Thus children who experienced more hours of care with caregivers who were less responsive and more detached and who provided less cognitive stimulation and less encouragement of exploration had more behavior problems than children who experienced more hours but higher quality care. The link with more hours of care in settings with many children can be understood from observations of such care settings. In settings with many children, children get less individual attention from adults (Blatchford, 2003), developmentally appropriate activities are less common, and caregivers are less sensitive and engage in more negative discipline (Howes et al., 1996). In addition, when more children are in the group, children tend to wander aimlessly and not engage with their peers in a positive fashion (Ruopp, Travers, Glantz, & Coelen, 1979; Vandell & Powers, 1983), and conflict and aggression among peers is more likely (Smith, McMillan, Kennedy, & Ratcliffe, 1989; Smith & Connolly, 1980). Caregivers are less likely to intervene in peer interactions in ways that help children become autonomous in negotiating successful interactions (Kemple, David & Hysmith, 1998). The importance of peer relationships in child care has also been highlighted by the findings that poor relations with peers in child care are associated with stress, as indicated by elevated cortisol in the children (Vermeer & van IJzendoorn, 2006).

Differential Susceptibility to Child Care: Child Temperament, Child Gender, and Poverty

The effects of child-care experiences and relationships in child care may depend on individual characteristics of children, such as temperamental qualities and gender, and on characteristics of the family, such as socioeconomic status. For example, longer hours in child care or more changes in care may be harmful for children with certain temperamental characteristics but beneficial or benign for others. Further, child-care quality may be more strongly associated with child outcomes for children with difficult temperaments and negative emotionality (Belsky, 1997; Bradley & Corwyn, 2008; Pluess & Belsky, 2009). Such effects were shown using data from the SECCYD: Lower quality child care was linked with more behavior problems, and higher quality care experience was related to fewer behavior problems, particularly among children with negative emotionality (Pluess & Belsky, 2009).

Boys have been considered to be at greater risk than girls in many developmental processes, including child care (Bornstein, Hahn, Gist, & Haynes, 2006; Desai, Chase-Lansdale, & Michael, 1989). Despite some support for this thesis, gender differences in the effects of child care have not been widespread, nor have they been consistent when found.

Differential susceptibility to the quality of caregiving in child care due to poverty has also been hypothesized, with high quality mattering more for children living in poverty who have fewer enriching experiences in their homes (Caughy, DiPietro, & Strobino, 1994). Positive results of high-quality child care for low-income children in experimental studies have supported this view, but the results are based on intensive early childhood programs, not community-based programs (Campbell & Ramey,

1994; Lazar & Darlington, 1982; Schweinhart, Weikart, & Larner, 1986). Nevertheless, several studies have reported larger effects of child-care quality in community-based programs for children from families with lower socioeconomic status (e.g., Baydar & Brooks-Gunn, 1991; Bryant, Burchinal, Lau, & Sparling, 1994). Others have failed to find more beneficial effects of higher quality child care for poor children. For example, contrary to the hypothesis that the quality of care mattered more for low-income children, Burchinal, Peisner-Feinberg, Bryant, and Clifford (2000) found that higher quality care, characterized by more appropriate and growth-promoting caregiving experiences, was associated with better development for children from all economic backgrounds.

Child Care and the Caregiver–Parent Partnership

The relationship between parent and child-care provider has become known as a "partnership," reflecting the widely acknowledged importance of positive connections between home and child care for healthy child development. This assumption has a strong theoretical basis in Bronfenbrenner's ecological theory, which hypothesizes that development is enhanced when linkages across developmental contexts are strong and demands on the child are compatible. Although efforts to increase parents' involvement in their children's day care are emphasized in the accreditation criteria of the National Association for the Education of Young Children (Ritchie & Willer, 2008) and in many articles oriented toward practitioners, research on the caregiver–parent relationship is relatively sparse. Research on parents' involvement in school is much more prevalent, as reviewed in the section on schools in this chapter.

Observational and interview studies have noted that parents and child-care providers typically spend little time together and exchange information about the child primarily during dropoff or pickup times, if at all (Endsley & Minish, 1991; Powell, 1989). Despite the general brevity of parent–caregiver contact, parents with more education and less authoritarian child-rearing beliefs do seek and share more information (Kontos & Wells, 1986; Owen, Ware, & Barfoot, 2000). Caregiver–parent communication, particularly concerning the behavior and experiences of the child, is a means of linking the home and child-care contexts and enriching the caregiver's and parent's supportive and sensitive care of the child (Powell, 1989). Supporting this contention, more communication between mother and caregiver about the child was related both to more positive caregiver–child interactions in child care and to more positive mother–child interactions (Owen et al., 2000).

Long-Term Effects of Child Care

The study of child care is also stimulated by interest in how early experiences in general may shape development over time. Most studies have focused on contemporaneous associations or have examined child-care effects over relatively short periods of time. Longer term outcomes, however, are beginning to emerge, and findings suggest that higher quality child care has lasting benefits in better academic and cognitive functioning that extend now through middle childhood and adolescence (Belsky et al., 2007; Campbell, Ramey, Pungello, Sparling, & Miller-Johnson, 2002; Peisner-Feinberg et al., 2001; Vandell, Belsky, Burchinal, Steinberg, Vandergrift, and the NICHD ECCRN, 2010). Higher achievement appears to be promoted by better preparation for school and greater school-readiness skills (Dearing, McCartney, & Taylor, 2009).

In addition, children who experience better relationships with their child-care providers subsequently have better relationships with their teachers in school (see the next section). Yet the positive effects of higher quality child care are often difficult to maintain, especially for ethnic-minority and low-income children. For example, Currie and Thomas (2000) reported that the effects of Head Start on standardized test scores fade out more rapidly among African American children than among other children, in part because they are more likely to attend lower quality elementary schools.

Recent provocative findings have linked lower waking cortisol levels in adolescence, an indicator of stress, to having had more center-based child-care experience and to lower maternal sensitivity in early childhood (Roisman et al., 2009). Given the findings linking center-based care with behavior problems, connections between center-based care and lower cortisol in adolescence are consistent with the theory that early interpersonal stressors result in down-regulation of basal cortisol levels (Susman, 2006; see also Carver & Tully, Chapter 2, this volume).

SCHOOL CONTEXT

The effect of schools and classrooms on children's academic achievement has been a central focus of education research for some time. An extensive body of work finds higher achievement test scores among children who attend better schools and classrooms (Betts, 1995; Rivkin, Hanushek, & Kain, 2005). More recently, however, children's sense of social relatedness in school has become a central focus in studies of academic success (Eccles, Wigfield, & Schiefele, 1998). Indeed, research has begun to focus on the type and quality of interactions (e.g., teacher–child, parent–teacher, and peer) that children experience in these settings as a predictor of both *social* and *academic* outcomes. A great deal of work has examined the role that positive teacher–child relationships, marked by high levels of closeness and low levels of conflict, as well as teacher sensitivity and responsivity, play in promoting children's social and academic development (Birch & Ladd, 1997; Hamre & Pianta, 2001). Others have focused on the role that the parent–teacher partnership, marked by active participation in a child's learning and positive parent–teacher relationships, plays in children's social and academic adjustment (Henderson & Mapp, 2002; Hill & Craft, 2003). Still others have focused on the role that peers at school play in children's adjustment (Buhs & Ladd, 2001; Gest, Welsh, & Domitrovich, 2005; Ladd, 1999) .

In the section that follows, we review the research concerning the effects of key relationships in school on children's social and academic development. In particular, we focus on the teacher–child relationship, the parent–teacher relationship, and the peer relationship.

School and the Teacher–Child Relationship

Children learn most effectively through positive social interactions with their teachers and peers (e.g., Landry, Smith, Swank, & Loncar, 2000). Not surprisingly, then, positive teacher–child relationships are increasingly recognized as essential for promoting social and academic outcomes (Bub, 2009; Hamre & Pianta, 2005). Positive teacher–child relationships are typically marked by high levels of closeness and low levels of conflict. More specifically, relationship quality tends to be high when children and teachers share a mutual sense of respect and when children perceive their teachers as trustworthy; in contrast, relationship quality tends to be low when interactions are discordant and there is little or no rapport between children and teachers (Pianta, 1999). High-quality teacher–child relationships contribute to the development of emotion regulation, social skills, and emotion understanding in young children and improve student learning (Birch & Ladd, 1998; Greenberg, Speltz, & Deklyen, 1993). Low-quality relationships diminish students' frustration tolerance, increase self-reported loneliness, and lower their work habits and school attendance (Birch & Ladd, 1997).

Attachment theory provides a useful framework for understanding the teacher–child relationship (Pianta, Nimetz, & Bennett, 1997). Attachment theory suggests that children develop internal working models through their early interactions with parents that then provide a foundation for future social interactions (Bowlby, 1983). Children appear to apply their parent–child relationship models to other supportive relationships, including those with their teachers (Thompson, 1999). Indeed, research suggests that the mother–child attachment relationship is associated with the quality of children's teacher–child relationships (O'Connor & McCartney, 2006), although it has been noted in early childhood that these relationships may be independent of each other (see earlier in the chapter). Children form models of effective and supportive teacher–child relationships that they then carry with them throughout elementary school (Howes, Phillipsen, & Peisner-Feinberg, 2000). These models are not based solely on early qualities of parent–child relationships but are influenced as well by children's relationships with their child-care providers. For example, a longitudinal study of children found that children formed relationships with their kindergarten teachers that were similar in quality and style to those with their preschool teachers (Howes et al., 2000).

In general, children who have higher quality relationships with their teachers exhibit better social and cognitive skills than do their peers with lower quality relationships (Birch & Ladd, 1997; Hamre & Pianta, 2001). For example, children who experience positive teacher–child relationships are rated by teachers as being more self-directed and as liking school more (Birch & Ladd, 1997). The positive effects of these relationships persist over time; this is especially true for positive effects on social competence, grade retention, achievement, and referrals to special education (Birch & Ladd, 1997, 1998; Hamre & Pianta, 2001). Furthermore, improvements in the teacher–child relationship over time are associated with better teacher–child relationships in subsequent grades (Pianta & Nimetz, 1991). In contrast, negative teacher–child relationships have detrimental effects on children's outcomes. Birch and Ladd (1997) found that dependency and conflict were strong negative predictors of school attitudes and liking, school engagement, and academic performance. Similarly, Pianta, Steinberg, and Rollins (1995) found that negative teacher–child relationships were associated with higher levels of problem behavior and lower levels of social competence in kindergarten.

High-quality teacher–child relationships may be particularly important for children at risk for social and academic difficulties. African American children who had high-quality relationships with their teachers gained more reading and receptive language skills between preschool and second grade than did European American children or children with low-quality relationships (Burchinal, Peisner-Feinberg, Pianta, & Howes, 2002). Moreover, positive teacher–child relationships in elementary school were found to buffer the negative effects of insecure parent–child attachments in early childhood on social and academic outcomes (O'Connor & McCartney, 2006).

We know very little, however, about how teachers foster these positive relationships, especially with challenging children. Importantly, the bulk of prior research in this area has focused on the contributions that children make to the student–teacher relationship through their classroom behaviors. Comparatively little attention has focused on teachers' emotional responses to children's behaviors or their awareness that their responses contribute to relationships and effectiveness with students (Sutton, Mudrey-Camino, & Knight, 2006). Yet teachers play a central role in shaping children's formal learning environments (Eccles & Roeser, 1999). Teachers who deal with children whose behaviors in the classroom are disruptive, demanding, or difficult to manage are subject to emotional distress and burnout (Raver et al., 2008). This emotional negativity challenges teachers' ability to behave with the warmth, support, and sensitivity that have consistently been linked to healthy child development.

School and the Parent–Teacher Partnership

There is considerable evidence that good schools, skilled teachers, and strong curricula are necessary but not sufficient to promote positive development among young children. A growing body of research suggests that the parent–teacher partnership, including parental involvement and positive parent–teacher relationships, is a powerful way to promote young children's adjustment throughout elementary school and beyond (Adelman & Taylor, 2000). Successful parent–teacher partnerships attend to families' interests and needs, engage in dialogue with families, tap families' local knowledge, and provide parents with leadership opportunities (Hemmeter, Ostrosky, & Fox, 2006). When parents and school staff collaborate and communicate, parents feel that their role is honored, and they gain a better understanding of what is expected of their children in school. As a result, they develop a caring and trusting relationship with school staff and are more likely to be involved in their children's educations. When the parent–teacher partnership works, children tend to receive consistent messages at home and school about acceptable social and academic behaviors, which foster positive developmental outcomes across multiple domains (Epstein, 1987).

Practices such as volunteering in the classroom, attending school events, and supporting learning at home, as well as parent–teacher relationships characterized by trust, open communication, and shared expectations, all confer benefits for children's learning and development (Fantuzzo, McWayne, & Bulotsky, 2003; Foster, Lambert, Abbott-Shim, McCarty, & Franze, 2005). These benefits include higher grades, better school attendance, higher graduation rates, and more positive attitudes about school (Henderson & Mapp, 2002). In addition, children whose parents are more involved in their schooling tend to have fewer behavioral problems, better academic performance, and better attendance; they enroll in more challenging academic programs; and they are more likely to complete secondary school than their peers whose parents are less involved (Henderson & Mapp, 2002). Better parent–teacher relationships are also associated with better socioemotional adjustment of children (Izzo, Weissberg, Kasprow, & Fendrich, 1999). In contrast, low parental involvement is associated with lower academic success, including lower grades and poorer classroom behavior (Miedel & Reynolds, 1999).

Parents' early contacts with the school system provide a critical opportunity to "set the stage" for the parent–teacher relationship throughout elementary school and beyond. These contacts help families develop habits and expectations regarding their children's educational experiences that set the stage for positive and sustained parental involvement throughout a child's academic career. Indeed, children who experience successful parent–teacher partnerships demonstrate gains in social and academic competencies over time (Hill & Craft, 2003). For instance, parental involvement in the Chicago Child–Parent Centers program during early childhood was associated with more parent involvement in the elementary school years, which in turn was related to positive youth outcomes in high school (Ou, 2005). Increases in parental school involvement over time have also been found to be associated with decreases in children's antisocial behavior and increases in their academic achievement over time (Jimerson, Egeland, & Teo, 1999). Yet the vast majority of studies examining the parent–teacher partnership indicate that parental involvement in school decreases as children get older. This is likely due, in part, to the fact that there are more opportunities for involvement at younger than at older ages (Dauber & Epstein, 1993). In addition to decreasing involvement, the quality of the parent–teacher relationship also appears to decline over time (Izzo et al., 1999).

School and Peer Relationships

As children age, the importance of peer groups and social networks increases, and the importance of relationships with teachers diminishes (Furman, 1989; Wentzel, 1993). Indeed, positive peer relationships in school are associated with more prosocial behaviors, greater school liking, higher motivation, and better achievement, whereas negative peer relations in school are generally associated with more antisocial behavior, aggression, and academic underachievement (Buhs & Ladd, 2001; Ladd, 1999). This shift is driven, in part, by the structure and organization of elementary schools. Children's desks are often arranged in small groups, and much of their schoolwork is group-based. Importantly, compared with child-care providers in early childhood, elementary school teachers spend far less time engaged in one-on-one interactions and more time in teacher-directed, group-based lessons. As a result, the school context becomes a social setting in which peers play a central role in daily interactions and learning. School-age children rely far less on adult direction and support to meet their needs than do preschool children.

Domains of peer relationships within the school context include friendship, social relatedness, peer acceptance or rejection, and popularity. *Friendship* is typically described as a dyadic interaction with a mutually agreed-on individual (Parker & Asher, 1987). *Social relatedness* refers to an individual's connectedness to specific social partners and is marked by feelings of support or loneliness (Furrer & Skinner, 2003). *Peer acceptance* is described as an individual's likability or positive regard within his or her peer group and thus is generally considered a group-based construct (Coie & Dodge, 1983). *Popularity* is a group-based construct that reflects the recognition among peers that an individual has achieved a high social status, but it does not necessarily reflect likability (Adler, Kless, & Adler, 1992).

Strong empirical evidence suggests that positive peer relationships in the school context are associated with better outcomes across a wide range of domains. For example, children who spend more time with peers with good emotional and behavioral regulation skills learn similar skills (Fabes, Hanish, & Martin, 2003). As a result, teachers tend to spend less time on behavior management and more time on task with these children. Importantly, children who have friends at school are more sociable and self-confident and exhibit fewer antisocial behaviors than peers without school friendships (Newcomb & Bagwell, 1995). Indeed, having at least one friend in school is positively related to grades, school liking, and school engagement (Wentzel & Caldwell,

1997). Thus peer groups provide an important context in which children learn the self-regulation and socialization skills necessary in more formal school settings. Children's social relatedness and peer acceptance also predict behavioral adjustment and academic achievement. More specifically, children who reported a greater sense of belonging within the school context demonstrated more school motivation and engagement than their peers who reported more loneliness (Coie, 1990). Similarly, children who were more accepted by their peers had higher achievement and motivation (Wentzel, 1991). Negative peer relationships have been associated with poorer adjustment in school. Researchers have posited that peer rejection actually interferes with the development of positive adjustment among young children (Parker & Asher, 1987), but the associations are likely reciprocal. Socially withdrawn and more aggressive children typically experience high levels of peer rejection and thus have fewer opportunities to collaborate with their peers on classroom activities (Ladd, Birch, & Buhs, 1999). Children's relations with their peers provide an important support for academic success and help to promote positive attitudes toward school. As a result children who are rejected by their peers are at greater risk of academic failure (Ladd et al., 1999).

Interestingly, popularity at school has been found to be associated with more aggressive behaviors and with engagement in risky behaviors, especially during adolescence (Estell, Cairns, Farmer, & Cairns, 2002). For example, popularity was positively correlated with aggression and school absences and negatively correlated with grade-point average once peer acceptance was taken into account (Schwartz, Gorman, Nakamoto, & McKay, 2006). Children who are considered popular by their peers but who also exhibit aggressive behaviors are often referred to as "aggressive popular" children (Estell, Farmer, Pearl, Van Acker, & Rodkin, 2003). Because aggression typically requires peer support in order to be maintained, aggressive popular children tend to be in classrooms with behaviorally difficult peers (Stormshak et al., 1999). The result is that teachers spend more time managing behaviors in the classroom and less time on instruction and learning.

Differential Effects of Salient Relationships: Child and Family Factors

The direct effects of student–teacher, parent–teacher, and peer relationships in school on the development of children's social and academic outcomes have been well established. More recent research has begun to examine differences in these relationships by particular child and family characteristics. With respect to the quality of the teacher–child relationship, teachers tend to report less positive relationships with boys and with African American children, as well as with children with disabilities (Murray & Greenberg, 2001; Saft & Pianta, 2001). Children from families with fewer economic resources also tend to have lower quality relationships with their teachers than do their more advantaged peers (Birch & Ladd, 1997). This is due, in part, to differences in social and academic school readiness that present different needs for the teacher's attention. Parental involvement also appears to be particularly important for children from less advantaged backgrounds. Children from low-SES families whose parents were more involved in their children's learning demonstrated higher-than-average achievement scores (Jimerson et al., 1999).

Children's adjustment appears to be a particularly strong predictor of the quality of the teacher relationship. For example, teachers of more aggressive and disruptive children report having a more conflictual relationship with these children than with other children (Birch & Ladd, 1998; Howes et al., 2000). Similarly, children who are more socially withdrawn appear to experience less closeness with their teachers than less socially withdrawn children (Buyse, Verschueren, Doumen, Van Damme, & Maes, 2008). Teachers often underestimate the intelligence of socially withdrawn children and fail to recognize the competencies of aggressive children (Rimm-Kaufman et al., 2002). As a result, they tend to provide difficult children with less instruction and less positive feedback (Arnold, 1997; Rimm-Kaufman, Pianta, & Cox, 2000), which leads to poorer teacher–child relationships over time.

Teacher characteristics, including education and experience, as well as the teacher–child racial–ethnic "match," have also been found to be associated with the quality of the student–teacher relationship. For example, more educated teachers report more positive relationships with their students than teachers with less education (Hearns, 1998). Interestingly, teachers with fewer years of experience tend to have more positive relationships with children (Stuhlman & Pianta, 2002). In addition, teachers and children with the same racial–ethnic background demonstrated more positive teacher–child interactions and relationships than teachers and children with different racial–ethnic backgrounds (Saft & Pianta, 2001). Researchers have posited that this occurs because teachers are more attuned to children of the same ethnic or racial background and thus better able to interpret their behaviors.

A somewhat less extensive body of work has shown that parent–teacher partnerships vary by a wide variety of child and family demographics, including gender, race–ethnicity, income, and education. Teachers report poorer quality parent–teacher interactions among parents of boys than among parents of girls (Izzo et al., 1999). African American and Latino families tend to be less involved in the school and experience less positive relationships with their children's teachers (Boethel, 2003). Additionally, positive parent–teacher relations appear to be less common among low-income and less educated families than among families with greater economic resources or more education (Entwistle & Alexander, 1988). There is also evidence to suggest that parental involvement is lower among urban than suburban or rural parents (Reynolds, Weissberg, & Kasprow, 1992).

Finally, a small body of work demonstrates that the effects of peer relationships in schools differ by child and family characteristics, though most of this research comes from studies of adolescents. For example, Schwartz and colleagues (2006) found that increases in popularity among peer groups in school were associated with increases in school absences and decreases in grade-point averages among highly aggressive individuals but not among those who were not aggressive. Gender differences in peer relationships among younger children within the school and classroom contexts appear such that interactions in girls' peer groups are more cooperative than interactions in boys' peer groups, which tend to be more arousing (Fabes et al., 2003). As such, girls are exposed to cooperative and regulated interactions at school earlier and more frequently than are boys.

PRESSING RESEARCH QUESTIONS
FOR CHILD-CARE AND SCHOOL CONTEXTS

From an ecological systems approach, studies of the child-care and school contexts of development have evolved to become rich studies of the nature and influences of children's early experiences and how experiences both inside and outside the home interact to influence children's development. Child care is no longer treated as an isolated entity that can be studied without considering features of the child's home experiences and also individual characteristics of the child that help to shape the child's experiences across child-care and home contexts. There is also growing recognition that features and qualities of child-care and school experiences may have differential influences on child outcomes depending on individual child characteristics and on past and current relationships with caregivers and peers. Many questions remain, however, about what characteristics of the child, concurrent home experiences, or history of experiences lead to greater susceptibility or diminished susceptibility to child-care and school experiences. Does a quality relationship with a nonmaternal caregiver or teacher in school matter more for some children than for others? Does poor-quality child care harm some children more than others? Answers to such questions can lead to a greater understanding of developmental processes and provide guidance for parents as they arrange child care best suited for their child and involve themselves in their children's school experiences.

Evidence clearly suggests that the caregiver–child and teacher–child relationships are important for positive development, but we know little about how those relationships are formed or about what aspects are important for which outcomes. Importantly, we know almost nothing about the role that teacher characteristics play in the development of this relationship. Thus studies focusing on the proximal processes within the classroom—and especially on the teacher–child relationship—are needed.

Although there is growing recognition that schools cannot—and should not—be solely responsible for producing child outcomes, more research is needed that uses an ecological contexts approach to understand development across multiple systems, including the home, child care, school, neighborhood, and so forth. Greater attention to the role of selection factors in determining child outcomes is necessary if we are to obtain the unbiased estimates of association needed to create policy and change practice. These selection factors must extend beyond family characteristics to include child and neighborhood characteristics as well.

Finally, if we are going to effectively meet our children's developmental needs across a wide range of outcomes and contexts, efforts are needed to develop training and professional development programs for child-care providers and teachers that emphasize children's socioemotional competencies and programs that foster partnerships with parents across these important relationship contexts for children. The generation of a common language across contexts will enhance children's developmental outcomes by providing consistency across the many settings children experience daily.

ACKNOWLEDGMENTS

Preparation of this chapter was supported by Grant Nos. R03-HD057351 (Margaret Tresch Owen, Principal Investigator) and 5U10HD027040-18 (Deborah Lowe Vandell, Principal Investigator) from the National Institute of Health and Human Development.

SUGGESTED READINGS

Ahnert, L., Pinquart, M., & Lamb, M. E. (2006). Security of children's relationships with nonparental care providers: A meta-analysis. *Child Development, 77,* 664–679.

Henderson, A.T., & Mapp, K. L. (2002). *A new wave of evidence: The impact of school, family, and community connections on student achievement: Annual synthesis 2002.* Austin, TX: Southeast Educational Development Laboratory, National Center for Family and Community Connections with Schools.

Ladd, G., Birch, S., & Buhs, E. (1999). Children's social and scholastic lives in kindergarten: Related spheres of influence? *Child Development, 70,* 1373–1400.

Love, J. M., Harrison, L., Sagi-Schwartz, A., van IJzendoorn, M. H, Ross, C., Ungerer, J. A., et al. (2003). Child care quality matters: How conclusions may vary with context. *Child Development, 74,* 1021–1033.

NICHD Early Child Care Research Network. (1997). The effects of infant child care on infant–mother attachment security: Results of the NICHD Study of Early Child Care. *Child Development, 68,* 860–879.

Pianta, R.C. (1992). Conceptual and methodological issues in research on relationships between children and nonparental adults. In R. Pianta (Ed.), *Beyond the parent: The role of other adults in children's lives* (pp. 121–129). San Francisco: Jossey-Bass.

REFERENCES

Adelman, H., & Taylor, L. (2000). Moving prevention from the fringes into the fabric of school improvement. *Journal of Educational and Psychological Consultation, 11,* 7–26.

Adler, P. A., Kless, S. J., & Adler, P. (1992). Socialization to gender roles: Popularity among elementary school boys and girls. *Sociology of Education, 65,* 169–187.

Ahnert, L., Pinquart, M., & Lamb, M. E. (2006). Security of children's relationships with nonparental care providers: A meta-analysis. *Child Development, 77,* 664–679.

Ainsworth, M. D. S. (1967). *Infancy in Uganda: Infant care and the growth of attachment.* Baltimore, MD: Johns Hopkins Press.

Arnold, D. H. (1997). Co-occurrence of externalizing behavior problems and emergent academic difficulties in high-risk boys: A preliminary evaluation of patterns and mechanisms. *Applied Developmental Psychology, 18,* 317–330.

Aviezer, O., & Sagi-Schwartz, A. (2008). Attachment and non-maternal care: Towards contextualizing the quantity vs. quality debate. *Attachment and Human Development, 10,* 275–285.

Bates, J., Marvinney, D., Kelly, T., Dodge, K., Bennett, R., & Pettit, G. (1994). Child care history and kindergarten adjustment. *Developmental Psychology, 30,* 690–700.

Baydar, N., & Brooks-Gunn, J. (1991). Effects of maternal employment and child care arrangements on preschoolers' cognitive and behavioral outcomes: Evidence from the National Longitudinal Survey of Youth. *Developmental Psychology, 27,* 932–945.

Belsky, J. (1986). Infant day care: A cause for concern? *Zero to Three, 6,* 1–9.

Belsky, J. (1997). Variation in susceptibility to rearing influences: An evolutionary argument. *Psychological Inquiry, 8,* 182–186.

Belsky, J. (1999). Quantity of nonmaternal care and boys' problem behavior/adjustment at 3 and 5: Exploring the meditating role of parenting. *Psychiatry: Interpersonal and Biological Processes, 62,* 1–21.

Belsky, J., & Rovine, M. (1988). Nonmaternal care in the first year of life and the security of infant–parent attachment. *Child Development, 59,* 157–167.

Belsky, J., Vandell, D. L., Burchinal, M., Clarke-Stewart, K. A., McCartney, K., Owen, M. T., et al. (2007). Are there long-term effects of early child care? *Child Development, 78,* 681–701.

Betts, J. R. (1995). Does school quality matter?: Evidence from the National Longitudinal Survey of Youth. *Review of Economics and Statistics, 77,* 231–247.

Birch, S. H., & Ladd, G. W. (1997). The teacher–child relationship and children's early school adjustment. *Journal of School Psychology, 35,* 61–79.

Birch, S. H., & Ladd, G. W. (1998). Children's interpersonal behaviors and the teacher–child relationship. *Developmental Psychology, 34,* 934–946.

Blatchford, P. (2003). A systematic observational study of teachers' and pupils' behavior in large and small classes. *Learning and Instruction, 13,* 569–595.

Boethel, M. (2003). *Diversity: School, family and community connections: Annual synthesis, 2003.*

Austin, TX: Southwest Educational Development Laboratory, National Center for Family and Community Connections with Schools.

Booth, C. L., Clarke-Stewart, K. A., Vandell, D. L., McCartney, K., & Owen, M. T. (2002). Child care usage and mother–infant "quality time." *Journal of Marriage and the Family, 64,* 16–26.

Bornstein, M. H., Hahn, C., Gist, N. F., & Haynes, O. M. (2006). Long-term cumulative effects of childcare on children's mental development and socioemotional adjustment in a nonrisk sample: The moderating effects of gender. *Early Child Development and Care, 176,* 129–156.

Bowlby, J. (1983). *Attachment and loss: Vol. 1. Attachment.* New York: Basic Books. (Original work published 1969).

Bradley, R. H., & Corwyn, R. F. (2008). Infant temperament, parenting, and externalizing behavior in first grade: A test of the differential susceptibility hypothesis. *Journal of Child Psychology and Psychiatry, 49,* 124–131.

Bronfenbrenner, U. (1979). Contexts of child rearing: Problems and prospects. *American Psychologist, 34,* 844–850.

Bryant, D. M., Burchinal, M., Lau, L. B., & Sparling, J. J. (1994). Family and classroom correlates of Head Start children's developmental outcomes. *Early Childhood Research Quarterly, 9,* 289–309.

Bub, K. L. (2009). Testing the effects of classroom supports on changes in children's social and behavioral skills using latent growth curve modeling. *Applied Developmental Science, 13,* 130–148.

Buhs, E. S., & Ladd, G. W. (2001). Peer rejection as an antecedent of young children's school adjustment: An examination of mediating processes. *Developmental Psychology, 37,* 550–560.

Burchinal, M. R., & Nelson, L. (2000). Family selection and child care experiences: Implications for studies of child outcomes. *Early Childhood Research Quarterly, 15,* 385–411.

Burchinal, M. R., Peisner-Feinberg, E., Bryant, D. M., & Clifford, R. (2000). Children's social and cognitive development and child-care quality: Testing for differential associations related to poverty, gender, or ethnicity. *Applied Developmental Science, 4,* 149–165.

Burchinal, M. R., Peisner-Feinberg, E., Pianta, R.C., & Howes, C. (2002). Development of academic skills from preschool through second grade: Family and classroom predictors of developmental trajectories. *Journal of School Psychology, 40,* 415–436.

Buyse, E., Verschueren, K., Doumen, S., Van Damme, J., & Maes, F. (2008). Classroom problem behavior and teacher–child relationships in kindergarten: The moderating role of classroom climate. *Journal of School Psychology, 46,* 367–391.

Campbell, F., & Ramey, C. T. (1994). Effects of early intervention on intellectual and academic achievement: A follow-up study of children from low-income families. *Child Development, 65,* 684–698.

Campbell, F. A., Ramey, C. T., Pungello, E. P., Sparling, J., & Miller-Johnson, S. (2002). Early childhood education: Young adult outcomes from the Abecedarian Project. *Applied Developmental Science, 6,* 42–57.

Caughy, M. O., DiPietro, J. A., & Strobino, D. M. (1994). Day-care participation as a protective factor in the cognitive development of low-income children. *Child Development, 65,* 457–471.

Clarke-Stewart, K. A. (1989). Infant day care: Maligned or malignant? *American Psychologist, 44,* 266–273.

Clarke-Stewart, K. A., Gruber, I. C., & Fitzgerald, L. M. (1994). *Children at home and in day care.* Hillsdale, NJ: Erlbaum.

Coie, J. D. (1990). Toward a theory of peer rejection. In S.R. Asher (Ed.), *Peer rejection in childhood* (pp. 365–401). Cambridge, UK: Cambridge University Press.

Coie, J. D., & Dodge, K. A. (1983). Continuities and changes in children's social status: A five-year study. *Merrill–Palmer Quarterly, 29,* 261–282.

Coleman, J. S. (1966). *Equality of educational opportunity.* Washington, DC: Office of Education, National Center for Educational Statistics.

Currie, J., & Thomas, D. (2000). School quality and the longer-term effects of Head Start. *Journal of Human Resources, 34,* 755–774.

Dauber, S. L., & Epstein, J. L. (1993). Parents' attitudes and practices of involvement in inner-city elementary and middle schools. In N.F. Chavkin (Ed.), *Families and schools in a pluralistic society* (pp. 53–72). Albany: State University of New York Press.

Dearing, E., McCartney, K., & Taylor, B. A. (2009). Does higher quality early child care promote low-income children's math and reading achievement in middle childhood? *Child Development, 80,* 1329–1349.

Desai, S. P., Chase-Lansdale, P. L., & Michael, R. (1989). Mother or market? The effect of maternal employment on the intellectual ability of four-year-old children. *Demography, 26,* 545–561.

Duncan, G. J., & Gibson-Davis, C. (2006). Connecting child care quality to child outcomes: Drawing policy lessons from nonexperimental data. *Evaluation Review, 30,* 611–630.

Eccles, J. S., & Roeser, R. W. (1999). School and community influences on human development. In M. H. Bornstein & M. E. Lamb (Eds.), *Developmental psychology: An advanced textbook* (4th ed., pp. 503–554). Hillsdale, NJ: Erlbaum.

Eccles, J. S., Wigfield, A., & Schiefele, U. (1998). Motivation to succeed. In W. Damon (Series Ed.) & N. Eisenberg (Vol. Ed.), *Handbook of child psychology: Vol. 4. Social and personality development* (pp. 1017–1095). New York: Wiley.

Endsley, R. C., & Minish, P. A. (1991). Parent–staff communication in day care centers during morning and afternoon transitions. *Early Childhood Research Quarterly, 6,* 119–135.

Entwisle, D. R., & Alexander, K. L. (1988). Factors affecting achievement test scores and marks of black and white first graders. *Elementary School Journal, 88,* 449–471.

Epstein, J. L. (1987). Toward a theory of family–school connections: Teacher practices and parent involvement. In K. Hurrelmann, F. Kaufmann, & F. Losel (Eds.), *Social intervention: Potential and constraints* (pp. 121–136). New York: DeGruyter.

Estell, D. B., Cairns, R. B., Farmer, T. W., & Cairns, B. D. (2002). Aggression in inner-city early elementary classrooms: Individual and peer group configurations. *Merrill–Palmer Quarterly, 48,* 52–76.

Estell, D. B., Farmer, T. W., Pearl, R., Van Acker, R., & Rodkin, P. C. (2003). Heterogeneity in the relationship between popularity and aggression: Individual, group, and classroom influences. *New Directions for Child and Adolescent Development, 101,* 75–85.

Fabes, R. A., Hanish, L. D., & Martin, C. L. (2003). Children at play: The role of peers in understanding the effects of child care. *Child Development, 74,* 1039–1043.

Fantuzzo, J., McWayne, C., & Bulotsky, R. (2003). Forging strategic partnerships to advance mental health science for vulnerable children. *School Psychology Review, 32*(1), 17–37.

Flouri, E., & Buchanan, A. (2003). What predicts fathers' involvement with their children? A prospective study of intact families. *British Journal of Developmental Psychology, 21,* 81–98.

Foster, E. M., & McLanahan, S. (1996). An illustration of the use of instrumental variables: Do neighborhood conditions affect a young person's chance of finishing high school? *Psychological Methods, 1*(3), 249–260.

Foster, M., Lambert, R., Abbott-Shim, M., McCarty, F., & Franze, S. (2005). A model of home learning environment and social risk factors in relation to children's emergent literacy and social outcomes. *Early Childhood Research Quarterly, 20,* 13–36.

Furman, W. (1989). The development of children's social networks. In D. Belle (Ed.), *Children's social networks and social supports* (pp. 151–172). New York: Wiley.

Furrer, C., & Skinner, E. (2003). Sense of relatedness as a factor in children's academic engagement and performance. *Journal of Educational Psychology, 95,* 148–162.

Gallagher, K. C., & Mayer, K. (2008). Enhancing development and learning through teacher–child relationships. *Young Children, 63,* 80–87.

Gest, S. D., Welsh, J. A., & Domitrovich, C. E. (2005). Behavioral predictors of changes in social relatedness and liking school in elementary school. *Journal of School Psychology, 43,* 281–301.

Goldberg, W. A., Greenberger, E., & Nagel, S. K. (1996). Employment and achievement: Mothers' work involvement in relation to children's achievement behaviors and mothers' parent behaviors. *Child Development, 67,* 1512–1527.

Greenberg, M. T., Speltz, M. L., & Deklyen, M. (1993). The role of attachment in the early development of disruptive behavior problems. *Development and Psychopathology, 5,* 191–213.

Hamre, B. K., & Pianta, R. C. (2001). Early teacher–child relationships and the trajectory of children's school outcomes through eighth grade. *Child Development, 72,* 625–638.

Hamre, B. K., & Pianta, R. C. (2005). Can instructional and emotional support in the first-grade classroom make a difference for children at risk of school failure? *Child Development, 76,* 949–967.

Harms, T., & Clifford, R. M. (1980). *Early Childhood Environment Rating Scale*. New York: Teachers College Press.

Hearns, S. (1998). Is child-related training or general education a better predictor of good quality care? *Early Child Development and Care, 141,* 31–39.

Hemmeter, L. L., Ostrosky, M., & Fox, L. (2006). Social and emotional foundations for early learning: A conceptual model for intervention. *School Psychology Reviews, 35*(4), 583–601.

Henderson, A. T., & Mapp, K. L. (2002). *A new wave of evidence: The impact of school, family, and community connections on student achievement. Annual synthesis 2002.* Austin, TX: Southeast Educational Development Laboratory, National Center for Family and Community Connections with Schools.

Hill, N. E., & Craft, S. A. (2003). Parent–school involvement and school performance: Mediated pathways among socioeconomically comparable African American and Euro-American families. *Journal of Educational Psychology, 95,* 74–83.

Howes, C., Galinsky, E., Shinn, M., Gulcur, L., Clements, M., Sibley, A., et al. (1996). *The Florida child care quality improvement study.* New York: Families and Work Institute.

Howes, C., & Hamilton, C. E. (1993). The changing experience of child care: Changes in teachers and in teacher–child relationships and children's social competence with peers. *Early Childhood Research Quarterly, 8,* 15–32.

Howes, C., Hamilton, C. E., & Phillipsen, L. C. (1998). Stability and continuity of child–caregiver and child–peer relationships. *Child Development, 69,* 418–426.

Howes, C., Matheson, C. C., & Hamilton, C. E. (1994). Maternal, teacher, and child care history correlates of children's relationships with peers. *Child Development, 55,* 257–273.

Howes, C., Phillipsen, L.C., & Peisner-Feinberg, E. (2000). The consistency of perceived teacher–child relationships between preschool and kindergarten. *Journal of School Psychology, 38,* 113–132.

Howes, C., Rodning, C., Galluzzo, D. C., & Myers, L. (1988). Attachment and child care: Relationships with mother and caregiver. *Early Childhood Research Quarterly, 3,* 703–715.

Howes, C., & Smith, E. W. (1995). Children and their child-care caregivers: Profiles of relationships. *Social Development, 15,* 574–590.

Howes, C., & Spieker, S. (2008). Attachment relationships in the context of multiple caregivers. In J. Cassidy & P. R. Shaver (Eds.), *Handbook of attachment* (2nd ed., pp. 313–332). New York: Guilford Press.

Izzo, C. V., Weissberg, R. P., Kasprow, W. J., & Fendrich, M. (1999). A longitudinal assessment of teacher perceptions of parent involvement in children's education and performance. *American Journal of Community Psychology, 27,* 817–839.

Jaeger, E., & Weinraub, M. (1990). Early nonmaternal care and infant attachment: In search of process. *New Directions for Child Development, 49,* 71–90.

Jimerson, S., Egeland, B., & Teo, A. (1999). A longitudinal study of achievement trajectories: Factors associated with change. *Journal of Educational Psychology, 91,* 116–126.

Kemple, K. M., David, G. M., & Hysmith, C. (1998). Teachers' interventions in preschool and kindergarten children's peer interactions *Journal of Research in Childhood Education, 12,* 34–47.

Kontos, S., Howes, C., Shinn, M., & Galinsky, E. (1995). *Quality in family child care and relative care.* New York: Teachers College Press.

Kontos, S., & Wells, W. (1986). Attitudes of caregivers and the day care experiences of families. *Early Childhood Research Quarterly, 1,* 47–67.

La Paro, K. M., & Pianta, R. C. (2003). *CLASS: Classroom Assessment Scoring System.* Charlottesville: University of Virginia.

Ladd, G. W. (1999). Peer relationships and social competence during early and middle childhood. *Annual Review of Psychology, 50,* 333–339.

Ladd, G., Birch, S., & Buhs, E. (1999). Children's social and scholastic lives in kindergarten: Related spheres of influence? *Child Development, 70,* 1373–1400.

Lamb, M. E. (1998). Nonparental child care: Context, quality, correlates, and consequences. In I. Sigel & K. Renniger (Eds.), *Handbook of child psychology: Vol. 4. Child psychology in practice* (5th ed., pp. 73–134). New York: Wiley.

Lamb, M. E., & Ahnert, L. (2006). Nonparental child care: Context, concepts, correlates, and consequences. In W. Damon, R. M. Lerner, K. A. Renninger, & I. E. Sigel (Eds.), *Handbook of child psychology: Vol. 4. Child psychology in practice* (6th ed., pp. 950–1016). New York: Wiley.

Landry, S. H., Smith, K. E., Swank, P. R., & Loncar, C. L. (2000). Early maternal and child influences on children's later independent cognitive and social functioning. *Child Development, 71,* 358–375.

Lazar, I., & Darlington, R. (1982). Lasting effects of early education: A report from the Consortium for Longitudinal Studies. *Monographs of the Society for Research in Child Development, 47*(2–3, Serial No. 195).

Loeb, S., Bridges, M., Bassok, D., Fuller, B., & Rumberger, R. W. (2007). How much is too much?: The influence of preschool centers on children's social and cognitive development. *Economics of Education Review, 26,* 52–66.

Magnuson, K., Meyers, M., Ruhm, C., & Waldfogel, J. (2004). Inequality in preschool education and school readiness. *American Educational Research Journal, 41,* 115–157.

Mayer, D. P., Mullens, J. E., & Moore, M. T. (2000). *Monitoring school quality: An indicators report* (NCES 2001-030). Washington, DC: National Center for Education Statistics.

McCartney, K., Burchinal, P., Clarke-Stewart, A., Bub, K. L., Owen, M. T., Belsky, J., et al. (2010). Testing a series of causal propositions relating time spent in child care to children's externalizing behavior. *Developmental Psychology, 46,* 1–17.

McCartney, K., & Phillips, D. (1988). Motherhood and child care. In B. Birns & D. F. Hays (Eds.), *The different faces of motherhood: Perspectives in developmental psychology* (pp. 157–183). New York: Plenum Press.

Miedel, W. T., & Reynolds, A. J. (1999). Parent involvement in early intervention for disadvantaged children: Does it matter? *Journal of School Psychology 37,* 379–402.

Morrissey, T. W. (2009) Multiple child-care arrangements and young children's behavioral outcomes. *Child Development, 80,* 59–76.

Murnane, R. J., Willett, J. B., Bub, K. L., & McCartney, K. M. (2006). Understanding trends in the black-white achievement gaps during the first years of school. In G. Burtless & J. Rothenberg Pack (Eds.), *Brookings-Wharton papers on urban affairs: 2006* (pp. 97–127). Washington, DC: Brookings Institution Press.

Murray, C., & Greenberg, M. T. (2001). Relationships with teachers and bonds with school: Social-emotional adjustment correlates for children with and without disabilities. *Psychology in the Schools, 38,* 24–41.

National Scientific Council on the Developing Child. (2004). Young children develop in an environment of relationships (Working Paper No. 1). Retrieved September 14, 2009, from *www. developingchild.harvard.edu.*

Newcomb, A. F., & Bagwell, C. L. (1995). Children's friendship relations: A meta-analytic review. *Psychological Bulletin, 117,* 306–347.

NICHD Early Child Care Research Network. (1996). Characteristics of infant child care: Factors contributing to positive caregiving. *Early Childhood Research Quarterly, 11,* 269–306.

NICHD Early Child Care Research Network. (1997a). Familial factors associated with characteristics of nonmaternal care for infants. *Journal of Marriage and the Family, 59,* 389–408.

NICHD Early Child Care Research Network. (1997b). The effects of infant child care on infant–mother attachment security: Results of the NICHD Study of Early Child Care. *Child Development, 68,* 860–879.

NICHD Early Child Care Research Network. (1998). Early child care and self-control, compliance, and problem behavior at 24 and 36 months. *Child Development, 69,* 1145–1170.

NICHD Early Child Care Research Network. (1999). Child care and mother–child interaction in the first three years of life. *Developmental Psychology, 35,* 1399–1413.

NICHD Early Child Care Research Network. (2000). Characteristics and quality of child care for toddlers and preschoolers. *Applied Developmental Science, 4,* 116–135.

NICHD Early Child Care Research Network. (2001). Child care and family predictors of preschool attachment and stability from infancy. *Developmental Psychology, 37,* 847–862.

NICHD Early Child Care Research Network. (2003a). Does amount of time spent in child care predict socioemotional adjustment during the transition to kindergarten? *Child Development, 74,* 976–1005.

NICHD Early Child Care Research Network. (2003b). The NICHD Study of Early Child Care: Contexts of development and developmental outcomes over the first seven years of life. In J. Brooks-Gunn & L.J. Berlin (Eds.), *Early childhood development in the 21st century* (pp. 182–201). New York: Teachers College Press.

NICHD Early Child Care Research Network. (2005). A day in third grade: A large-scale study of classroom quality and teacher and student behavior. *Elementary School Journal, 105*, 305–323.

NICHD Early Child Care Research Network. (2006). Child care effect sizes for the NICHD Study of Early Child Care and Youth Development. *American Psychologist, 61*, 99–116.

O'Connor, E., & McCartney, K. (2006). Testing associations between young children's relationships with mothers and teachers. *Journal of Educational Psychology, 98*, 87–98.

Oppenheim, D., Sagi, A., & Lamb, M. E. (1988). Infant–adult attachments on the kibbutz and their relation to socio-emotional development four years later. *Developmental Psychology, 27*, 727–733.

Ou, S. R. (2005). Pathways of long-term effects of an early intervention program on educational attainment: Findings from the Chicago longitudinal study. *Applied Developmental Psychology, 26*, 578–611

Owen, M. T., Ware, A. M., & Barfoot, B. (2000). Caregiver-mother partnership behavior and the quality of caregiver–child and mother–child interactions. *Early Childhood Research Quarterly, 15*, 413–428.

Parker, J. G., & Asher, S. R. (1987). Peer relations and later personal adjustment: Are low-accepted children "at risk"? *Psychological Bulletin, 102*, 357–389.

Peisner-Feinberg, E. S., & Burchinal, M. R. (1997). Relations between preschool children's child care experiences and concurrent development: The Cost, Quality and Outcomes Study. *Merrill-Palmer Quarterly, 43*, 451–477.

Peisner-Feinberg, E. S., Burchinal, M. R., Clifford, R.M., Culkin, M. L., Howes, C., Kagan, S. L., et al. (2001). The relation of preschool child-care quality to children's cognitive and social developmental trajectories through second grade. *Child Development, 72*, 1534–1553.

Phillips, D., McCartney, K., & Scarr, S. (1987). Childcare quality and children's social development. *Developmental Psychology, 23*, 537–543.

Pianta, R. C. (1999). *Enhancing relationships between children and teachers*. Washington, DC: American Psychological Association.

Pianta, R. C., & Nimetz, S. (1991). Relationships between teachers and children: Associations with behavior at home and in the classroom. *Journal of Applied Developmental Psychology, 12*, 379–393.

Pianta, R. C., Nimetz, S. L., & Bennett, E. (1997). Mother–child relationships, teacher–child relationships, and school outcomes in preschool and kindergarten. *Early Childhood Research Quarterly, 12*, 263–280.

Pianta, R. C., Steinberg, M. S., & Rollins, K. (1995). The first two years of school: Teacher–child relationships and deflections in children's classroom adjustment. *Development and Psychopathology, 7*, 295–312.

Pluess, M., & Belsky, J. (2009). Differential susceptibility to rearing experience: The case of childcare. *Journal of Child Psychology and Psychiatry, 50*, 396–404.

Powell, D. R. (1989). *Families and early childhood programs*. Washington, DC: National Association for the Education of Young Children.

Raikes, H. H., & Edwards, C. P. (2009). *Extending the dance in infant and toddler caregiving: Enhancing attachment and relationships*. Washington, DC: National Association for the Education of Young Children.

Rathbun, A., & West, J. (2004). *From kindergarten through third grade: Children's beginning school experiences* (NCES Publication No. 2004-007). Washington, DC: U.S. Government Printing Office.

Raver, C. C., Jones, S. M., Li-Grining, C. P., Metzger, M., Champion, K. M., & Sardin, L. (2008). Improving preschool classroom processes: Preliminary findings from a randomized trial implemented in Head Start settings. *Early Childhood Research Quarterly, 23*, 10–26.

Reynolds, A. J., Weissberg, R. P., & Kasprow, W. (1992). Predictions of early social and academic adjustment of children from the inner city. *American Journal of Community Psychology, 20*, 599–624.

Rimm-Kaufman, S. E., Pianta, R. C., & Cox, M. J. (2000). Teachers' judgments of problems in the transition to kindergarten. *Early Childhood Research Quarterly, 15*, 147–166.

Rimm-Kaufman, S. E., Early, D. M., Cox, M. J., Saluja, G., Pianta, R. C., Bradley, R. H., et al. (2002). Early behavioral attributes and teachers' sensitivity as predictors of competent behavior in the kindergarten classroom. *Applied Developmental Psychology, 23*, 451–470.

Ritchie, S., & Willer, B. (2008). *Relationships: A guide to the NAEYC early childhood program standards and related accreditation criteria.* Washington, DC: National Association for the Education of Young Children.

Rivkin, S. G., Hanushek, E. A., & Kain, J. F. (2005). Teachers, schools and academic achievement. *Econometrica, 73*(2), 417–458.

Roggman, L. A., Langlois, J. H., Hubbs-Tait, L., & Rieser-Danner, L. A. (1994). Infant day-care, attachment, and the "file drawer problem." *Child Development, 59*, 512–522.

Roisman, G. I., Susman, E., Barnett-Walker, K., Booth-LaForce, C., Owen, M. T., Belsky, J., et al. (2009). Early family and child-care antecedents of awakening cortisol levels in adolescence. *Child Development, 80*, 907–920.

Ruopp, R., Travers, J., Glantz, F., & Coelen, C. (1979). Children at the center: Final report of the National Day Care Study. Cambridge, MA: Abt.

Saft, E., & Pianta, R. C. (2001). Teachers' perceptions of their relationships with students: Effects of child age, gender, and ethnicity of teachers and children. *School Psychology Quarterly, 16*, 125–141.

Sameroff, A., Seifer, R., Barocas, R., Zax, M., & Greenspan, S. (1987). Intelligence quotient scores of 4-year-old children: Social–environmental risk factors. *Pediatrics, 79*, 343–350.

Schwartz, D., Gorman, A. H., Nakamoto, J., & McKay, T. (2006). Popularity, social acceptance, and aggression in adolescent peer groups: Links with academic performance and school attendance. *Developmental Psychology, 42*, 1116–1127.

Schweinhart, L. J., Weikart, D. P., & Larner, M. B. (1986). Consequences of three preschool curriculum models through age 15. *Early Childhood Research Quarterly, 1*, 15–45.

Smith, A. B., McMillan, B. W., Kennedy, S., & Ratcliffe, B. (1989). The effect of improving preschool teacher/child ratios: An "experiment in nature." *Early Child Development and Care, 41*, 123–138.

Smith, P. K., & Connolly, K. J. (1980). *The ecology of preschool behaviour.* London: Cambridge University Press.

Sroufe, L. A. (1988). A developmental perspective on day care. *Early Childhood Research Quarterly, 3*, 283–291.

Stormshak, E. A., Bierman, K. L., Bruschi, C. J., Dodge, K. A., Coie, J. D., & Conduct Problems Prevention Research Group. (1999). The relation between behavior problems and peer preference in different classroom contexts. *Child Development, 70*, 169–182.

Stuhlman, M., & Pianta, R. (2002). Teachers' narratives about their relationships with children: Associations with behavior in classrooms. *School Psychology Review, 31*, 148–163.

Susman, E. J. (2006). Psychobiology of persistent antisocial behavior: Stress, early vulnerabilities and the attenuation hypothesis. *Neuroscience and Biobehavioral Reviews, 30*, 376–389.

Sutton, R. E., Mudrey-Camino, R., & Knight, C. C. (2006). Teachers' emotion regulation and classroom management. *Theory into Practice, 48*, 130–137.

Thompson, R. (1999). Early attachment and later development. In J. Cassidy & P. R. Shaver (Eds.), *Handbook of attachment: Theory, research and clinical applications* (pp. 265–287). New York: Guilford Press.

Vandell, D. L., Belsky, J., Burchinal, M., Steinberg, L., Vandergrift, N., and the NICHD Early Child Care Research Network. (2010). Do effects of early child care extend to age 15 years? *Child Development, 81*, 737–756.

Vandell, D. L., & Powers, C. P. (1983). Day care quality and children's free play activities. *American Journal of Orthopsychiatry, 53*, 493–500.

van IJzendoorn, M. H., Sagi, A., & Lambermon, M. W. E. (1992). The multiple caregiver paradox: Data from Holland and Israel. *New Directions for Child Development, 57*, 5–27.

Vermeer, H. J., & van IJzendoorn, M. H. (2006). Children's elevated cortisol levels at daycare: A review and meta-analysis. *Early Childhood Research Quarterly, 21*, 390–401.

Wentzel, K. R. (1991). Relations between social competence and academic achievement in early adolescence. *Child Development, 62,* 1066–1078.

Wentzel, K. R. (1993). Social and academic goals at school: Motivation and achievement in early adolescence. *Journal of Early Adolescence, 13,* 4–20.

Wentzel, K. R., & Caldwell, K. (1997). Friendships, peer acceptance, and group membership: Relations to academic achievement in middle school. *Child Development, 68,* 1198–1209.

Whitebook, M., Howes, C., & Phillips, D. (1998). *Worthy work, unlivable wages: The National Child Care Staffing Study, 1988–1997.* Washington, DC: Center for the Child Care Workforce.

15

Culture

Thomas S. Weisner

THE IMPORTANCE OF CULTURE

Consider for a moment a thought experiment about the important influences that are going to shape social development. Imagine a neurologically healthy newborn. Bring that image up in your mind and think about that newborn. If you could do one thing that might well be the single most important thing that you could do to influence the life pathway and social development of that baby—what would that be? What comes first to mind?

There are biological and maturational requirements for growth and development that are essential for social development of children (Bogin, 1999; Konner, 1982; Small, 2001). These kinds of requirements will influence how parents in all cultures care for and socialize their children. For example, feeding practices and adequate nutrition will matter for the children. Providing adequate shelter and sufficient security and safety are essential. These requirements include providing the child with one or more caretakers who will give the child stability and primary attachments. A stimulating environment for the child is essential. Stimulation will require touching and holding, verbal and nonverbal communication, and responsiveness, particularly contingent responsiveness, by which the young child experiences reciprocal reaction to his or her own actions (Keller, 2007). Finally, resources are needed in order to provide these requirements and, as the child grows older, to provide the investments in the child that will assist him or her in learning essential skills for social competence. These features all matter as viewed from the point of view of the individual child and from the perspective of dyadic caretaker–child interactions.

However, it is worth considering that none of these specific influences taken separately, important as they are, would be the *most* important influence on social development. The community the child is born into, with its pattern of beliefs and practices, may be the most important influence. Hence, *it may well be that the most important thing you could do would be to determine where on Earth, in what household in what cultural community, that child is going to grow up.*

The same features (stimulation, nutrition, and resources) that we know are important for social development can also be viewed from the perspective of the cultural community in which the infant and his or her caregiver reside. The infant and caretaker are embedded in that cultural community (Weisner, 1996a, 2009). The parents share a cultural model for parenting (Harkness & Super, 1996). This model includes the features of physical security and safety, social stimulation, and resources needed, among others. A cultural model of parenting and social development is a shared set of goals, beliefs, practices, and experiences that organize socialization in that cultural community. This cultural model is both held in the minds of those in a community and visible in behaviors and the settings children will be in throughout childhood. This cultural community, therefore, organizes into a *pattern* all the specific features that matter for social development, directed at attaining specific goals that have moral value in that community (LeVine & New, 2008).

We might have found that baby in a homestead in rural western Kenya, perhaps among the Gusii (LeVine et al., 1994) or the Maragoli (Munroe & Munroe, 1997) or the Abaluyia in Kisa (Weisner, 1997). In these communities, women might have four to eight children, and they live in extended family compounds. They rely on shared caretaking and a mix of trade, subsistence farming, and remittances by kin from wage work for survival. Perhaps the baby lives among the Beng of the Ivory Coast in West Africa (Gottlieb, 2004), where parents want to draw their infants into the social world of the community and away from the spiritual world to which they believe their babies desire to return. The baby might be in North India, in a large Brahman extended family, also with multiple caretakers and a strong emphasis on familism, gender separation, hierarchy, family responsibility, and intergenerational economic and educational achievement (Seymour, 1999). He or she may begin life in a *favela*, an impoverished slum neighborhood in Rio in Brazil, in which threats from violence, drugs, and circumstances of poverty are powerful (Goldstein, 2003) or in a poor slum neighborhood in northeastern Brazil, in which structural poverty as a form of violence perpetrated on mothers and their children and high infant mortality exists (Scheper-Hughes, 1990). Perhaps the child arrives as the only child in a small nuclear household living in a high-rise apartment block in Japan, a complex civilization, an important part of the world economy that emphasizes academic achievement and social empathy and awareness (Holloway, 2000; Rothbaum, Pott, Azuma, Miyake, & Weisz, 2000; Shwalb & Shwalb, 1996). Perhaps the child is in a tragically war-torn region of Africa or Eastern Sri Lanka, with Muslim, Hindu, and Buddhist families interlocked and in conflict, with child soldiers and catastrophic violence and destruction (McGilvray, 2008; Trawick, 2007). These are only a tiny fraction of the thousands of communities into which this baby may have been born.

The richest accounts of children's social development in family and community context come from the remarkable holistic, comparative, community-based ethnographic studies of children's lives around the world, past and present (LeVine, 2007), including the rich accounts of the pluralistic worlds of children today (Shweder et al., 2009). Those cultural contexts vary widely and shape social development. The empirical evidence shows "that the conditions and shape of childhood tend to vary in central tendency from one population to another, are sensitive to population-specific contexts, and are not comprehensible without detailed knowledge of the socially and culturally organized contexts that give them meaning" (LeVine, 2007, p. 247).

This chapter on culture and social development proposes that the place in which we might have imagined that baby to be born is, if not the *most important influence we could imagine for that baby*, surely among the most important. The patterns of socialization the child experiences in his or her local ecology matters a great deal and will continue to be critical as the child grows into the juvenile period and adolescence.

The *cultural learning environment* is our focus. A cultural understanding of social development considers the child and the child's development as always occurring in a context. The context and the child codevelop. It is *analytically* useful for some purposes to think of the individual child in isolation—his or her temperament, genetic characteristics, and unique experiences. It is also analytically useful to think of a child in a dyadic relationship—mother and child interacting together in a mutual way, for example. However, these units for analysis do not exist in the real world. The basic unit for social development would always include the cultural context, the child, and the complex social relationships around the child. This is the cultural learning environment for the child.

OVERVIEW OF CHAPTER

I begin with a brief inventory of methods and references in this field to guide further reading, followed by a description of some ways to conceptualize cultural contexts, including cultural models for social development. I emphasize the developmental niche of the child and family, as well as the cultural learning environment and biosocial context. I then turn to infancy, middle childhood, and adolescence. For each developmental period, I illustrate some selective cultural influences on social development. For recent books providing an overview of children's social development in a range of cultures around the world, see, for example, Montgomery (2009), Lancy (2008), and Whiting and Edwards (1988).

Social development, as can be seen from the breadth of topics in this volume, is a very large subject indeed, and in this chapter, focused on culture, only some of the many topics can be covered. I touch on several: social responsibility and caretaking; gender; sociolinguistics and language; attachment; socioemotional patterns, such as shyness, aggression, and prosociality; play; and social intelligence.

Other chapters in this volume emphasize the diversity present in the child's community by class, by ethnicity, and in other ways. This chapter adds to these other sources of variation, offering a glimpse of the vast range of communities around the world children grow up in, with their patterned cultural learning environments.

METHODS OF CULTURAL RESEARCH

To appreciate the importance of cultural and contextual influences on social development and the diverse life pathways available to children around the world, leave the lab and the library and go out into some of those communities and observe, participate in, and experience them for yourself. Talk with others in those communities who have intimate, local knowledge about them. Focus on the settings children are in every day and the kinds of activities that organize the everyday routine of life of the child and family. Understand the cultural and ecological contexts of the child.

Methods of cultural research in social development also include those that address this question: What are the people in that community thinking about their own behavior and conduct? *What does their social world mean to them?* What are their own cultural models, reasons, and intentions for doing what they are doing? Considering their resources and ecology, why do they have those ethnotheories and practices? These are very useful questions to ask and are important complements to the use of standard research methods.

Methods of studying culture and the developmental niche are mentioned throughout the chapter. Understanding cultural activities and cultural models often requires mixed strategies, integrating qualitative and quantitative methods together (Weisner, 2005b; Yoshikawa, Weisner, Kalil, & Way, 2008). Qualitative methods are based on text, video, and photos. Qualitative methods represent the world through narratives, stories, vignettes, and visual modes and are person-centered as well as context-centered. Quantitative methods use numbers and variables. They represent the world in variable-centered ways. Most of the research summarized in this chapter used both qualitative and quantitative methods.

Ethnography—the study of the way of life of a community—is an important holistic method included throughout this chapter and key to cultural understanding. Ethnography includes participant observation by researchers in a community and in-depth, qualitative *conversations* (not question–answer–next question frames, and not circling numbers on questionnaire items) with children themselves, parents, and community members about their ethnopsychology and their scripts for activities. A key to all cultural data is to include the meanings of activities and of community life as evidence in research—to incorporate the experience and points of view of those whom we are studying. Ethnography can include a whole suite of methods in addition to qualitative ones, however, such as systematic behavior observations, community surveys and careful sampling, and the use of questionnaires and cognitive assessments (Bernard, 1998, 1995). Cross-cultural methods can also include biosocial indicators of stress and genetic relatedness and other physiological indicators (Worthman, 2010).

INTRODUCTION TO RESEARCH ON CULTURE AND HUMAN DEVELOPMENT

There is a wealth of reviews, texts, and handbooks reviewing the evidence on how culture shapes the learning environment. There is no reason that any claim about processes and outcomes in social development from a sample in one community cannot then be compared with evidence from communities around the world, because an extensive literature is available that can put those specific empirical findings from one population into extensive and well-documented comparative cultural context around the world. For example, extensive collections summarize social development and cultural contexts for children drawn from hundreds of cultures around the world in the Human Relations Area Files (HRAF; *www.yale.edu/hraf*). Summaries of adolescent development using the HRAF and other sources, for example, can be found in Schlegel and Barry (1991). Lancy (2008) frequently uses excerpts from the HRAF along with many other sources to provide a sharp and contemporary contrast between Western beliefs and practices concerning child care and parenting and those of the rest of the world.

Shweder et al. (2006) provide a scholarly overview and review of much of the literature of the field of cultural psychology, including many topics in social development. Shweder, Minow, and Markus (2002) introduce a range of contemporary moral, ethical, and legal dilemmas concerning families and children from immigrant groups now living together in nations that do not necessarily have the kinds of flexible and pluralistic legal systems available to deal with them. Shweder et al. (2009) edited *The Child*, a remarkable compendium of brief overviews of topics in the field, including many on social development, written by hundreds of experts in their fields; this is a highly recommended, beautiful, and accessible introduction to a pluralistic view of children and parenting around the world.

There are several textbooks and comparative overviews that provide excellent, accessible introductions to the cultural comparative study of children, including Werner (1979), Munroe and Munroe (1975), Cole (1996), Montgomery (2009), and Rogoff (2003). Lancy (2008) not only provides an overview of the rich cultural record on children assembled by anthropologists and other social scientists, but his introduction also compares cross-cultural evidence with that on contemporary childhood and parenting in the United States in interesting and provocative ways.

DeLoache and Gottlieb (2000) imagine advice books about how to raise children written from the points of view of seven different cultures and traditions. Imagine a parenting advice book written for parents on the island of Ifaluk in the Pacific, for example, or for parents during the American Puritan colonial era, or for parents among the Beng in the Ivory Coast. Kagitçibasi (1996, 2007) reviews cross-cultural evidence, as well as providing a rich autobiographical perspective from her own Turkish experiences. LeVine, Miller, and West (1988), Cole and Cole (1993), Ochs (1988), Bornstein (2010), Rubin and Chung (2006), and Tudge (2008) offer essays and collections of review articles covering a wide range of topics in this field.

Children of Different Worlds (Whiting & Edwards, 1988) compares 14 cultures in which comparable interview and observational data were collected on key dimensions of social development. *Children of Different Worlds* and its predecessor, *Children of Six Cultures* (Whiting & Whiting, 1975), offer fundamental empirical studies of social development in cultural context, with rich descriptions of the cultural learning environments of many of these children and parents as well, elaborated in Whiting (1963).

WAYS TO CONCEPTUALIZE CULTURAL COMMUNITIES

When we think of culture, we may begin by thinking of a particular "culture" as identified by a social address category: Italians, Samoans, Mexicans, the Gusii of western Kenya, Japanese. These are useful ways to identify communities, nation-states, or geographic locations that putatively share a common cultural learning environment and that are believed to have ethnotheories, resources, and social relationships that are on average similar (though not identical) across many households in that population and different (though not completely different) from other social addresses. Cultures can be identified by language, cultural history, geography, political status, or ethnic identity.

The cultural learning environment influences social development through multiple pathways, which I review in this chapter: values and goals, normative scripts for practice, organization of behavior settings and the learning environment, allocations of resources, and others. Social identity theory (Fuligni & Flook, 2005; Hogg, 2003) points to the centrality of cultural and ethnic group identification as an important definer of self and identity and therefore the cultural community. Families often are the context in which this identity is acquired and experienced due to coresidence, shared surnames, and physical appearance, among other features. The more this social identity functions to provide resources and support, and the more salient it is, whether due to external threats or opportunities or shared heritage, the greater the importance it has for human development.

THE CULTURAL CONTEXT: THE DEVELOPMENTAL NICHE AND CULTURAL LEARNING ENVIRONMENT

Ultimately, the social address or other categories that define a social identity group must be empirically related to influences on the local world and everyday life of the child, family, and community. If you are thinking of the social development of children in some particular setting or context, you are already on the way to a working definition of cultural context and the importance of this social identity. Super and Harkness (1986, 1999, 2002) describe the *developmental niche* of the child as comprising three core features: "the physical and social settings of development, the customary methods of child care, and the psychology of the caretakers" (Super & Harkness, 1996, p. 449). These three core features jointly structure the child's environment. Parental ethnotheories (shared patterns of beliefs and scripts for behavior that are both part of the psychology and part of local shared customs) are significant because they mediate the past history of that family and community, the current possibilities for what to do, and the shaping of the actual environment of the child's niche. Super and Harkness (1996) emphasize that parental ethnotheories contribute to the organization of children's early experience in several ways: through the choice of settings, the instantiation of customary caretaking behaviors, and guiding of moment-to-moment interaction.

These three core features of the developmental niche (setting, methods of care, caretaker psychology) are in turn organized by the cultural community. The child's and parents' *culture* is that network of beliefs, relationships, and resources (customs, actors, and settings) that the child is embedded in within the niche. It also includes the material products (toys, media, and clothing) of that niche that surround the child and family. When we think of a child, we would at the least also have in mind (in addition to the individual child) the community's beliefs about social development, patterns of child care, the resources and ecological context around that child and family, and the kinds of relationships in which the child is intertwined. The *cultural learning environment*, another useful construct, includes the child's active learning within his or her behavior settings, acquiring the cultural beliefs and practices of that niche (Edwards & Bloch, 2010; Lancy, Bock, & Gaskins, 2010).

Studies of cultural context that incorporate both the proximal learning environment (the behavior settings of everyday child and parental life) and the more distal ecological and physical environment are *ecocultural* theories (Weisner, 2002; Whiting, 1980; Worthman, 2010). A cultural study centers on the *beliefs* and *practices* learned in and shared by a community or a population. Cultural practices and activities are a familiar unit of culture to use: dinnertime, visiting relatives, doing homework, doing household work, hanging out with friends, organized play dates, bedtime, soccer practice, playing video games, going to church, going on a date, and many others. Activities such as these have certain features that are important in determining how they are done: their goals and values; the tasks that have to be accomplished in them; the norms, rules, and scripts for the right way or ways to do them; the people and relationships in them; our engagement, motives, and feelings in them; the resources it takes to do them; and how stable, familiar, and predictable they are in our lives. Cultures have many activities in common (e.g., all members of all communities visit relatives, eat meals, play with friends, have bedtime and sleeping arrangements), but these activities can vary widely as to how or why they are done. Those social activities are what the child experiences, and thereby they shape social development (Cole, 1996; Farver, 1999; Weisner, 2002).

Another very useful and well-known ecological conceptual framework is from Uri Bronfenbrenner (1979, 1995). Bronfenbrenner's Person/Process/Context/Time model, for instance, considers an active parent or child enmeshed in an equally active and dynamic social-ecological system, which includes everyday behavior settings, family and community context, structural institutions of society, and the wider cultural context.

It is fair to say that there is no single consensus theory of cultural influences on social development in our field. However, there is a broad consensus that some combination of these conceptual approaches will be required for a comprehensive account. Greenfield, Keller, Fuligni, & Maynard (2003) posit three universal tasks of human development: the formation of social relationships, the acquisition of knowledge, and the balance between autonomy and relatedness at adolescence. The interdependent, *contextual* study of these tasks is largely unelaborated in current developmental psychology, compared with the independent-dyadic model. Greenfield et al. (2003) argue that sociohistorical, ecocultural, and cultural values or models are all useful for understanding the roles of cultural context in the varied ways communities address the three universal developmental tasks.

INFANCY: CROSS-CULTURAL VARIATION IN THE DEVELOPMENTAL NICHE

Cultural beliefs and practices begin to influence social development well before birth and throughout infancy (Leiderman, Tulkin, & Rosenfeld, 1977). Super and Harkness (1996) and Harkness et al. (2007) observed middle-class professional Dutch parents and American parents (in Cambridge, Massachusetts), and their babies, interviewed parents about beliefs, customs, and relationships that varied between the two communities, and compared the ethnotheories. The Dutch (compared to U.S. and other communities) emphasized the importance of an infant and young child being calm, rested, relaxed, and regular. They valued an even-tempered child who did not change emotional and social patterns too much and who was rather tranquil. The Dutch community had an expression for their widely shared ethnotheory: *Rust, Regelmaat,* and *Reinheid*—the three R's (rest, regularity, and cleanliness). A related ethnotheory is the belief in innateness; whether some children are innately more regular in sleep than others, for example. Thirty percent of the U.S. sample believed this; almost all the Dutch parents did not (5%). So the Dutch more often believed that social and physical management of the context could give most babies the three R's most of the time if they followed up their ethnotheories with specific practices.

The psychologist–anthropologist team did daily routine studies, daily diaries, and observations of the babies' sleep and calm/resting time over a year or more. And sure enough, the Dutch babies, at around 6 months of age, in fact slept and rested 2 hours longer than the U.S. babies; they went to bed around an hour earlier, and they were less variable in sleep patterns as a group. They were more often calmly resting in their beds. The Dutch babies responded to the more scheduled rest and sleep times favored by Dutch parents by resting and sleeping more. In both Dutch and U.S. contexts, babies had separate cribs or sleeping places (unlike babies in most of the world). However, in most of the world, they would be cosleeping with their mothers and with others as they grew older (McKenna & McDade, 2005; Morelli, Rogoff, Oppenheim, & Goldsmith, 1992). Recall that there is pluralism within these communities, of course; some Dutch and American parents sleep with their young children (Okami, Weisner, & Olmstead, 2002). The modal custom is to sleep apart in both societies, however.

Socioeconomic status (SES) and other differences within each community could also have accounted for these differences (and often are related), but they did not account for them in this study. Rather, each community showed a patterned qualitative difference in their ethnotheories, which in turn influenced the organization of the niche of the child and family to promote rest, regularity, and cleanliness among the Dutch. The United States and the Netherlands are both complex, first-world economies with high levels of education, so the group differences cannot be attributed to levels of economic development or formal education. The U.S. babies experienced more verbal, touching, and other "stimulation" during interactions with parents and others compared with the Dutch (and compared with most other communities).

Super and Harkness (1996) worked with a team of researchers from several other countries, including Italy, Australia, Spain, and Sweden, to further compare ethnotheories. In Italy, for instance, parents wanted a baby who was *vivace*—lively, active, smiling, bright—which also described the social child most desired (Axia & Weisner, 2002). With that ethnotheory, Italian parents provided a much more socially engaged, variable social developmental world for infants. So the reason for the differences in social stimulation and routines was indeed cultural—that is, due to the beliefs, practices, and daily routines favored in each community. Abels (2008) compared ethnotheories about infant sleep and independence across 10 communities. German mothers believe that babies can sleep alone at 2.8 months and can be sleeping through the night before 5 months of age. Similarly low ages (well below 12 months) are reported by mothers in urban samples in Los Angeles, Athens, Crete, and Costa Rica. Mothers in Delhi and in rural Gujarat in India, as well as the rural Nso in Cameroon, however, describe ages for sleeping through the night ranging from more than 60 to more than 96 months. Mothers in Mexico, in urban China, and among the urban Nso report around 12–18 months (Abels, 2008).

Ethnotheories emphasizing independence (e.g., German), relatedness but with individual autonomy (e.g., Mexico), and interdependence (e.g., rural Nso), as well as greater concerns about child survival (e.g., among rural Nso and India samples), underlie these wide variations in beliefs and practices regarding early childhood care and sleep. Keller (2007) provides a rich comparative perspective on infancy, contrasting a prototypical autonomous-independent and interdependent pattern of raising infants and uses both prototypes with evolutionary and ecocultural perspectives:

> The model of independence prioritizes the perception of the individual as separate, autonomous, bounded, and self-contained. Socialization strategies focus on mental states and personal qualities to support self-enhancement and self-maximization.... The model of interdependence prioritizes the individual as interrelated with others and heteronomous (coagent). Socialization strategies focus on the acceptance of norms and hierarchies to contribute to the harmonic functioning of the social unit, in particular, the family.... The model of autonomous relatedness combines interpersonal relatedness with autonomous functioning. Socialization strategies focus on both harmonic integration into the family and autonomy as an agent. (Keller et al., 2006, p. 156)

In Keller et al. (2006), a version of this model is used for a comparative study of German, European American, and Greek middle-class women, representing the independent cultural model; Cameroonian Nso and Indian Gujarati farming women, representing the interdependent cultural model; and urban Indian, urban Chinese, urban Mexican, and urban Costa Rican women, representing a combination of these—the third, autonomous–relational model. Infant care beliefs vary along the lines of these prototypical models.

Gottlieb (2004) studied babies among the Beng of the Ivory Coast. The ethnotheory among Beng mothers and fathers was of a child who was highly social and who could be engaged with many others in their community. There is a connection between ethnotheories such as this and other cultural beliefs. In the Beng community, beliefs about the spiritual world were very important. Beng believe that children before birth live in a spiritual world called *wrugbe*, a wonderful world that children do not want to leave and have to enter the village world. The ethnotheory is that more caretakers and social relationships these babies establish in their early years of life, the more likely they are to be persuaded to fully exit *wrugbe* and live in their new social community. Beng communities are very poor and have few resources. Mothers have to work hard on farms that are often located far from their compact villages, and fathers are often away seeking work, and in any case are not involved in much infant and child care. There are few if any modern biomedical or educational resources available. Infant and young child mortality is unfortunately fairly high, adding to the pressures on mothers to find social support. The Beng also want to protect their children from harm through the use of charms and other body manipulations. They do so by immersing themselves in social relationships—orienting the child outward, toward others; encouraging a social child through socially distributed caretaking; and making sure that the child comes to know lots of other people. For this reason, "A member of every household in the village is expected to call on a newborn baby within hours after the birth" (DeLoache & Gottlieb, 2000, p. 12). Gottlieb (2004) observed infants and young children and found that they were regularly being cared for by three or four people in a 2.5-hour observation period and were typically in the presence of several people. Infants' and young children's anger and frustration are rather calmly accepted, partly because these are interpreted as signs that the child, of course, wants to return to *wrugbe*.

Ecological and Resource Influences on the Cultural Learning Environment and Ethnopsychology

Infant and early childhood contexts influence the physical survival, health, and motoric development of the young child (a "pediatric" emphasis) as in the Beng case. Other developmental contexts encourage language and cognitive and early social responsiveness in development (a "pedagogical" emphasis; LeVine et al., 1994). LeVine's team research among the Gusii of western Kenya found a strong emphasis on the pediatric model. Among families in this horticultural community mothers faced heavy workload pressures and had high fertility rates, with completed family sizes of around seven or eight children per woman during the period of their studies in the 1970s. The community had a history of high rates of infant and young child mortality as well. The ethnopsychology of the Gusii focused on signs of children's motoric development as indicators of physical robustness and health. Caretakers engaged in exercises to encourage walking and other skills, carried infants and young children close, and kept them well covered in infancy and early childhood.

The Gusii mothers also avoided directly gazing into the baby's eyes out of concern that they might inadvertently transfer dangerous threats from sorcery and from the envy of others over the baby to the child. Parents do not boast about their children directly, because this potentially would bring envy and attention to them. This general category of belief, described as the "evil eye" or by other terms, is a common one, channeling a kind of generalized social and spiritual concern for dangers lurking that could affect a child. Children are expected to be (and typically are) quiet and deferential, not boisterous or emotionally labile with one another (though they are somewhat more so with closer peers and siblings) and certainly not with adults and strangers (S. LeVine, 2009). This pattern is encouraged through calm, low-affect caretaker behaviors (Goldschmidt, 1975).

Early Attachment and Cultural Context

The development of social and psychological attachment shows strong cultural influences. Although the onset of separation anxiety and distress in infants begins around the similar age of 9–11 months or so, the timing of the resolution of this attachment distress varies widely, ranging up to 36 months or older in many communities. This occurs because of the wide variations in ethnotheories about the meaning of the child's attachment and separation behavior and variations in the caretaking practices that influence attachment, separation, and social trust. Indeed, the question that is important for many communities is not, "Is my child 'securely attached'?" but rather, "How can I ensure that my child knows whom to trust?" Parents are concerned that the child learns culturally appropriate social behaviors that display proper comportment and also show trust toward appropriate other people yet also remains respectful or vigilant toward others.

In the many communities around the world with multiple caretakers of infants and young children, the children clearly show attachment toward those other caretakers, as well as toward their mothers. There is strong evidence that children do need and benefit from having predictable caretakers available. A chaotic, changing, unpredictable social world does not promote early security in a young child. But those caretaking patterns do not need to consist of a single primary caretaker with dyadic, monomatric attachment in order for the child to be appropriately socially connected to others in their social world with a sense of emotional, social, and cultural security (Weisner, 2005a).

Nor do behaviors labeled as *secure* in standardized assessments necessarily always look the same or mean the same thing in other cultures. Secure attachment is found among children around the world who experience very different caretaking patterns, with different ethnotheories about social trust and emotional security (LeVine & Norman, 2001; Lewis & Takahashi, 2005; Weisner, 2005a). Further, the experience of being in the presence of strange and unfamiliar others, which varies across cultural learning environments, itself influences the onset and duration of separation anxiety (e.g., Chisholm, 1996, on the Navajo). Being very strongly attached to a single caretaker and fearful toward everyone else would not be a sign of secure attachment among the Beng, for example. The ability of a young child not to cry when separated from his or her mother and to be able to approach others in such situations may be interpreted as a sign of social intelligence and early interdependence. Attachment behaviors may well have both a universal patterning and an evolutionary basis early in development and, at the same time, be contextually variable and dependent on local cultural context for their expression and developmental meanings (Harwood, Miller, & Irizarry, 1995; van IJzendoorn, Bakermans-Kranenburg, & Sagi-Schwartz, 2006).

Beng infants, like all infants and young children around the world, are learning how to trust others and with whom. Parents shape their children's attentional processes by orienting attention and directing children's gaze outward toward others, not exclusively toward a single (maternal) caretaker. These patterns of very early infant and young child care are found in many parts of the world, such as in Polynesia (Ochs, 1988), in societies in which there often is elaborate social ranking by clans, chiefs, and senior elites as well, making the social hierarchy important and not easy to learn. In agrarian and pastoral communities in sub-Saharan Bantu Africa (Nsamenang & Lo-oh, 2010), there are strong cultural models and ecological and relational pressures on children to work and contribute to the family and household economy. Religious and political beliefs favor the control of those older over the younger, and usually men over women. All these ecocultural patterns share an emphasis on socially shared care of children and pluralistic attachments with those giving such care.

Early Language Socialization and Cultural Context

Language socialization in early childhood varies widely around the world, in the amount of talk directed at a child, the training in word naming and vocabulary enrichment directed at children, and the extent to which children are involved through language socialization in communication with adults and others, which is particularly relevant for social development (Ochs, 1988). Children learn most cultural knowledge, including language, through participation, mimicry, apprenticeship, and observation of others. Language socialization is closely related to young children's learning of appropriate emotional expression and of social rules about hierarchy and the right ways to talk with others (e.g., kin, religious leaders, men, women, elders). One important finding from such research across cultures is how relatively infrequent direct adult tuition of children mediated through language (so common in the Western middle-class family and society) is in many communities. Yet children learn the complexities of sociolinguistic worlds and pragmatics of language, often without such direct adult involvement. They learn through close watching and listening and through their gradual social incorporation into their local speech community with peers (Leon, 1998; Miller, Wiley, Fung, & Liang, 1997; Richman et al., 1988).

Multiparty speaking contexts are practically the only language-learning environment of young children in many African, Meso-American, and Pacific societies, or at least among large segments of those societies. Rabain-Jamin (2001) studied the polyvocal language socialization of 2-year-olds and older siblings (4–5 years old) among the Wolof of Senegal. Children learn at an early age their place in a complex social network, in which adults orient the child regarding how and when to respond appropriately. Conversational skills, social positioning and referencing, and prompting are key early sociolinguistic routines commonly found in such sociocentric social developmental learning environments. Rabain-Jamin found in her study of 2-year-olds, 4-year-olds, and mothers that

> appropriate phrases and structures are presented to the learning child in the form of prompts, which the child is expected to try to repeat. Discourse devices that require the involvement of other persons broaden the mother–child relationship and force the child to take part in multi-party dialogues [often directed at siblings and sibling caretakers]. (2001, p. 380)

Older siblings participate sociolinguistically to manage a sequence of acts that must be accomplished. These are culturally framed as positive for the children; they bring younger children into the community activity and recognize the child's active learning role, though not directly through the mother. Wolof mothers' speech to 2-year-olds is primarily directed "to get her child to carry out socially appropriate actions [rather than] teaching the baby to describe the state of the world by means of assertions" (Rabain-Jamin, 2001, p. 378).

Social Intelligence

Social intelligence is a key culturally valued competence linking many of these features of ethnopsychology and the cultural learning environment. An important conclusion from cross-cultural research is that "intelligence is appreciated only if it comes hand-in-hand with a socially cooperative disposition" (Rabain-Jamin, 2001, p. 379). "Participatory pedagogy" scaffolds the development of this social intelligence, because "[in much of Africa, the] attainment of intelligent capacities [in childhood] is not [from the principle of direct] instruction but participatory pedagogy.... children's developmental lessons [are] extracted ... from family routines, ethnic languages, institutional structures, cultural practices, ... and social encounters" (Nsamenang & Lo-oh, 2010, p. 397).

MIDDLE CHILDHOOD

Social intelligence becomes as or more central during middle childhood. Social development changes sharply as children make the 5-to-7 shift (Sameroff & Haith, 1996). This maturational change marks the transition into the juvenile, or *school-age*, period. Children are much better at self-regulation, and they can engage jointly in complex, collaborative social and task activities that require their understanding of shared goals, joint planning, and a clear grasp of the intentions of others. Attentional skills and focus are much stronger. Such beliefs regarding children's new abilities emerging at around these ages is very widespread around the world and suggests a maturational basis for the recognition of the *age of reason and responsibility*, or the time when children are seen as being able to take on joint and shared tasks for the household and for themselves and to do them reliably and in concert with others.

At this time in development, in fact, brain growth is slowed down, but there is intensified consolidation and synaptic maturation and an increase in the executive functioning areas of the brain. Growth slows down in height and weight, child mortality is relatively low, and, of course, the child is not yet sexually mature (Campbell, 2008). Children can help support a household by doing chores, assisting in child care, and helping with subsistence tasks. However, they will only rarely be living alone outside of a household and family context. If children are living outside a family context during middle childhood, this is almost certainly due to being orphaned or homeless due to family neglect, deep poverty, pathology, epidemics, or the consequences of war and violence.

Social Obligation and Responsibility

The socialization of social responsibility and respect is a domain of social behavior in which there are large cultural differences around the world and which fully emerges during middle childhood. Children learn a respectful awareness of others and a responsiveness to and anticipation of the needs of others. Children often are expected to do important, meaningful work for their families during this period of social development. Intelligence and cognitive ability are believed to increase as a result. Nsamenang and Lo-oh (2010, p. 397) comment that "within the African worldview, responsibility is more valued than cognition, per se, in the sense that one cannot be responsible without cognizing, whereas some people are cognitively alert but irresponsible."

Sibling Caretaking and Social Development

Older children, often beginning at the transition into the juvenile period, are assigned to take on the care of younger siblings or cousins in their household (Nuckolls, 1993; Serpell, 1993, 2008; Zukow, 1989). Middle childhood is also the time when many other chores, tasks, and social obligations and responsibilities are expected from children around the world (Rogoff, Sellers, Pirrotta, Fox, & White, 1975). In rural Gujarat and elsewhere, teenage girls will sometimes take care of babies, often beginning after they have started menstruating and therefore have to leave school due to some parents' concerns about the girl's safety and honor, and thus her marriageability. This is considered a type of training and preparation for marriage and for being a wife (Abels, October 2010, personal communication).

Sibling caretaking, or *socially distributed care*, experiences are a near cross-cultural universal for children in many parts of the world (Weisner & Gallimore, 1977). Caretaking is an example of what Margaret Mead called a pivot role: First, you are the recipient of the care from others, then you gradually age into being a caretaker yourself (Mead, 1949).

Certain ecological and demographic features of a community contribute to the likelihood that children are involved in these socially distributed caretaking responsibilities. These features include heavy maternal workload and resource pressures on the family, fathers who are absent or unavailable for caretaking, relatively large family sizes and households (or single caretakers without much social support for care), and joint or extended families living together. Girls are preferred for performing child care and other domestic tasks. Where there otherwise already is more gender-role segregation and specialization in a community, sibling care is often more common.

Children often will combine child care with concurrent mixed-age and mixed-sex play and work around the home with other children. There often is a shared cultural ethnotheory that children can do such work by middle childhood, that it is good for them to acquire valuable skills through family responsibilities, and that children learn well and rapidly during this time. A 4- to 5-year age gap between a child caretaker and his or her charge might be preferred, if possible. Children are under indirect monitoring and supervision in their care by parents and other adults, so they are not doing these social caretaking activities entirely on their own (Weisner, 1987, 1989).

Socially distributed caretaking may be linked to a common human attribute that underlies the evolution in *Homo sapiens* of sociality itself:

> Where did the human quest for intersubjective engagement [being interested in and responsive to others' mental states; caring about what others think, feel, and intend] come from? ... by focusing [in other theoretical models] on intergroup competition, we have been led to overlook factors such as childrearing that are at least as important (in my opinion, even more important) for explaining the early origins of humankind's peculiarly hypersocial tendencies. We have underestimated just how important shared care and provisioning of offspring by group members other than parents have been in shaping prosocial tendencies. (Hrdy, 2009, pp. 20, 29)

All social development—indeed, human culture itself—depends on the uniquely human ability for intersubjective engagement, which requires understanding the minds and intentions of others in our social world and then socially coordinating our behaviors based on that understanding. Selection for shared care of young children may well have gone along with selection for the ability for intersubjective engagement.

Play

Play is a universal feature of children's social development, although the kinds of play and the games, the participants, and the contexts of play vary widely in cultures around the world (Edwards, 2000). Western middle-class parental play encourages verbal and cognitive abilities, egalitarianism, providing choice for children's play, and a kind of child–adult protofriendship role and routines. In this reciprocal role, adults treat the child as a kind of coequal playmate and take on the playful, emotional roles of the child's level of play and understanding. Special toys, play areas, fantasy play, symbolic play and special scripts, media characters, films, videos, and so forth are used and marketed specifically for play (Berk, 2009). These commercial images, narratives, and marketed toys are themselves important symbolic partners in children's play.

One striking feature of cross-cultural research on play that is not fully appreciated in most Western research (and not reflected in our own ethnopsychology and theory about play) is that in most of the world, adults rarely or never engage in play with children in the ways that U.S. parents do (Lancy, 2007). U.S. parents might very actively get down on the floor with children and play or engage in sports and games with children. But in most of the world, parents and other adults do not do these types of play activities with children. Parents often engage children in work for the household, as we have seen, and do not see the value for them or their children of adult–child play (Lancy, 1996). In nearly all cultural learning environments described from around the world, regardless of adult involvement, children will seek out play with objects and others, make toys, fantasize, and play sports and games without adult management and intervention. But in most settings, parents do not view their roles, nor their ethnopsychological script for parenting and development, as including play (Gaskins, 1996). Nor are marketed commercial toys even necessarily available or affordable, if available. Children are exceedingly creative, however, in making their own toys (dolls, toy boats, toy cars, kites, pictures) from found objects in their environment—old plastic bottles or gourds, string, wire, bits of cloth, corn cobs, and so forth (ChildFund International, 2009).

Gender

Culture deeply influences gender development and play. For example, by middle childhood, it is more likely that boys and girls will play with same-sex groups (boys somewhat more likely than girls to form such groups; Whiting & Edwards, 1973). More generally, gender has "profound effects on most every aspect of behavior, prescribing how babies are delivered, how children are socialized, how children are dressed, what is considered intelligent behavior, what tasks children are taught, and what roles adult men and women will adopt.... Children grow up in the context of other people's [gendered, cultural] scripts" (Best, 2010, p. 211; Williams & Best, 1990). Culture is not the only influence on gendered differences in social development, of course, but studies from the Six Cultures research program and its successors (in communities in India, Kenya, Mexico, Okinawa, the Philippines, and the United States) show both universals and variations in gender and social behavior (Munroe & Munroe, 1997; Whiting & Edwards, 1988; Whiting & Whiting, 1975).

Cross-cultural evidence provides support for some broad pancultural differences by gender, as well as features that vary across cultures. Boys more often appear to display physical aggression toward others and, on average, to display less social nurturance and domestic and other task responsibility than girls (Whiting & Edwards, 1988; Whiting & Whiting, 1975). However, there are often local exceptions to these patterns, and they may not hold at all ages. These kinds of gender differences become more pronounced during middle childhood, when often quite sharp separation of the social contexts for boys and girls develops (Whiting & Edwards, 1973). Social and life pathway opportunities for girls vary dramatically across cultures and are reflected in family practices regarding task training, whom girls can be with socially, age of marriage, and many other domains (Schlegel, 1977; Seymour, 1999).

Children are more likely to seek out same-sex children to interact and play with and to prefer to play with same-sex children, if they are available, from ages 3–4 on. There often are differences, on average, in what boys do in interactions and groups of peers compared with girls: Boys typically engage in more rough play and aggressive, physical competitive activities, take more risks, are less likely to disclose weaknesses, talk less, and more often exclude others (Best, 2010; Whiting & Edwards, 1988; see also Leaper & Bigler, Chapter 12, this volume). Where both boys and girls are expected to take on household tasks and child-care responsibilities and do so about equally, some other social behaviors, in turn, are less likely to differ by gender (Ember, 1973). More often than not, however, girls in cultures in which they have significant child work and household task responsibility expectations were treated differently in many other domains as well, compared with boys in those societies (Edwards, 2000). Recall that these are averaged, generalized patterns across the ethnographic record. None are invariant across cultures, and there is always variation within cultures as well.

Peer Relationships and Aggression

Peers and peer relationships provide a rich context for cultural differences and variations (Edwards, deGuzman, Brown, & Kumru, 2006). Rubin, Cheah, and Menzer (2010) have reviewed some of the cross-cultural findings on social development and peers. Not all cultural communities provide open and ready access to peers (outside of schools or other institutional contexts) because families may worry about and fear (often with good reason) negative peer influences on children. Children may be needed for work within the household and family or peer contacts may be restricted to subgroups (ethnic groups, religious communities) that may be viewed as more similar to their natal family or group or more important than others.

Aggression (physical, relational, social, verbal) is not tolerated in many communities from younger children toward adults or even toward older peers—but it is not necessarily the other way around. Physical aggression is generally more common in male groups, though not absent in girls' groups (Goodwin, 2006). Bergeron and Schneider reviewed cross-national differences in peer aggression among children in school in 28 different countries and reported that "cultures characterized by collectivistic values, high moral discipline, a high level of egalitarian commitment, and high uncertainty avoidance ... [and with] heavily Confucian values showed lower levels of aggression towards peers" (quoted in Rubin et al., 2010, p. 227). Communities emphasizing the importance of social order, responsible and task-dedicated behavior, egalitarianism, voluntary cooperation, and moral restraint reported lower aggression levels among children as well.

In communities with few strangers or outsiders in them, consisting mostly of kin known to children and families, the task for children and others is not to meet strangers and form new friendships and groups, because everyone largely is known. Rather, the task is to differentiate among peers and others one knows already and then form closer relationships with some of them.

Desirable Emotional and Personality Attributes

Cultural ethnotheories of temperament and personality and, more generally, concepts of what patterns of social behavior are desirable can deeply influence not only how the behavior is evaluated but of course what parents and peers do about it (Kitayama & Markus, 2000). Cultures differ significantly in how they evaluate behaviorally inhibited or shy versus bold children, for example. Rubin et al. (2006) contrasted the influence of cultural beliefs about children who are shy and withdrawn, reserved, or very cautious and wary with that of beliefs about children who are gregarious, outgoing, exploratory, socially active, and bold. North American parents are very concerned about children with withdrawn behavior; peers may well victimize and reject such children in the United States. They have few friends and often feel lonely and depressed. However, in mainland China (at least until recently) such children might be seen as

> reverential, conforming, reserved, and compliant. These characteristics are considered typical and desirous. Given the significance attached to achieving and maintaining social order and interpersonal harmony with traditional Chinese culture, it makes sense that individuals are encouraged to restrain their personal desires and to behave in a sensitive, cautious, and inhibited fashion. Indeed, children who exhibit

such tendencies are described as *Guai Hai Zi* in Mandarin, which may be loosely translated as meaning "good" or "well-behaved." (Rubin et al., 2006, pp. 91–92).

Children who might be temperamentally more behaviorally inhibited or "shy" (vigilant in new settings; experiencing some negative anxiety; attention more often fixated on fearful events) but living in a community with more positive cultural beliefs about the meaning of such behaviors may well be less negatively affected as a result. The more general point is that variations in cultural beliefs about the positive or negative valence of different behaviors seen in children (such as being reserved or gregarious) can substantially influence the social and emotional consequences of those behaviors for the children and the family and on the other hopes and desires (educational, cognitive, affective, as well as social) parents have for those children:

> If a given behavior is viewed as acceptable [i.e. gregarious, *vivace*, bold children in the United States], then parents will attempt to encourage its development; if the behavior is perceived as maladaptive or abnormal [being overly shy in the United States, thus responded to with harshness and/or overprotectiveness], then parents (and significant others) will attempt to discourage its growth and development. (Rubin & Chung 2006, p. vii)

The existence of lexically marked terms identifying particular behaviors or psychological states, terms that are meaningful in their cultural context, is itself an important indicator that those behaviors and states are important themes in social development in that community. Xu, Farver, Chang, Yu, and Zhang (2006) describe the belief in and Chinese social practice of *ren*, or "forbearance," for example. *Ren* is a known, marked term, a mode of coping, relating, and confronting conflict among peers. It is not avoidance, because children attempt to elicit *ren* from others to encourage social harmony and group orientation and solidarity. It is a very socially competent practice, understood in those communities. Yet *ren* is not a category of behavior named, marked, or studied in the West. A reserved, respectful forbearance to encourage group social harmony might be a phrase that roughly translates *ren*, but this phrase certainly does not index an important socialization goal in the West, and there is no word for it.

Showing respect and anticipating the needs of others also illustrate the salience of culturally indexed and marked categories. The showing of respect for elders and kin living in a child's household is a named and expectable practice in many communities, such as in India, much of the Islamic world, Africa, and elsewhere (Gregg, 2005). Yet it is not to be found on most family or home environment scales developed in the West. Similarly, Tobin (2000) describes the Japanese term *kejime*, "correctly reading the context for what it is and acting accordingly" (p. 1157). An emphasis on "symbiotic harmony" in Japan (as contrasted with "generative tension" in relationships in the United States) and a concern for *amae*, or anticipating the needs of others and appropriately eliciting *amae* from others, are similar concepts widely admired and expected in Japan. All these can be said to characterize Japanese social relationships as a general cultural pattern and emphasis (though not as a rigid absolute by any means; Rothbaum et al., 2000; Shwalb & Shwalb, 1996). It is fair to say that the social development of children in most of the world is much more focused on some version of these kinds of behaviors, states, and abilities than would be true in the social development of contemporary middle-class children in the United States.

High- and Low-Threat Cultural Environments: Effects on Social Relationships and Parenting

Parental and community concerns over fears and threats to children, including the potential harsh treatment of children in such situations, have been mentioned earlier as shaping cultural ethnotheories, practices, and settings. The example of families and child care in an impoverished *favela* in Rio do Janiero, Brazil, shows the effects of such fear and much else on children of all ages, but particularly children in middle childhood and into adolescence (Goldstein, 1998, 2003). These sprawling slum communities are dangerous places, in which physical violence and threats, gang control of territory, drugs and alcohol abuse, often accompanied by deep poverty, are omnipresent and in which sheer survival requires sometimes harsh parental and sibling control over others, over resources, and over the household routine. Goldstein describes this world in great depth through the story of Graca, a single mother holding a large household together in just a couple of rooms. She works for a well-off middle-class family caring for their children and household during the days and then returns to the *favela* at night. Goldstein describes harsh punishments for children if they do not complete household tasks, if they are out when they should not be, or if they take the possessions of others. Graca believes that only through the use of harsh punishment sometimes can children be protected and survive in the *favela*. An emphasis on shared work and obedience required for sheer survival is strongly felt and emotionally emphasized.

Such fears exist in communities around the world, including, of course, in the United States. Kling, Liebman, and Katz (2005, p. 255) quotes a poor working mother living in a dangerous neighborhood in a city in the United States: "bullets got no name," she remarked. She had to keep her kids inside and instructed her children to crouch down below window level inside the house at night for safety. "We came to realize during our interviews that these mothers were more than simply concerned for their children. They had organized their entire lives around protecting their sons and daughters from the genuine dangers of ghetto life" (p. 255).

ADOLESCENCE

Initiation of boys and girls into new social positions and identities is a social practice found around the world in many forms, although some of these rites of passage are declining in frequency and in the participation of the wider community beyond family and close friends. Initiations at adolescence serve many purposes. One is to mark and regulate the maturation of girls and boys as they reach some stage of physical puberty. Initiation ceremonies often separate boys and girls completely for extended periods of time, offer them specialized and secret knowledge, and emphasize their induction into not only a new maturational stage but also new work and tasks. Adult religious knowledge, secret songs, and specialized knowledge are now presented to adolescents. The cohort, or convoy, of peers, adult leaders, and kin sponsors of these initiation or coming-of-age ceremonies can become available to the teen and parents for support throughout life, and children's participation in such groups can be sociopolitically important for parents. Boys might now be seen as ready to help defend their communities, and girls may now be ready for marriage or other family responsibilities. There are new responsibilities and privilege perhaps, but also new forms of adult hierarchical controls over the new youths (Schlegel & Barry, 1991)

Initiation ceremonies can also include adolescent circumcision for boys and for girls. Female genital surgery for girls varies widely in type, extent, and the age at which it occurs. Other scarification, or marking of the body, may be used to show the new social status, now literally inscribed on the bodies of youths. There are active debates and legal and political conflicts over whether such genital surgery should continue at all, and if so in what forms (Shweder, 2002).

In many communities around the world today, adolescence is a brief period in social development, because girls may be married well before 18. They may be forming a household, having children, moving to the households of in-laws, expected to take on significant responsibilities in their natal households for their parents, and in other ways beginning adult life (Herdt & Leavitt, 1998). Boys are less likely than girls to make this transition as quickly, but they also will find themselves more involved in adult roles. This is more often the case in poor families and neighborhoods, with expectations that require youths to support others and to fend for themselves, but it is also a normative pathway in life regardless of SES in many parts of the world. Generally speaking, the greater the economic, subsistence, and survival pressure on a household and community, the greater these kinds of normative, enforced expectations on social development during adolescence are likely to be. In addition, the cultural definition of the length of the developmental stage of adolescence is also likely to be briefer. At the same time, adolescence and young adult status are extended later and later in other settings, including in the more resource-rich first-world economies; this situation characterizes many U.S. middle-class youths today.

Family Patterns and Social Development

We have barely touched on some of the variations in family patterns that affect social development and that in many ways crystallize the variations in cultural pathways that matter for children's social development that we have described throughout this chapter. Therborn (2009) characterizes seven broad cross-cultural patterns: Christian European; Islamic West Asian/North African; South Asian Hindu; Confucian East Asian; sub-Saharan African; Southeast Asian; and Creole (U.S. South, Caribbean, Brazil, parts of South America). Each of these seven broad family patterns differs in social dimensions that have profound influences on the pathways of social development for children growing up within those family systems. These highly cultural variable dimensions of family systems include, for example, norms concerning inheritance (e.g., whether all children inherit equally, or only males, or only firstborn males) or descent rules (e.g., bilateral as in the United States or patrilineal); marriage customs that are preferred or permitted in different communities (e.g., whether there is an ideal norm of lifetime monogamy; whether divorce and serial monogamy are allowed or plural marriage is permitted). Beliefs about sexuality and gender and patterns of household formation (i.e., whether couples form independent households, live with parents, or form joint or extended households; whether children typically remain in one household or move between multiple households during childhood) also vary systematically across these family regions. Influences of religious practices on families and many other norms, laws, and customs that shape family life show such patterned variation, and so they deeply affect the developmental pathways of children and youths.

Other family dimensions that can strongly influence children's social development include variations in family values: Is it appropriate and even normative for children to live with adults other than parents, for example? How important is showing public and private respect for parents? Do parents invest in and sacrifice for children, or are children expected to invest in household and family just as much or more so as they grow up? How important is it for children to show obedience and respect versus showing their independence? Family goals and the moral socialization of all these values and other dimensions of family life have powerful influences on the social development of children growing up in each of these seven prototypical family systems. As Therborn comments about the widely varying families around the world, and the lives of children in them, "The boys and girls of the world enter many different childhoods and depart them through many different doors" (2009, p. 338).

HETEROGENEITY IN CULTURAL CONTEXTS

Cultural influences do not constitute homogeneous, unchanging influences. The fact that beliefs are not completely shared in a cultural community is not evidence that this is not a cultural community. A cultural analysis assumes and predicts some internal *heterogeneity* within every community; cultures are constantly changing, and there is argument and disagreement about many beliefs and practices in most every community (Weisner, 2009). Cultural norms and practices create social and psychological conflicts and frustrations and envy of others. There are always tensions across generations, family groups, neighborhoods, and ethnic groups. There are also differences in temperament and other characteristics between individual children that lead to differences in each person's degree of shared knowledge and his or her sense of comfort living in their cultural community. Socially learned and transmitted shared beliefs and practices in an ecocultural niche are a criterion for those beliefs and practices being cultural—but cultural knowledge is not just uniformly "faxed" into the minds of children. To the contrary: Such knowledge is acquired *selectively* and becomes a part of shared, as well as unique individual, models. The extent to which features of the settings in a cultural learning environment are similar and shared by those in a defined population is an *empirical* question to be investigated and shown in a study, not an assumption to make based only on a shared social address.

CULTURAL MODELS AND THEIR ACQUISITION

Children acquire their cultural models, scripts for behavior, and shared ethnopsychology; it is not present in their minds at birth formed by experiences in utero. The *anthropology of learning* is an important part of understanding social development in context (Lancy et al., 2010). The cultural models in a community are very much a part of the social world of the classroom and of the school, as well. This social curriculum varies widely around the world, even as schools have spread nearly everywhere (Tobin, Wu, & Davidson, 1989). There are some general indicators in a cultural community that suggest which features of that culture's practices are particularly intended to be acquired by children and matter to that community (Schönpflug, 2009). We have already touched on several of these in this chapter, such as evidence of a fairly widely shared ethnotheory; similar ecocultural contexts for children; similar relationship models and people to interact with across settings; the "redundant control" or repetition of a desired pattern (Levy, 1973) of some behaviors and practices, created by adults, peers, and others; and repeating certain ideas across many settings, across age periods, and so forth. More generally, when there is repeated emphasis and repetition of family and community patterns in a child's cultural learning environment, it is then more likely that these in fact are shared, important cultural beliefs and scripts.

These shared patterns are marked as the culturally meaningful practices that the community and parents want to inculcate in their children as part of their project of rearing children to be culturally valued adults. They reflect desired personal qualities and cultural goals (Quinn, 2006, p. 478):

> First, such [cultural models for raising children] universally incorporate practices that maximize the constancy of the child's experience around the learning of important lessons about what is valued. Second, such models universally include practices that make the child's experience of learning these lessons emotionally arousing. Third, such models universally attach these lessons to more global evaluations of the child's behavior, and of the child, as approved or disapproved. Fourth, and finally, such models universally train children first in some emotional predisposition, the strategic role of which is to prime the child for subsequent lessons about what is desired and expected of him or her as an adult.

CONCLUSION

Throughout this volume you will read a wide range of hard-won summaries of evidence and theory about social development. You might extend the culture framework to those summaries from other chapters by asking: In what ecocultural context, developmental niche, and cultural learning environment were those data collected? Would a particular empirical finding or generalization (likely studied in only one context, in one cultural community) hold up in others? As we have seen, cultural evidence can lead to findings of cross-cultural generalizations that hold quite widely, if not universally. In other cases, such evidence leads to the conclusion that context and culture make a major difference. There often can be universal processes in social development (attachments, dealing with aggression or shyness, early language acquisition) but with widely varying beliefs, practices, and outcomes from those processes, for both children and parents, across cultures. A continuing core scientific question for this field is to disentangle possible universal processes from their varying expressions in local cultural contexts.

The importance of a cultural-comparative database and theory for understanding human behavior and psychology is not limited to social development. The same urgency for developing a global database comes from the fields of visual perception, spatial reasoning, moral reasoning, styles of thinking, variations in self-concepts around the world, and almost any topic in social development. There is a long way to go to fully incorporate the world's children into developmental research. For example, 96% of people studied in the top journals in six subdisciplines of psychology from 2003 through 2007 were from North America, Europe, Australia, and Israel: "this means that 96% of psychological samples come from countries with only 12% of the world's population" (Henrich, Heine, & Norenzayan, 2010, p. 63). Furthermore, the great majority of these samples are composed solely of undergraduates in psychology courses. "A randomly selected American undergraduate is more than 4000 times more likely to be a research participant than is a randomly selected person from outside of the West" (Henrich et al., 2010, p. 65). So we need a much more representative database for social development; this means greater pluralism in whom we talk with and observe and in the settings around the world to which we go to study. The next generations of scholars—including those reading this volume—are the ones to do this cross-cultural field research. Of the many questions and research programs important for future research in social development, this goal is probably the single most important.

The world is changing rapidly today, and globalization, modernization, and global economic development, underdevelopment, and disparities are important features influencing children's social lives, families, and cultural learning environments (Weisner & Lowe, 2005). Understanding how these changes shape social development is another critical question for the future. Globalization is, among other things, the reducing of barriers to the flow of information, objects, people, and capital around the world. The result has been to give youths, children, parents—everyone—access to incredible new experiences shared regionally or globally and encourage the rise in immigration and mixing of cultural and family traditions in new places. But it is an empirical matter as to how much children's social experiences will become homogeneous as a result of rapid change (Casey & Edgerton, 2005; Edwards & Whiting, 2004). Perhaps the more affluent share more of this global experience and benefit from it more than the poor. There is resistance and pushback to global influences, as well. Family life and parenting are relatively more conservative aspects of life and more difficult to change in many respects than media consumption or work roles, for example. With due regard to the process of globalization, there are still *very* substantial variations in children's cultural learning environments around the world today, and this variation is definitely not about to be eliminated in the next generations. Understanding the influences on social development of these very diverse, pluralistic, and ever-changing cultural learning environments and developmental niches in the coming generations is going to be a fascinating research topic for the future.

SUGGESTED READINGS

Bornstein, M. H. (Ed.). (2010). *Handbook of cultural developmental science*. New York: Psychology Press.

Lancy, D. F. (2008). *The anthropology of childhood: Cherubs, chattel, changelings*. Cambridge, UK: Cambridge University Press.

LeVine, R. A., Levine, S., Dixon, S., Richman, A., Leiderman, P. H., & Keefer, C. (1994). *Child care and culture: Lessons from Africa*. Cambridge, UK: Cambridge University Press.

Shweder, R. A., Bidell, T. R., Dailey, A. C., Dixon, S., Miller, P. J. & Modell, J. (Eds.). (2009). *The child: An encyclopedic companion*. Chicago: University of Chicago Press.

Whiting, B., & Edwards, C. P. (1988). *Children of different worlds: The formation of social behavior*. Cambridge, MA: Harvard University Press.

REFERENCES

Abels, M. (2008). Kulturvergleichende Grundlagen frühkindlicher Selbstregulationsprozesse [Cross-cultural bases of self-regulation processes in infancy]. In J. Borke & A. Eickhorst (Eds.), *Systemische Entwicklungsberatung in der frühen Kindheit* (pp. 44–59). Stuttgart, Germany: UTB.

Axia, V. D., & Weisner, T. S. (2002). Infant stress reactivity and home cultural ecology of Italian infants and families. *Infant Behavior and Development, 25*(3), 1–14.

Berk, L. E. (2009). Social development. In R. Shweder, T. R. Bidell, A. C. Dailey, S. Dixon, P. J. Miller, & J. Modell (Eds.), *The child. An encyclopedic companion* (pp. 920–924). Chicago: University of Chicago Press.

Bernard, H. R. (1995). *Research methods in anthropology: Qualitative and quantitative approaches.* Walnut Creek, CA: AltaMira Press.

Bernard, H. R. (1998). *Handbook of methods in cultural anthropology.* Walnut Creek, CA: Alta-Mira Press.

Best, D. L. (2010). Gender. In M. H. Bornstein (Ed.), *Handbook of cultural developmental science* (pp. 209–222). New York: Psychology Press.

Bogin, B. (1999). *Patterns of human growth.* Cambridge, UK: Cambridge University Press.

Bornstein, M. H. (Ed.). (2010). *Handbook of cultural developmental science.* New York: Psychology Press.

Bronfenbrenner, U. (1979). *The ecology of human development: Experiments by nature and design.* Cambridge, MA: Harvard University Press.

Bronfenbrenner, U. (1995). Developmental ecology through space and time: A future perspective. In P. Moen, G. H. Elder, K. Luscher, & U. Bronfenbrenner (Eds.), *Examining lives in context: Perspectives on the ecology of human development* (pp. 619–647). Washington, DC: American Psychological Association.

Campbell, B. (2008, November). *Middle childhood, adrenarche and brain development.* Paper presented at the meeting of the American Anthropological Association.

Casey, C., & Edgerton, R. B. (2005). *A companion to psychological anthropology. Modernity and psychocultural change.* Oxford, UK: Blackwell.

ChildFund International. (2009). Toys made by children around the world on display at Museum of Tolerance. *www.latimes.com/entertainment/news/la-ca-toys13–2009dec13, 0,6098403.story; www.washingtonpost.com/wp-dyn/content/article/2009/11/10/AR200911 1017222.html*

Chisholm, J. S. (1996). *Navajo infancy: An ethological study of child development.* New York, NY: Aldine de Gruyter.

Cole, M. (1996). *Cultural psychology: A once and future discipline.* Cambridge, MA: Harvard University Press.

Cole, M., & Cole, S. R. (1993). *The development of children.* New York: Scientific American Books.

DeLoache, J., & Gottlieb, A. (2000). If Dr. Spock were born in Bali: Raising a world of babies. In J. DeLoache & A. Gottlieb (Eds.), *A world of babies. Imagined childcare guides for seven societies* (pp. 1–27). New York: Cambridge University Press.

Edwards, C. P. (2000). Children's play in cross-cultural perspective: A new look at the Six Culture Study. *Cross Cultural Research, 34,* 318–338.

Edwards, C. P., & Bloch, M. (2010). The Whitings' concepts of culture and how they have fared in contemporary psychology and anthropology. *Journal of Cross-Cultural Psychology, 41*(4), 485–498.

Edwards, C. P., deGuzman, M. T., Brown, J., & Kumru, A. (2006). Children's social behaviors and peer interactions in diverse cultures. In X. Chen, D. French, & B. Schneider (Eds.), *Peer relations in cultural context* (pp. 23–51). New York: Cambridge University Press.

Edwards, C. P., & Whiting, B. B. (Eds.). (2004). *Ngecha: A Kenyan village in a time of rapid social change.* Lincoln: University of Nebraska Press.

Ember, C. R. (1973). Feminine task assignment and the social behavior of boys. *Ethos, 1*(4), 424–439.

Farver, J. A. (1999). Activity settings analysis: A model for examining the role of culture in development. In A. Goncu (Ed.), *Children's engagement in the world: Sociocultural perspectives* (pp. 99–127). Cambridge, UK: Cambridge University Press.

Fuligni, A. J., & Flook, L. (2005). A social identity approach to ethnic differences in family relationships during adolescence. In R. Kail (Ed.), *Advances in child development and behavior* (pp. 125–152). New York: Academic Press.

Gaskins, S. (1996). How Mayan parental theories come into play. In S. Harkness & C. Super (Eds.), *Parents' cultural belief systems* (pp. 345–361). New York: Guilford Press.

Goldschmidt, W. (1975). Absent eyes and idle hands: Socialization for low affect among the Sebei. *Ethos, 3*(2), 157–163.

Goldstein, D. M. (1998). Nothing bad intended: Child discipline, punishment, and survival in a shantytown in Rio de Janiero, Brazil. In N. Scheper-Hughes & C. Sargent (Eds.), *Small wars: The cultural politics of childhood* (pp. 389–415). Berkeley: University of California Press.

Goldstein, D. M. (2003). *Laughter out of place: Race, class, violence, and sexuality in a Rio shantytown.* Berkeley: University of California Press.

Goodwin, C. (2006). *The hidden life of girls: Games of stance, status, and exclusion.* Oxford, UK: Blackwell.

Gottlieb, A. (2004). *The afterlife is where we come from: The culture of infancy in West Africa.* Chicago: University of Chicago Press.

Greenfield, P. M., Keller, H., Fuligni, A., & Maynard, A. (2003). Cultural pathways through universal development. *Annual Review of Psychology, 54,* 461–490.

Gregg, G. S. (2005). *The Middle East: A cultural psychology.* New York: Oxford University Press.

Harkness, S., & Super, C. M. (Eds.). (1996). *Parents' cultural belief systems: Their origins, expressions, and consequences.* New York: Guilford Press.

Harkness, S., Super, C. M., Moscardino, U., Rha, J.-H., Blom, M. J. M., Huitrón, B., et al. (2007). Cultural models and developmental agendas: Implications for arousal and self-regulation in early infancy. *Journal of Developmental Processes, 1*(2), 5–39.

Harwood, R., Miller, J., & Irizarry, N. L. (1995). *Culture and attachment. Perceptions of the child in context.* New York: Guilford Press.

Henrich, J., Heine, S. J., & Norenzayan, A. (2010). The weirdest people in the world? *Behavioral and Brain Sciences, 33,* 61–135.

Herdt, G., & Leavitt, S. C. (Eds.). (1998). *Adolescence in Pacific Island societies.* Pittsburgh, PA: University of Pittsburgh Press.

Hogg, M. A. (2003). Social identity. In M. R. Leary & J. P. Tangney (Eds.), *Handbook of self and identity* (pp. 462–479). New York: Guilford Press.

Holloway, S. D. (2000). *Contested childhood: Diversity and change in Japanese preschools.* New York: Routledge.

Hrdy, S. B. (2009). *Mothers and others: The evolutionary origins of mutual understanding.* Cambridge, MA: Harvard University Press.

Kagitçibasi, C. (1996). *Family and human development across cultures. A view from the other side.* Mahwah, NJ: Erlbaum.

Kagitçibasi, C. (2007). *Family, self and human development across countries: Theory and applications* (2nd ed.). Hillsdale, NJ: Erlbaum

Keller, H. (2007). *Cultures of infancy.* Mahwah, NJ: Erlbaum.

Keller, H., Lamm, B., Abels, M., Yovsi, R., Borke, J., Jensen, H., et al. (2006). Cultural models, socialization goals, and parenting ethnotheories: A multicultural analysis. *Journal of Cross-Cultural Psychology, 37*(2), 155–172.

Kitayama, S., & Markus, H. R. (2000). The pursuit of happiness and the realization of sympathy: Cultural patterns of self, social relations, and well-being. In E. Diener & E. Suh (Eds.), *Subjective well-being across cultures* (pp. 113–161). Cambridge, MA: MIT Press.

Kling, J., Liebman, J. B., & Katz, L. F. (2005). Bullets got no name: Consequences of fear in the ghetto. In T. S. Weisner (Ed.), *Discovering successful pathways in human development: Mixed methods in the study of childhood and family life* (pp. 243–281). Chicago: University of Chicago Press.

Konner, M. (1982). *The tangled wing: Biological constraints on the human spirit.* New York: Holt, Rinehart, & Winston.

Lancy, D. F. (1996). *Playing on the mother-ground: Cultural routines for children's development.* New York: Guilford Press.

Lancy, D. F. (2007). Accounting for variability in mother–child play. *American Anthropologist, 109*(2), 273–284.

Lancy, D. F. (2008). *The anthropology of childhood: Cherubs, chattel, changelings.* Cambridge, UK: Cambridge University Press.

Lancy, D. F., Bock, J., & Gaskins, S. (Eds.). (2010). *The anthropology of learning in childhood.* Walnut Creek, CA: AltaMira Press.

Leiderman, P. H., Tulkin, S., & Rosenfeld, A. (1977). *Culture and infancy.* New York: Academic Press.

Leon, L. D. (1998). The emergent participant: Interactive patterns in the socialization of Tzotzil (Mayan) infants. *Journal of Linguistic Anthropology, 8*(2), 131–161.

LeVine, R. A. (2007). Ethnographic studies of childhood: A historical overview. *American Anthropologist, 109*(2), 247–260.

LeVine, R. A., LeVine, S., Dixon, S., Richman, A., Leiderman, P. H., & Keefer, C. (1994). *Child care and culture: Lessons from Africa*. Cambridge, UK: Cambridge University Press.

LeVine, R. A., Miller, P. M., & West, M. M. (1988). *Parental behaviors in diverse societies*. San Francisco: Jossey-Bass.

LeVine, R. A., & New, R. S. (2008). *Anthropology and child development: A cross-cultural reader*. Malden, MA: Blackwell.

LeVine, R. A., & Norman, K. (2001). The infant's acquisition of culture: Early attachment reexamined in anthropological perspective. In C. C. Moore & H. F. Mathews (Eds.), *The psychology of cultural experience* (pp. 83–104). New York: Cambridge University Press.

LeVine, S. (2009). Formality and fun in kinship relations among the Gusii. In R. Shweder et al. (Eds.), *The child: An encyclopedic companion* (p. 82). Chicago: University of Chicago Press.

Levy, R. (1973). *The Tahitians: Mind and experience in the Society Islands*. Chicago: University of Chicago Press.

Lewis, M., & Takahashi, K. (Eds.). (2005). Beyond the dyad: Conceptualization of social networks. *Human Development, 48*(1–2), 5–7.

McGilvray, D. B. (2008). *Crucible of conflict: Tamil and Muslim society on the East Coast of Sri Lanka*. Durham, NC, & London: Duke University Press.

McKenna, J. J., & McDade, T. (2005). Why babies should never sleep alone: A review of the co-sleeping controversy in relation to SIDS, bedsharing and breast feeding. *Paediatric Respiratory Reviews, 6*(2), 134–152.

Mead, M. (1949). *Coming of age in Samoa: A study of adolescence and sex in primitive society*. New York: New American Library.

Miller, P. J., Wiley, A. R., Fung, H., & Liang, C. H. (1997). Personal storytelling as a medium of socialization in Chinese and American families. *Child Development, 68*(3), 557–568.

Montgomery, H. (2009). *An introduction to childhood: Anthropological perspectives on children's lives*. Oxford, UK: Wiley-Blackwell.

Morelli, G. A., Rogoff, B., Oppenheim, D., & Goldsmith, D. (1992). Cultural variation in infants' sleeping arrangements: Questions of independence. *Developmental Psychology, 28*(4), 604–613.

Munroe, R. L., & Munroe, R. H. (1975). *Cross-cultural human development*. Monterey, CA: Brooks/Cole.

Munroe, R. L., & Munroe, R. H. (1997). Logoli childhood and the cultural reproduction of sex differentiation. In T.S. Weisner, C. Bradley, & P. L. Kilbride (Eds.), *African families and the crisis of social change* (pp. 299–314). Westport, CT: Bergin & Garvey.

Nsamenang, A. B., & Lo-oh, J. L. (2010). Afrique Noire. In M.H. Bornstein (Ed.), *Handbook of cultural developmental science* (pp. 383–407). New York: Psychology Press.

Nuckolls, C. W. (Ed.). (1993). *Siblings in South Asia: Brothers and sisters in cultural context*. New York: Guilford Press.

Ochs, E. (1988). *Culture and language development: Language acquisition and language socialization in a Samoan village*. New York: Cambridge University Press.

Okami, P., Weisner, T. S., & Olmstead, R. (2002). Outcome correlates of parent–child bedsharing: An 18-year longitudinal study. *Journal of Developmental and Behavioral Pediatrics, 23*(4), 244–253.

Quinn, N. (2006). Universals of child rearing. *Anthropological Theory, 5*(4), 475–514.

Rabain-Jamin, J. (2001). Language use in mother–child and young sibling interactions in Senegal. *First Language, 21*(63), 357–385.

Richman, A. L., LeVine, R. A., New, R. S., Howrigan, G. A., Wells-Nystrom, B., & LeVine S. E. (1988). Maternal behavior to infants in five cultures. In R. A. LeVine, P. M. Miller, & M. W. Maxwell (Eds.), *Parental behavior in diverse societies* (pp. 81–98). San Francisco: Jossey-Bass.

Rogoff, B. (2003). *The cultural nature of human development*. Oxford, UK: Oxford University Press.

Rogoff, B., Sellers, M. J., Pirrotta, S., Fox, N., & White, S. H. (1975). The age of assignment of roles and responsibilities to children: A cross-cultural survey. *Human Development, 18*(5), 353–369.

Rothbaum, F., Pott, M., Azuma, H., Miyake, K., & Weisz, J. (2000). The development of close relationships in Japan and the United States: Paths of symbiotic harmony and generative tension. *Child Development, 71*(5), 1121–1142.

Rubin, K. H., Cheah, C., & Menzer, M. M. (2010). Peers. In M. H. Bornstein (Ed.), *Handbook of cultural and development science* (pp. 223–237). New York: Psychology Press.

Rubin, K. H., & Chung, O. B. (2006). *Parenting beliefs, behaviors, and parent–child relations: A cross-cultural perspective.* New York: Psychology Press.

Rubin, K. H., Hemphill, S. A., Chen, X., Hastings, P., Sanson, A., Lococo, A., et al. (2006). Parenting beliefs and behaviors: Initial findings from the International Consortium for the Study of Social and Emotional Development (ICSSED). In K. H. Rubin & O. B. Chung (Eds.), *Parenting beliefs, behaviors, and parent–child relations: A cross-cultural perspective* (pp. 81–103). New York: Psychology Press.

Sameroff, A. J., & Haith, M. M. (1996). *The five- to seven-year shift: The age of reason and responsibility.* Chicago: University of Chicago Press.

Scheper-Hughes, N. (1990). Mother love and child death in Northeast Brazil. In J.W. Stigler, R.A. Shweder, & G. Herdt (Eds.), *Cultural psychology: Essays on comparative human development* (pp. 542–565). Cambridge, UK: Cambridge University Press.

Schlegel, A. (Ed.). (1977). *Sexual stratification: A cross-cultural view.* New York: Columbia University Press.

Schlegel, A., & Barry, H., III. (1991). *Adolescence: An anthropological inquiry.* New York: Free Press.

Schönpflug, U. (2009). *Cultural transmission. Psychological, developmental, social, and methodological aspects.* New York: Cambridge University Press.

Serpell, R. (1993). *The significance of schooling: Life-journeys in an African society.* New York: Cambridge University Press.

Serpell, R. (2008, July). *African socialization: Goals, practices, and policies.* Invited lecture at the 20th biennial meeting, International Society for the Study of Behavioural Development, Wuerzburg, Germany.

Seymour, S. (1999). *Women, family and child care in India.* New York: Cambridge University Press.

Shwalb, D. W., & Shwalb, B. J. (1996). *Japanese child rearing: Two generations of scholarship.* New York: Guilford Press.

Shweder, R. A. (2002) "What about female genital mutilation?" and why understanding culture matters in the first place. In R. Shweder, M. Minow, & H. R. Markus (Eds.), *Engaging cultural differences* (pp. 216–251). New York: Russell Sage Foundation.

Shweder, R. A., Bidell, T. R., Dailey, A. C., Dixon, S., Miller, P. J., & Modell, J. (Eds.). (2009). *The child: An encyclopedic companion.* Chicago: University of Chicago Press

Shweder, R. A., Goodnow, J. J., Hatano, G., LeVine, R. A., Markus, H. R., & Miller, P. J. (2006). The cultural psychology of development: One mind, many mentalities. In W. Damon & R. Lerner (Eds.), *Handbook of child psychology: Vol. 1. Theoretical models of human development* (6th ed., pp. 716–792). New York: Wiley.

Shweder, R., Minow, M., & Markus, H. R. (2002). *Engaging cultural differences.* New York: Russell Sage Foundation.

Small, M. F. (2001). *Kids: How biology and culture shape the way we raise our children.* New York: Doubleday.

Super, C. M., & Harkness, S. (1986). The developmental niche: A conceptualization at the interface of child and culture. *International Journal of Behavioral Development, 9*(4), 545–569.

Super, C. M., & Harkness, S. (1996). The "three R's" of Dutch child rearing and the socialization of infant state. In S. Harkness & C. M. Super (Eds.), *Parents' cultural belief systems: Their origins, expressions, and consequences* (pp. 447–466). New York: Guilford Press.

Super, C. M., & Harkness, S. (1999). The environment as culture in developmental research. In S. L. Friedman & T. D. Wachs (Eds.), *Measuring environment across the life span: Emerging methods and concepts* (pp. 279–323). Washington, DC: American Psychological Association.

Super, C. M., & Harkness, S. (2002). Culture structures the environment for development. *Human Development, 45*, 270–274.

Therborn, G. (2009). Family. In R. A. Shweder, T. R. Bidell, A. C. Dailey, S. Dixon, P. J. Miller, & J. Modell (Eds.), *The child: An encyclopedic companion* (pp. 333–338). Chicago: University of Chicago Press.

Tobin, J. (2000). Using "the Japanese problem" as a corrective to the ethnocentricity of Western theory. *Child Development, 71*(5), 1155–1158.

Tobin, J., Wu, D., & Davidson, D. (1989). *Preschool in three cultures: Japan, China, and the United States.* New Haven, CT: Yale University Press.

Trawick, M. (2007). *Enemy lines: Warfare, childhood, and play in Batticaloa.* Berkeley: University of California Press.

Tudge, J. (2008). *The everyday lives of young children: Culture, class, and child rearing in diverse societies.* New York: Cambridge University Press.

van IJzendoorn, M. H., Bakermans-Kranenburg, M. J., & Sagi-Schwartz, A. (2006). Attachment across diverse sociocultural contexts: The limits of universality. In K. H. Rubin & O. B. Chung (Eds.), *Parenting beliefs, behaviors, and parent–child relations: A cross-cultural perspective* (pp. 107–142). New York: Psychology Press.

Weisner, T. S. (1987). Socialization for parenthood in sibling caretaking societies. In J. Lancaster, A. Rossi, J. Altmann, & L. Sherrod (Eds.), *Parenting across the lifespan* (pp. 237–270). New York: Aldine.

Weisner, T. S. (1989). Cultural and universal aspects of social support for children: Evidence among the Abaluyia of Kenya. In D. Belle (Ed.), *Children's social networks and social supports* (pp. 70–90). New York: Wiley.

Weisner, T. S. (1996a). Why ethnography should be the most important method in the study of human development. In R. Jessor, A. Colby, & R. A. Shweder (Eds.), *Ethnography and human development: Context and meaning in social inquiry* (pp. 305–324). Chicago: University of Chicago Press.

Weisner, T. S. (1996b). The 5–7 transition as an ecocultural project. In A. J. Sameroff & M. M. Haith (Eds.), *The five- to seven-year shift: The age of reason and responsibility* (pp. 295–326). Chicago: University of Chicago Press.

Weisner, T. S. (1997). Support for children and the African family crisis. In T. S. Weisner, C. Bradley, & P. Kilbride (Eds.), *African families and the crisis of social change* (pp. 20–44). Westport, CT: Greenwood Press/Bergin & Garvey.

Weisner, T. S. (2002). Ecocultural understanding of children's developmental pathways. *Human Development, 45*(4), 275–281.

Weisner, T. S. (2005a). Attachment as a cultural and ecological problem with pluralistic solutions. *Human Development, 48*(1–2), 89–94.

Weisner, T. S. (2005b). *Discovering successful pathways in children's development: Mixed methods in the study of childhood and family life.* Chicago: University of Chicago Press.

Weisner, T. S. (2009). Culture, development, and diversity: Expectable pluralism, conflict, and similarity. *Ethos, 37*(2), 181–196.

Weisner, T. S., & Gallimore. R. (1977). My brother's keeper: Child and sibling caretaking. *Current Anthropology, 18*, 169–190.

Weisner, T. S., & Lowe, E. (2005). Globalization and the psychological anthropology of childhood and adolescence. In C. Casey & R. Edgerton (Eds.), *A companion to psychological anthropology: Modernity and psychocultural change* (pp. 315–336). Oxford, UK: Blackwell.

Werner, E. E. (1979). *Cross-cultural development.* Monterey, CA: Brooks/Cole.

Whiting, B.B. (Ed.). (1963). *Six cultures: Studies of child rearing.* New York: Wiley.

Whiting, B. (1980). Culture and social behavior: A model for the development of social behavior. *Ethos, 8*, 95–116.

Whiting, B., & Edwards, C. P. (1973). A cross-cultural analysis of sex differences in the behavior of children aged 3–11. *Journal of Social Psychology, 91*, 171–188.

Whiting, B., & Edwards, C. P. (1988). *Children of different worlds: The formation of social behavior.* Cambridge, MA: Harvard University Press.

Whiting, J., & Whiting, B. (1975). *Children of six cultures: A psychocultural analysis.* Cambridge, MA: Harvard University Press.

Williams, J. E., & Best, D. L. (1990). *Measuring sex stereotypes: A multi-nation study*. Newbury Park, CA: Sage.

Worthman, C. M. (2010). The ecology of human development: evolving models for cultural psychology. *Journal of Cross-Cultural Psychology, 41*(4), 546–562.

Xu, Y., Farver, J., Chang, L., Yu, L., & Zhang, Z. (2006). Culture, family contexts, and children's coping strategies in peer interactions. In X. Chen, D. French, & B. H. Schneider (Eds.), *Peer relationships in cultural context* (pp. 264–280). New York: Cambridge University Press.

Yoshikawa, H., Weisner, T. S., Kalil, A., & Way, N. (2008). Mixing qualitative and quantitative research in developmental science: Uses and methodological choices. *Developmental Psychology, 44*(2), 344–354.

Zukow, P. G. (1989). Siblings as effective socializing agents: Evidence from Central Mexico. In P.G. Zukow (Ed.), *Sibling interaction across cultures* (pp. 70–105). New York: Springer Verlag.

Part V

Risk and Resilience

16

Child Maltreatment and Social Relationships

Penelope K. Trickett
Sonya Negriff

Different forms of child abuse and neglect, or *child maltreatment*, as these are often collectively termed, are inherently social phenomena. That is to say, these terms refer to behavioral and verbal interchanges between parents and their minor offspring. As such, it would be reasonable to consider all the social development topics of this book as likely affecting and being affected by child maltreatment and thus as being appropriate foci for this review of research. Such a comprehensive review, however, would require a book of its own. Instead, the focus here is on the impact of child maltreatment on one especially important aspect: social or interpersonal relationships examined from a developmental perspective. Thus we review, in turn, research on the impact of different forms of child maltreatment on attachment relationships of infants and young children with their parents; on peer relationships and friendships of school-age children; on romantic and sexual relationships of adolescents and emerging adults; and on parenting of the next generation.

HISTORY OF THE PROBLEM

Prior to beginning this review, it is important to provide a brief history of how child abuse and neglect became recognized as an important social problem in the United States. and how the subsequent involvement of the federal government influenced how child maltreatment is identified, defined, and addressed. This involvement affected how and when social and behavioral science research on this topic in the United States has progressed.

Awareness of Child Abuse

Society has been aware of the existence of child neglect since the earliest years of the 20th century. On the other hand, societal awareness of the physical and sexual abuse of children has been more recent—within the past 40 years. With physical abuse this came about in the 1960s when medical doctors "discovered" that children were being physically injured by their parents and then coined the phrase *battered child syndrome* (Kempe, Silverman, Steele, Droegemueller, & Silver, 1962). About a decade after that came recognition of the frequency of sexual abuse, which had previously been considered an extremely rare phenomenon.

Out of this awareness came federal legislation in 1974, in the form of the Child Abuse Prevention and Treatment Act (CAPTA) and the establishment of the National Center on Child Abuse and Neglect (NCCAN) within the Children's Bureau, Administration for Youth and Families, U.S. Department of Health and Human Services. This 1974 legislation was amended most recently as the Keeping Children and Families Safe Act of 2003. The primary purpose of this federal legislation was to ensure the development by the states of programs and services for abused children and their families. Four main categories of abuse and neglect were identified, although the exact definitions of these types was a task left explicitly to the states, and thus they vary somewhat from locale to locale. Generally, state statutes' definitions are as follows (see Child Welfare Information Gateway, 2007):

Physical abuse: This type of maltreatment is generally defined as any nonaccidental physical injury to a child (resulting from such acts as striking, kicking, burning) perpetrated by a parent or caregiver.

Sexual abuse: A type of maltreatment that refers to the involvement of the child in sexual activity to provide sexual gratification or financial benefit to the perpetrator, including molestation, statutory rape, prostitution, pornography, exposure, incest, or other sexually exploitative activities.

Psychological or emotional maltreatment: This type of maltreatment refers to acts or omissions, other than physical abuse or sexual abuse, that caused, or could have caused, conduct, cognitive, affective, or other mental disorders. This frequently occurs as verbal abuse or excessive demands on a child's performance.

Neglect: A type of maltreatment that refers to the failure by the parent or caregiver to provide needed, age-appropriate care although financially able to do so or offered financial or other means to do so. This includes deprivation of adequate food, clothing, shelter, medical care, or supervision. In many states this also includes failure to educate.

Note that all these definitions, except for that of sexual abuse, describe negative and extreme forms of dimensions of parenting or child rearing (e.g., harsh physical punishment, low nurturance, rejection) that have been identified for years as detrimental to competent development of children (Maccoby & Martin, 1983). Note, too, that these definitions of the different forms of child abuse and especially neglect tend to be vague. Further, as stated previously, they vary from state to state, and thus, because many research studies recruit samples from public child protective service agencies, there has been considerable variability in the operational definitions of the maltreatment. Thus, for example, a study of neglected children taking place in one locale could well include children not considered neglected in an adjacent state. These sorts of definitional problems contribute to the complexity and oftentimes inconsistency in results of child maltreatment research (Feerick, Knutson, Trickett, & Flanzer, 2006).

Studies of Child Abuse

One important function of NCCAN (now called OCAN, Office of Child Abuse and Neglect) was to sponsor studies to determine the incidence of abuse and neglect in the United States. Four such national incidence studies have been conducted, published in 1980 (Burgdorf, 1980), 1988 (National Center on Child Abuse and Neglect [NCCAN], 1988), 1996 (NCCAN, 1996), and 2010 (Sedlak et al., 2010). The data in these annual incidence studies derive from a national representative sample of U.S. counties. Using a "sentinel survey methodology," the study team was provided with reports on all children who were reported as being abused or neglected to child protection agencies and also from other "sentinels"—community professionals, such as staff in police departments, public schools, day-care centers, and so forth, who have contact with children and families. The data were then "unduplicated" to ensure that each maltreated child was reported only once (Sedlak, et al, 2010). All of these studies indicate that a very large number of children in the United States are victims of abuse and neglect (or, more accurately, are known to authorities to have been victims of abuse or neglect or both). These rates increased from the first to the second study and from the second to third. The fourth study, just released, indicates a reduction in the annual incidence rate since the third study, but the numbers are still very large.

As Table 16.1 indicates, the Fourth National Incidence Study of Child Abuse and Neglect (NIS-4; Sedlak et al., 2010) found that, using the more stringent *harm standard* (i.e., evidence that the child *had been harmed* by the maltreatment), the annual incidence of child abuse and neglect in the United States was about 1.25 million (a rate of 17.2 per 1,000 children). Using the less stringent *endangerment standard* (i.e., evidence that the child *had been harmed or was in danger of being harmed* by the maltreatment), the accrued incidence of all forms of abuse and neglect was almost 3 million annually (a rate of 40 per 1,000). Table 16.1 also indicates the percentage of maltreated children labeled as physically abused, sexually abused, emotionally abused, or neglected. The majority of maltreated children were neglected, and the increase in cases seen with the endangerment standard, as compared with the harm standard, is due to the disproportionate increases in neglect. Other important information coming from this study (and supported by the findings of the prior incidence studies) include the following:

• The rates of all different forms of maltreatment are lowest for infants and very young children and then rise before leveling off and remaining relatively steady throughout childhood and adolescence. The rise may reflect the importance of school

TABLE 16.1. Annual Incidence of Child Maltreatment

Type of maltreatment	Harm standard	Endangerment standard
All maltreatment	1,256,600	2,905,800
Abuse		
Physical	26%	16%
Sexual	11%	6%
Emotional	12%	10%
Neglect	61%	77%

Note. Data are from NIS-4 (Sedlak et al., 2010).

entry in detection of child maltreatment. Thus, despite the stereotype of the neglected child in particular as an infant or a very young child, the rates are equally high or higher for school-age children and adolescents. Similarly, it is important to recognize that victims of sexual abuse can be infants or toddlers. (The mean age of sexual abuse victims as reported in NIS-3 (NCCAN, 1996) is about 8 years of age.)

• With the exception of sexual abuse, for which rates are about 3 times greater for girls than boys, no gender differences are found. That is, boys and girls are equally likely to be reported as neglected or abused.

• Although child abuse and neglect occur among all social classes, abuse and especially neglect occur with greater frequency in low-socioeconomic-status (SES) households, as indexed by household income, participation in poverty programs, and parents' education. In fact, children in such households are found to experience some type of maltreatment at rates 5 times greater than children growing up in more advantaged households.

What is not clear from the data reported in the national incidence studies is that there is much evidence that many children experience more than one type of maltreatment, experienced either simultaneously or sequentially (Claussen & Crittenden, 1991). In our current study, for example, we found that in a sample of about three hundred 9- to 12-year-old maltreated children recruited from a large urban child protection agency, 54% had experienced at least two types of maltreatment. Additionally, neglect co-occurred with physical abuse in 50% of the sample and with emotional abuse in 61% of the sample (Mennen, Kim, Sang, & Trickett, 2010; Trickett, Mennen, Kim, & Sang, 2009) . Furthermore, the average number of separate reports to the child welfare agencies for these children was almost 5, with a range from 1 to 17. Thus, although from a child development perspective it is logical to assume that different forms of child maltreatment—as different as injuring a child by striking or burning and failing to provide adequate food or medical care—would have different developmental outcomes, the complexity of the maltreatment experience and the definitional problems mentioned previously often make this difficult, if not impossible, to ascertain.

THE IMPACT OF CHILD MALTREATMENT
ON SOCIAL DEVELOPMENT

In the mid-1990s, Trickett and McBride-Chang (1995) published a review of research that had been conducted at the behest of the National Academy of Sciences' Panel on Research on Child Abuse and Neglect. This review attempted to integrate research knowledge about the impact of different forms of child maltreatment—physical abuse, sexual abuse, and neglect—on the development of children and, as they grew up, adolescents and adults. (Emotional maltreatment was not included because studies were rare.) It examined not only social and emotional development but physical and cognitive development, as well. This review noted that much of the early research, conducted within a decade or so of the passage of CAPTA, was weak. Often the samples were very small, definitions of maltreatment were especially vague, no appropriate control or comparison groups were used, and measures used had little or no evidence of reliability or validity. A "second generation," if you will, of research studies with stronger designs were conducted in the mid-1980s and later, and these were reviewed in

Trickett and McBride-Chang (1995). Compared with the earlier studies, these studies usually had larger samples, with clearer operational definitions of maltreatment, comparison groups, and outcome measures with established reliability and validity. What follows is a brief summary of those studies that pertain to the impact of maltreatment on social relationships and then a review of more recently published studies.

Attachment Relationships in Infancy and Early Childhood

One of the earliest foci of studies on the impact of child maltreatment on social development concerned attachment styles of very young children maltreated by parents and the social behaviors of these children. One of these early studies, which had a profound influence on the field, was that of George and Main (1979). Using observational methodology in a child-care setting, this study linked disturbed attachment relationships to odd and negative social interactions (especially what they termed "harassment" and approach–avoidance behaviors) with both peers and teachers in physically abused 1- to 3-year-olds as compared with matched controls. Many other studies addressing attachment relationships of young maltreated children followed this seminal study. The findings of these studies reinforced the prevalence of insecure attachment among maltreated children and identified an unusual form of attachment, initially labeled disorganized/disoriented, among young children who were physically abused (Crittenden, 1981; Erickson & Egeland, 1987) and neglected or otherwise maltreated (Carlson, Cicchetti, Barnett, & Braunwald, 1989; Lyons-Ruth, Connell, & Zoll, 1989). In these early studies, attachment relationships were not examined in young sexually abused children.

In a recent meta-analysis, Baer and Martinez (2006) reviewed the findings of eight studies (all but one of which were published prior to 1993) involving children 48 months of age or younger who were either physically abused or neglected (including some samples labeled "failure to thrive"). These authors confirmed that the maltreated children were significantly more likely to show insecure attachment, especially of the "disorganized" type. They also found that the effect size was greater for the physically abused children—as compared, especially, with those labeled "failure to thrive"—and recommended that further research be conducted to clarify the relationships between different forms of maltreatment and insecure attachment relationships. In another recent review, Cicchetti and Toth (2005) also conclude that maltreated infants are at very high risk of developing insecure attachment relationships. They also note that, in the few studies that have examined attachment in school-age maltreated children (e.g., Lynch & Cicchetti, 1991), the same risk for insecure attachments has been found. (See also Roisman & Groh, Chapter 5, this volume).

Peer Relations and Friendships

Establishing successful peer relations is considered to be a central developmental task of childhood. There is substantial evidence that all types of maltreatment are linked to problems with peers and friendships (for a summary of studies, see Table 16.2). Early clinical studies found that maltreated children behaved in one of two ways toward peers: with excessive aggression or with excessive withdrawal and avoidance of other children (Mueller & Silverman, 1989). As noted earlier, George and Main (1979) found that very young abused children were more likely to exhibit aggressiveness, avoidance, and approach–avoidance conflict behaviors. They were often observed to

TABLE 16.2. Studies of Maltreatment and Peer Relations and Friendships

Source	Sample characteristics	Main findings
Anthonysamy & Zimmer-Gembeck (2007)	• 25 maltreated, 375 nonmal-treated • Ages 4–8 yr (M = 6.6) from urban Australia • 46% female • Maltreated sample referred to child protective services • All had experienced physical abuse and emotional neglect	Maltreated children were significantly more disliked, physically/verbally aggressive, withdrawn, and less prosocial. Maltreatment had indirect associations with peer likeability and peer rejection via maltreated children's relatively higher levels of physical/verbal aggression and, in some cases, withdrawal and relatively lower prosocial behavior.
Bolger, Patterson, & Kupersmidt (1998)	• 107 maltreated, 107 comparison • 112 male, 104 female • Ages 8–10 yr, followed for 4 yr • 60% European American, 40% African American • 65% multiple types of maltreatment: physical abuse, failure to provide, lack of supervision, emotional maltreatment, sexual abuse • Maltreated sample drawn from the statewide central registry of all substantiated child maltreatment cases in Virginia	Heightened difficulties in peer relationships were associated with greater severity and chronicity of maltreatment. Children who experienced chronic maltreatment were less popular with peers than children who did not; the more chronic the maltreatment, the less popular a child was likely to be. Physically abused children whose maltreatment was chronic started out with higher friendship quality scores at grades 2–3, but their scores then declined over time, ending up lower than other children's by grades 6–7. Children who experienced emotional maltreatment had fewer reciprocated playmates.
Bolger & Patterson (2001)	• 107 maltreated, 107 comparison • 112 male, 104 female • Ages 8–10 yrs, followed for 4 yr • 60% European American, 40% African American • 65% multiple types of maltreatment: physical abuse, emotional maltreatment, neglect, sexual abuse	Chronic maltreatment was associated with heightened risk of rejection by peers; also, chronically maltreated children were more likely to be rejected by peers repeatedly across multiple years from childhood to early adolescence. Maltreatment chronicity was also associated with higher levels of children's aggressive behavior, as reported by peers, teachers, and children themselves. Aggressive behavior accounted in large part for the association between chronic maltreatment and rejection by peers.
Egeland, Yates, Appleyard, & Van Dulmen (2002)	• 140 children, followed from 12 months to 17 yr • Identified as physically abused or emotionally neglected • From the Minnesota Longitudinal Study of High-Risk Parents and Children	Alienation and dysregulation helped explain the relation between early maltreatment and later antisocial behavior. Physical abuse in early childhood, not emotional neglect, led to alienation in preschool, which then predicted early-onset externalizing problems in the elementary school years, ultimately resulting in antisocial behavior in adolescence.

TABLE 16.2. (*continued*)

Source	Sample characteristics	Main findings
Feiring, Rosenthal, & Taska (2000)	• 56 sexually abused adolescents (42 girls, 14 boys; ages 12–15 yr) • 30% African American, 38% European American, 20% Hispanic • Abuse was confirmed using at least one of the following criteria: specific medical findings, confession by the offender, abuse validated by an expert, abuse substantiated by child protective services, and conviction of the offender in family or criminal court.	Higher self-blame attributional style for the abuse was related to more satisfaction with other-sex friends and less satisfaction with same-sex friends. More shame was related to less satisfaction with same-sex friends and to having a larger number of other-sex friends. Higher self-blame attributional style was related to perceptions of poorer peer acceptance and close friendship and to perceptions of poorer romantic appeal. More shame was related to lower perceptions of peer acceptance and close friendship.
Howe & Parke (2001)	• 35 severely abused, 43 matched • Ages 4.3–11.6 yr ($M = 8.7$) • Abused children were from a residential treatment center for severely abused and neglected children: abused: 51% European American, 20% African American, 9% Latino Nonabused: 73% European American, 3% African American, 19% Latino	Abused children were not rated significantly lower sociometrically, nor did they differ significantly from control children on several measures of friendship quality. Abused children were observed to be more negative and less proactive in their interactions. Abused children reported their friendships as being more conflictual and as higher on betrayal and lower on caring.
Kim & Cicchetti (2009)	• 215 maltreated, 206 nonmaltreated • Ages 6–12 yr ($M = 8.11$, $SD = 1.77$) • 64% boys • 61% African American, 30% European American, 7% Latino • Maltreatment coded from case records (physical and sexual abuse, emotional maltreatment, neglect)	Maltreatment was related to emotion dysregulation, which was related to higher externalizing behavior, which contributed to later peer rejection. However, emotional maltreatment was the only type (neglect, physical, sexual) directly related to peer rejection.
Parker & Herrera (1996)	• 16 abused (7 girls), 32 nonabused (15 girls) • Ages 9–14 yr ($M = 10.32$, $SD = 1.32$) • Abused: 62% European American, 25% African American • Nonabused: 81% European American, 9% African American • Substantiated physical abuse by a household member within the past 2.5 yr	Abused children and their friends displayed less overall intimacy than nonabused children and their friends, although peak levels of intimacy were similar for the two groups. Dyads containing an abused child were more conflictual than dyads without abused children, especially during game-playing activities. Abused boys and their friends also displayed more negative affect during game playing than did dyads of nonabused friends. Abused girls and their friends displayed less positive affect than other friendship dyads during activities involving primarily conversation and discussion.

(*continued*)

TABLE 16.2. (*continued*)

Source	Sample characteristics	Main findings
Salzinger, Feldman, Hammer, & Rosario (1993)	• 87 physically abused, 87 nonabused • Ages 8–12 yr (M = 10.2) • 71% boys • Abused: 52% African American, 43% Hispanic • Nonabused: 42% African American, 49% Hispanic • Confirmed cases on the New York State Child Abuse and Maltreatment Register	Abused children had lower peer status and less positive reciprocity with peers chosen as friends; they were rated by peers as more aggressive and less cooperative and by parents and teachers as more disturbed; and their social networks showed more insularity, atypicality, and negativity.

respond to a peer's distress with fear, threats, and angry behavior (including physical attack; Main & George, 1985). The review by Trickett and McBride-Chang (1995) indicated that for physically abused children, whether of school age or younger, peer problems included disruptiveness and aggression toward peers (e.g., Dodge, Bates, & Pettit, 1990; Trickett, 1993), whereas for sexually abused children social relationships were more sexualized, and these children showed more inappropriate sexual behavior, as well as isolated and withdrawn behavior (Friedrich, Beilke, & Urquiza, 1987; White, Halpin, Strom, & Santilli, 1988).

In the more recent review by Cicchetti and Toth (2005), it was found that, in general, maltreated youngsters evidence elevated aggression toward or withdrawal from peers and that they are more likely than nonmaltreated children to bully others. Studies show that even as young as toddlerhood, maltreated children are more aggressive, less prosocial, and more disturbed in their responses to others' distress than are children who have not been abused or neglected (Youngblade & Belsky, 1989). This trend continues into late childhood and early adolescence, in which it has been shown that physically abused children have more conflictual friendships and display less positive affect in activities within friendship dyads (Parker & Herrera, 1996). Similarly, Salzinger, Feldman, Hammer, and Rosario (1993) found that physically abused children had lower peer status and were rated by peers as more aggressive and less cooperative than nonabused children.

Although the early work unequivocally demonstrates the detrimental impact of maltreatment on social functioning, more recent studies have moved toward defining more specific characteristics of maltreatment, as well as mediational models, to pinpoint the source of disturbances in social relationships. For example, Feiring, Rosenthal, and Taska (2000) showed that specific attributional styles of sexually abused adolescents were related to their peer relationships. More shame was associated with less satisfaction with same-sex friends, having a larger number of other-sex friends, and lower perceptions of peer acceptance and close friendships. The authors also found that higher self-blame as an attributional style was also related to perceptions of poorer peer acceptance and less satisfaction with same-sex friends (Feiring et al., 2000). In a study with a sample of mixed maltreatment (physical abuse and emotional neglect), maltreated children were found to be significantly more disliked, more physically and verbally aggressive, more withdrawn, and less prosocial (Anthonysamy & Zimmer-Gembeck, 2007). Maltreatment was found to have indirect associations with peer likeability and rejection through maltreated children's higher levels of physical and verbal aggression and, in some cases, withdrawal and lower prosocial behavior.

Another study found that abused children did not differ significantly from nonabused children on friendship quality, but they were observed to be more negative and less proactive in their interactions (Howe & Parke, 2001). Additionally, it has been found that greater severity and chronicity of maltreatment was associated with heightened difficulties in peer relationships and that, in particular, chronic physical abuse was associated with a decline in friendship quality scores from grades 2 through 7 (Bolger, Patterson, & Kupersmidt, 1998). In a subsequent paper, Bolger and Patterson (2001) found that chronically maltreated children were more likely to be rejected by peers repeatedly across childhood to adolescence. In addition, aggressive behavior accounted for most of the association between chronic maltreatment and peer rejection.

A longitudinal study of physically abused or emotionally neglected children found that physical abuse in early childhood, but not emotional neglect, led to alienation in preschool, which then predicted early-onset externalizing problems in the elementary school years, culminating in antisocial behavior in adolescence (Egeland, Yates, Appleyard, & Van Dulmen, 2002). Conversely, a study by Kim and Cicchetti (2009) that compared physical abuse, sexual abuse, emotional maltreatment, and neglect found that only emotional maltreatment was directly related to peer rejection. The mediational model indicated that maltreatment was related to emotional dysregulation, which was related to higher externalizing problems, which contributed to later peer rejection.

Not only are maltreated children at risk for problematic peer relations, but studies also find that negative peer networks influence the antisocial behavior of maltreated adolescents. For abused adolescents, associating with delinquent peers was found to increase the risk for antisocial/delinquent behavior (Perkins & Jones, 2004). Similarly, in a sample of physically abused adolescents, abused youths with delinquent close friends were at highest risk for antisocial and delinquent behavior (Salzinger, Rosario, & Feldman, 2007). In a sample of mixed maltreatment, exposure to peer delinquency was found to predict higher self-report delinquency 1 year later (Negriff, Ji, & Trickett, 2011), and maltreated adolescents reported more exposure to peer delinquency (Negriff & Trickett, 2010).

Overall, these studies support the detrimental impact of maltreatment on the development of healthy peer relations and friendships. All types of maltreatment have been found to negatively affect the formation of friendships, as well as to increase peer rejection, which in turn can lead to more behavior problems. In terms of mediational mechanisms, aggression and emotion regulation seem to link maltreatment with later problems with peers. Of importance is that poor peer relations are not isolated to childhood but are the basis of poor dating and romantic relationships in adolescence and adulthood. Thus the deficiencies in healthy peer networks continue to affect individuals in their subsequent relationships.

Romantic Relationships and Dating Violence

Peer relationships are the building blocks for romantic relationships in adolescence and adulthood (Connolly, Craig, Goldberg, & Pepler, 2004; Connolly, Furman, & Konarski, 2000; see also Connolly & McIsaac, Chapter 8, this volume). Compromised peer relations may lead to unsatisfying and unhealthy sexual and romantic relationships

(Ehrensaft et al., 2003; Feiring & Furman, 2000). Evidence shows that maltreatment is associated with poor peer relationships and that this trend continues in romantic relationships (for a summary of studies, see Table 16.3). Sexual abuse in particular is linked to risky sexual activity and maladaptive attitudes about sex. Studies have shown that child sexual abuse victims are more likely to be sexually precocious than nonvictims (Beitchman, Zucker, Hood, & DaCosta, 1991; Goldston, Turnquist, & Knutson, 1989; Mayall & Gold, 1995) and to engage in harmful or high-risk sexual behaviors, such as sexual activity with multiple partners (Greenberg et al., 1999), in early-onset sexual behavior (Noll, Trickett, & Putnam, 2003; Wilsnack, Vogeltanz, Klassen, & Harris, 1997), in sexual aggression (Lodico, Gruber, & DiClemente, 1996), in unprotected sex (Lodico & DiClemente, 1994), and in prostitution (Beitchman et al., 1991; Fergusson, Horwood, & Lynskey, 1997; Lodico et al., 1996; Polusny & Follette, 1995; Senn, Carey, Vanable, Coury-Doniger, & Urban, 2006; Simons & Whitbeck, 1991; Springs & Friedrich, 1992). Women who were sexually abused in childhood have also been shown to have higher incidence of sexually transmitted diseases (Wingood & DiClemente, 1997), higher rates of teenage pregnancy (Fergusson et al., 1997; Noll, Shenk, & Putnam, 2009; Noll et al., 2003), and a greater number of lifetime sexual partners (Randolph & Mosack, 2006) than their nonabused peers.

Sexual abuse appears to interfere with both the development of adaptive and healthy romantic relationships and the victims' internalized beliefs about sexual behavior. For example, studies have shown that although sexually abused girls did not differ from comparison girls on a number of social network characteristics (i.e., number of peers, number of male peers, happiness with peer relationships), they were more preoccupied with sex, were younger at first consensual intercourse, were more likely to be teen mothers, and reported lower birth control efficacy (Noll, Trickett, & Putnam, 2000; Noll et al., 2003). Additionally, sexually abused girls were found to show more coy behaviors in an interaction with an unfamiliar male adult, and more coy behaviors predicted earlier sexual intercourse and unhealthy attitudes about sex 7 years later (Negriff, Noll, Shenk, Putnam, & Trickett, 2010). Lastly, sexual abuse victims are highly likely to be revictimized in their romantic relationships. Evidence shows that sexual abuse doubles the risk of sexual and physical revictimization in young adulthood (Barnes, Noll, Putnam, & Trickett, 2009).

The effects of maltreatment on romantic relationships are not limited to just sexual abuse. All types of maltreatment have been linked to compromised romantic relationships. Studies have found that maltreated females report a greater fear of intimacy in past relationships and that their current relationships lacked closeness, feelings of affection, and personal disclosure (DiLillo, Lewis, & Loreto-Colgan, 2007). Abused females were also less likely to have positive perceptions of their current romantic partners and to be sexually faithful (Colman & Widom, 2004). Additionally, in adulthood both males and females reported higher rates of walking out and divorce (Colman & Widom, 2004). Not only are maltreated individuals' romantic relationships unsatisfying and unhealthy, but there also tends to be physical aggression in these relationships (Wekerle & Wolfe, 1998). A study by Cyr, McDuff, and Wright (2006) found that over 45% of sexually abused females had experienced physical aggression in a dating relationship. In addition, duration of sexual abuse contributed to dating violence above and beyond other known risk factors. Dating violence has been widely linked not only to sexual abuse but also to other forms of maltreatment, although these effects seem to vary by gender in different studies.

TABLE 16.3. Studies of Maltreatment and Romantic Relationships or Dating Violence

Source	Sample characteristics	Main findings
Colman & Widom (2004)	• 676 abused, 520 nonabused • $M = 28.7$, $SD = 3.84$ yr • 49% female • 62% European American, 33% African American • Substantiated cases of abuse (physical or sexual) or neglect that occurred prior to age 11 yr	Male and female abuse and neglect victims reported higher rates of cohabitation, walking out, and divorce than controls. Abused and neglected females were also less likely than female controls to have positive perceptions of current romantic partners and to be sexually faithful.
Cyr, McDuff, & Wright (2006)	• 126 females, ages 13–17 yr, from Quebec • $M = 14.4$, $SD = 1.4$ yr • All had substantiated cases of sexual abuse; details of abuse gathered by self-report.	Duration of sexual abuse and the presence of violence or completed intercourse significantly contributed to dating violence above and beyond other known risk factors.
DiLillo, Lewis, & Loreto-Colgan (2007)	• 174 college students • $M = 19.9$, $SD = 1.87$ yr • 117 females, 57 males • 88% European American • Self-reported child maltreatment (physical and sexual abuse, emotional and physical neglect)	Females, but not males, with a history of child maltreatment reported greater levels of psychological and relationship difficulties than did nonmaltreated women. Females with a history of maltreatment reported more psychological distress than nonabused women, as well as a greater fear of intimacy in past relationships and current relationships that were lacking in closeness, feelings of affection, and personal disclosure. Female victims also tended to hold negative beliefs about sexuality (e.g., "Sex is power to control another person") and were more likely to respond to sexual overtures with disgust, fear, or shame. Finally, physical aggression occurred more often in female survivors' couple relationships.
Negriff, Noll, Shenk, Putnam, & Trickett (2010)	• Time 1: 133 girls (71 sexually abused, 62 comparison); mean age = 11.11, $SD = 3.02$ yr • Time 4: 144 girls (77 sexually abused); mean age = 18.52, $SD = 3.52$ yr • 49% European American, 46% African American • Sexual abuse cases referred from child protective services	Sexually abused girls showed more coy behaviors at Time 1. Coy behavior was related to earlier age at first intercourse 7 years later.

(continued)

TABLE 16.3. (*continued*)

Source	Sample characteristics	Main findings
Noll, Trickett, & Putnam (2000)	• Time 1: 141 girls (71 abused, 70 comparison); mean age = 11.3, *SD* = 2.9 yr • Time 4: 120 girls (60 abused, 60 comparison); mean age = 18.4, *SD* = 3.4 yr • 53% African American • Sexual abuse cases referred from child protective services	No difference between abused and comparison group on social network variables: number of peers, number of male or female peers, happiness with male or female peers, number of nonpeers, happiness with nonpeers, having a boyfriend > 1 yr older. Sexually abused girls had younger age at first intercourse.
Noll, Trickett, & Putnam (2003)	• 159 girls (77 abused); mean age = 18.53, *SD* = 3.2 yr • 53% African American • Sexual abuse cases referred from child protective services	Abused participants were more preoccupied with sex, younger at first voluntary intercourse, more likely to have been teen mothers, and endorsed lower birth control efficacy than comparison participants.
O'Keefe (1998)	• 232 participants ages 14–19 yr (138 girls, 94 boys); mean age = 16.9, *SD* = 1.13 yr • 60% Latino, 12% European American, 15% African American • Self-reported physical abuse	For females, child abuse increased the risk for inflicting and sustaining dating violence, but not for males.
Wekerle & Wolfe (1998)	• 321 participants ages 14–20 yr (*M* = 15.24, *SD* = 1.35); (128 males; 193 females) • 80% European American • Self-reported domestic violence, physical and sexual abuse	Maltreatment alone emerged as the most consistent predictor, accounting for 13–18% of the variance in males' physically, sexually, and verbally abusive behaviors; in contrast, it was not highly predictive of female's abusive behaviors. Maltreatment was predictive of victimization experiences for both males and females.
Wolfe, Wekerle, Reitzel-Jaffe, & Lefebvre (1998)	• 132 maltreated, 227 non-maltreated (218 girls, 151 boys) • Mean age = 15.24, *SD* = 1.34 yr • 70% white Canadian • Self-reports of witnessing violence between parents/caregivers, physical abuse, sexual abuse	Maltreated youths reported significantly more verbal and physical abuse both toward and by their dating partners and were seen by teachers as engaging in more acts of aggression and harassment toward others. In regression analyses, the significant association between maltreatment and dating conflict for males was strengthened by including adjustment dimensions in the equation; for females, adjustment variables mediated the association between maltreatment and dating conflict.

(*continued*)

TABLE 16.3. (*continued*)

Source	Sample characteristics	Main findings
Wolfe, Scott, Wekerle, & Pittman (2001)	• 1,419 high school students ages 14–19 yr; (mean age = 16.1, *SD* = 1.1) • 55% female • 79% white Canadian • Self-reports of emotional, physical, sexual abuse; emotional and physical neglect	For girls, maltreatment did not predict dating violence, but it did so for boys. Boys with histories of maltreatment were 2.5 to 3.5 times as likely to report clinical levels of depression, posttraumatic stress, and overt dissociation as were boys without a maltreatment history. They also had a significantly greater risk of using threatening behaviors (OR = 2.8) or physical abuse (OR = 3.4) against their dating partners.
Wolfe, Wekerle, Scott, Straatman, & Grasley (2004)	• 1,317 high school students ages 14–19 yr; (mean = 16.1, *SD* = 1.1) • 55% female • 79% white Canadian • Self-reports of emotional, physical, sexual abuse; emotional and physical neglect	Child maltreatment is a distal risk factor for adolescent dating violence, and trauma-related symptoms act as a significant mediator of this relationship. For girls, longitudinal analyses indicated that anger-specific trauma symptoms predicted change in dating violence over time.

Several studies show that maltreatment predicts males' but not females' physically, sexually, and verbally abusive behaviors and that maltreated boys had significantly greater risk of using threatening behaviors or physical abuse against their dating partners (Wekerle & Wolfe, 1998; Wolfe, Scott, Wekerle, & Pittman, 2001). Regarding females, there is evidence that maltreatment predicts not only being a victim of dating violence but also being a perpetrator: in a sample of both males and females, physical abuse increased the risk of both inflicting and sustaining dating violence only for females (O'Keefe, 1998).

Several studies have examined mediation effects in an attempt to explain the association between maltreatment and dating violence. In a study by Wekerle and colleagues (2001), posttraumatic stress disorder (PTSD) symptoms were found to mediate the relationship between maltreatment and dating violence, but only for females. Another study found that interpersonal sensitivity mediated the association between maltreatment and dating conflict, again only for females (Wolfe, Wekerle, Reitzel-Jaffe, & Lefebvre, 1998). Lastly, in another study by Wolfe and colleagues (Wolfe, Wekerle, Scott, Straatman, & Grasley, 2004) trauma-related symptoms were found to mediate the relationship between maltreatment and dating violence. Specifically for girls, anger-related trauma symptoms predicted change in dating violence over time (Wolfe et al., 2004).

Overall, these studies demonstrate the maladaptive patterns of social relationships that are formed during adolescence and continue into adulthood. The evidence shows that maltreatment of various types compromises an individual's ability to form normative romantic and sexual relationships, the mechanism being maladaptive cognitions and behaviors. Maltreatment also increases the risk of violence in intimate relationships and reduces the ability to maintain healthy social relationships.

Intergenerational Continuity of Maltreatment and Parenting

Much of the early writings that were concerned with how the experience of child maltreatment influences adults' relationships with their own offspring focused on what was termed "intergenerational transmission." In particular, this focus was on the degree to which children who were physically abused later became physically abusive parents (for a summary of studies, see Table 16.4). There was much evidence that experiencing physical abuse as a child increased the likelihood of being an abusive parent but also that this link was not inevitable. In fact, several reviews showed evidence that about 30% of physically abused children become abusive parents, and thus more than two-thirds do not (Kaufman & Zigler, 1987; Kolko, 2002). The emphasis of the early studies that created controversy was specifically on the likelihood of the "transmission" of physical abuse from generation to generation and not on any other forms of maltreatment, nor on possible mechanisms underlying this transmission. Thus, although this linkage was generally attributed to modeling or to other aspects of social learning theory, generally there was no assessment of parent's child-rearing practices or attitudes supporting such a conclusion.

Note also that for physical abuse, intergenerational transmission meant that being a victim of abuse as a child led to being a victimizer or perpetrator as a parent. Early on it was also realized that there was an intergenerational association between mothers' childhood sexual abuse histories and their daughters' (Kaufman & Zigler, 1987). It was very rare for the mother to be the perpetrator of this abuse. Rather, in this instance, the intergenerational association was between having been a victim as a child and being the parent of a victim. It was hard to see how the same social learning theory tenets that were proposed for physical abuse would apply to the intergenerational continuity of sexual abuse.

Recent studies have added to the knowledge about intergenerational continuity by examining other forms of child abuse, especially sexual abuse and neglect, and by looking more generally at continuity, examining whether experiencing certain forms of abuse as a child was associated with perpetrating not only the same but also different forms of abuse as a parent. One recent study examining intergenerational transmission used data from the National Longitudinal Study of Adolescent Health (Kim, 2009). In Wave 3 of this study, almost 3,000 participants were parents who had reported on both their own physical or sexual abuse or neglect and their physical abuse or neglect of their own children. Kim found evidence of intergenerational transmission and some support for "type-to-type" correspondence in that the parents who reported that they were neglected as children were most likely to report neglecting their own children, and those reporting being physically abused as children were most likely to report physically abusive behavior to their own children—in this case, 5.5 times more likely than parents not abused as children. Note, however, that, as is often the case in this research, the participants reported retrospectively on their own childhood experiences and also reported on their abusive behavior to their children. Using similar retrospective self-reports, Ball (2009) examined an infrequently studied group, incarcerated fathers, and found, similar to Kim (2009), that those who reported being physically abused as children were 5.5 times more likely to report their own physically abusive behavior toward their offspring. Pears and Capaldi (2001) found continuity between parents' own physical abuse and their abuse of their children in a rare longitudinal study in which parents reported on their own childhood experiences and, 10 years later, at age 20, their offspring reported on their physical abuse in childhood.

TABLE 16.4. Studies of Intergenerational Transmission/Continuity of Maltreatment and Parenting

Source	Sample characteristics	Main findings
Ball (2009)	• Incarcerated fathers; 53% white, 42% nonwhite; mean age about 30 ($N = 414$). • Retrospective self-reports of experience of physical abuse as children and perpetrating physical abuse as parents	Experiencing physical child abuse associated with perpetrating physical abuse—odds ratio greater than 5.5. Experiencing mild abuse stronger predictor than experiencing severe abuse.
Bert, Guner, & Lanzi (2009)	• First-time teen mothers of infants (18 or younger, $N = 369$) and first-time adult (over 21) mothers of infants ($N = 386$). • Retrospective self-reports on Childhood Trauma Questionnaire	Very high rates of childhood abuse reported (46–82%) and high correlations between different forms of abuse. In general, childhood abuse predicted scores on the Child Abuse Potential Inventory and on indices of parenting style (responsivity/empathy, use of physical punishment, authoritarian style) but did not predict scores on knowledge of infant development. No differences found in general for teen mothers and adult mothers, and type of abuse experienced did not differentially predict parenting styles.
DiLillo, Tremblay, & Peterson (2000)	• Community sample of low-SES participants that included 138 mothers classified as having experienced childhood sexual abuse, and a comparison group of 152 non-sexually abused mothers • Retrospective report of physical or sexual abuse as children	Examined link between childhood sexual abuse and later child abuse potential. With maternal history of physical abuse as a covariate, maternal childhood sexual abuse predicted increased potential for physical abuse of own children. Maternal anger mediated this link.
Dixon, Browne, & Hamilton-Giachritsis (2005)	• Families ($N = 4351$) of newborn children in Essex, England; approx. 95% white. • Data collected during home visits by community nurses. • Retrospective self-reports of experiencing physical or sexual abuse as children. • Referrals to child protective services or physical, sexual, or emotional abuse or neglect during 13 months.	In 13 months after birth of child, significantly more family members who reported experiencing abuse as children were referred to child protective services than those not reporting childhood abuse. Three risk factors were found to mediate, partially, this intergenerational continuity: youth of parent (under 21), history of mental illness or depression, residing with a violent adult.
Dubowitz, Black, Kerr, Hussey, Morrel, Everson, et al. (2001)	• 419 mothers and their children from 2 sites: a southern state and an eastern city • Children at risk of developmental problems due to poverty or other risk factors • Retrospective self-reports of physical and sexual victimization in childhood/adolescence and adulthood	Mothers victimized in both childhood and adulthood reported more harsh parenting practices (verbal aggression and "minor" violence) than others. Generally, those reporting both sexual and physical victimization report harsher parenting.

(continued)

TABLE 16.4. (*continued*)

Source	Sample characteristics	Main findings
Kim, J. (2009)	• Included participants in National Longitudinal Study of Adolescent Health who, at Wave 3, reported being parents ($N = 2,977$) • Median age 23 yr, 67% female, 48% non-Hispanic white, 28% African American, 19% Hispanic • Self-reports of own physical or sexual abuse or neglect as children and of neglect or physical abuse of children.	45% of parents reported never experiencing any abuse or neglect in childhood. Young parents who reported being neglected were 2.6 times more likely to report their own neglectful parenting and twice as likely to report physically abusive parenting as those who did not. Those who reported being physically abused as children were five times more likely to report their own physically abusive parenting. Author concludes that results suggest a "type-to-type" correspondence of intergenerational transmission of maltreatment.
Kim, Noll, Putnam, & Trickett (2007); Kim, Chung, & Trickett (2007); Kim, Trickett, & Putnam (2011); Trickett & Kim (2007)	• 72 mothers of sexually abused girls, and 55 mothers of nonabused comparison group girls • Retrospective self-reports by mothers of sexual abuse	Mothers of abused girls significantly more likely to report childhood sexual abuse than mothers of comparison girls (45 vs. 16%). Mothers of sexually abused daughters who themselves reported sexual abuse also report most physical and emotional abuse in childhood; poor peer relationships as children; most separation from own mothers; and lowest provision of positive structure and satisfaction with children as parents.
Kwako, Noll, Putnam, & Trickett (2010)	• Sexually abused mothers ($N = 16$) and nonabused comparison mothers ($N = 19$) of young children • Participants in longitudinal study • Abuse substantiated by child protection agency at Time 1 (median age 11). Follow-up at median age 25.	Attachment relations of mothers and young children assessed via Strange Situation. Both groups had high levels of anxious attachment, but sexually abused mothers and their children were more likely to have extreme strategies of attachment.
Newcomb & Locke (2001)	• Community sample of parents (mothers and fathers), $N = 383$ • Retrospective self-reports of childhood abuse (physical, sexual, emotional) and neglect using Child Trauma Questionnaire. • Parenting assessed using Parental Acceptance and Rejection Questionnaire.	Using structural equation modeling, it was found that child maltreatment of parents predicted a general factor of poor parenting (low warmth, high aggression, rejection, and neglect). Some differences were found for mothers and fathers in relation to sexual abuse. For mothers, sexual abuse was related to experiencing other types of familial abuse and was independently associated with aggressive parenting. For fathers, sexual abuse was distinct from other forms of familial abuse and related to parental rejection.

(*continued*)

TABLE 16.4. (*continued*)

Source	Sample characteristics	Main findings
Noll, Trickett, & Putnam (2009)	• Mothers who were sexually abused females, substantiated by protective services (age 11 at entry into study), followed longitudinally until median age 25 (N = 60). • Comparison group of nonabused mothers in longitudinal study (N = 68).	Significantly more abuse-group mothers reported to child protection than comparison mothers (18% vs. 2%), mostly for neglect. Significantly more risk factors known to be associated with poor child development found in abused mothers, as compared with comparison mothers (e.g., teen parenthood, depression, substance abuse, lower educational attainment).
Pears & Capaldi (2001)	• Parents (106 mothers, 73 fathers) of 109 male youths at risk for delinquency. • Childhood physical abuse of parents assessed by 20-item self-report scale (with good reliability). • When youths were mean age 20, reported on their own physical abuse using modification of same scale	Parents who reported having been physically abused in childhood were significantly more likely to engage in abusive behaviors toward their offspring. This relationship was partially mediated by parents' use of inconsistent discipline and parents' depression plus PTSD.

Other recent studies have looked at transmission or continuity differently. For example, Kim, Noll, Putnam and Trickett (2007) found that 45% of (nonoffending) mothers of sexually abused girls reported being sexually abused themselves as compared with 16% of comparison group mothers. DiLillo, Tremblay and Peterson (2000) found, in a community sample, that mothers who had been sexually abused as children were more likely to exhibit potential for physical child abuse than comparison mothers. Dixon, Browne, and Hamilton-Giachritsis (2005) found that new parents who reported experiencing either sexual or physical abuse as children were more likely to be reported to child protective services in the following 13 months. In the 6th assessment of a longitudinal study, Noll, Trickett, and Putnam (2009) found that mothers known to have experienced substantiated sexual abuse approximately 15 years earlier at median age 11 were significantly more likely to have been reported to child protective services, mostly for child neglect, as compared with the nonabused mothers in the study.

A number of these studies examined possible mediators of intergenerational continuity. Those identified include parents' use of inconsistent discipline and parents' depression and PTSD (Pears & Capaldi, 2001), becoming a parent before age 21, having a mental illness, residing with a violent adult (Dixon et al., 2005), and parental anger (DiLillo et al., 2000). Although not examining mediators per se, several other studies identified characteristics that place parents at greater risk for maltreatment. For example, Kim and colleagues (Kim, Chung, & Trickett, 2007; Kim, Noll, et al., 2007) found that mothers of sexually abused daughters who were themselves abused reported the most physical and emotional abuse in childhood, the most separation from their own mothers and residential instability, and the lowest levels of emotional–informational support as adults, as compared with either nonabused mothers of sexually abused girls or comparison group mothers. Noll et al. (2009) report that the sexually abused mothers followed longitudinally since childhood had significantly more risk factors known to be associated with parenting problems (e.g., teen parenthood, depression, substance abuse, low educational attainment) as compared with the nonabused mothers.

Several studies have focused on the parenting beliefs and practices of parents who report maltreatment as children. Bert, Guner, and Lanzi (2009) found that first-time teen and adult mothers who report childhood abuse, as compared with those without such experiences, had higher scores on the Child Abuse Potential Inventory and on indices of parenting style (e.g., low responsiveness/empathy and authoritarian parenting) but not on knowledge of infant development. Dubowitz et al. (2001) found that low-income mothers victimized in both childhood and adulthood and those reporting both sexual and physical victimization had the highest rates of harsh parenting practices (verbal aggression and "minor" violence). Kim, Noll, et al. (2007) found that mothers of sexually abused daughters who were themselves abused report the lowest provision of positive structure and the lowest satisfaction with their children as parents. In a community sample, Newcomb and Locke (2001) found that parental experience of child abuse and neglect predicted a general factor of poor parenting (low warmth, high aggression, rejection, and neglect). In a rare observational study using variants of the Strange Situation paradigm, Kwako, Noll, Putnam, and Trickett (2010) found more extreme attachment styles for sexually abused mothers and their young children than for comparison mother–child dyads.

CONCLUSIONS

All the research reviewed here indicates that child maltreatment in all forms is detrimental to the development of healthy social relationships across childhood, adolescence, and adulthood. As presented in this chapter, there is an apparent developmental coherence in that insecure attachment relationships between maltreating parents and young children set up individuals to be unable to establish normative peer relations later. This outcome is perhaps mediated by aggression and emotion dysregulation, which subsequently affect the adolescent's ability to engage in healthy romantic relationships and that of the young adult to parent effectively. And yet there is greater complexity than this. It is still correct to say, as we did 10–15 years ago (Trickett, Allen, Schellenbach, & Zigler, 1998; Trickett & McBride-Chang, 1995), that our knowledge of the impact of child abuse and neglect on later development, including social development, is at a generic level. We know that for many, maybe most, victims, child maltreatment is associated with maladaptive development, but we still know little about how different forms of maltreatment in different combinations at different developmental stages put in motion these developmental problems. Much of our knowledge to date is still based on cross-sectional studies examining "main effects" and relies on retrospective and self-report methodology. There are inherent limitations with retrospective reports, namely the distortions of memory that can occur with the passage of time and with experience. These problems can be magnified when the past experiences being reported on involve child maltreatment (Trickett & McBride-Chang, 1995). Recent research, however, has improved on these older designs and includes better identification of the complex nature of child maltreatment experiences (Feerick et al., 2006); prospective longitudinal studies from childhood into adulthood (e.g., Noll, Trickett, & Putnam, 2009; Pears & Capaldi, 2001); examination of mediational processes (Feiring et al.,

2000) and resilience (Trickett, Kurtz, & Pizzigati, 2003) as predictors of variability of outcomes; and assessment of stress and trauma using psychobiological, as well as psychological, tools (Cicchetti & Rogosch, 2001a, 2001b; Trickett, Noll, Susman, Shenk, & Putnam, 2010).

In a recent *Annual Review of Psychology* article titled "Social bonds and post-traumatic stress disorder," Charuvastra and Cloitre (2008) review research indicating that (1) traumatic events that are caused by humans, in contrast to, for example, natural disasters, are most likely to lead to PTSD and (2) that certain characteristics of social networks and supports act as mediators of the connection between the trauma and the likelihood of PTSD. In this article, they note that child maltreatment is an especially pernicious form of interpersonal trauma because it is "a circumstance in which the child's source of safety is also a source of danger. A traumatizing parent clearly influences a child's ability to interact effectively with a social network" (pp. 310–311). Although the focus of these authors was on PTSD per se, one can generalize their conclusions to other maladaptive behavior and mental health outcomes of child maltreatment. It is thus reasonable to conclude that the focus of scientific efforts to understand more fully the impact of child maltreatment experiences should be on clarifying variations in the nature of this particular trauma—perpetrated on the developing child by a parent—and on the nature of the "social mediators" that can buffer adverse outcomes. Only then can more effective prevention and intervention efforts take place. (See also Gest & Davidson, Chapter 17, this volume.)

SUGGESTED READINGS

Child Welfare Information Gateway. (2009). *Definitions of child abuse and neglect: Summary of state laws.* Washington, DC: U.S. Department of Health and Human Services. Available online at *www.childwelfare.gov/systemwide/laws_policies/statutes/define.cfr*

Feerick, M. M., Knutson, J. F., Trickett, P. K., & Flanzer, S. M. (2006). *Child abuse and neglect: Definitions, classifications, and a framework for research.* Baltimore: Brookes.

Myers, J. E. B., Berliner, L., Briere, J. N., Hendrix, C. T., Reid, T. A., & Jenny, C. A. (Eds.), *The APSAC handbook on child maltreatment* (2nd ed.). Thousand Oaks, CA: Sage.

Sedlak, A. J., Mettenburg, J., Basena, M., Petta, I., McPherson, K., Greene, A., et al. (2010). *Fourth National Incidence Study of Child Abuse and Neglect (NIS-4): Report to Congress.* Washington, DC: U.S. Department of Health and Human Services, Administration for Children and Families.

REFERENCES

Anthonysamy, A., & Zimmer-Gembeck, M. J. (2007). Peer status and behaviors of maltreated children and their classmates in the early years of school. *Child Abuse and Neglect, 31,* 971–991.

Baer, J. C., & Martinez, C. D. (2006). Child maltreatment and insecure attachment: A meta-analysis. *Journal of Reproductive and Infant Psychology, 24*(3), 187–197.

Ball, J. (2009). Intergenerational transmission of abuse of incarcerated fathers: A study of the measurement of abuse. *Journal of Family Issues, 30*(3), 371–390.

Barnes, J. E., Noll, J. G., Putnam, F. W., & Trickett, P. K. (2009). Sexual and physical revictimization among victims of severe childhood sexual abuse. *Child Abuse and Neglect, 33,* 412–420.

Beitchman, J. H., Zucker, K. J., Hood, J. E., & DaCosta, G. A. (1991). A review of the short-term effects of child sexual abuse. *Child Abuse and Neglect, 15*(4), 537–556.

Bert, S. C., Guner, B. M., & Lanzi, R. G. (2009). The influence of maternal history of abuse on parenting knowledge and behavior. *Family Relations, 58*, 176–187.

Bolger, K. E., & Patterson, C. J. (2001). Developmental pathways from child maltreatment to peer rejection. *Child Development, 72*(2), 549–568.

Bolger, K. E., Patterson, C. J., & Kupersmidt, J. B. (1998). Peer relationships and self-esteem among children who have been maltreated. *Child Development, 69*(4), 1171–1197.

Burgdorf, K. (1980). *Recognition and reporting of child maltreatment: Summary findings from the National Study of the Incidence and Severity of Child Abuse and Neglect.* Washington, DC: U.S. Department of Health and Human Services.

Carlson, V., Cicchetti, D., Barnett, D., & Braunwald, K. (1989). Disorganized/disoriented attachment relationships among maltreated infants. *Developmental Psychology, 25*(4), 525–531.

Charuvastra, A., & Cloitre, M. (2008). Social bonds and posttraumatic stress disorder. *Annual Review of Psychology, 59*, 301–328.

Child Welfare Information Gateway. (2009). *Definitions of child abuse and neglect: Summary of state laws.* Washington, DC: U.S. Department of Health and Human Services. Available online at *www.childwelfare.gov/systemwide/laws_policies/statutes/define.cfr*

Cicchetti, D., & Rogosch, F. (2001a). Diverse patterns of neuroendocrine activity in maltreated children. *Development and Psychopathology, 13*, 677–693.

Cicchetti, D., & Rogosch, F. (2001b). The impact of child maltreatment and psychopathology on neuroendocrine functioning. *Development and Psychopathology, 13*, 783–804.

Cicchetti, D., & Toth, S. L. (2005). Child maltreatment. *Annual Review of Clinical Psychology, 1*, 409–438.

Claussen, A. H., & Crittenden, P. M. (1991). Physical and psychological maltreatment: Relations among types of maltreatment. *Child Abuse and Neglect, 15*(1–2), 5–18.

Colman, R. A., & Widom, C. S. (2004). Childhood abuse and neglect and adult intimate relationships: A prospective study. *Child Abuse and Neglect, 28*, 1133–1151.

Connolly, J., Craig, W., Goldberg, A., & Pepler, D. (2004). Mixed-gender groups, dating, and romantic relationships in early adolescence. *Journal of Research on Adolescence, 14*(2), 185–207.

Connolly, J., Furman, W., & Konarski, R. (2000). The role of peers in the emergence of heterosexual romantic relationships in adolescence. *Child Development, 71*(5), 1395–1408.

Crittenden, P. M. (1981). Abusing, neglecting, problematic, and adequate dyads: Patterns of interactions. *Merrill-Palmer Quarterly, 27*, 201–218.

Cyr, M., McDuff, P., & Wright, J. (2006). Prevalence and predictors of dating violence among adolescent female victims of child sexual abuse. *Journal of Interpersonal Violence, 21*(8), 1000–1017.

DiLillo, D., Lewis, T., & Loreto-Colgan, A. D. (2007). Child maltreatment history and subsequent romantic relationships: Exploring a psychological route to dyadic difficulties. *Journal of Aggression, Maltreatment and Trauma, 15*(1), 19–36.

DiLillo, D., Tremblay, G. C., & Peterson, L. (2000). Linking childhood sexual abuse and abusive parenting: The mediating role of maternal anger. *Child Abuse and Neglect, 24*(6), 767–779.

Dixon, L., Browne, K., & Hamilton-Giachritsis, C. (2005). Risk factors of parents abused as children: A mediational analysis of the intergenerational continuity of child maltreatment (Part I). *Journal of Child Psychology and Psychiatry, 46*(1), 47–57.

Dodge, K. A., Bates, J. E., & Pettit, G. S. (1990). Mechanisms in the cycle of violence. *Science, 250*, 1678–1683.

Dubowitz, H., Black, M. M., Kerr, M. A., Hussey, J. M., Morrel, T. M., Everson, M. D., et al. (2001). Type and timing of mother's victimization: Effects on mothers and children. *Pediatrics, 107*(4), 728–735.

Egeland, B., Yates, T., Appleyard, K., & Van Dulmen, M. (2002). The long-term consequences of maltreatment in the early years: A developmental pathway model to antisocial behavior. *Children's Services: Social Policy, Research, and Practice, 5*(4), 249–260.

Ehrensaft, M. K., Cohen, P., Brown, J., Smailes, E., Chen, H., & Johnson, J. G. (2003). Intergenerational transmission of partner violence: A 20-year prospective study. *Journal of Consulting and Clinical Psychology, 71*(4), 741–753.

Erickson, M. F., & Egeland, B. (1987). A developmental view of the psychological consequences of maltreatment. *School Psychology Review, 16*(2), 156–168.

Feerick, M. M., Knutson, J. F., Trickett, P. K., & Flanzer, S. M. (2006). *Child abuse and neglect: Definitions, classifications, and a framework for research.* Baltimore: Brookes.

Feiring, C., & Furman, W. C. (2000). When love is just a four-letter word: Victimization and romantic relationships in adolescence. *Child Maltreatment, 5*(4), 293–298.

Feiring, C., Rosenthal, S., & Taska, L. (2000). Stigmatization and the development of friendship and romantic relationships in adolescent victims of sexual abuse. *Child Maltreatment, 5*(4), 311–322.

Fergusson, D. M., Horwood, L. J., & Lynskey, M. T. (1997). Childhood sexual abuse, adolescent sexual behaviors and sexual revictimization. *Child Abuse and Neglect, 21*(8), 789–803.

Friedrich, W. N., Beilke, R. L., & Urquiza, A. J. (1987). Children from sexually abusive families: A behavioral comparison. *Journal of Interpersonal Violence, 2,* 391–402.

George, C., & Main, M. (1979). Social interactions of young abused children: Approach, avoidance, and aggression. *Child Development, 50*(2), 306–318.

Goldston, D. B., Turnquist, D. C., & Knutson, J. F. (1989). Presenting problems of sexually abused girls receiving psychiatric services. *Journal of Abnormal Psychology, 98*(3), 314–317.

Greenberg, J., Hennessy, M., Lifshay, J., Kahn-Krieger, S., Bartelli, D., Downer, A., et al. (1999). Childhood sexual abuse and its relationship to high-risk behavior in women volunteering for an HIV and STD prevention intervention. *AIDS and Behavior, 3*(2), 149–156.

Howe, T. R., & Parke, R. D. (2001). Friendship quality and sociometric status: Between-group differences and links to loneliness in severely abused and nonabused children. *Child Abuse and Neglect, 25,* 585–606.

Kaufman, J., & Zigler, E. (1987). Do abused children grow up to become abusive parents? *American Journal of Orthopsychiatry, 57*(2), 186–192.

Kempe, C. H., Silverman, F. N., Steele, B. F., Droegemueller, W., & Silver, H. K. (1962). The battered-child syndrome. *Journal of the American Medical Association, 181,* 17–24.

Kim, J. (2009). Type-specific intergenerational transmission of neglectful and physically abusive parenting behaviors among young parents. *Children and Youth Services Review, 31,* 761–767.

Kim, J., & Cicchetti, D. (2009). Longitudinal pathways linking child maltreatment, emotion regulation, peer relations, and psychopathology. *Journal of Child Psychology and Psychiatry,* 1–11.

Kim, K., Chung, I., & Trickett, P. K. (2007). Social support characteristics among mothers with and without childhood sexual abuse trauma. *Korean Journal of Social Welfare Studies, 35,* 215–237.

Kim, K., Noll, J. G., Putnam, F. W., & Trickett, P. K. (2007). Psychosocial characteristics on nonoffending mothers of sexually abused girls: Findings from a prospective, multigenerational study. *Child Maltreatment, 12*(4), 338–361.

Kim, K., Trickett, P. K., & Putnam, F. W. (2011). Attachment representations and anxiety: Differential relationships among mothers of sexually abused and comparison girls. *Journal of Interpersonal Violence, 26,* 498–521.

Kolko, D. J. (2002). Child physical abuse. In J. E. B. Myers, L. Berliner, J. N. Briere, C. T. Hendrix, T. A. Reid, & C. A. Jenny (Eds.), *The APSAC handbook on child maltreatment* (2nd ed., pp. 21–54). Thousand Oaks, CA: Sage.

Kwako, L., Noll, J. G., Putnam, F. W., & Trickett, P. K. (2010). Childhood sexual abuse and attachment: An intergenerational perspective. *Journal of Child Psychology and Psychiatry, 15*(3), 407–422.

Lodico, M. A., & DiClemente, R. J. (1994). The association between childhood sexual abuse and prevalence of HIV-related risk behaviors. *Clinical Pediatrics, 33*(8), 498–502.

Lodico, M. A., Gruber, E., & DiClemente, R. J. (1996). Childhood sexual abuse and coercive sex among school-based adolescents in a midwestern state. *Journal of Adolescent Health, 18*(3), 211–217.

Lynch, M., & Cicchetti, D. (1991). Patterns of relatedness in maltreated and nonmaltreated children: Connections among multiple representational models. *Development and Psychopathology, 3,* 207–226.

Lyons-Ruth, K., Connell, D., & Zoll, D. (1989). Patterns of maternal behavior among infants at risk for abuse: Relations with infant attachment behavior and infant development at 12 months of age. In D. Cicchetti & V. Carlson (Eds.), *Child maltreatment: Theory and research on the causes and consequences of child abuse and neglect* (pp. 464–493). New York: Cambridge University Press.

Maccoby, E. E., & Martin, J. A. (1983). Socialization in the context of the family: Parent–child interaction. In E. M. Hetherington (Ed.), *Mussen manual of child psychology* (4th ed., Vol. 4, pp. 1–102). New York: Wiley.

Main, M., & George, C. (1985). Responses of abused and disadvantaged toddlers to distress in agemates: A study in the day care setting. *Developmental Psychology, 21*(3), 407–412.

Mayall, A., & Gold, S. R. (1995). Definitional issues and mediating variables in the sexual revictimization of women sexually abused as children. *Journal of Interpersonal Violence, 10*(1), 26–42.

Mennen, F. E., Kim, K., Sang, J., & Trickett, P. K. (2010). Child neglect: Definition and identification of adolescents' experiences. *Child Abuse and Neglect, 34*(9), 647–658.

Mueller, E., & Silverman, N. (1989). Peer relations in maltreated children. In D. Cicchetti & V. Carlson (Eds.), *Child maltreatment: Theory and research on the causes and consequences of child abuse and neglect* (pp. 529–578). New York: Cambridge University Press.

National Center on Child Abuse and Neglect. (1988). *Study findings: Study of national incidence and prevalence of child abuse and neglect: 1988.* Washington, DC: U.S. Department of Health and Human Sciences.

National Center on Child Abuse and Neglect. (1996). *Study findings: Study of national incidence and prevalence of child abuse and neglect: 1993.* Washington, DC: U.S. Department of Health and Human Sciences.

Negriff, S., Ji, J., & Trickett, P. K. (2011). Exposure to peer delinquency as a mediator between self-report pubertal timing and delinquency: A longitudinal study of mediation *Development and Psychopathology, 23,* 293–304.

Negriff, S., Noll, J. G., Shenk, C. E., Putnam, F. W., & Trickett, P. K. (2010). Associations between nonverbal behaviors and subsequent sexual attitudes and behaviors of sexually abused girls. *Child Maltreatment, 15*(2), 180–189.

Negriff, S., & Trickett, P. K. (2010, March). *Characteristics of friendship networks as mediators between pubertal timing and delinquency.* Paper presented at the meeting of the Society for Research on Adolescence, Philadelphia, PA.

Newcomb, M. D., & Locke, T. F. (2001). Intergenerational cycle of maltreatment: A popular concept obscured by methodological limitations. *Child Abuse and Neglect, 25,* 1219–1240.

Noll, J. G., Shenk, C. E., & Putnam, K. T. (2009). Childhood sexual abuse and adolescent pregnancy: A meta-analytic update. *Journal of Pediatric Psychology, 34*(4), 366–378.

Noll, J. G., Trickett, P. K., & Putnam, F. W. (2000). Social network constellation and sexuality of sexually abused and comparison girls in childhood and adolescence. *Child Maltreatment, 5*(4), 323–337.

Noll, J. G., Trickett, P. K., & Putnam, F. W. (2003). A prospective investigation of the impact of childhood sexual abuse on the development of sexuality. *Journal of Consulting and Clinical Psychology, 71*(3), 575–586.

Noll, J. G., Trickett, P. K., & Putnam, F. W. (2009). The cumulative burden borne by offspring whose mothers were abused as children: Descriptive results from a multigenerational study. *Journal of Interpersonal Violence, 24*(3), 736–746.

O'Keefe, M. (1998). Factors mediating the link between witnessing interparental violence and dating violence. *Journal of Family Violence, 13*(1), 39–57.

Parker, J. G., & Herrera, C. (1996). Interpersonal processes in friendship: A comparison of abused and nonabused children's experiences. *Developmental Psychology, 32*(6), 1025–1038.

Pears, K. C., & Capaldi, D. M. (2001). Intergenerational transmission of abuse: A two-generational study of an at-risk sample. *Child Abuse and Neglect, 25,* 1439–1461.

Perkins, D. F., & Jones, K. R. (2004). Risk behaviors and resiliency within physically abused adolescents. *Child Abuse and Neglect, 28,* 547–563.

Polusny, M. A., & Follette, V. M. (1995). Long-term correlates of child sexual abuse: Theory and review of the empirical literature. *Applied and Preventive Psychology, 4,* 143–166.

Randolph, M. E., & Mosack, K. E. (2006). Factors mediating the effects of childhood sexual abuse on risky sexual behavior among college women. *Journal of Psychology and Human Sexuality, 18*(1), 23–41.

Salzinger, S., Feldman, R. S., Hammer, M., & Rosario, M. (1993). The effects of physical abuse on children's social relationships. *Child Development, 64*(1), 169–187.

Salzinger, S., Rosario, M., & Feldman, R. S. (2007). Physical child abuse and adolescent violent delinquency: The mediating and moderating roles of personal relationships. *Child Maltreatment, 12*, 208–219.

Sedlak, A. J., Mettenburg, J., Basena, M., Petta, I., McPherson, K., Greene, A., et al. (2010). *Fourth National Incidence Study of Child Abuse and Neglect (NIS-4): Report to Congress.* Washington, DC: U.S. Department of Health and Human Services, Administration for Children and Families.

Senn, T. E., Carey, M. P., Vanable, P. A., Coury-Doniger, P., & Urban, M. A. (2006). Childhood sexual abuse and sexual risk behavior among men and women attending a sexually transmitted disease clinic. *Journal of Consulting and Clinical Psychology, 74*(4), 720–731.

Simons, R. L., & Whitbeck, L. B. (1991). Sexual abuse as a precursor to prostitution and victimization among adolescent and adult homeless women. *Journal of Family Issues, 12*(3), 361–379.

Springs, F., & Friedrich, W. N. (1992). Health risk behavior and medical sequelae of child sexual abuse. *Mayo Clinic Proceedings, 67*, 527–532.

Trickett, P. K. (1993). Maladaptive development of school-aged, physically abused children: Relationships with child-rearing context. *Journal of Family Psychology, 7*(1), 134–147.

Trickett, P. K., Allen, L., Schellenbach, C., & Zigler, E. F. (1998). Integrating and advancing the knowledge base about violence against children: Implications for intervention and prevention. In P. K. Trickett & C. Schellenbach (Eds.), *Violence against children in the family and the community* (pp. 419–437). Washington, DC: American Psychological Association.

Trickett, P. K., & Kim, K. (2007, July). *Multigenerational familial sexual abuse: Perspectives from longitudinal research.* Paper presented at the International Family Violence and Child Victimization Research Conference, Portsmouth, NH.

Trickett, P. K., Kurtz, D., & Pizzigati, K. (2003). Resilient outcomes in abused and neglected children: Bases for strength-based interventions and policies. In K. Maton, C. Schellenbach, B. Leadbeater, & A. Solarz (Eds.), *Investing in children, youth, families, and communities: A strengths-based approach to research and policy.* Washington, DC: American Psychological Association.

Trickett, P. K., & McBride-Chang, C. (1995). The developmental impact of different forms of child abuse and neglect. *Developmental Review, 15*(3), 311–337.

Trickett, P. K., Mennen, F. E., Kim, K., & Sang, J. (2009). Emotional abuse in a sample of multiply maltreated, urban young adolescents: Issues of definition and identification. *Child Abuse and Neglect, 33*(1), 27–35.

Trickett, P. K., Noll, J. G., Susman, E. J., Shenk, C. E., & Putnam, F. W. (2010). Attenuation of cortisol across development for victims of sexual abuse. *Development and Psychopathology, 22*(1), 165–175.

Wekerle, C., & Wolfe, D. A. (1998). The role of child maltreatment and attachment style in adolescent relationship violence. *Development and Psychopathology, 10*, 571–586.

Wekerle, C., Wolfe, D. A., Hawkins, D. L., Pittman, A. L., Glickman, A., & Lovald, B. E. (2001). Childhood maltreatment, posttraumatic stress symptomatology, and adolescent dating violence: Considering the value of adolescent perceptions of abuse and a trauma mediational model. *Development and Psychopathology, 13*, 847–871.

White, S., Halpin, B. M., Strom, G. A., & Santilli, G. (1988). Behavioral comparisons of young sexually abused, neglected, and nonreferred children. *Journal of Clinical Child Psychology, 17*, 53–61.

Wilsnack, S. C., Vogeltanz, N. D., Klassen, A. D., & Harris, T. R. (1997). Childhood sexual abuse and women's substance abuse: National survey findings. *Journal of Studies on Alcohol, 58*(3), 264–271.

Wingood, G. M., & DiClemente, R. J. (1997). Child sexual abuse, HIV sexual risk, and gender relations of African-American women. *American Journal of Preventive Medicine, 13*(5), 380–384.

Wolfe, D. A., Scott, K., Wekerle, C., & Pittman, A. L. (2001). Child maltreatment: Risk of adjustment problems and dating violence in adolescence. *Journal of the American Academy of Child and Adolescent Psychiatry, 40*(3), 282–289.

Wolfe, D. A., Wekerle, C., Reitzel-Jaffe, D., & Lefebvre, L. (1998). Factors associated with abusive relationships among maltreated and nonmaltreated youth. *Development and Psychopathology, 10,* 61–85.

Wolfe, D. A., Wekerle, C., Scott, K., Straatman, A. L., & Grasley, C. (2004). Predicting abuse in adolescent dating relationships over 1 year: The role of child maltreatment and trauma. *Journal of Abnormal Psychology, 113*(3), 406–415.

Youngblade, L. M., & Belsky, J. (1989). Child maltreatment, infant–parent attachment security, and dysfunctional peer relationships in toddlerhood. *Topics in Early Childhood Special Education, 9,* 1–15.

17

A Developmental Perspective on Risk, Resilience, and Prevention

Scott D. Gest
Alice J. Davidson

Why is it that some children who experience major stress or trauma in life struggle to adapt, whereas others are seemingly unaffected and even thrive? The question is a simple one, but the situations to which it applies are diverse. Why do some children whose parents have schizophrenia experience major mental health problems as adults (perhaps even developing schizophrenia themselves), whereas others experience no such difficulties? Why do some children born to poor, young, single mothers drop out of school and display high levels of delinquency, whereas others graduate high school, develop productive work careers, and establish their own stable families? Why do some youths meet the challenges of adolescent autonomy with academic and social success, whereas others are derailed by serious problems with drugs and alcohol? These questions are sometimes motivated by purely scientific interest, based on the premise that understanding the diverse developmental pathways of seemingly similar children will reveal something important about basic developmental processes. But they often have a more practical and applied motivation: If only we could understand why some children succeed where others fail, perhaps we could do something to create conditions in our communities to help more children succeed. These questions and motivations are at the heart of the fields of *risk, resilience* and *prevention science*. In this chapter, our goal is to provide a brief overview of how research on these topics has developed over the past several decades and where it is going, providing a guide to important concepts and terminology along the way so that interested readers can delve deeper into these topics with additional reading.

We organize this chapter using the historical framework proposed by Masten (2007), a major contributor to research on risk and resilience research, to characterize progress in risk, resilience, and prevention research. Masten describes three "waves" of resilience research. After introducing some basic terminology, we summarize the main findings of the first wave of resilience research, which focused on identifying the individual, family, or contextual characteristics associated with resilience. Next we focus on the second wave of resilience research, which focused on clarifying the developmental processes that may account for the role of these protective factors (i.e., these processes may function as mediators). Building on the accumulating findings of these efforts, the third wave involved developing and testing the impact of intervention programs that were intended to promote resilience and positive development. We conclude with some thoughts on important emerging trends in resilience and prevention research (including what Masten calls the "fourth wave"), and highlight some readings that provide additional background and details on important concepts and trends.

Consistent with the broader themes of this volume, a central theme of this chapter is the critical importance of adaptive social relationships to every aspect of risk, resilience, and prevention research. We will see that from birth through adolescence, the absence of adaptive social relationships represents a major threat to development, that naturally occurring supportive relationships account for many instances of resilience, and that many of the most effective preventive intervention programs focus on increasing the availability of or capacity to develop supportive social relationships.

RISK AND RESILIENCE:
SOME BASIC CONCEPTS AND TERMINOLOGY

Resilience is defined as "good outcomes in spite of serious threats to adaptation or development" (Masten, 2001, p. 228) or as "a dynamic process encompassing positive adaptation within the context of significant adversity" (Luthar, Cicchetti, & Becker, 2000, p. 543). These deceptively simple definitions entail two distinct judgments, each of which requires some elaboration. (See Table 17.1 for brief definitions of key terms in risk and resilience research.)

A *good outcome* or *positive adaptation* can be conceptualized in many ways. It could mean simply the absence of disorder or maladaptation, such as not developing a mental health disorder or not being arrested. But resilience researchers have been especially interested in characterizing variability in developmental outcomes beyond the mere absence of bad outcomes. For example, physical health can be measured by strength, flexibility, and endurance; psychological wellness by feelings of satisfaction, well-being and happiness; and civic competence by engagement and participation in civic affairs. The point is that the researcher has considerable flexibility in defining the good outcomes that define resilience.

Similarly, there is variation in what constitutes the *serious threat* to adaptation or development. Threat is often defined statistically by the presence of a *risk factor*, defined as any measurable characteristics of an individual, family or the social context associated with an increased probability of some undesired developmental outcome. For example, early resilience researchers noted that children of parents with schizophrenia were more likely to develop schizophrenia than other children, so having a parent with schizophrenia was considered a risk factor for schizophrenia (Garmezy,

TABLE 17.1. Important Concepts and Terms in Risk, Resilience, and Prevention Science

Risk and Resilience

Risk factors	Measurable attributes of people, their relationships, or contexts associated with an elevated probability of a negative or undesirable outcome in the future
Cumulative risk	Measure of the presence of multiple risk factors in an individual's life
Developmental assets, resources, compensatory or promotive factors	Measurable attributes of people, their relationships, or contexts generally associated with positive outcomes or development *regardless of* adversity or risk level
Protective factor	Measurable attributes of people, their relationships, or contexts associated with positive outcomes or development *especially in the context of* adversity or risk level
Resilience	Good outcomes in spite of serious threats to adaptation or development
Psychosocial competence	Adaptive use of personal and contextual resources to achieve important developmental tasks
Developmental tasks	Accomplishments expected by society of individuals of different ages (often vary across cultures and historical time)

Intervention theory

Developmental (or causal) theory	Theory of how risk and protective factors unfold over time to lead to the developmental outcome of interest, including the role of moderators
Program theory	Theory of how intervention techniques and strategies produce changes in the risk and protective factors highlighted by the developmental theory, including the role of moderators
Logic model	The combination of the developmental theory and the program theory
Causal risk factor	A risk factor that is thought to play a causal role in the development of the outcome of interest
Modifiable risk factor	A risk factor that is at least potentially changeable through intervention efforts
Mediator	A risk factor, protective factor, or competency that developmentally precedes and is thought to lead to the outcome of interest
Moderator	Something that may alter the impact of the intervention or the developmental process linking mediators to outcomes

Intervention paradigms and spectrum

Risk reduction	Prevention strategy focused on reducing levels of risk factors and reducing rates of negative developmental outcomes
Competence promotion	Intervention delivered to all individuals in a setting regardless of their risk status and focused entirely on promoting positive competencies or developmental assets or increasing rates of positive developmental outcomes; also called health promotion
Universal prevention	Intervention delivered to all individuals in a setting regardless of their risk status; may include any combination of risk-reduction and competence-promotion strategies
Selective prevention	Intervention delivered to individuals in a setting who have been identified as at risk for a particular undesired outcome (by virtue of a single risk factor or a measure of cumulative risk), but who are not yet showing signs of the problem to be prevented

(continued)

TABLE 17.1. (*continued*)

Indicated prevention	Intervention delivered to individuals in a setting who are showing early signs of the problem to be prevented but who do not yet display the full problem

Design and evaluation

Randomized controlled trial (RCT)	An experimental research design in which participants are randomly assigned to receive either the intervention to be tested or one or more comparison conditions (typically either the "usual practice" for that setting or a previously studied intervention)
Efficacy	The extent to which an intervention shows evidence of a positive impact when it is tested under ideal conditions with extensive control by the program developer
Effectiveness	Extent to which an intervention shows evidence of a positive impact when it is tested under more "real-world" conditions with less extensive control by the program developer or researcher
Evidence-based programs	Specific intervention programs that have demonstrated evidence of efficacy and effectiveness in randomized controlled trials
Best practices	General intervention principles, strategies, and practices typically identified through a detailed statistical analysis of the results of many RCTs, often with a technique called meta-analysis

Research to practice

Fidelity	Adherence to the specific intervention procedures and content used in the RCTs that established a program's efficacy and effectiveness
Adaptation	Practice of adapting an evidence-based program by altering specific procedures or content to increase acceptability or fit with a specific community population
Sustainability	Extent to which an evidence-based program continues to be implemented with high quality over an extended period of time
Dissemination	Process by which evidence-based interventions are implemented on a large scale as part of routine practice in communities

1974). Research on children of depressed mothers was based on similar observations (Zahn-Waxler, Cummings, McKnew, & Radke-Yarrow, 1984).

Sometimes the concept of serious threat is broadened to include *cumulative risk*, defined as the number (or temporal persistence) of risk factors to which an individual is exposed. In a frequently cited longitudinal study of children in the United Kingdom, Rutter (1979) argued that it was not any specific risk factor but the number of risk factors in a child's environment that increased the likelihood of a psychiatric disorder. The six risk factors examined in Rutter's study included severe marital distress, low socioeconomic status (SES), overcrowding or large family size, paternal criminality, maternal psychiatric disorder, and admission of the child into the care of the local authorities for any reason. Rutter found that psychiatric risk for a sample of 10-year-olds rose from 2% in families with zero or one risk factor to 20% in families with four or more risk factors. Similarly, Sameroff, Seifer, Baldwin, and Baldwin (1993) studied the effect of social and family risk factors on children's intelligence in a longitudinal study of children from preschool through adolescence. They calculated an environmental risk score for each child by counting the number of high-risk conditions from

10 risk factors similar to those used in Rutter's study. Sameroff and colleagues found that the multiple environmental risk score predicted children's IQs at 4 and 13 years of age, such that higher risk scores were associated with lower IQs. A persistent finding in studies of cumulative risk is that it is generally the sheer number of risk factors, rather than the specific profile of risks faced by a given individual, that best predicts future problems.

Although resilience has a relatively simple and intuitive general meaning, resilience research has taken many forms, mostly due to variations in the definition of good outcomes or positive adaptation, in what constitutes the threat to adaptation or development, and in the statistical approaches to analyzing data. These varying definitions and research strategies have led to some challenges and controversies in interpreting the broad range of resilience research (for discussions of these issues, see Luthar, Cicchetti, & Becker, 2000; Masten, 2001). For the purposes of this chapter, however, we focus on the most widely used concepts and terms and the most broadly consistent research findings.

THE FIRST WAVE: IDENTIFYING THE CORRELATES OF RESILIENCE

With these basic concepts in mind, early resilience researchers set out to identify characteristics of children, their families, or their social environments that were correlated with (or associated with) resilience (Garmezy, 1985). A classic study that illustrates the basic logic of this first wave of research and that produced many findings that have been replicated in other studies is Werner and Smith's study of children born on the island of Kauai in 1955 (Werner & Smith, 1982, 1992, 2001). Werner and Smith studied the economically and ethnically diverse sample of 698 children born that year and conducted follow-up studies at 1, 2, 10, 18, 32, and 40 years of age.

They began by creating an index of perinatal risk (or threat to adaptation) based on measures of birth complications and examined the roles of chronic poverty, parental psychopathology, and early parenting interactions in relation to measures of developmental outcomes at age 10 years. They found that when birth complications were severe (i.e., leading to major central nervous system damage), rearing conditions did not make a difference in outcomes at age 10 years. But when birth complications were in the mild to moderate range, early complications were associated with poor developmental outcomes only if they were accompanied by persistently poor rearing conditions (as indexed by parental psychopathology, chronic poverty, and poor parenting). In other words, these early rearing conditions were identified as correlates of resilient outcomes.

Building on this finding, Werner and Smith (2001) defined a new index of early risk by combining the index of birth complications with the measures of poor rearing conditions. At ages 10 and 18 years, they defined good outcomes in terms of school adaptation (grades, absence of behavior problems) and adjustment in the community (absence of legal problems). To identify the correlates of resilience, they considered the 30% of youths who experienced significant developmental risk in the first 2 years and sought to identify characteristics that distinguished those who were resilient (achieving good outcomes at ages 10 and 18) from those who appeared troubled at those ages. They found that youths classified as resilient at ages 10 and 18 had several distinct personal characteristics (such as average intelligence and sociable personalities), close relationships with parent substitutes (such as grandparents), and community support that rewarded competence and provided a sense of coherence and faith (such as through community centers and faith-based youth groups). In similar analyses following these same individuals to ages 32 and 40 years, Werner and Smith (2001) found additional correlates of resilience, such as marriage to a stable partner and experience in the armed services. This study is important for several reasons: It was the first large-scale study of resilience that brought attention to the subject, it illustrates the basic logic of using longitudinal developmental studies to identify the correlates of resilience, and it produced findings that anticipated the results of many studies conducted in subsequent decades.

In summarizing findings from the first wave of resilience research, which includes research encompassing a wide range of definitions of risk and good developmental outcomes, Masten and Coatsworth (1998) identified a short list of correlates of resilience that recur across many studies. At the individual level, resilient children are characterized by (1) good intellectual functioning; (2) appealing, sociable, easygoing dispositions; (3) self-efficacy, self-confidence, and high self-esteem; (4) talents; and (5) faith. At the family level, resilient children and adolescents are characterized by (1) close relationships with caring parent figures; (2) authoritative parenting (providing warmth, structure, and high expectations); (3) socioeconomic advantages; and (4) connections to extended supportive family networks. Beyond the family, resilient children and adolescents tend to have bonds to prosocial youths outside the family and connections to prosocial organizations and to attend effective schools. Note that prominent correlates of resilience include individual characteristics that facilitate the establishment of adaptive relationships (sociability and interpersonal appeal) and the presence of such relationships with parents, extended family, and peers.

Interestingly, Masten and Coatsworth's (1998) summary of resilience research also highlights the importance of putting resilience research in the context of research on child and adolescent development in nonrisk environments. They point out the distinction between: (1) characteristics associated with good developmental outcomes for all youths, regardless of their risk status—variously called *assets* or *compensatory* or *promotive* factors—and (2) characteristics that are especially associated with good developmental outcomes in the context of risks or threats to development, typically called *protective factors*. The former can be considered facilitators of good development in all circumstances, whereas the latter have a facilitating role that is restricted to or enhanced in the context of risk. Many early resilience researchers proceeded on the assumption that the correlates of resilience would often be unique and different from the correlates of good developmental outcomes in nonrisk situations. That is, they expected to find many protective factors and fewer assets, compensatory, or promotive factors. However, Masten and Coatsworth (1998) concluded that the correlates of resilience bore a striking resemblance to the correlates of competence under low-risk conditions. We return to this point in the context of research on the developmental processes that account for the correlates of resilience.

THE SECOND WAVE: IDENTIFYING DEVELOPMENTAL PROCESSES THAT ACCOUNT FOR RESILIENCE

The second wave of resilience research focused on clarifying the developmental processes that may account for the correlates of resilience (Masten, 2007). For example,

Rutter (1987) claimed that *protective processes* were involved when individuals were able to positively respond to risk and when life trajectories changed from risk to adaptation. Rather than focusing on identifying the correlates of resilience, he argued that researchers should focus on processes or mechanisms, which involve interactions and changes in life trajectory. He suggested several types of protective processes that could be relevant: (1) those that reduce the impact of risk by their effect on riskiness itself or by modifying exposure to or involvement in the risk (e.g., effective parental monitoring of children's peer involvement, such that parents encourage and guide children toward involvement with prosocial vs. risky peers); (2) those that reduce the likelihood of a negative chain of reactions that stem from risk (e.g., supportive single parenting in the aftermath of the death of or divorce from the other parent); (3) those that promote self-worth through the availability of supportive relationships or task accomplishment (e.g., secure attachment to supportive caregivers); and (4) those that open up opportunities (e.g., postponement of pregnancy for teenage girls living in poverty). More specifically, Rutter (1987) observed that protection operated through the ways in which people dealt with life changes and with stress and adversity.

Luthar and colleagues (2000) provide a thoughtful analysis of challenges facing research on developmental processes related to resilience. First, it is difficult to integrate results of different studies due to variations in how researchers define risk, good outcomes, and resilience and in how they label different resilience processes (such as those described by Rutter). Second, some individuals display a mixed profile of adaptation in the context of risk: Are youths who attend school in high-risk urban environments resilient if they display a profile of high academic achievement but also high levels of internalizing distress (Luthar, 1991)? Luthar and colleagues argue that the best way to meet these and other challenges is to anchor resilience research in basic developmental theories and research.

In that regard, recall that Masten and Coatsworth (1998) concluded that the correlates of resilience are very often the same individual, family, and extrafamilial characteristics associated with good developmental outcomes in low-risk contexts. Masten (2001) returned to this finding to consider its implications for resilience and prevention research. She concluded that the early presumption that resilience research would identify many protective factors (i.e., many attributes that have special importance in the context of adversity) has largely not been supported by the last three decades of resilience research. What are the implications of this pattern of findings? Masten (2001) argues that the recurring appearance of the same attributes on the "short list" of correlates of resilience and the correlates of good adaptation in low-risk contexts suggests that the same fundamental human adaptational systems are implicated in positive development regardless of the risk context. These fundamental adaptational systems include intellectual functioning, behavioral self-regulation, and caregiver–child relationships.

Masten (2001) proposes that researchers interested in processes associated with resilience should therefore turn their attention to how the fundamental human adaptational systems are affected by risk factors and other threats to development. A positive way to frame this interpretation is that resilience appears to be a common phenomenon that arises spontaneously from ordinary human adaptive processes and that we do not need to discover and foster special magical qualities to promote resilience. In fact, Masten argues that this new perspective on resilience can support a move toward an integrated science of basic human adaptation and development and intervention efforts to enhance the adaptation of high-risk children and adolescents.

From this perspective, Masten's argument is similar to those made by other researchers who conceptualize prevention efforts as attempts to minimize cumulative risk (e.g., Yoshikawa, 1994) or to maximize cumulative protection (e.g., Yates, Egeland, & Sroufe, 2003). In arguing that promoting resilience requires protecting, nurturing, and restoring basic adaptational systems in the lives of children, Masten echoes the views of those from the cumulative risk tradition who claim that optimal functioning can be achieved only by attending to the broader constellation of ecological adaptive systems in which children and their families are embedded (Sameroff, 1999), and that seeking promotive influences that facilitate everyday competence in all children may be most efficient (Yates et al., 2003).

Research on risk and resilience underscores the critical role of supportive social relationships in several ways. First, risk itself is often defined on the basis of the absence of an adaptive caregiver–child relationship (e.g., Werner & Smith, 2001, defined poor parenting at age 2 as a risk factor for subsequent development) or in terms of the presence of factors that may undermine the parent's ability to provide a supportive caregiving relationship (e.g., parental psychopathology). Second, lists of the correlates of resilience either include supportive social relationships (with caregivers, extended family, nonparenting adults, and prosocial peers) or describe individual attributes that facilitate the development of such relationships (sociability, interpersonal appeal, capacity for behavioral self-regulation). Not surprisingly, interventions designed to promote positive development and resilience share a similar emphasis on fostering adaptive social relationships.

THE THIRD WAVE: FROM RISK AND RESILIENCE RESEARCH TO PREVENTION SCIENCE

Models of risk and resilience have always been motivated by the goal of arriving at insights into developmental processes that could lead to more effective efforts to intervene on behalf of children and youth. In the past two decades, insights from risk and resilience research have been integrated with developments in several complementary lines of scientific research to make major strides in this direction (Luthar & Cicchetti, 2000; Masten, 2001). The rapidly emerging multidisciplinary field of prevention science is the focus of the remainder of this chapter. As with the topic of risk and resilience, we begin by outlining some key conceptual issues and related terminology (summarized in Table 17.1). Next we illustrate these concepts by describing several successful preventive intervention programs. We conclude by highlighting several emerging directions of research on risk, resilience, and preventive interventions.

Origins of Prevention Science

Prevention science is an interdisciplinary field with roots in multiple disciplines such as developmental, community and clinical psychology, developmental psychopathology, psychiatry, public health, and epidemiology (Coie et al., 1993; Institute of Medicine, 2009; Kellam, Koretz & Moscicki, 1999; Weissberg & Greenberg, 1998). Recent milestones in the emergence of prevention science include the publication of the first Institute of Medicine report, *Reducing Risks for Mental Disorders: Frontiers for Preventive Intervention Research* (1994); a series of interrelated federal prevention research initiatives in the late 1990s; the initiation of the journal *Prevention Science* in 2000; and the publication of a new Institute of Medicine report, *Preventing Mental, Emotional and Behavioral Disorders Among Young People* (2009).

The Role of Theory in Intervention Development

We define an intervention as any organized attempt to alter individual functioning or developmental trajectories in some desired direction. By using *organized*, we emphasize that interventions are planned activities delivered in a similar way to multiple individuals (or groups of individuals), typically under the auspices of a social institution such as a social service agency, school, or community organization. This organized quality of interventions distinguishes them from informal attempts at individual helping. By including *developmental trajectories* in the definition, we recognize that preventive interventions are often concerned with outcomes that may be measured months or even years after the intervention itself concludes. In prevention science, the full theoretical model specifying the processes by which a particular intervention is thought to achieve its goals is called the *logic model* of the intervention (Baldwin, Caldwell, & Witt, 2005).

A logic model consists of two overlapping parts (Baldwin et al., 2005). First, there is a *developmental theory* (sometimes called *theory of the problem* or *causal theory*) that specifies how, in the absence of intervention efforts, particular risk factors, protective factors, or competencies unfold over time to produce the outcome of interest. Developmental theories emerge from both basic developmental research and from risk and resilience research. For reasons that should be obvious, intervention developers focus on *causal* and *malleable* risk factors: that is, risk factors that are thought to play a causal role in the development of the longer term outcome and that are at least potentially changeable through intervention efforts. Second, there is a *theory of the intervention* (sometimes called the *program theory or action theory*) that details how the specific techniques and activities of the intervention bring about change in one or more risk or protective factors, that play a key role in the developmental theory. The risk factors, protective factors or competencies that are the targets of intervention efforts are called *mediators* because they occupy an inter*mediate* point in time between the intervention efforts and the outcomes of interest.

The basic form of a logic model is illustrated in Figure 17.1. Note that both the developmental theory and the theory of the intervention should identify potential *moderators*: Moderators are factors that might alter the impact of the intervention or the developmental process. For example, if an intervention were expected to work differently for boys and girls, then gender would be considered a moderator of intervention effects. Similarly, if a particular risk factor were thought to relate to the outcome differently for youths in urban and in rural environments, then urban–rural status would be considered a moderator of the developmental process. Note, also, that when the intervention is designed to prevent an outcome many years in the future, or when a developmental theory is especially well developed, a logic model may contain a developmental chain of mediators (i.e., risk factors, protective factors, or competencies) that precede the longer term outcome. In such instances, the mediators that are closest in time to the intervention are described as *proximal* outcomes of the intervention, whereas those closer in time to the longer term outcome are described as *distal*.

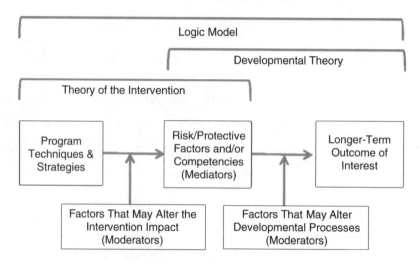

FIGURE 17.1. A logic model consists of a developmental theory that specifies how risk factors, protective factors, and competencies are related to an outcome of interest and a program theory that specifies how intervention techniques and strategies produce desired changes in those risk factors, protective factors, or competencies (known collectively as mediators). Logic models also clarify the role of potential moderators that are expected to alter the impact of the intervention or the links between mediators and outcomes.

Two Paradigms: Risk Reduction and Competence Promotion

Intervention logic models vary in their relative emphasis on two different sorts of changes, both of which are sensible strategies from the perspective of risk and resilience research. Some interventions focus exclusively on *risk reduction* (i.e., preventing specific developmental problems by reducing risk factors for the problem). For example, the Back to Sleep public health education program was based on research indicating that rates of sudden infant death syndrome (SIDS) were nearly 50% higher in countries (such as the United States) in which infants were traditionally put to sleep on their stomachs (American Academy of Pediatrics, 1992); within 4 years, rates of SIDS in the United States were reduced by over 38% simply by encouraging parents to put their infants to sleep on their backs instead of on their stomachs (Willinger et al., 1998). In this example, both the long-term outcome and the short-term intervention strategy were focused exclusively on reducing a risk factor and rates of a problem. Risk reduction and problem prevention are prominent themes in epidemiology, public health, and mental health research (Institute of Medicine, 2009).

Other interventions focus exclusively on *competence* or *health promotion* (i.e., promoting competence, health, or protective factors; Hawkins, Catalano, Kosterman, Abbott, & Hill, 1999). For example, schools may require students to engage in community service activities to foster feelings of community bonding and to promote longer term habits of civic engagement. Several lines of theory and research have converged to increase such promotion efforts (Wyman, Sandler, Wolchik, & Nelson, 2000), including the second wave of resilience and its focus on basic human protective systems (Masten, 2001), positive psychology and its focus on concepts of wellness (Seligman & Csikszentmihalyi, 2000), and the positive youth development movement, which has emphasized positive dimensions of adaptation and the potential contributions of youths and adolescents to counterbalance the traditional emphasis on behavior problems and maladjustment (Benson, Scales, Hamilton, & Sesma, 2006; Benson, Scales, Leffert, & Roehlkepartain, 1999; Damon, 2004).

In practice, most interventions include a combination of risk-reduction and health-promotion strategies and outcomes. For example, an intervention focused on physical health may eliminate junk food from school vending machines (risk reduction) and increase physical education time (health promotion) in an effort to both reduce obesity rates (risk reduction) and improve cardiovascular health (health promotion). This sort of combined approach is supported by empirical research indicating that risk factors and protective factors each make unique contributions to the prediction of important developmental outcomes in adolescence (Catalano, Hawkins, Berglund, Pollard, & Arthur, 2002).

Intervention Spectrum

Interventions can be placed along an intervention spectrum according to their goals and the populations that they target. Interventions that focus exclusively on competence promotion are offered to all members of a setting (e.g., increasing physical education time for all students at a school). All preventive interventions share the feature of being offered to individuals who have not yet displayed or experienced the problem to be prevented, but they can vary in the specific populations they target (Offord, 2000). *Universal* prevention efforts are offered to all members of a setting (e.g., a school) regardless of their level of risk. *Selective* prevention programs are offered only to individuals who have one or more risk factors for the problem of interest. *Indicated* prevention programs are offered to individuals who have begun to display early signs of the problem behavior. Consider the example of high school dropout prevention: A universal program might focus on all youths at the school (regardless of their risk status) by restructuring the school to create multiple smaller teams that provide all students with closer peer and teacher relationships (Felner et al., 2001). A selective program might focus on students with a history of behavior problems in middle school (a risk factor for dropout) and offer such students extra levels of advising support. Finally, an indicated approach might restrict such extra advising support to students who are beginning to show signs of truancy (an early sign of dropout behavior).

A critical issue in developing a prevention program is deciding on the level of prevention: universal, selective, or indicated. Note that because universal approaches include everyone in a setting, they subsume the selective and indicated subpopulations (see Figure 17.2). Offord (2000) identified several important potential advantages and disadvantages of universal approaches relative to *targeted* approaches (an umbrella term referring to both selective and indicated programs). Universal interventions have the potential to bring positive changes to the broader context in which all individuals (including high-risk individuals) develop. For example, in the FAST Track intervention focused on highly aggressive young children at risk for conduct disorder, researchers decided to include a universal classroom intervention to improve the social-emotional skills of all children in the classroom in the hopes that this would provide a more supportive peer context for the high-risk youths (Conduct Problems Prevention Research Group, 1999). But universal interventions are often relatively low in intensity out of financial necessity, suggesting that they may bring relatively small benefits to each individual; and they involve spending scarce intervention resources on many low-risk

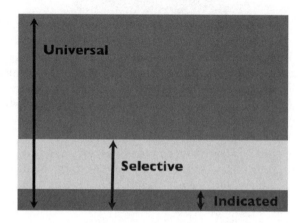

FIGURE 17.2. Levels of prevention. Universal prevention programs include all individuals in a setting; selective prevention programs include individuals who have one or more risk factors for the problem of interest; and indicated prevention programs include only individuals who have begun to demonstrate early signs of the problem. Note that universal programs include everyone in the setting, including the selective and indicated subpopulations.

youths who are very unlikely to develop the problem outcome. In contrast, targeted approaches allow for relatively more intensive interventions, suggesting that scarce intervention resources can produce larger gains among youths who are at highest risk to develop the problem outcome. However, targeted approaches have their own limitations: identifying the youths at highest risk is an imperfect and often expensive process, there is potential for labeling and stigmatization, and the broader social context of the high-risk youth is not addressed (Offord, 2000).

Some of the trade-offs between universal and selective interventions become clearer by considering a hypothetical school with 50 students (Figure 17.3). Assume that you know from past research that about 32% of all students (16 of 50) will experience a particular problem outcome. You have identified two risk factors, each of which nearly doubles the probability of the problem: 6 of 10 students with each risk factor (60%) develop the problem. The small number of students who have both risk factors have an even higher rate of the problem (4 of 5 = 80%). You could consider several prevention strategies. One option is a selective prevention program in which you focus on the 5 highest-risk youths because you know that 80% of them will develop the problem. But note that even if your intervention is completely effective with those youths, you will have prevented only 4 of the 16 eventual problem cases, because most youths who develop the problem (the filled circles in Figure 17.3) have only one or no risk factors. You can broaden your selective approach to include the 15 youths who have at least one risk factor, but you still would not reach the 8 future-problem youths who do not show any risk factors. To reach those youths you would have to adopt a universal intervention, delivering the intervention to all 50 youths at the school. This example is hypothetical but fairly typical of the situation faced by intervention developers: Universal interventions are the only way to ensure that all youths who might otherwise develop a problem are reached but targeted interventions are appeal-

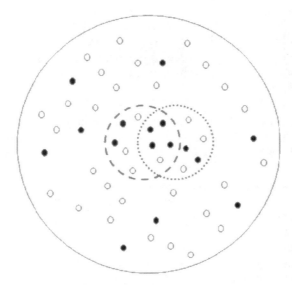

FIGURE 17.3. Choosing among universal, selective, or indicated prevention strategies involves difficult trade-offs. Consider the hypothetical situation of 50 students (smallest circles) within a school (largest circle). You know from past research that 16 of these students (32%; filled circles) will go on to develop a particular problem. You have identified two risk factors (medium-sized circles) that are each associated with a 60% chance of developing the problem. As explained in the text, universal interventions are the only way to ensure that all youths who might otherwise develop the problem are reached, but selective approaches are appealing because of their potential to bring greater benefits to students facing the highest risk.

ing because of their potential efficiency in bringing greater benefits to students facing the highest risk.

Evaluating Intervention Programs

There is broad agreement that for prevention efforts to qualify as a science, rigorous standards of evidence must be applied in evaluating intervention efforts. Given the challenges of conducting tightly controlled research studies in real-world settings (e.g., schools and communities), specific standards of evidence relevant to prevention efforts have been articulated only relatively recently (Society for Prevention Research, 2004; Institute of Educational Sciences, 2003). Ideally, evidence comes from *randomized controlled trials* (RCTs), experimental designs in which participants are randomly assigned to receive either the intervention or some comparison condition (e.g., the current "usual practice" for dealing with the issue at hand or an older intervention approach). These studies should demonstrate benefits that are statistically significant, of a magnitude that is of practical importance, and sustained for a meaningful period of time (e.g., 1 year). There are several phases in the evaluation of an intervention. First, a small-scale *pilot* study tests the components of the intervention to determine whether they show some promise for having the desired impact. Second, a larger scale *efficacy* study is conducted to test whether the intervention produces the desired outcomes when it is implemented under ideal conditions (e.g., delivered by highly trained staff supervised by the program developer). Finally, an *effectiveness* study tests whether the same intervention produces the desired outcomes when it is implemented under real-world conditions (e.g., delivered by staff at the social service agency that would potentially adopt the program).

The number of published reports of RCTs of prevention programs has exploded in the past 20 years. In the 1980s, there were fewer than 5 such reports per year; that number rose to 25 per year by 2000 and to 40 per year by 2005 (Institute of Medicine, 2009). This rapid expansion of data on prevention program effects has led to two sorts of efforts to summarize and synthesize findings. First, several organizations have attempted to identify *evidence-based programs*, programs that have met rigorous standards of evidence for efficacy and effectiveness. For example, the U.S. federal government's Substance Abuse and Mental Health Services Administration (SAMHSA) has created the National Registry of Evidence-based Programs and Practices (NREPP), a searchable website database with information on 159 (as of this writing) programs that met specific standards of evidence (*www.nrepp.samhsa.gov*). Second, researchers have identified *best practices* in interventions by combining the results of multiple RCTs. Results of these *meta-analyses* (i.e., a special type of statistical analysis that combines the results of multiple studies) can reveal patterns that are not evident in the results of any single RCT. For example, one meta-analysis revealed that youth substance use prevention programs that use interactive lesson formats are generally more effective than those that use more didactic formats (Tobler et al., 2000).

Issues in Moving from Research to Practice

After a program has demonstrated evidence of positive outcomes under both ideal conditions (efficacy) and real-world conditions (effectiveness), important challenges remain in adopting the program in real-world settings. One important issue involves balancing *fidelity* (adherence to program procedures) against the desire to make *adaptations* (changes that are hoped to optimize the fit of a program to the local community). From a strict scientific perspective, it is critical to implement the program under the exact same conditions under which it was proved effective. This means that communities should maximize fidelity (e.g., adhering to procedures regarding the number, format, and content of sessions and the training and qualification of program staff; Elliott & Mihalic, 2004). However, a social agency may wish to make adaptations to the program to maximize its acceptability and impact given the local community culture and available resources (e.g., altering the number or format of sessions or the qualifications of program staff). Ideally, decisions about balancing fidelity and adaptations should be guided by the program's logic model; small changes to program features that do not play a prominent role in the logic model are less concerning than major omissions or modifications to features that play a key role in the logic model (Castro, Barrera, & Martinez, 2004).

A second set of challenges in moving from research to practice concerns the dissemination and sustainability of evidence-based programs. *Dissemination* refers to the widespread adoption of an evidence-based program after it has met high standards of efficacy and effectiveness. Unfortunately, very few programs that have met standards of efficacy and effectiveness are implemented broadly. Moreover, some programs that are known to be ineffective (e.g., Drug Abuse Resistance Education, DARE; Lynam et al., 1999) are disseminated very broadly. The reasons for this state of affairs are not well understood (Society for Prevention Research, 2004; Institute of Medicine, 2009), but two likely contributing factors are the absence of clear channels of communication between researchers and practitioners and funding systems for social service providers that do not provide incentives to adopt evidence-based programs (Institute of Medicine, 2009). *Sustainability* refers to maintaining high-quality implementation of a program over an extended period of time. In many instances, evidence-based programs that are adopted are not sustained due to the discontinuation of funding or the departure of key staff members who first adopted the program. Researchers are beginning to study more systematically how to promote the broad dissemination and sustainability of evidence-based programs (Durlak & DuPre, 2008).

Examples of Evidence-Based Prevention Programs from Birth through Adolescence

In this section, we use the concepts introduced in the previous sections to describe several prevention programs. We devote the most space to the Nurse–Family Partnership program in infancy because it has been researched so thoroughly (e.g., Kitzman et al., 1997; Olds, 2006) and illustrates virtually all of the issues we have discussed previously. We then provide briefer descriptions of a range of other evidence-based programs across childhood and adolescence.

Infancy: The Nurse–Family Partnership

In the late 1960s, David Olds enrolled at Johns Hopkins University planning to study international relations, but his interests gradually shifted to urban poverty and what could be done to support the development of poor young children (Robert Wood Johnson Foundation, 2006). After working as a Baltimore preschool teacher for 2 years, Olds decided he needed to reach children and their families earlier in development. Under the mentorship of Urie Bronfenbrenner at Cornell University, Olds began to develop the logic model for what became the Nurse–Family Partnership (NFP) intervention. From existing developmental research, Olds noted that rates of adolescent crime and delinquency were especially high among youths who were born to poor, single, teenage first-time mothers. Research also suggested that during the preschool period, children who later became delinquents were characterized by neuropsychological impairments (e.g., impulsiveness and attention problems), conflictual parent–child relationships, and inadequate preparation for formal schooling (e.g., poor language and emergent literacy skills). Olds developed NFP prior to Masten's (2001) summary of risk and resilience research, but note that the preschool risk factors he identified represent failures to master key developmental tasks of infancy: biological self-regulation, parent–infant attachment, and language.

Olds developed a selective prevention program, focusing on poor, young, single, first-time mothers. He aimed to begin working with these mothers as soon as possible during their pregnancies until their children were 2 years old. He reasoned that the most likely way to engage vulnerable young pregnant women was to offer them support from a trusted source of authority on pregnancy—a nurse. In considering how he wanted nurses to engage these young mothers, Olds drew upon several theories, including self-efficacy theory (building mothers' confidence and skills; Bandura, 1977), human ecology theory (fostering positive connections to family and community; Bronfenbrenner, 1979), and attachment theory (fostering sensitive mother–infant interactions; Bowlby, 1969). The resulting program was the NFP (Olds, 2006).

In NFP, qualifying women are invited to join the program as soon as their pregnancies are identified (they are typically referred by a doctor's office). During the pregnancy, a nurse visits the expectant mother at her home every week for the first 4 weeks, then every other week until birth, then every week for 6 weeks, then every 2 weeks until the child is 20 months old, then every month until 24 months. Detailed manuals guide nurses through a predetermined series of topics for each visit. Each visit addresses developmentally appropriate topics in several areas—maternal health (e.g., substance use, nutrition, exercise), environmental safety, maternal life course development (e.g., family planning, work), the maternal role (e.g., physical and emotional care of infant), and family and friends (e.g., building supportive, positive relationships)—and links the mother to relevant social services. The manuals describe a standard curriculum, but the impact of the program depends on the development of a close and supportive relationship between the nurse and the young mother. Because of the unique features of the program, nurses receive a week of specialized training and ongoing mentoring to become certified NFP providers.

NFP includes both risk-reduction and competence-promotion components. Risk-reduction components include the effort to reduce maternal substance use during pregnancy, the consistent emphasis on eliminating physical risks from the home environment during infancy, and the emphasis on family planning to reduce unwanted or closely spaced pregnancies. Competence-promotion components include efforts to encourage maternal employment, foster sensitive mother–infant interactions, and promote supportive relationships with extended family. NFP is typical of many successful prevention programs in integrating risk-reduction and competence-promotion efforts into a single comprehensive program.

There is strong evidence that NFP produces important and long-lasting benefits to both mothers and their children. The evidence comes from three separate RCTs: one focused on white mothers in rural areas around Elmira, New York (Olds et al., 1997), one focused on primarily African American mothers in Memphis, Tennessee (Kitzman et al., 1997), and another one focused on a multiethnic group of mothers (including many Latinas) in Denver, Colorado (Korfmacher, O'Brien, Hiatt, & Olds, 1999). All three trials demonstrated desired program effects, both proximal (during the intervention) and distal (long after the intervention ended). For example, NFP participants demonstrated improved prenatal health behavior (less smoking, better nutrition), better birth outcomes (increased birth weight), improved parenting (more sensitive), reduced child abuse (decreased reports of abuse, fewer emergency room visits), improved parental life course (increased employment, fewer subsequent pregnancies), and improved child outcomes (fewer arrests; Kitzman et al., 1997; Olds, 2006; Olds, Henderson, Tatelbaum, & Chamberlin, 1986). By including multiple experimental conditions in each of these trials, Olds was able to compare his full program with two less expensive alternative programs: for example, the Elmira trial revealed that the combination of pre- and postnatal visits had stronger impacts than prenatal-only visits, and the Denver trial revealed that nurses had stronger impacts than trained paraprofessionals recruited from the mothers' own communities.

Olds soon began to receive requests to help start NFP programs in local communities throughout the United States, leading him to establish the NFP national office to coordinate the process of disseminating the NFP program to local communities (*www.nursefamilypartnership.org*). Olds is convinced that NFP will succeed only if local communities implement the program with fidelity—that is, by adhering to the same procedures that he used in the three RCTs. Accordingly, the NFP national office provides specialized training to local nurses to certify them in NFP procedures and requires local communities to submit paperwork from nurses to monitor program fidelity (e.g., number of visits completed and topics covered at each visit). Several state governments worked with the national center to develop state-sponsored NFP initiatives, resulting in dozens of new NFP sites within a single state. For several years in the mid-2000s, these state-level initiatives stretched the resources of the national center to the point that new communities from other states could not receive initial NFP training and support. Olds could have met this demand simply by mailing the NFP manuals to interested communities, but he opted to limit the growth of NFP to ensure that each NFP community implemented the program with fidelity. More recently, the national center has greatly expanded its capacity, but the NFP experience illustrates the growing pains associated with disseminating and sustaining an effective program on a large scale with fidelity.

Another challenge faced by communities interested in NFP is financial. NFP costs approximately $9,100 per family, mostly in the form of salaries for nurses and nurse-supervisors (Aos, Lieb, Mayfield, & Pennucci, 2004). Either these funds must be shifted from an existing program or new funds must be obtained. Some states, such as Pennsylvania, provide short-term funding (e.g., 3 years) for a local community to initiate an NFP program, but the local community must sustain the program beyond that point. If new funds cannot be obtained from other outside sources, communities face difficult decisions about how to reallocate resources away from other existing programs to sustain NFP. Because so many communities face these pressures, the NFP national office supports communities by helping to document and market their successes with NFP and by identifying potential sources of ongoing funding.

Overall, NFP illustrates many key concepts that link research on risk and resilience to prevention science and highlights the critical role of adaptive social relationships in development. Beginning with a focus on a specific set of problem behaviors in adolescence, Olds used existing theory and research to build a logic model specifying how specific risk-reduction and competence-promotion efforts could help vulnerable young mothers to establish more supportive relationships with their infants, resulting in greater mastery of developmental tasks in infancy and improved long-term outcomes. Evidence from RCTs provided strong support for the program's impact and led to increasing demands for program dissemination to local communities. The NFP national office expanded rapidly to support the broad dissemination of NFP, while working to ensure high-fidelity implementation and to support sustained implementation despite financial pressures. Next we provide briefer descriptions of several additional evidence-based programs.

Middle Childhood: Promoting Alternative Thinking Strategies and Big Brothers Big Sisters

The Promoting Alternative THinking Strategies (PATHS) program is a classroom-based curriculum that is typically offered as a universal prevention program to students across the elementary school grades. The program is based on a theory of the development of self-regulation that emphasizes the need for children making the transition to middle childhood to bring their emotional experiences under cognitive and linguistic control as a prerequisite for engaging in effective social problem solving

(Greenberg, Kusche, Cook, & Quamma, 1995). Consequently, at each grade level, PATHS places special emphasis on helping children learn developmentally appropriate skills in labeling, understanding, and communicating about emotions, as well as positive social interaction skills and effective self-control and social problem-solving skills (Conduct Problems Prevention Research Group, 1999). The classroom teacher presents two to three 20-minute lessons per week on these topics (e.g., introducing a new emotion word and concept) and also looks for opportunities to generalize lesson concepts and skills throughout the day (e.g., labeling examples of emotions, modeling social skills, scaffolding children's attempts to use new problem-solving skills). Randomized trials evaluating the impact of a single year of the PATHS curriculum indicate a range of positive effects, such as increased fluency and comfort in discussing basic feelings (Greenberg et al., 1995), reductions in peer reports of aggression and hyperactive–impulsive behavior, and improvements in observer ratings of classroom atmosphere (Conduct Problems Prevention Research Group, 1999).

Big Brothers Big Sisters of America (BBBSA) is the nation's largest and oldest youths mentoring program, with a century-long history of providing adult support and friendship programs to youths . The contemporary version of BBBS is a selective prevention program: It targets youths ages 6–18 from single-parent, low-income homes (McGill, Mihalic, & Grotpeter, 1998). The local BBBS agency screens and trains volunteer mentors and assesses potential youths mentees, then establishes mentor–mentee pairings or *matches* based on the needs of the youths, the abilities of the mentor, and parental preferences. A premise of the BBBS program is that supportive relationships between youths and nonparenting adults can foster a sense of social relatedness (Baumeister & Leary, 1995) and increase community engagement (Grossman & Bulle, 2006). Mentors interact regularly with a youths in a one-to-one relationship, with ongoing follow-ups conducted by the local BBBS agency. BBBS programs operate in either community- or school-based settings. In community-based mentoring (CBM), mentors meet with youths in community settings for 4–8 hours per week for at least one year. In school-based mentoring (SBM), mentors meet with youths for 1 hour per week during or after school for at least one 9-month school year (Herrera et al, 2007; Rhodes, 2008).

CBM programs provide considerable freedom to the mentor and the mentee to decide how and where they want to spend their time together (Karcher, Kuperminc, Portwood, Sipe, & Taylor, 2006). Evaluations of BBBS in CBM contexts found that when certain conditions were met (e.g., relationships lasted longer than 1 year), mentoring relationships were associated with small positive youths outcomes, including increases in self-worth, peer acceptance, academic competence, parent relationship quality, school attendance, and school value and decreases in substance use (e.g., Grossman & Rhodes, 2002; LoSciuto, Rajala, Townsend, & Taylor, 1996). Initial results of a large, randomized evaluation of BBBS in SBM contexts were mixed: At the end of the first school year, youths assigned to receive mentoring showed significant improvements in academic adjustment relative to a control group, but most differences were no longer significant a year later (Herrera et al., 2007). Further analyses revealed that mentees who experienced longer, higher quality relationships received greater benefits than those in shorter or weaker relationships and that those involved in weaker relationships actually showed declines in functioning in the second year. Recent growth in SBM programs reflects a rapid increase in *cross-age peer mentoring*, in which high school youths provide mentoring to elementary-age children (Herrera, Kauh, Cooney, Grossman, & McMaken, 2008); indeed, teens now represent a quarter of BBBS volunteer mentors. There is some evidence that children benefit when they are paired with teen mentors in BBBS SBM programs, especially when disconnected youths are paired with teen mentors who hold positive attitudes toward youths in the community (Karcher, Davidson, Rhodes, & Herrera, 2010).

Early Adolescence: Life Skills Training and Iowa Strengthening Families Program

A major developmental task in early adolescence is the responsible management of individual behavior in the context of increasing autonomy. As youths move from relatively small elementary schools with self-contained classrooms to larger middle schools with multiple teachers, they experience greater freedom to select and manage their own peer relationships (Eccles et al., 1993), and they experience increased opportunities to spend time outside of direct adult supervision at home and in the community (Larson, Wilson, Brown, Furstenberg, & Verma, 2002). Prevention programs in this period typically focus on helping youths manage increased autonomy in ways that promote positive peer relationships and responsible decision making, measured in part by the avoidance of early use of tobacco, alcohol, and other drugs.

The Life Skills Training program (LST; *lifeskillstraining.com*; Botvin, 1998) is a universal school-based program with the goal of preventing early substance use. LST is a classroom curriculum delivered over the 3 middle school (or junior high school) years. Each lesson is approximately 45 minutes and is typically delivered as part of the school's regular health curriculum, with 15 lessons in Year 1, 10 lessons in Year 2, and 5 lessons in Year 3. The LST logic model presumes that early substance use is most likely to arise when youths have weak self-management skills (e.g., difficulty coping with anxiety and anger/frustration, vulnerability to media influences, poor problem-solving skills), when they lack the social skills to form positive peer relationships (e.g., excessive shyness, low assertiveness), and when they possess inaccurate or maladaptive attitudes about drug use. Accordingly, the majority of LST lessons focus on promoting personal and social competencies to improve personal management skills and skills for establishing supportive peer relationships (e.g., strategies for managing upsetting emotions, steps for solving social problems and making decisions, skills for initiating and sustaining friendships). About one-third of the lessons deal more explicitly with issues related to drug use and try to reduce risks in that area (e.g., reducing positive perceptions of drugs, reducing the tendency to choose friends who use drugs). Multiple RCTs indicate that student-reported drug use is lower in schools in which students experience the LST curriculum than in schools that continue their usual practice (Botvin, Baker, Dusenbury, Botvin, & Diaz, 1995; Botvin & Griffin, 2004). There is even some evidence that the benefits of LST may extend to other behavioral domains in which personal management and social skills are relevant (e.g., HIV risk behavior, car accidents; e.g., Griffin, Botvin, & Nichols, 2006).

Efforts to address the developmental needs of early adolescents also include family-based prevention programs. The Strengthening Families Program for 10–14-year-olds (SFP 10–14) is a family skills program with particularly extensive evidence of positive impact (Spoth, Redmond, & Shin, 2001; *www.extension.iastate.edu/sfp*). The SFP 10–14 program is designed as a universal program for youths enrolled in sixth grade, although fewer than 30% of families at the school typically choose to attend sessions. The program consists of seven 2-hour sessions. In the first hour, youths and parents meet separately in small groups; in the second hour, youths and parents come together to meet as families. The youths' sessions reflect some of the same themes of personal and social management emphasized in LST, but with much greater emphasis on the role of family communication skills. The parent sessions are built around the theme of "Love and Limits," reflecting the findings of basic developmental research on the importance of these dimensions of parenting for adolescent development (Steinberg, 2001). For example, parent session topics include making house rules, encouraging good behavior, implementing consequences, learning to listen to teens, and preventing substance use. Group leaders use videotaped vignettes to illustrate important concepts and to generate group discussions about parenting strategies. An RCT has documented impressive benefits associated with SFP 10–14 (Spoth, Redmond, & Lepper, 1999; Spoth et al., 2001; Spoth, Redmond, Shin, & Azevedo, 2004). For example, SFP 10–14 was associated with lower rates of alcohol, tobacco, and marijuana use 1 year after the intervention ended, and the differences between the SFP 10–14 group and the control group actually increased over the next several years, suggesting that the skills promoted by the program continued to influence behavior long after the program ended (Spoth et al., 2001, 2004). Communities interested in implementing SFP 10–14 may pay to obtain training for group leaders to promote fidelity to standard program practices.

Adolescence: School Transition Environment Program and the Teen Outreach Program

The School Transition Environment Program (STEP; Felner et al., 2001) is a universal prevention program motivated by research documenting that the transition to high school is often a period of increased risk for social and academic difficulties; academic demands increase, while opportunities for supportive interactions with teachers and peers decrease due to the large school environment and hourly changes of classes. The STEP program seeks to reduce these risks by restructuring large high schools into smaller units in which subsets of teachers work together to teach a more limited number of students who take all of their classes together and in which each teacher is assigned a formal advising role to a limited set of students. These structural and role changes are designed to enhance collaborative relationships among teachers (reducing their own social alienation) and to provide more opportunities for the development of close teacher–student and student–student relationships. In a randomized trial testing the impact of implementing the STEP program in urban school districts during the first year of high school (but not in subsequent years), attendance rates increased, and high school dropout rates were reduced by 50%. In subsequent trials evaluating STEP programs implemented in middle and junior high schools, students reported greater feelings of social connectedness at school and displayed improved academic and behavioral adjustment.

The Teen Outreach Program (TOP) takes a very different approach to enhancing adolescent adjustment (Allen, Kuperminc, Philliber, & Herre, 1994; Allen, Philliber, Herrling, & Kuperminc, 1997). The program, which is designed to be offered as a universal program (i.e., as a "health" elective course at the high school), provides youths in grades 9–12 with supervised volunteer experiences in the community (at least 20 hours per year) and weekly classroom-based activities (e.g., structured discussions, group exercises, role plays) focused on either youths' volunteer experiences or important adolescent developmental tasks. Discussions of service-learning experiences were used as opportunities to deal with common challenges (e.g., lack of self-confidence, assertiveness, or self-discipline), and teachers were given flexibility to address whichever other developmental issues were of greatest interest to students (e.g., handling close friendships, academic and employment issues). In a randomized trial involving 695 youths who participated in TOP or a control condition, results indicated decreased rates of pregnancy, school failure, and academic suspension among TOP participants (Allen et al., 1997). In a separate study, analyses indicated that the effects of TOP were greatest at schools in which TOP students were provided with more opportunities for peer interaction, in which students had greater autonomy to select their volunteer experiences, and in which volunteer opportunities taught students new skills (Allen et al., 1994). TOP is an excellent example of a program that achieves reductions in problem behaviors through strategies that focus entirely on competence promotion.

Conclusions

Given the prominence of supportive social relationships in risk and resilience research, it is not surprising that these relationships play a central role in the logic models of the intervention programs just described. Direct attempts to enhance caregiver–child relationships lie at the heart of some programs (NFP, SFP 10–14). Other programs focus on increasing youths' access to close relationships with supportive nonparenting adults (BBBS, TOP) or with teachers and peers (STEP). Finally, some programs aim to enhance youths' self-regulatory and social skills (PATHS, LST), thereby enhancing their capacity to develop and maintain supportive peer relationships. Note, however, that none of these programs attempts to enhance all types of supportive social relationships across all developmental periods in all ecological contexts. Rather, each program is built on a logic model that outlines how enhancing a specific relationship (or set of underlying relationship skills) at a specific point in development in a specific social context can produce enduring developmental benefits.

FUTURE DIRECTIONS IN RISK, RESILIENCE, AND PREVENTION RESEARCH

In the past 30 years researchers have made major strides in translating basic research on risk and resilience into intervention programs (such as those described in the preceding section) that have a meaningful positive impact on the lives of children and families. Despite this important progress, many major challenges remain. Here we highlight three issues that are likely to play a prominent role in the next two decades of research on risk, resilience and prevention science: multilevel analyses that integrate biological processes, research on how to facilitate high-quality implementation and sustainability of intervention efforts, and the development of public policies that provide incentives for communities to adopt evidence-based programs and that consider both the benefits and the costs of interventions.

Multilevel Analyses

In Masten's (2007) description of waves of resilience research, she suggests that the emerging fourth wave of resilience research will be characterized by multilevel analysis of risk and resilience processes, including a prominent focus on how biological systems (e.g., genes, stress hormones) interact with social systems. (Recall that the first wave was defined by the classic studies that identified key risk and protective factors, the second wave by studies of mediators of risk, and the third wave by the development and testing of interventions built on resilience models.) For example, there is emerging evidence that children with different variants of the same gene may be differentially sensitive to particular environmental experiences such as child maltreatment (Caspi et al., 2002). Increasing knowledge of such gene–environment interactions could help to provide more sensitive measures of individual developmental risk that could be used to define the population targeted for intervention or perhaps to alter the form of the intervention. A major challenge in this area is clarifying the specificity of the risk associated with a particular genetic variant (Belsky, Bakermans-Kranenburg, & van IJzendoorn, 2007; Rutter, Moffitt, & Caspi, 2006). Other multilevel research focuses on the dynamics linking environmental stress, biological stress hormones, cellular functioning, and physical and mental health (Sliwinski, Almeida, Smyth, & Stawski, 2009). Multilevel perspectives on development are not new, but recent advances in the measurement of biological systems and in the statistical analysis of complex systems point to more rapid gains in these areas in the coming years.

Best Practices and Evidence–Based Interventions

A second major direction of future research is the development of a science focused on facilitating the use of best practices and evidence-based interventions in local communities. Identifying and refining best practices will increasingly depend on meta-analyses of the many RCTs published every year; and, as the list of individual programs that meet strict standards of evidence grows over time, it will be increasingly important to develop ways to link local communities to up-to-date scientific knowledge regarding effective intervention practices and programs. One way to do this is through websites that maintain searchable databases of programs that have been vetted to meet some minimal standard of evidence (e.g., the National Registry for Evidence-based Programs and Practices, *www.nrepp.samhsa.gov*; and the What Works Clearinghouse, *ies.ed.gov/ncee/wwc*). Websites are more accessible and interpretable to community leaders than are scientific journals reporting results of RCTs, but they are not always updated as new research emerges; different sites employ different standards of evidence; and few sites provide guidance to communities regarding how to begin implementing a program. Alternative approaches focus on supporting community members with the broader decision-making process about prevention efforts. For example, the Getting to Outcomes system is a printed guide that contains a 10-step process designed to walk community leaders through a process of needs assessment, program selection, evaluation, and continuous improvement (Hunter et al., 2009).

An alternative system involving more sustained technical support is the Communities That Care (CTC) system (Hawkins et al., 2009). CTC staff provide initial training and ongoing technical support to a board of community leaders as the board learns basic concepts of prevention science, conducts a survey of risk and protective factors existing in the community, uses results of the survey to inform decisions about which risk and protective factors to target with interventions, chooses from an up-to-date list of evidence-based programs that address the prioritized risk and protective factors, obtains relevant support in implementing the programs they choose, and monitors changes in risk and protective factors over time. The CTC staff provides training, information, and technical support, but community leaders make the final decisions about which programs to implement. In the first-ever RCT evaluating the effectiveness of the CTC process, communities that used the CTC process had lower rates of adolescent substance use than communities that continued with their previous (non-CTC) approach (Hawkins et al., 2009). All CTC materials are available for free download through a U.S. federal agency website (*preventionplatform.samhsa.gov*). Other systems are also emerging to link experts on current intervention research with local community decision makers and service agencies, such as a program to link university researchers to local schools and community mental health agencies through the University Cooperative Extension system (Spoth, Greenberg, Bierman, & Redmond, 2004). A critical focus of research in the next two decades will be identifying factors that effectively link local communities and service agencies to current scientific knowledge and lead to the high-quality implementation and sustainability of best practices and evidence-based programs (Durlak & DuPre, 2008).

Benefit–Cost Analyses

Finally, there is an emerging trend to document the benefits and the costs of different preventive intervention programs and to formulate public policies that provide incentives to state and local governments to consider these benefits and costs when allocating scarce social services resources. Currently, social programs that are popular among constituents may persist even in the face of scientific evidence that they do not produce the desired benefits. For example, the DARE program continues to be implemented in the majority of U.S. school systems despite a scientific consensus that it does not lead to lower rates of substance use (Lynam et al., 1999). But a new federal law that required schools seeking Safe and Drug-Free Schools money to use programs that have scientific evidence of efficacy appears to have increased the number of schools implementing these programs (Payne, Gottfredson, & Gottfredson, 2006). The field of benefit–cost analysis has the potential to play a major role in these dynamics in the coming years. A benefit–cost analysis of a prevention program involves *monetizing* (assigning a dollar value to) all costs and all benefits of a program. Monetizing costs is relatively straightforward, although it includes some nonobvious steps such as putting a dollar value on participants' time investment. Putting a dollar value on the benefits of a prevention program can be much more difficult. Some benefits emerge very quickly and are easy to monetize (e.g., decreased payment of federal welfare funds to NFP mothers), but other benefits take many years to emerge (e.g., lower juvenile detention expenses for 19-year-olds whose mothers received NFP) or are difficult to monetize (e.g., fewer sexual partners among 19-year-olds whose mothers received NFP). It is also possible that some benefits are never documented because researchers did not test for them.

Despite these limitations, benefit–cost analysis is already having a significant impact on discussions of public policies related to prevention. For example, in an influential analysis, Aos and colleagues (2004) compared the benefits and costs of several dozen prevention programs targeting different problem behaviors in childhood and adolescence. They found that DARE cost only $99 per child to implement but had $0 dollars in benefits per child, so the program's *net benefits* (benefits minus costs) were negative (–$99), and the *benefit-to-cost ratio* (benefits divided by costs) was zero (0/99 = 0.00), suggesting that the community got no monetary benefit for each dollar it invested in DARE. In contrast, they found that LST cost $29 per child and brought $746 in benefits per child, indicating a net benefit of $717 per child, and a benefit-to-costs ratio of $25.61, suggesting that the community received more than $25 in benefits for each dollar it invested in LST. Other evidence-based substance use prevention programs have similarly positive benefit–cost numbers. (NFP had costs of $9,100 per family, with benefits of $26,300 per child, indicating that the community experiences $2.88 in benefits for every dollar it invests in the programs, mostly due to reduced maternal welfare dependency and reduced juvenile court and detention costs; Aos et al., 2004.) Given that financial resources to pay for prevention programs are certain to remain scarce and the intuitive appeal of using benefit–cost analysis (net benefits or benefits-to-costs ratios) to guide choices about how to allocate these scarce resources, it seems likely that research on the relative benefits and costs of different prevention programs will increase in quantity and in policy impact in the coming years.

CONCLUSION

We have organized this chapter according to historical waves of resilience research (Masten, 2007), but it is important not to take the metaphor of sequential waves too literally. New studies of the correlates of resilience and the processes accounting for resilience continue to be published, even as new prevention programs are developed and as new studies of gene–environment interactions, implementation processes, and benefit–cost analyses emerge. In fact, the waves of resilience research interact with and inform each other. For example, researchers evaluating new intervention programs are considering how to collect DNA samples from participants (Society for Prevention Research, 2009), which could lead to new insights into the biological correlates of resilience and a better understanding of how intervention strategies interact with biological processes. This, in turn, could inspire new interventions that gain efficiency by customizing intervention techniques for different subgroups of a population, perhaps by identifying the optimal developmental times and contexts for the promotion of supportive social relationships. The broader point is that risk, resilience, and prevention continues to be a vibrant area of research that requires us to bring the full range of developmental theories and research findings to bear on questions of great practical importance to social institutions concerned with the development of youths and families.

SUGGESTED READINGS

Aos, S., Lieb, R., Mayfield, J., Miller, M., & Pennucci, A. (2004). *Benefits and costs of prevention and early intervention programs for youth.* Olympia, WA: Washington State Institute for Public Policy. Available at *www.wsipp.wa.gov/rptfiles/04-07-3901.pdf.*

Baldwin, C. K., Caldwell, L. L., & Witt, P. A. (2005). Deliberate programming with logic models: From theory to outcomes. In P. A. Witt & L. L. Caldwell (Eds.), *Recreation and youth development* (pp. 219–239). State College, PA: Venture.

Institute of Medicine. (2009). *Preventing mental, emotional, and behavioral disorders among young people: Progress and possibilities.* Washington, DC: National Academies Press.

Luthar, S. S., & Cicchetti, D. (2000). The construct of resilience: Implications for interventions and social policies. *Development and Psychopathology, 12,* 857–885.

Masten, A. S. (2001). Ordinary magic: Resilience processes in development. *American Psychologist, 56*(3), 227–238.

Werner, E. E., & Smith, R. S. (2001). *Journeys from childhood to midlife: Risk, resilience and recovery.* Ithaca: Cornell University Press.

REFERENCES

Allen, J. P., Kuperminc, G., Philliber, S., & Herre, K. (1994). Programmatic prevention of adolescent problem behaviors: The role of autonomy, relatedness, and volunteer service in the Teen Outreach Program. *American Journal of Community Psychology, 22,* 617–638.

Allen, J. P., Philliber, S., Herrling, S., & Kuperminc, G. (1997). Preventing teen pregnancy and academic failure: Experimental evaluation of a developmentally based approach. *Child Development, 68,* 729–742.

American Academy of Pediatrics Task Force on Infant Positioning and SIDS. (1992). Positioning and SIDS. *Pediatrics, 89,* 1120–1126.

Aos, S., Lieb, R., Mayfield, J., Miller, M., & Pennucci, A. (2004). *Benefits and costs of prevention and early intervention programs for youth.* Olympia, WA: Washington State Institute for Public Policy. Available at *www.wsipp.wa.gov/rptfiles/04-07-3901.pdf.*

Baldwin, C. K., Caldwell, L. L., & Witt, P. A. (2005). Deliberate programming with logic models: From theory to outcomes. In P. A. Witt & L. L. Caldwell (Eds.), *Recreation and youth development* (pp. 219–239). State College, PA: Venture.

Bandura, A. (1977). Self-efficacy: Toward a unifying theory of behavioral change. *Psychological Review, 84,* 191–215.

Baumeister, R. F., & Leary, M. R. (1995). The need to belong: Desire for interpersonal attachments as a fundamental human motivation. *Psychological Bulletin, 117*(3), 497–529.

Belsky, J., Bakermans-Kranenburg, M. J., & van IJzendoorn, M. H. (2007). For better *and* for worse: Differential susceptibility to environmental influences. *Current Directions in Psychological Science, 16,* 300–304.

Benson, P., Scales, P. C., Hamilton, S. F., & Sesma, A., Jr. (2006). Positive youth development: Theory, research, and applications. In R. M. Lerner & W. Damon (Eds.), *Handbook of child psychology: Vol. 1. Theoretical models of human development* (6th ed., pp. 894–941). Hoboken, NJ: Wiley.

Benson, P. L., Scales, P. C., Leffert, N., & Roehlkepartain, E. C. (1999). *A fragile foundation: The state of developmental assets among American youth.* Minneapolis, MN: Search Institute.

Botvin, G. J. (1998). Preventing adolescent drug abuse through life skills training: Theory, methods, and effectiveness. In J. Crane (Ed.), *Social programs that work* (pp. 225–257). New York: Russell Sage Foundation.

Botvin, G. J., Baker, E., Dusenbury, L., Botvin, E. M., & Diaz, T. (1995). Long-term follow-up results of a randomized drug abuse prevention trial in a white middle-class population. *Journal of the American Medical Association, 273,* 1106–1112.

Botvin, G. J., & Griffin, K. W. (2004). Life skills training: Empirical findings and future directions. *Journal of Primary Prevention, 25,* 211–232.

Bowlby, J. (1969). *Attachment and loss: Vol. 1. Attachment.* New York: Basic Books.

Bronfenbrenner, U. (1979). *The ecology of human development: Experiments by nature and design.* Cambridge, MA: Harvard University Press.

Caspi, A., McClay, J., Moffitt, T. E., Mill, J., Martin, J., Craig, I. W., et al. (2002). Role of genotype in the cycle of violence in maltreated children. *Science, 297,* 851–854.

Castro, F. G., Barrera, M., Jr., & Martinez, C. R. (2004).The cultural adaptation of prevention interventions: Resolving tensions between fidelity and fit. *Prevention Science, 5,* 41–45.

Catalano, R. F., Hawkins, J. D., Berglund, L. M., Pollard, J. A., & Arthur, M. W. (2002). Prevention science and positive youth development: Competitive or cooperative frameworks? *Journal of Adolescent Health, 31*(Suppl. 6), 230–239.

Coie, J. D., Watt, N. F., West, S. G., Hawkins, J. D., Asarnow, J. R., Markman, H. J., et al. (1993). The science of prevention: A conceptual framework and some directions for a national research program. *American Psychologist, 48,* 1013–1022.

Conduct Problems Prevention Research Group. (1999). Initial impact of the Fast Track prevention trial for conduct problems: II. Classroom effects. *Journal of Consulting and Clinical Psychology, 67,* 648–657.

Damon, W. (2004). What is positive youth development? *Annals of the American Academy of Political and Social Science, 591,* 13–24.

Durlak, J. A., & DuPre, E. P. (2008). Implementation matters: A review of research on the influence of implementation on program outcomes and the factors affecting implementation. *American Journal of Community Psychology, 41*, 327–350.

Eccles, J. S., Midgley, C., Wigfield, A., Buchanan, C. M., Reuman, D., Flanagan, C., et al. (1993). Development during adolescence: The impact of stage–environment fit on young adolescents' experiences in schools and in families. *American Psychologist, 48*, 90–101.

Elliott, D. S., & Mihalic, S. (2004). Issues in disseminating and replicating effective prevention programs. *Prevention Science, 5*, 47–53.

Felner, R. D., Favazza, A., Shim, M., Brand, S., Gu, K., & Noonan, N. (2001). Whole school improvement and restructuring as prevention and promotion: Lessons from STEP and the project on high-performance learning communities. *Journal of School Psychology, 39*(2), 177–202.

Garmezy, N. (1974). The study of competence in children at risk for severe psychopathology. In A. Koupernik (Ed.), *The child in his family: Children at psychiatric risk* (Vol. 3, pp. 77–97). New York: Wiley.

Garmezy, N. (1985). Stress-resistant children: The search for protective factors. In J. E. Stevenson (Ed.), *Recent research in developmental psychopathology* (pp. 213–233). Oxford, UK: Pergamon Press.

Greenberg, M. T., Kusche, C. A., Cook, E. T., & Quamma, J. P. (1995). Promoting emotional competence in school-aged children: The effects of the PATHS curriculum. *Development and Psychopathology, 7*, 117–136.

Griffin, K. W., Botvin, G. J., & Nichols, T. R. (2006). Effects of a school-based drug abuse prevention program for adolescents on HIV risk behavior in young adulthood. *Prevention Science, 7*, 103–112.

Grossman, J. B., & Bulle, M. J. (2006). Review of what youth programs do to increase the connectedness of youth with adults. *Journal of Adolescent Health, 39*(6), 788–799.

Grossman, J. B., & Rhodes, J. E. (2002). The test of time: Predictors and effects of duration in youth mentoring programs. *American Journal of Community Psychology, 30*, 199–206.

Hawkins, J. D., Catalano, R. F., Kosterman, R., Abbott, R. D., & Hill, K. G. (1999). Preventing adolescent health-risk behavior by strengthening protection during childhood. *Archives of Pediatrics and Adolescent Medicine, 153*, 226–234.

Hawkins, J. D., Oesterle, S., Brown, E. C., Arthur, M. W., Abbott, R. D., Fagan, A. A., et al. (2009). Results of a Type 2 translational trial to prevent adolescent drug use and delinquency. *Archives of Pediatric and Adolescent Medicine, 163*, 789–798.

Herrera, C., Grossman, J. B., Kauh, T. J., Feldman, A. F., McMaken, J., & Jucovy, L. Z. (2007). *Making a difference in schools: Big Brothers Big Sisters school-based mentoring impact study.* Philadelphia: Public/Private Ventures.

Herrera, C., Kauh, T. J., Cooney, S. M., Grossman, J. B., & McMaken, J. (2008). *High school students as mentors: Findings from the Big Brothers Big Sisters school-based mentoring impact study.* Philadelphia: Public/Private Ventures.

Hunter, S. B., Chinman, M., Ebener, P., Imm, P., Wandersman, A., & Ryan, G. W. (2009). Technical assistance as a prevention capacity-building tool: A demonstration using the Getting to Outcomes framework. *Health Education and Behavior, 36*, 810–828.

Institute of Educational Sciences. (2003). Identifying and implementing educational practices supported by rigorous evidence: A user-friendly guide. Washington, DC: U.S. Department of Education. Available at *www.ed.gov/about/offices/list/ies/news.html#guide.*

Institute of Medicine. (1994). Reducing risks for mental disorders: Frontiers for preventive intervention research (P. J. Mrazek & R. J. Haggerty, Eds.). Washington, DC: National Academies Press.

Institute of Medicine. (2009). *Preventing mental, emotional, and behavioral disorders among young people: Progress and possibilities.* Washington, DC: National Academies Press.

Karcher, M. J., Davidson, A. J., Rhodes, J. E., & Herrera, C. (2010). Pygmalion in the program: The role of teenage peer mentors' attitudes in shaping their mentees' outcomes. *Applied Developmental Science, 14*(4), 212–227.

Karcher, M. J., Kuperminc, G. P., Portwood, S. G., Sipe, C. L., & Taylor, A. S. (2006). Mentoring programs: A framework to inform program development, research, and evaluation. *Journal of Community Psychology, 34*(6), 709–725.

Kellam, S. G., Koretz, D., & Moscicki, E. K. (1999). Core elements of developmental epidemiologically based prevention research. *American Journal of Community Psychology, 27*, 463–482.

Kitzman, H., Olds, D. L., Henderson, C. R., Jr., Hanks, C., Cole, R., Tatelbaum, R., et al. (1997). Effect of prenatal and infancy home visitation by nurses on pregnancy outcomes, childhood injuries, and repeated childbearing: A randomized controlled trial. *Journal of the American Medical Association, 278,* 644–652.

Korfmacher, J., O'Brien, R., Hiatt, S., & Olds, D. (1999). Differences in program implementation between nurses and paraprofessionals providing home visits during pregnancy and infancy: A randomized trial. *American Journal of Public Health, 89,* 1847–1851.

Larson, R., Wilson, S., Brown, B. B., Furstenberg, F. F., & Verma, S. (2002). Changes in adolescents' interpersonal experiences: Are they being prepared for adult relationships in the 21st century? *Journal of Research on Adolescence, 12,* 31–68.

LoSciuto, L., Rajala, A. K., Townsend, T. N., & Taylor, A. S. (1996). An outcome evaluation of across ages: An intergenerational mentoring approach to drug prevention. *Journal of Adolescent Research, 11,* 116–129.

Luthar, S. S. (1991). Vulnerability and resilience: A study of high-risk adolescents. *Child Development, 62,* 600–616.

Luthar, S. S., & Cicchetti, D. (2000). The construct of resilience: Implications for interventions and social policies. *Development and Psychopathology, 12,* 857–885.

Luthar, S. S., Cicchetti, D., & Becker, B. (2000). The construct of resilience: A critical evaluation and guidelines for future work. *Child Development, 71*(3), 543–562.

Lynam, D. R., Milich, R., Zimmerman, R., Novak, S. P., Logan, T., Martin, C., et al. (1999). Project DARE: No effects at 10-year follow-up. *Journal of Consulting and Clinical Psychology, 67,* 590–593.

Masten, A. S. (2001). Ordinary magic: Resilience processes in development. *American Psychologist, 56*(3), 227–238.

Masten, A. S. (2007). Resilience in developing systems: Progress and promise as the fourth wave rises. *Development and Psychopathology, 19,* 921–930.

Masten, A. S., & Coatsworth, J. D. (1998). The development of competence in favorable and unfavorable environments: Lessons from successful children. *American Psychologist, 53,* 205–220.

Masten, A. S., Hubbard, J. J., Gest, S. D., Tellegen, A., Garmezy, N., & Ramirez, M. L. (1999). Competence in the context of adversity: Pathways to resilience and maladaptation from childhood to late adolescence. *Developmental Psychopathology, 11,* 143–169.

McGill, D. E., Mihalic, S. F., & Grotpeter, J. K. (1998). *Blueprints for violence prevention: Book 2. Big Brothers Big Sisters of America.* Boulder, CO: Center for the Study and Prevention of Violence.

Offord, D. R. (2000). Selection of levels of prevention. *Addictive Behaviors, 25,* 833–842.

Olds, D. L. (2006). The Nurse–Family Partnership: An evidence-based preventive intervention. *Infant Mental Health Journal, 27,* 5–25.

Olds, D. L., Eckenrode, J., Henderson, C. R., Kitzman, H., Powers, J., Cole, R., et al. (1997). Long term effects of home visitation on maternal life course and child abuse and neglect: Fifteen-year follow up of a randomized trial. *Journal of the American Medical Association, 278,* 637–643.

Olds, D. L., Henderson, C. R., Tatelbaum, R., & Chamberlin, R. (1986). Improving the delivery of prenatal care and outcomes of pregnancy: A randomized trial of nurse home visitation. *Pediatrics, 77,* 16–28.

Payne, A. A., Gottfredson, D. C., & Gottfredson, G. D. (2006). School predictors of implementation of school-based prevention programs: Results from a national study. *Prevention Science, 7,* 225–237.

Rhodes, J. E. (2008). Improving youth mentoring interventions through research-based practice. *American Journal of Community Psychology, 41,* 35–42.

Robert Wood Johnson Foundation. (2006). The story of David Olds and the Nurse–Family Partnership program. Available at *www.rwjf.org/files/publications/other/DavidOldsSpecialReport0606.pdf*

Rutter, M. (1979). Protective factors in children's responses to stress and disadvantage. In M. W. Kent & J. E. Rolf (Eds.), *Primary prevention of psychopathology: Vol. 3. Social competence in children* (pp. 49–74). Hanover, NH: University Press of New England.

Rutter, M. (1987). Psychosocial resilience and protective mechanisms. *American Journal of Orthopsychiatry, 57,* 316–331.

Rutter, M., Moffitt, T. E., & Caspi, A. (2006). Gene–environment interplay and psychopathology: Multiple varieties but real effects. *Journal of Child Psychology and Psychiatry, 47,* 226–261.

Sameroff, A. J. (1999). Ecological perspectives on developmental risk. In J. D. Osofsky & H. E. Fitzgerald (Eds.), *WAIMH handbook of infant mental health: Vol. 4. Infant mental health in groups at high risk* (pp. 233–248). New York: Wiley.

Sameroff, A. J., Seifer, R., Baldwin, A., & Baldwin, C. (1993). Stability of intelligence from preschool to adolescence: The influence of social and family risk factors. *Child Development, 64*, 80–97.

Seligman, M. E., & Csikszentmihalyi, M. (2000). Positive psychology: An introduction. *American Psychologist, 55*, 5–14.

Sliwinski, M. J., Almeida, D. M., Smyth, J., & Stawski, R. S. (2009). Intraindividual change and variability in daily stress processes: Findings from two measurement-burst diary studies. *Psychology and Aging, 24*, 828–840.

Society for Prevention Research. (2004). Standards of evidence: Criteria for efficacy, effectiveness, and dissemination. Available at *www.preventionresearch.org/sofetext.php.*

Society for Prevention Research. (2009, May). *How to add genetics to your studies.* Preconference workshop held at the annual meeting of the Society for Prevention Research.

Spoth, R., Greenberg, M., Bierman, K., & Redmond, C. (2004). PROSPER community–university partnership model for public education systems: Capacity building for evidence-based, competence-building prevention. *Prevention Science, 5*(1), 31–39.

Spoth, R., Redmond, C., & Lepper, H. (1999). Alcohol initiation outcomes of universal family-focused preventive interventions: One- and two-year follow-ups of a controlled study. *Journal of Studies on Alcohol, 13*, 103–111.

Spoth, R.L., Redmond, C., & Shin, C. (2001). Randomized trial of brief family interventions for general populations: Adolescent substance use outcomes 4 years following baseline. *Journal of Consulting and Clinical Psychology, 69*(4), 627–642.

Spoth, R., Redmond, C., Shin, C., & Azevedo, K. (2004). Brief family intervention effects on adolescent substance initiation: School-level curvilinear growth curve analyses six years following baseline. *Journal of Consulting and Clinical Psychology, 72*(3), 535–542.

Steinberg, L. (2001). We know some things: Parent–adolescent relationships in retrospect and prospect. *Journal of Research on Adolescence, 11*(1), 1–19.

Tobler, N. S., Roona, M. R., Ochshorn, P., Marshall, D. G., Streke, A. V., & Stackpole, K. M. (2000). School-based adolescent drug prevention programs: 1998 meta-analysis. *Journal of Primary Prevention, 20*, 275–336.

Weissberg, R. P., & Greenberg, M. T. (1998). Prevention science and collaborative community action research: Combining the best from both perspectives. *Journal of Mental Health, 7*, 479–492.

Werner, E. E., & Smith, R. S. (1982). *Vulnerable but invincible: A study of resilient children.* New York: McGraw-Hill.

Werner, E. E., & Smith, R. S. (1992). *Overcoming the odds: High-risk children from birth to adulthood.* Ithaca, NY: Cornell University Press.

Werner, E. E., & Smith, R. S. (2001). *Journeys from childhood to midlife: Risk, resilience and recovery.* Ithaca: Cornell University Press.

Willinger, M., Hoffman, H. J., Wu, K. T., Hou, J., Kessler, R. C., Ward, S. L., et al. (1998). Factors associated with the transition to nonprone sleep positions of infants in the United States: The National Infant Sleep Position Study. *Journal of the American Medical Association, 280*, 329–335.

Wyman, P. A., Sandler, I., Wolchik, S., & Nelson, K. (2000). Resilience as cumulative competence promotion and stress protection: Theory and intervention. In D. Cicchetti, J. Rapport, I. Sandler, & R. P. Weissberg (Eds.), *The promotion of wellness in children and adolescents* (pp. 133–184). Washington, DC: Child Welfare League of America Press.

Yates, T. M., Egeland, B., & Sroufe, L. A. (2003). Rethinking resilience: A developmental process perspective. In S. S. Luthar (Ed.), *Resilience and vulnerability: Adaptation in the context of childhood adversities* (pp. 243–266). New York: Cambridge University Press.

Yoshikawa, H. (1994). Prevention as cumulative protection: Effects of early family support and education on chronic delinquency and its risks. *Psychological Bulletin, 115*, 28–54.

Zahn-Waxler, C., Cummings, E. M., McKnew, D., & Radke-Yarrow, M. (1984). Altruism, aggression, and social interaction in young children with a manic-depressive parent. *Child Development, 55*, 112–122.

Author Index

Abbott, R. D., 436
Abbott-Shim, M., 359
Abecassis, M., 165
Abels, M., 379, 384
Aboud, F., 167
Acker, M. M., 137
Acock, A. C., 128
Adamczyk-Robinette, S., 140
Adams, G. R., 84, 85, 86, 88, 89, 92
Adams, R. E., 189, 190
Adamson, L., 73
Adamson, L. B., 270, 272
Addy, C. L., 335
Adelman, H., 359
Adler, K. K., 79
Adler, N. E., 325
Adler, P. A., 222, 360
Adolphs, R., 40
Adorno, T. W., 238
Afrank, J., 15
Ahnert, L., 37, 350, 351, 353
Aikins, J. W., 91, 168, 169, 196, 222
Ainsworth, B. E., 335
Ainsworth, M. D. S., 82, 101, 106, 107, 109, 110, 353
Aksan, N., 45, 56
Albersheim, L., 114
Albus, K. E., 114
Alexander, K. L., 362
Alisat, S., 279
Allen, G., 186, 187
Allen, J. G., 88
Allen, J. P., 446, 447
Allen, L., 420
Allen, N. B., 53
Allen, V. L., 188
Almas, A. N., 274
Almeida, D. M., 140, 448
Aloise, P. A., 17
Alpert, R., 7
Amatya, K., 165
Amsterdam, B., 75
Anbar, S., 190
Anderson, C. A., 214
Anderson, D. R., 279

Anderson, G. M., 31
Anderson, K. J., 292, 300, 303, 305
Anderson, M. C., 40
Anderson, N. B., 318
Anderson, V. D., 317
Andreas, D., 55
Andrews, D. M., 170, 276
Anthonysamy, A., 408, 410
Aos, S., 443, 449
Appleyard, K., 408, 411
Aquan-Assee, J., 165
Archer, J., 208, 209, 219, 221, 300
Archer, S. L., 85, 86, 87, 89
Ardelt, M., 332
Argyle, M., 328
Aries, P., 4
Arnett, J. J., 86, 326
Arnold, D. H., 211, 212, 218, 362
Arnold, D. S., 137
Aro, H., 169
Aronoff, J., 305
Arthur, A. E., 307
Arthur, M. W., 437
Asencio, M., 306
Asendorph, J., 162
Asher, S. R., 156, 162, 168, 300, 360, 361
Astone, N. M., 322, 325
Atkinson, L., 115
Auslander, B. A., 192
Avery-Leaf, S., 305
Aviezer, O., 353
Axia, V. D., 379
Ayala, A., 31
Ayres, M. M., 292
Azevedo, K., 446
Aziz-Zadeh, L., 91
Azmitia, M., 86, 155, 304
Azuma, H., 373

Bachner-Melman, R., 269
Baer, J. C., 407
Bagwell, C. L., 156, 165, 169, 360
Bakeman, R., 270, 272

Baker, C., 304
Baker, E., 445
Bakermans-Kranenburg, M. J., 102, 110, 117, 118, 119, 382, 448
Baldwin, A., 430
Baldwin, C., 430, 435
Ball, J., 416, 417
Bandura, A., 6, 14, 15, 90, 293, 294, 302, 441
Banks, W. C., 238
Barber, B. K., 138, 139, 141
Barefoot, J. C., 335
Barfoot, B., 356
Bargh, J. A., 250, 253
Barker, E. T., 140
Barlett, C. P., 306
Barnes, J. E., 412
Barnett, D., 57, 407
Barnett, R. C., 324
Barocas, R., 349
Baron, R. M., 56
Baron-Cohen, S., 40
Barraza, V., 36, 135
Barrera, M., Jr., 440
Barry, C., 169
Barry, C. M., 276
Barry, C. T., 79
Barry, H., III., 375, 389
Barry, R. A., 31, 32, 33
Barthel, M., 37
Bartle-Haring, S., 191
Bartsch, K., 245
Bassen, C. R., 292, 305
Bassett, H. H., 273
Bassok, D., 354
Batenhorst, C., 277
Bates, B., 114
Bates, E., 76
Bates, J., 354
Bates, J. A., 331
Bates, J. E., 45, 46, 47, 49, 51, 156, 210, 213, 214, 273, 410
Bauer, P. M., 38
Baumeister, R. F., 79, 87, 444

455

Baumgartner, T., 36
Baumrind, D., 131, 132, 133,
    145, 210
Baydar, N., 356
Bear, G. G., 208, 219
Beauchaine, T. P., 119
Beauregard, M., 53, 62
Bebeau, M. J., 237
Beck, J., 56
Becker, B., 428, 431
Beilke, R. L., 410
Beitchman, J. H., 412
Belding, M., 215
Bell, R. Q., 14
Belsky, J., 108, 113, 117, 323,
    351, 355, 356, 410, 448
Bem, D. J., 187
Bem, S. L., 293, 303
Bender, H. L., 141
Benenson, J. F., 161
Bennett, C., 298
Bennett, E., 358
Bennion, L. D., 84, 85
Benson, P. L., 437
Bent, N., 335
Berdan, L. E., 52
Berenbaum, S. A., 90, 292
Berg, C. A., 300
Berglund, L. M., 437
Bergman, A., 7
Berk, L. E., 385
Berlin, L. J., 134
Bernard, H. R., 375
Berndt, T. J., 82, 164, 165, 167,
    168, 169, 170
Bernzweig, J., 58
Beron, K. J., 207, 217
Berry, J. W., 90
Bersoff, D. M., 265, 280
Bert, S. C., 417, 420
Berzonsky, M. D., 89
Best, D. L., 291, 292, 296, 386
Betts, J. R., 357
Beyers, W., 86
Bhullar, N., 160
Bichard, S. L., 240
Biederman, J., 273
Biehl, M. C., 194
Bierman, K., 44, 168, 449
Biesecker, G., 133
Biesta, G., 276
Bigbee, M. A., 208, 218
Bigelow, B. J., 158, 164
Bigler, R. S., 90, 160, 289, 292,
    293, 294, 297, 298, 299,
    301, 302, 305, 307, 335,
    386
Billingsley, A., 331
Birch, H. G., 45
Birch, S. H., 357, 358, 361
Biringen, Z., 271
Birns, B., 297
Bjorklund, D. F., 22
Bjorklund, F., 251
Bjorkqvist, K., 208, 209, 212,
    216, 221
Black, M. M., 417
Blacklund, E., 323
Blair, C., 59, 60

Blair, K. A., 57, 58
Blakemore, J. E. O., 292, 295
Blandon, A. Y., 53, 58
Blasi, A., 236, 250, 254
Blatchford, P., 355
Blehar, M. C., 101
Bloch, M., 377
Bloom, P., 252, 253
Blustein, D. L., 86
Boergers, J., 223
Boethel, M., 362
Boggiano, A. K., 78
Bogin, B., 372
Bohn, K., 296
Boisvert, M., 80
Boivin, M., 44, 161, 165, 169,
    216
Bokhorst, C. L., 118
Boldizar, J. P., 292, 299
Bolger, K. E., 408, 411
Bonham, V. L., 318
Bonica, C., 195, 212
Booth, C. L., 352
Booth-LaForce, C., 120, 167, 168
Borden, M. G., 156
Borelli, J. L., 169
Borker, R., 298
Bornstein, M. H., 23, 129, 131,
    133, 376
Bosma, H., 324
Bosma, H. A., 86, 87, 89
Bosquet, M., 115
Bost, K. K., 111, 112, 117
Boston, T., 325
Bosworth, K., 163
Botvin, E. M., 445
Botvin, G. J., 445
Bouchey, H. A., 83, 193
Bouffard, T., 80
Boulton, M. J., 165
Bourdieu, P., 327
Bourgeois, M. J., 88, 89
Bowker, J. C., 162
Bowlby, J., 12, 17, 21, 22, 81,
    101, 102, 103, 104, 105,
    106, 107, 109, 110, 111,
    112, 114, 116, 130, 358,
    442
Boyd, D. R., 239
Boylan, A., 55
Brabeck, M., 306
Bradley, R. H., 129, 355
Bradley, S. J., 90
Brame, B., 220
Brand, S., 189
Branje, S. J. T., 169, 190
Braungart, J. M., 46
Braungart-Rieker, J. M., 55
Braunwald, K., 407
Breed, L., 299
Brendgen, M., 154, 165, 170,
    194, 216, 217, 218
Bresnick, S., 83
Bretherton, I., 81, 110
Brewer, M. B., 84
Bridges, M., 354
Brillon, L., 331
Brinthaupt, T. M., 73, 74, 76
Britner, P. A., 105

Brodersen, L., 37
Brody, G. H., 144, 331
Broidy, L. M., 213
Bromley, D. B., 275
Bronfenbrenner, U., 24, 128, 184,
    316, 349, 378, 442
Bronson, M. B., 46
Brooks-Gunn, J., 74, 75, 76, 278,
    328, 329, 356
Broom, D. H., 324
Brown, A., 54
Brown, B. B., 185, 445
Brown, B. S., 335
Brown, C., 217
Brown, C. H., 214
Brown, C. S., 84, 90, 293, 298,
    304, 305, 328
Brown, G. L., 112
Brown, J., 387
Brown, J. D., 73, 74, 78, 82
Brown, M. M., 44
Brown, P., 168
Brown, S. A., 218
Browne, K., 417, 419
Brumbaugh, C. C., 116
Bruner, J. S., 273
Brunner, E., 324
Bryant, D. M., 356
Bub, K. L., 347, 350, 357
Buchanan, A., 352
Buchanan, C. M., 217
Buchanan, N. R., 158
Buck, M., 135
Buck, R., 271
Buehler, C., 144
Bugental, D. B., 36, 135, 141,
    147
Buhrmester, D., 86, 153, 155,
    158, 165, 166, 167, 168,
    169, 186, 190, 196, 211,
    303
Buhs, E. S., 357, 360, 361
Bukowski, W. M., 44, 86, 153,
    154, 156, 162, 164, 165,
    169, 170, 186, 196, 211,
    275, 303
Bulle, M. J., 444
Bulotsky, R., 359
Burchard, E., 318
Burchinal, M. R., 170, 348, 349,
    350, 356, 358
Burgdorf, K., 405
Burgess, K. B., 167, 168, 211,
    215
Burgy, L., 82
Burleson, B. R., 213, 304
Burns, A., 328
Burt, K. B., 44, 53
Burts, D. C., 143, 210
Bushman, B. J., 214
Buss, A. H., 46, 48, 52, 55, 60,
    208, 210
Buss, D. M., 21, 22
Buss, K. A., 37, 45, 56
Busseri, M. A., 223
Bussey, K., 90, 293, 294, 302
Buswell, B. N., 304
Butterworth, G., 74
Buyse, E., 362

Caetano, R., 335
Cairns, B., 167
Cairns, B. D., 208, 214, 222, 361
Cairns, R. B., 167, 208, 214, 216, 222, 361
Caldera, Y. M., 301
Caldwell, C., 435
Caldwell, C. H., 329
Caldwell, K., 360
Calkins, S. D., 44, 46, 47, 48, 49, 50, 51, 52, 53, 54, 55, 56, 57, 58, 59, 61, 62
Caltran, G., 74
Camarena, P. M., 304
Camodeca, M., 163
Campbell, A., 33, 90
Campbell, B., 384
Campbell, E., 86
Campbell, F., 355
Campbell, F. A., 356
Campbell, J. D., 79
Campbell, S. B., 213
Campione-Barr, N., 275
Campos, J. J., 46, 52, 116
Camras, L., 52
Capaldi, D. M., 208, 221, 416, 419, 420
Capella, E., 224
Caplan, M. Z., 265
Caprara, G. V., 187
Card, N. A., 165, 209, 216, 219, 222, 223, 225, 307
Carey, M. P., 412
Carlo, G., 275, 276, 277
Carlson, E. A., 12, 101, 113
Carlson, V., 306, 407
Carlson, W., 170, 186, 307
Carmody, D. P., 91
Carson, M., 304
Carstensen, L., 24
Carter, C. S., 31
Carter, D. B., 293, 299
Cartrite, B., 319
Carver, K., 182, 183, 187, 188, 190
Carver, L. J., 29, 39, 40, 50, 357
Casas, J. F., 162, 207
Cascardi, M., 305
Casey, A. E., 128, 143
Casey, C., 393
Casey, D. M., 278
Casey, E. C., 160
Casey, R. J., 248
Caspi, A., 45, 51, 187, 210, 213, 220, 225, 448
Cassano, M., 52
Cassidy, J., 81, 91, 101, 102, 109, 110, 115, 271
Castellazzo, G., 325
Castro, F. G., 440
Catalano, R. F., 436, 437
Caughy, M. O., 334, 355
Cavanagh, S. E., 188, 189, 192
Caygill, L., 90
Chacko, M. R., 183
Chadwick, A., 161
Chakrabarti, B., 269
Chalmers, H., 223
Chamberlain, P., 223, 224

Chamberlin, R., 442
Chambers, J. C., 274
Champagne, F. A., 34
Chang, L., 164, 388
Chang-Schneider, C., 80
Chao, R. K., 306, 327, 331
Chapman, J. W., 80
Chapman, M., 248, 271
Charles, C. Z., 326, 329
Charlesworth, R., 154
Charlton, K., 191
Charuvastra, A., 421
Chase-Lansdale, P. L., 355
Chassin, L., 78
Chau, C., 165
Chavous, T. M., 335
Cheah, C. S., 169, 387
Chen, L., 334
Chen, X., 171
Cheng, C., 167
Cherney, I. D., 299, 300, 302
Chernoff, J. J., 91
Cherry, K. E., 53
Chess, S., 45, 46, 48
Childs, J., 161, 211
Chisholm, J. S., 382
Chomsky, N., 14
Chow, J., 330
Christopher, F. S., 275
Chugani, H. T., 38
Chung, I., 418, 419
Chung, O. B., 376, 388
Cicchetti, D., 12, 36, 38, 54, 57, 76, 82, 407, 409, 410, 411, 421, 428, 431, 434
Cillessen, A. H. N., 156, 208, 222
Clancy, S. M., 88
Clark, C., 335
Clark, R. A., 306
Clarke-Stewart, K. A., 348, 351, 352
Clausen, J. A., 7
Claussen, A. H., 406
Clements, M. S., 324
Clifford, R. M., 350, 356
Cloitre, M., 421
Clore, G. L., 189
Close, G. C., 35
Clyman, R. B., 271
Coan, J. A., 120
Coates, B., 154
Coatsworth, J. D., 432, 433
Cobb, R., 195
Coelen, C., 355
Cogburn, C., 335
Cohen, D. J., 12
Cohen, J., 291
Cohen, J. D., 251
Cohen, L., 278
Coie, J. D., 44, 156, 163, 168, 207, 208, 209, 211, 214, 215, 221, 360, 361, 434
Cok, F., 86
Colburne, K. A., 159, 211
Colby, A., 238, 239, 255, 256
Cole, M., 20, 376, 378
Cole, P. M., 51, 54, 59
Cole, S. R., 376
Coleman, J. S., 349

Collins, A., 4
Collins, F. S., 318
Collins, N. L., 188
Collins, W. A., 12, 101, 115, 133, 184, 187, 191, 194
Colman, R. A., 412, 413
Colwell, M. J., 274
Compian, L., 194
Comstock, G., 214, 215, 302, 306
Conger, K. J., 316
Conger, R. D., 316, 332
Conley, D., 316, 324, 329
Connell, D., 407
Connolly, J. A., 166, 167, 180, 181, 182, 183, 185, 186, 187, 188, 189, 190, 192, 193, 195, 304, 305, 411
Connolly, K. J., 355
Conroy, D. E., 307
Consolacion, T. B., 183
Cook, E. T., 444
Cooley, C. H., 82
Cooney, S. M., 444
Cooper, C. R., 86, 306
Cooper, M. L., 188
Cooper, S. M., 328, 329
Copeland-Linder, N., 335
Coplan, R. J., 50, 162
Corbett, M., 135
Corey, J. M., 59
Cornell, A. H., 273
Cornew, L., 40
Corwyn, R. F., 355
Costa, M., 192
Costigan, K. A., 47
Côté, J. E., 87
Cote, S., 212
Coulton, C. J., 330
Coury-Doniger, P., 412
Covatto, A. M., 300
Cowan, P. A., 133, 246
Cox, M. J., 362
Coyne, S. M., 208, 218, 219, 221
Cozzarelli, C., 328
Craft, S. A., 357, 360
Craig, W. M., 167, 181, 182, 185, 187, 192, 193, 304, 305, 411
Cramer, A., 15
Crawford, J. K., 306
Cribbie, R., 189
Crick, N. R., 24, 162, 164, 168, 207, 208, 209, 211, 212, 213, 216, 217, 218, 219, 221, 222, 223, 265
Crissey, S. R., 188
Crittenden, P. M., 82, 406, 407
Crocetti, E., 84
Crocker, J., 80
Crockett, L. J., 53, 59, 140
Croft, C. M., 118
Crompton, R., 320
Crosby, L., 208, 221
Cross, D., 137
Cross, H. J., 88
Cross, T. B., 336
Cross, W. E., 326, 335, 336
Crouter, A. C., 140, 144, 183, 332

Crowell, J. A., 109, 114
Csikszentmihalyi, M., 165, 436
Culang, M. E., 86
Cullerton-Sen, C., 213, 217
Cummings, E. M., 116, 213, 430
Cundick, B., 188
Cunradi, C. B., 335
Currie, J., 357
Cushman, F., 252
Cyr, M., 412, 413

DaCosta, G. A., 412
Dahrendorf, R., 320
Daley, S. E., 195
Dalrymple, J., 276
Damon, W., 74, 75, 77, 246, 255, 256, 437
Danaher, D. L., 300
D'Angelo, S. L., 139
Daniels, T., 218
Daood, C., 266
D'Arcy, H., 195
D'Argembeau, A., 91
Darley, J. M., 251
Darling, N., 130
Darlington, R., 356
Darwin, C., 5, 6, 7, 22, 73
Datson, N. A., 35
Dauber, S. L., 360
David, G. M., 355
Davidov, M., 269, 270, 272
Davidson, A. J., 421, 427, 445
Davidson, D., 391
Davidson, R. J., 38, 50
Davies, B., 155
Davies, P. T., 195, 196, 213
Davila, J., 192, 194, 195
Davis, E. P., 50
Davis, K., 320, 321, 324
Davis, M. H., 186
Davis-Kean, P. E., 304
Day, W. H., 136
de Kloet, E. R., 35
de Vries, B., 240, 244
de Wiede, M., 190
De Wolff, M. S., 32, 102, 113
Deane, K. E., 107
Dearing, E., 356
Deater-Deckard, K., 129, 145, 210
DeBaryshe, B. D., 137, 213, 224
Debiec, J., 91
Dedmon, S. E., 46, 48, 52, 54, 55, 59
Degnan, K. A., 52, 58
deGuzman, M. T., 387
Deklyen, M., 358
Dell'Angelo, T., 337
DeLoache, J., 376, 380
Delveaux, K. D., 218
deMause, L., 4, 5
Demo, D. H., 128
DeNavas-Walt, C., 337
Denham, S. A., 44, 57, 273
Dennis, T. A., 51
Denton, N. A., 129
DeRosier, M., 156
Derryberry, D., 46
Desai, S. P., 355

Dettling, A. C., 212
Deutsch, F. M., 301
DeWolf, D. M., 143, 210
Dhariwal, A., 187
Di Loreto-Colgan, A. D., 412, 413
Diamond, L. M., 304
Diaz, T., 445
Dickens, C., 5
Dickson, J. W., 195
DiClemente, R. J., 140, 412
Diekman, A. B., 299
Diener, M. L., 56, 57
DiLalla, L. F., 45, 269
DiLillo, D., 412, 413, 417, 419
Dionne, J., 88
DiPietro, J. A., 47, 355
Dirks, E., 276
Dishion, T. J., 53, 140, 167, 169, 170, 196, 216, 276
Dix, T., 136, 141
Dixon, L., 417, 419
Dixon, W. E., 101
Dobbs, J., 218
Dobbs, T., 142
Dobson, J., 145
Dobson, W. R., 86
Doctoroff, G. L., 218
Dodge, K. A., 24, 44, 145, 156, 163, 167, 168, 207, 208, 209, 210, 211, 213, 214, 216, 219, 220, 221, 224, 331, 360, 410
Doise, W., 155
Dollard, J., 7
Dollinger, S. J., 88
Domes, G., 33
Domjan, M., 143
Dondi, M., 74
Donlan, C., 335
Donnellan, M. B., 80
Donzella, B., 212
Dornbusch, S. M., 82, 132, 185, 217
Douglas, L., 24
Doumen, S., 362
Doussard-Roosevelt, J. A., 49, 57, 59
Dovidio, J. F., 250
Dowling, T., 289
Downey, G., 195
Doyle, A. B., 194
Doyle, A. E., 273
Dozier, M., 114
Dragan, W. L., 269
Droegemueller, W., 404
D'Souza, R. M., 324
Dubé, E. M., 304
DuBois, W. E. B., 329
Dubowitz, H., 417, 420
Duckett, E., 275
Dumas, C., 80
Duncan, G. J., 322, 328, 332, 349
Duncan, J., 142
Dunn, J., 169
Dunphy, D., 166, 167
Dunsmore, J. C., 160
Dunston, K., 335
DuPre, E. P., 441, 449

Dupree, D., 336
Durlak, J. A., 80, 441, 449
Dusenbury, L., 445
Dwyer, K. M., 110

Eagly, A. H., 291, 292, 300
Earls, F., 329
Eastenson, A., 161
Easterbrooks, M. A., 76
Eaton, W. O., 300
Eccles, J. S., 279, 304, 332, 357, 359, 445
Eddy, J. M., 137
Edelen, M. O., 209
Eder, D., 163, 186
Eder, R. A., 77
Edgerton, R. B., 393
Edwards, C. P., 347, 374, 376, 377, 385, 386, 387, 393
Egan, S. K., 90
Egeland, B., 12, 101, 110, 113, 114, 115, 116, 360, 407, 408, 411, 434
Eggebeen, D., 323
Ehlert, U., 36
Ehrensaft, M. K., 412
Eisen, M., 76, 77, 78
Eisenberg, N., 44, 51, 52, 58, 60, 163, 237, 249, 269, 272, 274, 275, 300
Eisenberg-Berg, N., 17
Eisenbud, L., 296
Eisenhower, A., 156
Elam, K. K., 269
Elder, G. H., 8, 187, 316, 332
Ellickson, P. L., 209
Elliott, D. S., 221, 440
Ellis, B. J., 22, 188
Ellis, W. E., 214, 218, 276
Else-Quest, N., 295, 300
El-Sheikh, M., 59
Ely, R., 295
Ely, R. J., 91
Ember, C. R., 386
Emde, R. N., 11, 82, 116, 268, 271, 274
Emmons, R. A., 276
Endsley, R. C., 356
Engels, R. C. M. E., 84
Englund, M., 298
Enke, J. L., 163
Ennett, S. T., 219
Enns, L. R., 300
Entwisle, D. R., 322, 325, 362
Epel, E. S., 325
Epps, S. R., 324
Epstein, J. L., 167, 359, 360
Erickson, K., 32
Erickson, M. F., 37, 115, 407
Erikson, E. H., 7, 12, 74, 84, 86, 87, 336
Eron, L. D., 214
Eslea, M., 219, 221
Espelage, D. L., 163, 214, 222
Estell, D. B., 361
Ethier, K. A., 79
Evans, D. W., 274
Evans, G. W., 329
Evans, M. D. R., 337

Evans, S. M., 296
Everson, M. D., 417

Fabes, R. A., 44, 58, 160, 161, 163, 211, 269, 272, 274, 275, 276, 296, 298, 300, 360, 362
Fagbemi, J., 212
Fagot, B. I., 137, 143, 160, 211, 297, 298
Fantuzzo, J., 359
Faraone, S. V., 273
Farmer, T. W., 215, 361
Farver, J., 161, 164, 388
Farver, J. A., 378
Farver, J. M., 161, 164, 211
Feagans, L., 298
Fearon, R. M. P., 102, 115, 118, 120
Featherman, D. L., 324
Feeney, B. C., 91
Feerick, M. M., 404, 420
Fegley, S., 255
Fein, G., 163
Feinberg, M., 144
Feingold, A., 304
Feiring, C., 114, 182, 186, 187, 188, 189, 190, 409, 410, 412, 420
Feldman, E., 168
Feldman, N. S., 78
Feldman, R., 33, 36
Feldman, R. S., 410, 411
Feldman, S. S., 190
Felner, R. D., 437, 446
Felsman, D. E., 86
Felson, R. B., 82
Fendrich, M., 359
Ferguson, C. J., 302, 306
Fergusson, D. M., 220, 412
Ferrer-Wreder, L., 133
Feshbach, N. D., 208
Festinger, L., 82
Fhagen-Smith, P., 336
Fielding, B. A., 35
Fife, J., 306
Fincham, F., 192, 195
Fine, G. A., 221
Fine, M., 328
Fineran, S., 307
Finkel, D., 118
Finkelstein, B., 165
Finkenauer, C., 84
Fisher, G. M., 322
Fisher, J. D., 264
Fisher, P. A., 273
Fisher, P. H., 212
Fitch, S. A., 88
Fitzgerald, L. M., 348
Fitzsimons, C. P., 35
Fivush, R., 76
Flanagan, O., 256
Flanzer, S. M., 404
Flavell, J. H., 16, 17, 18
Fletcher, A. C., 140
Flook, L., 377
Flor, D. L., 331
Flores, G., 183
Flouri, E., 352

Fogel, A., 24
Follette, V. M., 412
Fonagy, P., 114
Forbes, D., 300
Ford, L. H., 77
Fortuna, K., 110
Foshee, V. A., 219
Foster, E. M., 350
Foster, M., 359
Fox, L., 359
Fox, N. A., 38, 46, 49, 50, 51, 52, 54, 55, 56, 59, 61, 162, 384
Frable, D. E. S., 321
Frabutt, J. M., 274
Fraley, R. C., 101, 102, 108, 113, 114, 116, 118, 120
Francis, S. J., 35
Frankel, C. B., 52
Franze, S., 359
Franzoi, S. L., 186
Fraser, E., 86
Fredricks, J., 279
French, D., 171
Frenkel-Brunswik, E., 238
Freud, A., 12
Freud, S., 7, 10, 11, 12, 22, 103, 237
Frey, K. S., 82, 83
Frick, P. J., 223, 224, 273
Friedl, S., 32
Friedlander, L. J., 185, 188, 195
Friedlmeier, W., 280
Friedman, C. K., 295, 297
Friedrich, W. N., 410, 412
Friend, R., 297
Frimer, J. A., 8, 18, 235, 239, 243, 255, 256
Frodi, A., 208
Froh, J. J., 276
Frosch, C. A., 56, 117
Fry, M. D., 277
Frydenberg, E., 304
Fukumoto, A., 248
Fulcher, M., 296
Fuligni, A. J., 84, 306, 333, 334, 377, 378
Fuller, B., 323, 354
Fultz, J., 275
Fung, H., 382
Furman, W., 120, 155, 165, 166, 168, 181, 184, 186, 187, 190, 191, 193, 194, 360, 411, 412
Furnham, A., 328
Furrer, C., 360
Furstenberg, F. F., 331, 445

Gådin, K. G., 305
Gaertner, S. L., 250
Galambos, N. L., 140, 323
Galen, B. R., 207, 208
Galinsky, E., 348
Gallagher, K. C., 347
Galliher, R. V., 183, 195
Gallimore. R., 384
Gallup, G. G., 75
Galluzzo, D. C., 354
Galotti, K. M., 218
Galperin, M. B., 217
Galvin, K. B., 160

Ganiban, J. M., 48, 57
Gannon-Rowley, T., 331
Gano-Overway, L. A., 277
Garber, J., 188
Garcia Coll, C. T., 316, 326, 327, 328, 329, 331, 334
Gardner, W., 84
Gareis, K. C., 324
Gariépy, J., 167, 208
Garmezy, N., 428, 431
Garner, P. W., 160, 271, 273
Gaskins, S., 386
Gauvain, M., 273
Gauze, C., 165
Gavinski-Molina, M. H., 162
Ge, X., 194
Gelfand, D. M., 273
Gelles, M., 49
Gelman, S. A., 294, 297, 302
Gentsch, J. K., 217
George, C., 407, 410
Gerard, J. M., 144
Gershoff, E., 133, 136, 141, 145, 146
Gershoni, R., 166
Gesell, A., 6
Gest, S. D., 167, 208, 421, 427
Gettman, D. C., 191
Giammarino, M., 215
Gibbs, J., 239
Gibson, N. M., 144
Gibson-Davis, C., 349
Giesler, R. B., 91
Giles, J. W., 209, 211
Gill, K. L., 46, 54, 55
Gilligan, C., 237, 242, 243, 244, 245, 250
Gillihan, S. J., 306
Gilliom, M., 56
Giordano, P. C., 182, 189, 193, 195
Giuliani, C., 192
Glantz, F., 355
Glazer, J. A., 154
Gleason, J. B., 295
Glick, P., 304
Glover, J. A., 183
Golbeck, S. L., 155
Gold, P. W., 31
Gold, S. R., 412
Goldberg, A., 167, 181, 182, 185, 188, 304, 411
Goldberg, S., 120
Goldberg, W. A., 352
Golding, G., 243
Goldschmidt, W., 381
Goldsmith, D., 379
Goldsmith, H. H., 45, 46, 48, 52, 54, 55, 60, 295
Goldstein, D. M., 373, 389
Goldstein, S. E., 304, 307
Goldston, D. B., 412
Goldwyn, R., 110, 113
Gooden, A. M., 299
Gooden, M. A., 299
Goodman, M., 3, 103, 127
Goodnow, J. J., 134, 142, 278
Goodwin, C., 387
Goodwin, M. H., 298, 303

Goossens, F. A., 163
Goossens, L., 139
Gordon, A. K., 276
Gordon, I., 30, 34
Gordon, T., 139
Gorman, A. H., 361
Gorman-Smith, D., 209, 221
Gosling, S. D., 83
Gotlib, I. H., 79
Gottfredson, D. C., 449
Gottfredson, G. D., 449
Gottfried, N. W., 53
Gottlieb, A., 373, 376, 380
Gottman, J., 50, 158, 159, 161, 163, 166, 214, 221
Goudena, P. P., 161
Gould, L., 289
Gowen, L. K., 191, 194
Grabe, S., 306, 307
Grafeman, S. J., 79
Grafen, A., 267
Graham, P. B., 320, 321
Graham, S., 164, 214, 317
Gralen, S., 185
Gralinski, J. H., 76
Granic, I., 24, 53
Grasley, C., 415
Gray, M. R., 147
Graziano, P. A., 44, 52, 54, 59
Green, M. G., 303
Greenberg, J., 412
Greenberg, M. T., 220, 224, 358, 361, 434, 444, 449
Greenberger, E., 352
Greene, J. D., 251, 252
Greene, M. L., 329
Greene, R. W., 156
Greener, G., 265
Greenfield, P. M., 378
Greenspan, S. I., 49, 59, 349
Gregg, G. S., 388
Greulich, F., 82
Griffin, K. W., 445
Griffin, N., 78, 79
Griffin, T., 335
Grimm, K. J., 58
Groh, A. M., 12, 101, 111, 120, 134, 353, 407
Grosbras, M.-H., 155
Gross, J. J., 51, 62
Grossman, J. B., 444
Grossmann, K. E., 37, 101, 114, 115
Grotevant, H. D., 84, 86, 306
Grotpeter, J. K., 168, 208, 216, 218, 219, 444
Grover, R. L., 194
Gruber, E., 412
Gruber, I. C., 348
Gruber, J. E., 307
Grundy, E., 325
Grusec, J. E., 21, 120, 131, 134, 142, 249, 263, 265, 269, 270, 272, 274, 275, 278
Guastella, A. J., 34
Guerra, N. G., 44, 163
Guivernau, M. R., 277
Gulko, J., 159, 211, 292
Gunderson, B. H., 195

Guner, B. M., 417, 420
Gunnar, M. R., 36, 37, 49, 50, 54, 56, 158, 212, 271
Gustafson, P., 239
Gustafsson, P. A., 37
Guthrie, I. K., 44, 58, 161, 211
Guyer, B., 128

Haas, B., 320
Haas, E., 169
Hacker, A., 324, 326, 330
Haden, C. A., 19
Hagan, R., 211
Hagele, S., 253
Haidt, J., 236, 237, 250, 251, 252
Haith, M. M., 383
Halfon, N., 135
Hall, G. S., 6, 139
Halpin, B. M., 410
Haltiwanger, J., 83
Halverson, C. F., 293
Hamilton, C. E., 114, 354, 358
Hamilton, S. F., 437
Hamilton, W. D., 266
Hamilton-Giachritsis, C., 417, 419
Hammer, M., 410
Hamre, B. K., 348, 357, 358
Hand, L. S., 181
Haney, C., 238
Haney, P., 80
Hanish, L. D., 44, 160, 163, 360
Hanrock, S., 211
Hanson, J. L., 38
Hanushek, E. A., 357
Harachi, T. W., 221
Hardaway, C. R., 328
Hardy, S. A., 88
Harel, S., 186
Harger, J., 59
Harkness, S., 373, 377, 378, 379
Harley, K., 76
Harlow, H. F., 14, 22, 101, 103
Harman, C., 54
Harmon, R. J., 76
Harmon, T., 305
Harmon, Y., 189
Harms, T., 350
Harpalani, V., 337
Harper, M. S., 195
Harré, R., 208
Harris, J. D., 272
Harris, J. R., 133, 140, 294, 298
Harris, T. R., 412
Harris-Britt, A., 335
Harrison, H. M., 195
Harrison, M. S., 317
Harrison-Hale, A. O., 329
Hart, C. H., 143, 162, 207, 210, 212, 213
Hart, D., 74, 75, 77, 255
Hart, J., 36
Harter, S., 17, 74, 75, 77, 78, 79, 80, 81, 82, 83
Hartman, S. G., 73
Hartman, T., 336
Hartmann, D. P., 163, 273
Hartup, W. W., 58, 154, 155, 158, 161, 162, 165, 167

Harwood, R., 306, 382
Haselager, G. J. T., 165, 167
Hastings, P. D., 131
Hatzinger, M., 189
Haugen, P. T., 190
Hauser, M., 252
Hauser, R. M., 324, 325
Hawkins, J. D., 436, 437, 448, 449
Hawley, P. H., 162
Hay, D. F., 158, 161, 162, 211, 265, 271
Haydel, K. F., 302
Haydon, K. C., 114, 194
Hayes, R., 277
Haynie, D. L., 195
Hayward, C., 194
Hazan, C., 184
Head, M. R., 140
Hearns, S., 362
Heatherton, T. F., 91
Heaton, T. B., 328
Hebebrand, J., 32
Hediger, K., 34
Hedrick, A. M., 19
Heim, C., 35, 36
Heine, S. J., 392
Heinrichs, M., 33, 34, 36
Helfand, M., 189
Helms, J. E., 318, 335, 336
Helsen, M., 89
Hemingway, H., 324
Hemmeter, L. L., 359
Henderson, A. T., 357, 359
Henderson, C. R., 442
Henderson, H. A., 46, 49, 162
Henkel, R. R., 214
Henley, N. M., 302
Hennig, K. H., 240, 254
Hennighausen, K. H., 191
Henrich, J., 392, 393
Herdt, G., 389
Herman-Stahl, M. A., 332
Hernandez, D. J., 129
Hernandez, M. D., 160
Herre, K., 446
Herrera, C., 409, 410, 444, 445
Herrling, S., 446
Hershey, K., 46
Hertsgaard, L., 37
Hertzig, M., 45
Hesse, E., 108, 110, 111
Hetherington, E. M., 133, 144
Heyman, G. D., 209, 211
Hiatt, S., 442
Hickman, L. J., 305
Higley, J. D., 31
Hill, A., 44, 51, 52
Hill, K. G., 436
Hill, N. E., 89, 316, 317, 319, 321, 326, 327, 331, 332, 337, 357, 360
Hill, P. L., 250
Hill-Soderlund, A. L., 58
Hilt, L., 304
Hinde, R. A., 157
Hines, M., 292
Hinney, A., 32
Hinshaw, S. P., 51

Hirschfeld, L. A., 318
Ho, A. Y., 317
Ho, M. J., 194
Hodges, E. V. E., 44, 155, 163, 165
Hodgson, D. M., 47
Hoegh, D. G., 88, 89
Hoehl, S., 30
Hoeksma, J., 276
Hofer, C., 51
Hoff, E., 320, 323, 331, 332, 335
Hoffman, C. L., 31
Hoffman, L., 299
Hoffman, M. L., 248, 271, 272, 275
Hofman, J., 166
Hofstede, G., 298
Hogg, M. A., 377
Hogue, A., 167
Holden, G. W., 127, 131, 135, 138, 142, 144, 146, 210, 332
Holland, A., 110
Holland, R., 223
Hollenstein, T., 53, 160
Holliday, H., 304, 307
Holloway, S. D., 373
Holmbeck, G., 275
Holsboer-Trachsler, E., 189
Holt, G., 325
Holt, M. K., 214
Holub, S. C., 276
Hood, J. E., 412
Hopkins, J. R., 84
Hopps, J., 335
Hornung, K., 38
Horowitz, F. D., 127
Horsch, E., 161, 211
Horwood, L. J., 220, 412
Howe, M. L., 76
Howe, T. R., 409, 411
Howes, C., 157, 158, 159, 160, 161, 162, 208, 348, 353, 354, 355, 358, 361
Hoyle, S. G., 165
Hoza, B., 164, 186
Hrdy, S. B., 385
Hubbard, J., 187
Hubbard, J. A., 58
Hubbs-Tait, L., 351
Hübscher, R., 273
Hudley, C. A., 214
Huesmann, L. R., 214
Hughes, D., 90, 331, 333, 334
Hughes, J. M., 307
Hugo, V., 5
Huizinga, D., 221
Hull, C., 103
Humphreys, A., 163
Hunsberger, B., 279
Hunter, S. B., 448
Hunter, W., 243
Hussey, J. M., 417
Huston, A. C., 278, 279, 298, 301, 303, 324
Huynh, V., 333, 334
Hyde, J. S., 243, 244, 245, 291, 294, 295, 302, 303, 306, 307

Hyman, C., 156
Hymel, S., 162, 166, 303, 304
Hysmith, C., 355

Iacoboni, M., 91
Iafrate, R., 192
Ialongo, N., 214
Ichise, M., 31
Ickovics, J. R., 325
Iedema, J., 89
Inkelas, M., 135
Insel, T. R., 34
Irizarry, N. L., 382
Ispa, J., 158
Israel, S., 268, 269, 273
Izard, C. E., 59, 62
Izzo, C. V., 359, 360, 362

Jacklin, C. N., 208
Jackson, J. S., 329
Jackson, S., 187
Jackson-Newsom, J., 144
Jacob, M. N., 187
Jacobson, D., 251
Jacobson, K. C., 140
Jacoris, S., 34
Jaeger, E., 351
Jaffe, D., 238
Jaffee, S., 243, 244, 245
Jambor, E. E., 280
James, W., 74
Jaskir, J., 75
Jaycox, L. H., 305
Jencks, C., 329, 330
Jenkins, J. M., 120
Jensen, L. C., 188
Jernigan, M., 318
Jessor, R., 223
Jessor, S. L., 223
Ji, J., 411
Jimerson, S., 360, 361
Jin, R. K.-X., 252
Jin, R. L., 323
Jin, S., 212
Johann, M., 31
Johnson, A. M., 182, 186, 189, 190, 193
Johnson, D. J., 334
Johnson, L., 46
Johnson, M. C., 54, 55
Johnson, M. L., 236
Johnson, M. S., 307
Johnson, N. J., 323
Johnson, S., 130
Johnson, T. R. B., 47
Joiner, T. E., 91
Jones, D. C., 271, 306
Jones, F. L., 320, 323
Jones, K. R., 411
Jones, R. M., 89
Jones, S., 45
Josephs, R. A., 91
Josselson, R., 89
Jouriles, E. N., 144
Joussemet, M., 139
Joyner, K., 182, 194
Julian, T. W., 331
Juvonen, J., 164

Kachadourian, L., 195
Kagan, J., 7, 46, 48, 49, 117, 248
Kagitçibasi, C., 376
Kahn, J. H., 191
Kahn, V., 48
Kahneman, D., 253
Kain, J. F., 357
Kalil, A., 375
Kalpidou, M. D., 53
Kamkar, K., 194
Kan, M. L., 183, 192
Kandel, D. B., 167
Kant, I., 236, 239, 264
Kao, G., 326
Kaplan, J. T., 91
Kaplan, N., 110
Karbon, M., 58
Karcher, M. J., 444, 445
Karpathian, M., 74
Karriker-Jaffe, K. J., 219
Kashdan, T. B., 276
Kasprow, W. J., 359, 362
Kassel, J. D., 79
Katainen, S., 48
Katz, L. F., 389
Katz, P. A., 293, 303
Kaufman, J., 416
Kauh, T. J., 444
Kaukiainen, A., 208, 209, 219
Kawabata, Y., 207
Kawaguchi, M. C., 195
Kawakami, K., 250
Keane, S. P., 44, 52, 53, 54, 58
Kearns, K. T., 160
Keating, D. P., 83
Keating, L., 89
Keefe, K., 168, 169, 170
Keehn, D., 140
Keenan, K., 51
Keith, J. G., 279
Kellam, S. G., 214, 434
Keller, A., 77
Keller, H., 20, 76, 372, 378, 379, 380
Kelly, J., 337
Kelly, J. B., 17
Keltikangas-Jarvinen, L., 48
Kemmelmeier, M., 280
Kempe, C. H., 404
Kemple, K. M., 355
Kennedy, E., 163
Kennedy, S., 355
Kennel, J. H., 116
Kenney, G. W., 81
Kenny, D. A., 56
Kenny, M. E., 306
Kerig, P. K., 217
Kerns, K. A., 109, 110, 168
Kerr, M., 133, 140
Kerr, M. A., 417
Kestenbaum, R., 54
Khatri, P., 164
Kiang, L., 120
Kielburger, C., 263
Killen, M., 305
Killoren, S. E., 144
Kilpatrick, S. D., 276
Kim, J., 409, 411, 416, 418
Kim, K., 406, 418, 419, 420

Kim, M., 277
Kindermann, T. A., 214
Kingston, L., 210
Kingston, R. S., 324
Kirschbaum, C., 36
Kirtland, K. A., 335
Kisling, J. W., 88
Kitayama, S., 280, 387
Kitzman, H., 441, 442
Klagsbrun, M., 110
Klassen, A. D., 412
Klaus, M. H., 116
Klaver, P., 34
Klein, D. J., 209
Klemencic, N., 135
Kless, S. J., 360
Klessinger, N., 191
Kling, J., 389
Kling, K. C., 303
Knafo, A., 268, 269, 273
Knickman, J., 329
Knight, C. C., 359
Knutson, J. F., 404, 412
Kobak, R., 121
Kobielski, S. J., 190
Kochanek, K. D., 128
Kochanoff, A., 57
Kochanska, G., 31, 136, 248, 249
Kochenderfer, B., 165
Kohlberg, L., 8, 11, 17, 237, 238,
    239, 240, 241, 242, 243,
    245, 246, 250, 251, 254,
    257, 292
Kohn, M. L., 320, 324, 332
Kokko, L., 215, 216
Kolko, D. J., 416
Konarski, R., 166, 186, 187, 411
Konner, M., 372
Kontos, S., 348, 356
Koopman, R. F., 88
Kopp, C. B., 47, 56, 76
Korbin, J. E., 330
Korda, R. J., 324
Koretz, D., 434
Korf, J., 33
Korfmacher, J., 442
Korn, S., 45
Koskenvuo, M., 335
Kosterman, R., 436
Kraatz-Keily, M., 156
Kraemer, H. C., 302
Krage, M., 266
Krehbiel, G., 215
Krettenauer, T., 240
Kreuger, J. I., 79
Kreutzer, R., 116
Krieger, N., 317, 318, 322, 323,
    326
Kroger, J., 84, 86, 87, 88, 89, 92
Krogh, H. R., 302
Krull, D. S., 82, 91
Ksansnak, K. R., 293, 303
Kuczynski, L., 136, 275
Kuhn, B., 145
Kumru, A., 387
Kunnen, E. S., 86, 87
Kupanoff, K., 275, 276
Kuperminc, G. P., 444, 446

Kupersmidt, J. B., 156, 164, 170,
    215, 221, 408, 411
Kurian, J. R., 34
Kurtz, D., 421
Kurtz-Costes, B., 335
Kusche, C. A., 224, 444
Kusel, S. J., 163
Kuttler, A. F., 163, 186, 193, 304
Kutz-Costes, B., 298
Kwako, L., 418, 420

La Greca, A. M., 163, 186, 193,
    195, 304
La Paro, K. M., 350
Labrie, G., 171
Lacourse, E., 215
Ladd, G. W., 162, 165, 211, 213,
    215, 357, 358, 360, 361
Ladouceur, C. D., 53
Lagace-Seguin, D., 162
Lagattuta, K. H., 57
Lagerspetz, K., 209
Lahey, B. B., 220
Laible, D. J., 20, 275, 276
Lakatos, K., 118
Lam, M., 306
Lamb, M. E., 37, 292, 305, 348,
    349, 350, 351, 354
Lamb, R., 208
Lambermon, M. W. E., 354
Lambert, R., 359
Lamborn, S. D., 82, 132, 140
Lamere, T. G., 183
Lamey, A. V., 24
Lan, W., 79
Lancy, D. F., 374, 375, 385, 391
Landman-Peeters, K., 187
Landry, S. H., 357
Lang, S., 54, 290
Langlois, J. H., 351
Lansford, J. E., 129, 131, 210,
    216
Lanthier, R., 79
Lanting, A., 187
Lanzi, R. G., 417, 420
Lapsley, A., 102
Lapsley, D. K., 250, 253
Lareau, A., 316, 320, 328, 331,
    332, 333, 337
Larkin, J., 305
Larner, M. B., 356
Larson, D. B., 276
Larson, R., 165, 168, 189, 275,
    445
Larzelere, R. E., 133, 145
Lasky, B., 253
Lau, L. B., 356
Lau, M., 183
Laupa, M., 246
Laursen, B., 161, 165, 189, 190,
    191, 193, 320
Lay, K. L., 109
Lazar, I., 356
Le Guin, U. K., 290
Leadbeater, B. J., 88
Leaper, C., 90, 160, 289, 292,
    294, 295, 296, 297, 298,
    299, 300, 301, 303, 304,
    305, 306, 307, 386

Leary, M. R., 74, 444
Leavitt, S. C., 389
LeDoux, J. E., 91
Lee, H., 33
Lee, J. M., 195
Lee, K., 138
Lee, L., 157, 158
Lee-Shin, Y., 164
Lefebvre, L., 414, 415
Leffert, N., 437
Leiderman, P. H., 378
Leinbach, M. D., 211, 297
Lemery, K. S., 45, 54
Lengua, L. J., 48
Lengua, L. L., 210
Leon, L. D., 382
Lepper, H., 446
Lepper, M., 272
Lerner, J., 323
Lerner, R. M., 316
Leroux, L., 244
Lesser, I. M., 88
Letner, J., 280
Levant, R. F., 303, 305, 307
Leve, L. D., 137, 143, 223, 224
Leventhal, T., 329
Levesque, J., 53
Levin, H., 7
Levine, A., 33
Levine, C., 87, 239
Levine, M. P., 185
LeVine, R. A., 373, 374, 376,
    381, 382
LeVine, S., 381
Levinson, D. J., 238
Levran, E., 190
Levy, R., 391
Lewinsohn, P. M., 195
Lewis, C., 133
Lewis, M., 23, 24, 52, 53, 61, 74,
    75, 76, 91, 114, 382
Lewis, R., 304, 335
Lewis, T., 412, 413
Leyendecker, B., 306
Liang, C. H., 382
Liben, L. S., 90, 292, 293, 294,
    299, 302
Lieb, R., 443
Lieberman, M., 239
Liebman, J. B., 389
Lim, L. L-Y., 324
Lin, H., 183
Lindahl, K. M., 213
Lindberg, S. M., 307
Lindell, S. G., 31
Lindsey, E. W., 274
Linebarger, D. L., 279
Ling, X., 214
Linver, M. R., 278
Lipka, R. P., 73, 74, 76
Little, J. K., 296
Little, T. D., 209, 307
Liu, W. M., 318, 325, 327, 334,
    335, 336, 337
Livesley, W. J., 275
Lochman, J. E., 156, 224
Locke, J., 5, 133
Locke, L. M., 134
Locke, T. F., 418, 420

Lodico, M. A., 412
Loeb, S., 354
Loeber, R., 209, 211, 221
Loebl, J. H., 78
Lohrfink, K. F., 334
Lokken, G., 158
Lollis, S. P., 158, 244
Lomax, L., 46
Lomax, R., 306
Lonardo, R. A., 193, 196
Loncar, C. L., 357
London, K., 299, 300, 302
Long, J. D., 44, 187, 296
Longley, S., 54
Longmore, M. A., 182, 189, 193, 195
Lo-oh, J. L., 382, 383, 384
Lord, S., 332
Lorenz, K. Z., 21
LoSciuto, L., 444
Low, S., 194
Lowe, E., 393
Luethi, M., 189
Lukon, J., 56
Luria, Z., 298, 300
Luster, T., 320, 324, 332
Luthar, S. S., 331, 333, 337, 428, 431, 433, 434
Luzzo, D. A., 335
Lynam, D. R., 163, 207, 440, 449
Lynch, J. H., 306
Lynch, M., 407
Lynskey, M. T., 412
Lyons, C. K., 34
Lyons-Ruth, K., 407
Lytton, H., 21, 297, 301
Lyxell, B., 73

Mac Iver, D., 80
Macartney, S. E., 129
Macaulay, J., 208
Macbeth, A. H., 33
Maccoby, E. E., 4, 7, 14, 130, 132, 133, 143, 160, 208, 211, 217, 272, 295, 296, 298, 404
MacDorman, M. F., 128
Macfie, J., 82
MacGeorge, E. L., 306
Machmian, M., 37
MacKinnon-Lewis, C., 274
Mackler, J. S., 44
Madsen, S. D., 121, 191, 192, 276
Maes, F., 362
Maestripieri, D., 31, 32, 33, 36
Magnuson, K. A., 332, 354
Magnusson, D., 188, 195
Magyar, T. M., 277
Mahler, M., 7, 12
Main, M., 101, 108, 109, 110, 113, 407, 410
Maita, A. K., 57
Major, B., 80
Malanchuk, O., 304
Malik, N. M., 213
Malone, M. J., 155
Malone, P. S., 220
Maltz, D. N., 298

Mangelsdorf, S., 37, 54, 56, 117
Manning, W. D., 182, 189, 193, 195
Mapp, K. L., 357, 359
Marchand, J. F., 195
Marcia, J. E., 74, 84, 85, 86, 88, 89, 91, 336
Marcoen, A., 81
Marcovitch, S., 61
Marcus, N. E., 213
Mares, M. L., 275, 299
Marin, B. V., 331
Marin, G., 331
Markell, M., 298
Markham, C., 183
Markiewicz, D., 194
Markovits, H., 80
Marks, P. E. L., 221
Markstrom-Adams, C., 86, 337
Markovits, H. R., 280, 376, 387
Marmot, M. G., 324, 325
Marsee, M. A., 223
Marsh, H. W., 83
Marshall, L. A., 144
Marshall, M. A., 73
Marshall, P. J., 46, 162
Marshall, R. E., 49
Marshall, T. R., 46
Martin, B., 191
Martin, C. L., 90, 160, 161, 211, 292, 293, 295, 296, 298, 301, 302, 360
Martin, J., 128
Martin, J. A., 132, 404
Martin, P., 335
Martin, S., 190
Martin, S. E., 51
Martinez, C. D., 407
Martinez, C. R., 440
Martino, S. C., 209, 220
Martorell, G. A., 36, 135, 141
Marttunen, M., 169
Marvin, R. S., 105, 109
Marx, K., 320
Mascher, J., 318
Massey, D. S., 330, 337
Masten, A. S., 44, 187, 428, 431, 432, 433, 434, 436, 441, 447, 450
Maszk, P., 58
Matheny, A. P., 49, 118
Mather, M., 326
Matheson, C. C., 158, 354, 358
Mathews, F., 34
Matsuba, M. K., 254
Maughan, S. L., 138, 139
Maumary-Gremaud, A., 44
Mayall, A., 412
Mayer, B., 280
Mayer, D. P., 348
Mayer, K., 347
Mayer, S., 329, 330
Mayeux, L., 222
Mayfield, J., 443
Maynard, A., 378
May-Plumlee, T., 275
Mayseless, O., 191, 192
Mazzella, R., 304
Mazziotta, J. C., 38

McAdams, D. P., 255
McAdoo, H. P., 329
McAndrew, F. T., 267
McBride, B. A., 112
McBride-Chang, C., 406, 407, 410, 420
McCabe, M. P., 306
McCaffrey, D., 209
McCartney, K., 348, 350, 351, 352, 354, 356, 358
McCarty, F., 359
McClarty, K., 80
McClaskey, C. L., 44, 168
McCord, J., 170
McCormack, K., 31
McCullough, M. E., 276
McDade, T., 379
McDonald, K., 168
McDougall, P., 166, 303, 304
McDuff, P., 412, 413
McElwain, N. L., 120
McFadyen-Ketchum, S., 51
McGill, D. E., 444
McGilvray, D. B., 373
McGinley, M., 249, 277
McGinnis, M., 329
McGuire, S., 81
McHale, J., 144
McHale, J. L., 56
McHale, S. M., 144, 183, 332
McInnes, L., 335
McIsaac, C., 180, 182, 187, 190, 195, 411
McKay, H. D., 329, 330
McKay, S., 223
McKay, T., 361
McKelvey, M. W., 331
McKenna, J. J., 379
McKenney, K. S., 187
McKenry, P. C., 331
McKnew, D., 430
McKown, C., 318, 328, 329
McLanahan, S., 350
McLoyd, V. C., 316, 328, 329, 331, 332
McMahon, R. J., 140
McMaken, J., 444
McMaster, L. E., 304, 305
McMillan, B. W., 355
McMillan, J., 320, 323
McNeilly-Choque, M. K., 207, 212
McNelles, L. R., 166, 304
McNulty, J. K., 190
McWayne, C., 359
Meacham, J. A., 77
Mead, G. H., 155
Mead, M., 384
Mealey, L., 266
Meaney, M. J., 34
Meehl, P. E., 108
Meeus, W., 84, 89
Meeus, W. H. J., 169, 190
Mehta, T. G., 91
Meier, A., 186, 187
Meijer, O. C., 35
Meilman, P., 85, 86
Meinlschmidt, G., 35, 36
Melchior, A., 279

Meltzoff, A. N., 74
Mendelson, M., 167
Mennen, F. E., 406
Menzer, M. M., 387
Merisca, R., 214
Merrick, S., 114
Messner, M. A., 303, 307
Mettetal, G., 214, 221
Metz, E. C., 279
Metzger, A., 275
Meyer, E., 331
Meyer, F., 169
Meyer, S., 61, 249
Meyer-Bahlburg, H. F., 189
Meyers, M., 354
Michael, R., 355
Michels, S., 134
Mick, E., 273
Miedel, W. T., 359
Mihalic, S. F., 440, 444
Mikhail, J., 252
Mikulincer, M., 81, 102
Miles, S., 215
Milevsky, A., 140
Milgram, S., 238
Miller, A., 306
Miller, J., 382
Miller, J. G. E., 265, 280
Miller, J. T., 212
Miller, M., 443
Miller, N. E., 7
Miller, P. C., 131
Miller, P. H., 9, 10, 17, 18, 23
Miller, P. J., 382
Miller, P. M., 300, 376
Miller, S. A., 18
Miller-Johnson, S., 44, 221, 356
Minish, P. A., 356
Minow, M., 376
Mistry, R., 298
Mitchell, P. B., 34
Miyake, K., 115, 373
Moffitt, T. E., 210, 213, 220,
    224, 448
Mohajeri-Nelson, N., 221
Moilanen, K. L., 53, 54
Moise-Titus, J., 214
Moller, L. C., 159, 166, 211, 296
Monahan, K. C., 195
Moneta, G., 275
Monroe, S. M., 195
Monroe, W. S., 157
Monsour, A., 79
Montemayor, R., 76, 77, 78, 303
Montgomery, H., 374, 376
Montgomery, R., 155
Mooney, K. S., 191
Moore, G. E., 236
Moore, K., 279
Moore, K. J., 223
Moore, M. T., 348
Moore, W. E., 320, 321, 324
Morelius, E., 37
Morelli, G. A., 115, 379
Morenoff, J. D., 331
Moretti, M. M., 222, 223
Morrel, T. M., 417
Morris, A. S., 52, 57, 58, 59, 275
Morris, P. A., 24, 128, 316

Morrissey, T. W., 354
Morrongiello, B. A., 135
Mosack, K. E., 412
Moscicki, E. K., 434
Mosher, M., 162, 207
Moss, H. A., 7
Moss, N. E., 317, 330
Motzoi, C., 169
Moulson, M. C., 38
Mounts, N. S., 82, 132
Moyer, D., 56
Mudrey-Camino, R., 359
Mueller, E., 407
Mugny, G., 155
Mullen, B., 82
Mullens, J. E., 348
Muller, C., 188
Muller, P. A., 141
Munholland, K. A., 81
Munro, G., 92
Munroe, R. H., 373, 376, 386
Munroe, R. L., 373, 376, 386
Muraven, M., 87
Murnane, R. J., 350
Murnen, S. K., 299, 307
Murphy, B. C., 58, 274
Murray, C., 361
Murray-Close, D., 217, 218, 221
Murry, V. M., 317
Musher-Eizenman, D. R., 276
Mussen, P., 17
Myers, B. J., 116
Myers, L., 354
Myers, S. B., 304
Myers, S. S., 52

Nachmias, M., 37, 56
Nadler, A., 264
Nagel, S. K., 352
Nagin, D. S., 215, 220
Nakamoto, J., 361
Nakao, K., 324
Nangle, D. W., 194
Narvaez, D., 237, 251, 253
Nash, A., 158, 271
Natsuaki, M. N., 194
Neblett, E., 335
Neckerman, H. J., 167, 208
Neemann, J., 187, 188
Negriff, S., 403, 411, 412, 413
Neiderhiser, J. M., 48
Neiss, M. B., 81
Nelson, C. A., 38
Nelson, C. S., 279
Nelson, D. A., 164, 212
Nelson, K., 76, 111, 436
Nelson, L., 349, 350
Nelson, L. J., 207, 276
Nelson, N., 37
Netter, S., 140
Nettles, S. M., 334
New, R. S., 373
Newcomb, A. F., 156, 164, 165,
    169, 360
Newcomb, M. D., 418, 420
Newcomer, R. R., 307
Newmann, F., 279
Newton, M., 277
Nguyen, S. P., 294

Nichols, T. R., 445
Nickerson, K. J., 318, 334
Nielsen, M., 75
Niemela, P., 208
Nimetz, S. L., 358
Noble, P. L., 34
Noguchi, R. J. P., 160
Nolen-Hoeksema, S., 304
Noll, J. G., 412, 413, 414, 418,
    419, 420, 421
Norenzayan, A., 392
Norman, K., 382
Nsamenang, A. B., 382, 383, 384
Nucci, L., 247
Nuckolls, C. W., 384
Nystrom, L. E., 251

Oakes, J. M., 318, 320, 321, 322,
    325
Oakes, R., 325
O'Boyle, C., 297
Obradovic, J., 44
O'Brien, M., 53, 58, 301
O'Brien, R., 442
Obsuth, I., 222
O'Campo, P. J., 334
Ochs, E., 376, 382
Ochsner, K. N., 40, 62
O'Connor, E., 358
O'Connor, T. G., 118
Odgers, C. L., 222
Offord, D. R., 437, 438
Ogbu, J., 326
Ojanen, T., 82
Okami, P., 379
O'Keefe, M., 414, 415
Okin, S. M., 247
Oldenburg, C., 168
Olds, D. L., 441, 442, 443
O'Leary, K. D., 190, 305
O'Leary, S. G., 137
Oliner, S. P., 255
Ollendick, T. H., 156
Olmedo, E. L., 90
Olmstead, R., 379
Olsen, J. A., 138, 139, 188, 212
Olsen, S. F., 207, 212
Olster, D. H., 141, 147
Olweus, D., 163, 164
Omar, H. A., 139
Oniszczenko, W., 269
Ontai, L. L., 20
Oosterwegel, A., 83, 84
Oppenheim, D., 271, 354, 379
Oppenheimer, L., 83
Oppliger, P. A., 299
Orlofsky, J. L., 88, 89
Ornstein, P. A., 4, 19
Ortiz, C., 211
Osterman, K., 208, 209
Ostfeld, A. M., 335
Ostrosky, M., 359
Ostrov, J. M., 207, 213, 218, 219
O'Sullivan, L. F., 189
Ou, S. R., 360
Owen, M. T., 347, 352, 356

Paciello, M., 187
Padilla-Walker, L. M., 276

Padrón, E., 110
Pagani, J. H., 33
Pahl, K., 329
Paiement, D., 171
Paik, H., 214, 302, 306
Paine, H., 142
Palmer, D. J., 271
Pancer, S. M., 279
Papillo, A., 279
Papini, D. R., 86
Paquette, J. A., 207, 208
Paquette, V., 53
Parad, H. W., 215
Parham, T. A., 335, 336
Park, J. H., 217
Parke, R. D., 4, 213, 409, 411
Parker, J. G., 156, 162, 163, 167, 168, 193, 360, 361, 409, 410
Parpal, M., 272
Parritz, R. H., 37, 56
Partlow, M. E., 273
Pascarella, E., 87
Patenaude, R., 217
Patterson, C. J., 156, 170, 293, 296, 299, 408, 411
Patterson, G. R., 15, 137, 167, 170, 210, 213, 224, 273, 276
Patterson, M. M., 73, 307, 336
Patterson, S. J., 84
Pauli-Pott, U., 32
Pavlov, I., 13
Payne, A., 161
Payne, A. A., 449
Payne, J. D., 301
Pearl, R., 215, 361
Pears, K. C., 416, 419, 420
Pedersen, J., 158, 271
Pedersen, S., 304
Peevers, B. H., 164, 275
Peisner-Feinberg, E. S., 348, 356, 358
Pelham, B. W., 82, 91
Pelkonen, M., 169
Pellegrini, A. D., 163, 187, 296
Pennucci, A., 443
Pepler, D., 167, 181, 182, 185, 187, 192, 193, 304, 305, 411
Perez, L., 331
Perkins, D. F., 411
Perlman, C. A., 299
Perry, D. G., 82, 90, 155, 302
Perry, L. C., 163, 302
Perry-Parrish, C., 52
Petersen, A. C., 304
Peterson, L., 264, 417, 419
Pettit, G. S., 44, 156, 210, 213, 214, 273, 331, 410
Phelps, M. E., 38
Philibert, R. A., 31
Philip, C., 335
Philliber, S., 446
Phillips, D., 332, 348, 351, 354
Phillipsen, L., 161, 162, 354
Phinney, J. S., 89, 90, 317, 319, 336

Phinney, V. G., 188
Piaget, J., 8, 9, 11, 15, 16, 17, 18, 23, 155, 237, 239, 240, 246, 247, 250, 254, 294
Pianta, R. C., 134, 348, 350, 357, 358, 361, 362
Pickard, J. D., 79
Pickett, T., 335
Piehler, T. F., 196
Pierson, R. K., 38
Pike, R., 83
Pinderhughes, E. E., 331, 332
Pine, F., 7
Pinker, S., 248
Pinquart, M., 351
Pipp, S., 76
Pirrotta, S., 384
Pittman, A. L., 415
Pitts, R. C., 254
Pizarro, D. A., 252, 253
Pizzigati, K., 421
Plomin, R., 48, 210, 268, 269
Pluess, M., 355
Podolski, C. L., 214
Polanichka, N., 209, 211
Pollak, S. D., 34, 36, 38, 225
Pollard, J. A., 437
Polusny, M. A., 412
Pomerantz, E. M., 81, 82
Popaleni, K., 305
Porges, S. W., 49, 50, 57, 59
Portales, A. L., 49, 59
Porter, F. L., 49
Portwood, S. G., 444
Posada, G., 109
Posner, M. I., 40, 47, 54, 55
Pott, M., 115, 373
Potter, J., 83
Poulin, F., 161, 169, 170, 304
Powell, D. R., 356
Power, T. G., 53
Powers, C. P., 355
Powlishta, K. K., 159, 211, 292
Prager, K., 166
Pratt, M. W., 243, 279
Prescott, A., 54
Presser, H. B., 324
Price, D. A., 35
Price, J. M., 162, 211
Prillentensky, I., 328
Prinstein, M. J., 167, 169, 186, 196, 208, 222, 223, 304
Prinz, R. J., 134
Prior, M., 210
Proctor, B. D., 337
Puckett, M. B., 222
Puddy, R. W., 319
Pungello, E. P., 356
Puntambekar, S., 273
Putnam, F. W., 412, 413, 414, 418, 419, 420, 421
Putnam, K. T., 412
Putnam, S. P., 48
Pychyl, T. A., 88

Quamma, J. P., 444
Quinn, N., 392
Quintana, S. M., 318, 334

Raag, T., 297
Rabain-Jamin, J., 382, 383
Rabbitt, P., 335
Rackliff, C. L., 297
Radke-Yarrow, M., 248, 271, 430
Radmacher, K., 304
Raffaelli, M., 53, 59
Raikes, H. H., 347
Raikkonen, K., 48
Raine, A., 210, 213
Rajala, A. K., 444
Raley, R. K., 188
Ramey, C. T., 355, 356
Ramsay, D., 75, 76
Ramsey, E., 137, 213, 224
Randolph, M. E., 412
Randolph, S. M., 334
Rankin, D. B., 163
Ratcliffe, B., 355
Rathbun, A., 348
Rau, L., 7
Raudenbush, S. W., 329
Raver, C. C., 359
Razza, R. P., 60
Redler, E., 275
Redmond, C., 445, 446, 449
Reebye, P., 222
Reed, A., 38
Reed, D. C., 257
Reese, E., 76
Reese-Weber, M., 191, 195
Reeve, R. E., 134
Regalado, M., 135, 137
Reid, J. B., 223
Reid, V. M., 30
Reijntjes, A., 58
Reilly, J., 54
Reinherz, H. Z., 79
Reiser, J. J., 4
Reiser, M., 44
Reiss, D., 48
Reitzel-Jaffe, D., 414, 415
Renshaw, P., 168
Resnick, S., 46
Rest, J. R., 237, 241, 242, 250
Reynolds, A. J., 359, 362
Reznick, J. S., 49
Rheingold, H., 265, 271
Rhoades, K., 320
Rhodes, J. E., 444, 445
Ricciardelli, L. A., 306
Ricciuti, A. E., 118
Richards, M. H., 168, 275
Richman, A. L., 382
Richmond, M. K., 192, 193
Ridgeway, D., 110
Riese, M. L., 49
Rieser-Danner, L. A., 351
Rigatuso, J., 37
Riksen-Walraven, J., 167
Rimmele, U., 34
Rimm-Kaufman, S. E., 362
Rincón, C., 195
Riordan, K., 46
Ripke, M., 278
Risch, N., 318
Rispens, J., 161
Risser, S. D., 217
Ritchie, J., 142

Ritchie, S., 356
Rivas-Drake, D., 334, 335
Rivkin, S. G., 357
Rizzo, C. J., 195
Roberts, J. E., 79
Roberts, M. C., 319
Robertson, J., 103, 104
Robins, R. W., 80, 83
Robinson, B. E., 303
Robinson, C. C., 207, 212
Robinson, J. L., 268
Robinson, L. R., 52
Robinson, T. N., 302
Rochat, P., 74
Rodkin, P. C., 215, 361
Rodning, C., 354
Rodrigues-Doolabh, L., 111
Rodriguez, J., 334
Roehlkepartain, E. C., 437
Roesch, S. C., 276
Roeser, R. W., 359
Roggman, L. A., 351
Rogoff, B., 19, 20, 376, 379, 384
Rogow, A. M., 84
Rohde, P., 195
Roisman, G. I., 12, 101, 102, 108, 109, 110, 111, 114, 115, 116, 118, 120, 121, 134, 191, 353, 357, 407
Rollins, K., 358
Romney, D. M., 297, 301
Ronai, Z., 31
Rosario, M., 410, 411
Rose, A. J., 166, 170, 186, 222, 295, 299, 300, 303, 304, 305, 307
Rose, H., 296
Rose-Krasnor, L., 167, 168
Rosemond, J., 145
Rosen, L. H., 73, 127, 207, 210, 332, 336
Rosenberg, M., 76, 83
Rosenberg, N. A., 318
Rosenbloom, S. R., 329
Rosenblum, G. D., 53
Rosenbluth, D., 104
Rosenfeld, A., 378
Rosen-Reynoso, M., 189, 305
Rosenthal, N., 121
Rosenthal, S., 114, 409, 410
Rosenthal, S. L., 192
Roseth, C., 296
Rosicky, J., 47
Rosnati, R., 192
Ross, A. O., 74, 75
Ross, G., 273
Ross, H. S., 138, 158, 244, 301
Rossi, P. H., 318, 320, 321, 322, 325
Rostosky, S. S., 195
Roth, G., 277
Roth, J. L., 278
Roth, M. A., 193
Rothbart, M. K., 40, 45, 46, 47, 48, 49, 51, 54, 55, 56, 60
Rothbaum, F., 129, 373, 388
Rothbaum, R., 115
Rousseau, J. J., 5

Rovine, M., 351
Rowe, I., 88
Rowley, S. J., 298, 335
Rubin, K. H., 50, 162, 163, 166, 167, 168, 376, 387, 388
Rubini, M., 84
Ruble, D. N., 78, 82, 83, 84, 90, 136, 292
Rudolph, K. D., 166, 295, 299, 300, 304, 305
Rueda, M. R., 40
Ruff, H., 47
Ruhm, C., 354
Rumberger, R. W., 79, 354
Ruopp, R., 355
Rushton, J. P., 275
Russell, S. T., 183
Rutten, E., 276
Rutter, M., 430, 431, 433, 448
Rutter, R., 279
Ryan, R. M., 306
Rys, G. S., 208, 219

Sadovsky, A., 237
Saegert, S., 330
Saft, E., 361, 362
Sagi, A., 271, 354
Sagi-Schwartz, A., 107, 112, 112–113, 115, 353, 382
Salisch, M. V., 59
Salvaterra, F., 111
Salzinger, S., 410, 411
Sameroff, A. J., 46, 349, 383, 430, 431, 434
Sampson, R. J., 243, 329, 331
Samter, W., 167, 306
Sanchez, M. M., 31
Sanders, P., 292
Sandler, I. N., 210, 436
Sandstrom, M. J., 156, 218
Sanford, R. N., 238
Sang, J., 406
Santilli, G., 410
Saphir, M. N., 302
Sareen, H., 135
Sarigiani, P. A., 304
Saucier, D. A., 306
Saudino, K. J., 48
Savin-Williams, R. C., 167, 304
Sawalani, G. M., 209, 307
Saxon, J. L., 81
Scales, P. C., 437
Scaramella, L. V., 137
Scarr, S., 348
Schacter, D. L., 250
Schafer, J., 335
Schafer, M., 164
Schank, R., 111
Scharf, M., 182, 183, 186, 189, 191, 192, 193
Schellenbach, C., 420
Scheper-Hughes, N., 373
Schiefele, U., 357
Schiller, M., 46
Schiro, K., 268
Schlabach, J. H., 279
Schlechter, M., 140
Schlegel, A., 375, 386, 389
Schmader, T., 80

Schmidt, L. A., 50
Schmidt, M., 169
Schmitt, K. L., 279
Schmitz, S., 268
Schneider, B. H., 115, 171
Schneider, R., 54
Schneider, W., 250
Schneider-Rosen, K., 76
Schoefs, V., 81
Scholte, R. H. J., 165
Schonberg, M., 56
Schönpflug, U., 391
Schuengel, C., 118, 163, 276
Schwartz, D., 164, 361, 362
Schwartz, S. H., 256
Schweinhart, L. J., 356
Scott, K., 415
Scottham, K. M., 336
Seal, J., 167
Sears, R. R., 7, 208
Seaton, E. K., 329, 335, 336
Sebanc, A. M., 160
Secord, P. E., 275
Secord, P. F., 164
Sedikides, C., 81
Sedlak, A. J., 405
Seeley, J. R., 195
Seifer, R., 46, 55, 349, 430
Seiffge-Krenke, I., 186, 189, 190, 191, 193
Selfhout, M. H. W., 169
Seligman, M. E., 436
Sellers, M. J., 384
Sellers, R. M., 329, 335, 336
Selman, R. L., 8, 17, 158, 166
Senior, K., 158
Senn, T. E., 412
Serbin, L. A., 159, 211, 221, 225, 292, 296
Serpell, R., 384
Servis, L. J., 301
Sesma, A., Jr., 437
Seymour, S., 373, 386
Shackman, A. J., 38
Shackman, J. E., 38
Shaffer, L., 193
Shah, C. P., 323
Shakespeare, W., 5
Shanahan, L., 144
Shanahan, M. J., 88
Shannon, C., 31, 32
Shapiro, T., 326, 330
Shapka, J. D., 83
Sharabany, R., 166
Shaver, P., 184
Shaver, P. R., 101, 102, 115, 188
Shaw, C. R., 329, 330
Shaw, D., 56
Sheese, B. E., 60
Shekele, R. B., 335
Shelton, J. N., 335
Shen, Y., 53, 59
Shenk, C. E., 412, 413, 421
Shepard, S. A., 58, 161, 211
Sherman, A., 263
Sherrill, M. R., 216
Sherry, D. F., 250
Shields, A., 54, 59
Shiffrin, R. M., 250

Shin, C., 445, 446
Shin, N., 112
Shiner, R., 45, 51
Shinn, M., 348
Shipman, K., 54
Shirley, L., 90
Shirtcliff, E. A., 36
Shomaker, L. B., 190
Shonkoff, J. P., 332
Short, M. B., 192
Showers, C. J., 303
Shulman, S., 182, 183, 186, 189, 190, 191, 193, 298
Shute, R., 191
Shwalb, B. J., 373, 388
Shwalb, D. W., 373, 388
Shweder, R. A., 373, 376, 389
Shyu, S., 167
Siebenbruner, J., 187
Sifers, S. K., 319
Sigman, M., 53
Signorella, M. L., 293
Signorielli, N., 299
Silk, J., 52, 132, 139, 140
Silva, J. M., 307
Silver, H. K., 404
Silverman, F. N., 404
Silverman, N., 407
Simion, F., 74
Simon, T. R., 163
Simon, V. A., 169, 184, 190, 193, 196
Simoni, J. M., 331
Simons, R. L., 412
Simpson, J. A., 113, 194
Simutis, Z. M., 275
Singh-Manoux, A., 325
Singleton, L. C., 162
Sinha, P., 38
Sinnott-Armstrong, W., 251
Sipe, C. L., 444
Sippola, L. K., 164, 165, 186, 275
Skinner, B. F., 6, 13, 14, 237
Skinner, E., 130, 360
Skinner, M., 167
Slaughter, V., 75
Slep, A. M. S., 190, 305
Sliwinski, M. J., 448
Slugoski, B. R., 84, 88
Small, M. F., 372
Smalls, C., 335
Smedley, A., 318, 319
Smedley, B., 318, 319, 329
Smetana, J. G., 140, 191, 246, 247, 275
Smiler, A. P., 189
Smith, A. B., 355
Smith, C. L., 54, 55, 273, 275
Smith, E. P., 334
Smith, E. W., 353
Smith, J. C., 337
Smith, J. P., 324
Smith, K. E., 357
Smith, L. B., 23, 24
Smith, M. A., 335
Smith, M. D., 138
Smith, P. K., 163, 355
Smith, R. S., 431, 432, 434
Smith, T., 144

Smith, T. E., 292, 295, 297, 300, 303, 320, 321
Smolak, L., 185, 307
Smolen, A., 269
Smyth, J., 448
Sneed, J. R., 86
Snidman, N., 46, 48, 49
Snyder, J. R., 15, 161, 163, 211, 213, 217
Snyder, T., 130
Soby, B. A., 79
Sochting, I., 84
Soleck, G., 335
Sollors, W., 321
Solomon, J., 108
Sommerville, R. B., 251
Sorlie, P. D., 323
Spangler, G., 31, 32, 37
Sparling, J. J., 356
Speltz, M. L., 358
Spencer, M. B., 336, 337
Spencer, R., 189, 305
Spencer, S., 80
Spera, C., 140
Spieker, S. J., 101, 108, 113, 118, 353
Spinrad, T. L., 58, 163, 237, 269, 272
Spitz, R., 7, 12
Spoth, R. L., 445, 446, 449
Spracklen, K. M., 170, 276
Springs, F., 412
Sroufe, A. L., 57, 61
Sroufe, L. A., 12, 101, 110, 113, 114, 115, 116, 117, 184, 191, 298, 300, 351, 434
Stahl, D., 30
Stams, G., 276
Stangor, C., 305
Stanley-Hagan, M., 144
Stansbury, K., 49, 50, 53
Stansfeld, S., 324
Stattin, H., 133, 140, 188, 195
Stawski, R. S., 448
Steele, B. F., 404
Steele, H., 114
Steele, M., 114
Stegall, S., 52
Stegge, H., 58
Steinberg, L., 52, 53, 82, 130, 132, 133, 139, 140, 147, 167, 275, 356, 446
Steinberg, M. S., 358
Steinberg, S. J., 192, 195
Stein-Seroussi, A., 91
Stephen, J., 86
Sterk, S. M., 34
Sternberg, R. J., 181, 188
Stevens, J., 317
Stevens, N., 154
Stevenson, H. C., 336
Stevenson, J., 81
Stewart, A. D., 136
Stewart, M. I., 161
Stifter, C. A., 46, 48, 49, 55, 56, 59
Stipek, D., 76, 80, 215
Stocker, C. M., 192, 193
Stolberg, A. L., 192

Stone, L., 4
Stoneman, Z., 144
Stoolmiller, M., 167
Stormshak, E. A., 215, 361
Stovall, K. C., 114
Stowe, R. M., 211
Straatman, A. L., 415
Strack, F., 254
Strassberg, Z., 213
Straus, M., 137, 138, 141, 145
Strazdin, L., 324
Striano, T., 30, 74
Striepe, M., 189, 305
Strobino, D. M., 128, 355
Strohschein, L., 129
Strom, G. A., 410
Strough, J., 300
Stucky, B. D., 209, 307
Stuhlman, M., 362
Su, M., 330
Succop, P. A., 192
Suchindran, C., 219
Suddendorf, T., 75
Suftin, E. L., 296
Suizzo, M.-A., 129, 131
Sullivan, H. S., 155, 156, 158, 165, 166, 168, 169, 218
Suls, J., 82
Sunstein, C. R., 252
Super, C. M., 373, 377, 378, 379
Susman, E. J., 188, 357, 421
Sutton, R. E., 359
Svedja, M. J., 116
Svoboda, T. J., 323
Swank, P. R., 357
Swann, W. B., 80, 82, 91
Sweet, M., 39
Swenson, L. P., 222
Swift, D. J., 222
Swingler, M. M., 39
Szkrybalo, J., 90, 292

Tagler, M. J., 328
Tajfel, H., 294, 335
Takahashi, K., 382
Takaki, R., 327
Talbott, E., 219
Talwar, V., 138
Tang, H., 318
Tangney, J. P., 74
Taradash, A., 192, 193
Tardif, C., 115
Tardiff, T., 320
Taska, L., 409, 410
Tatelbaum, R., 442
Tatum, B. D., 336
Taylor, A. S., 444
Taylor, A. Z., 317
Taylor, B. A., 356
Taylor, L., 359
Taylor, M. G., 294
Tenenbaum, H. R., 301
Teo, A., 360
Terenzini, P., 87
Terry, R., 156
Terwogt, M. M., 58, 163
Thelen, E., 23, 24
Therborn, G., 389, 391
Thoma, S. J., 237, 245

Thomas, A., 45, 46, 48
Thomas, D., 357
Thomas, J. J., 291, 292, 296
Thomas, K. M., 317
Thome, P., 208
Thompson, C. J., 279
Thompson, E. E., 144
Thompson, J., 330
Thompson, J. S., 326
Thompson, R. A., 3, 18, 20, 51, 52, 57, 61, 103, 120, 127, 249, 358
Thompson, T. L., 299
Thorndike, E. L., 142
Thorne, B., 166, 298, 300
Timmerman, G., 307
Tinsley, B. R., 162
Tisak, M. S., 246
Tobin, J., 388, 391
Todd, R. M., 61
Tolman, D. L., 189, 305
Topolinski, S., 254
Tops, M., 33, 34
Toth, S. L., 82, 407, 410
Tourelle, L., 142
Townsend, T. N., 444
Townsend Betts, N., 165
Towsley, S., 48
Tracy, J. L., 83
Tran, S., 194
Tranel, D., 40
Travers, J., 355
Trawick, M., 373
Treas, J., 324
Treboux, D., 114
Tremblay, G. C., 417, 419
Tremblay, R. E., 207, 209, 210, 212, 215, 216, 220
Trentacosta, C. J., 59
Tresch, M., 363
Trevethan, S. D., 244
Trickett, P. K., 403, 404, 406, 407, 410, 411, 412, 413, 414, 418, 419, 420, 421
Trimble, J. E., 90
Trivers, R., 266
Trommsdorff, G., 280
Trueman, M., 165
Trzesniewski, K. H., 79, 80, 83
Tsang, J., 276
Tseng, V., 306
Tucker, C. J., 144
Tucker, D. M., 33
Tudge, J., 376
Tulkin, S., 378
Tully, L., 29, 50, 357
Tunmer, W. E., 80
Turiel, E., 244, 246, 250, 257
Turner, H. A., 141
Turner, J. C., 294, 325
Turner, K. L., 84
Turnquist, D. C., 412
Tuval-Mashiach, R., 186, 188, 190
Twenge, J. M., 80, 304

Uddin, L. Q., 91
Udry, J. R., 182, 194
Uhlmann, E., 253

Ulbricht, H., 48
Umaña-Taylor, A., 334
Underwood, M. K., 86, 153, 166, 196, 207, 208, 209, 211, 215, 217, 218, 221, 303, 307
Updegraff, K. A., 144
Urban, J., 298
Urban, M. A., 412
Urberg, K., 167
Urquiza, A. J., 410
Usher, B. A., 59

Vaillancourt, T., 212, 216, 217, 221
Valente, E., 214
Valiente, C., 272
Valrie, C., 335
Van Acker, R., 215, 361
Van Damme, J., 362
van den Oord, E. J. C. G., 161
van der Valk, I., 190
Van Dulmen, M., 408, 411
Van Hulle, C., 295
van IJzendoorn, M. H., 32, 102, 107, 110, 112, 113, 114, 115, 117, 118, 119, 120, 354, 355, 382, 448
Van Lieshout, C. F. M., 165, 167
Van Peer, J. M., 33
Van Ryzin, M., 296
van Schaick, K., 192
van Zeijl, J., 136
Vanable, P. A., 412
Vandell, D. L., 158, 352, 355, 356, 363
Vandenberg, B., 163
Vandergrift, N., 356
Varady, A., 302
Varma, S., 445
Vasquez-Suson, K. A., 186
Vaughan, J., 51
Vaughn, B. E., 117
Veríssimo, M., 111
Verma, S., 445
Vermande, M., 161
Vermeer, H. J., 355
Vernberg, E. M., 223
Vernon, S. W., 335
Verschueren, K., 81, 362
Vezeau, C., 80
Vinik, J., 274
Vitaro, F., 44, 154, 161, 165, 169, 170, 215
Vittrup, B., 127, 135, 136, 138, 142, 143, 146, 210, 332
Vleioras, G., 89
Vogeltanz, N. D., 412
Vohs, K. D., 79
Vollebergh, W., 89
von Dawans, B., 33
von Planta, A., 189
Vowels, C. L., 306
Vreugdenhil, E., 35
Vygotsky, L. S., 18, 19, 20, 155, 271, 273

Wacquant, L. J. D., 330
Wagner, E., 248
Waldfogel, J., 354

Walker, B. W., 307
Walker, L. J., 8, 18, 235, 239, 240, 242, 243, 244, 245, 254, 255, 256
Wall, S., 101
Waller, E., 170
Waller, E. M., 222, 307
Waller, N. G., 108
Wallerstein, J. S., 17
Walsh, S., 186
Walters, R. H., 6, 14
Wanner, B., 170
Ward, L. F., 320
Ward, L. M., 306
Ward, S. A., 291
Ware, A. M., 356
Warren, J. S., 319
Warren, M. R., 330
Warshauer-Baker, E., 318
Waterman, A. S., 84, 87, 89
Waters, E., 101, 107, 109, 111, 114, 116, 119
Waters, H. S., 111
Waters, P., 82
Watson, J., 6, 13, 137
Watson, J. B., 6, 7, 13, 14, 127, 132, 147
Watson, P., 335
Way, N., 329, 334, 375
Weber, E. K., 247
Wegner, D. M., 250, 253
Wehner, E., 184, 191, 193
Weikart, D. P., 356
Weimer, B., 168
Weinfield, N. S., 113, 114, 116
Weinraub, M., 351
Weinstein, R., 224
Weisner, T. S., 20, 87, 89, 129, 334, 372, 373, 375, 377, 378, 379, 381, 382, 384, 385, 391, 393
Weiss, R. J., 302
Weissberg, R. P., 359, 362, 434
Weist, M. D., 156
Weisz, J., 115, 373
Weitzman, N., 297
Wekerle, C., 412, 414, 415
Weller, A., 33
Wellman, H. M., 137
Wells, K. C., 224
Wells, W., 356
Welsh, D. P., 190, 195
Welsh, J. D., 59
Wentzel, K. R., 169, 360, 361
Wentzel, M., 272
Wenzlaff, R. M., 91
Werner, E. E., 376, 431, 432, 434
Werner, H., 257
Werner, N. E., 164, 218, 219, 223
West, J., 348
West, M. M., 376
West, S. G., 210
Whalley, S., 289
Whipp, B. J., 291
Whipple, B., 57
Whitbeck, L. B., 412
Whitbourne, S. K., 86
Whitcher-Alagna, S., 264
White, S., 410

White, S. H., 384
Whitebook, M., 354
Whitehand, C., 165
Whitehead, E., 218
Whitesell, N. R., 82, 83
Whiting, B. B., 280, 374, 376,
    377, 386, 393
Whiting, J. W. M., 280, 376, 386
Whitson, S. M., 59
Wichmann, C., 162
Widom, C. S., 412, 413
Wigfield, A., 74, 357
Wiggins, G., 243
Wijers, A. A., 33
Wilder, D., 189
Wiley, A. R., 382
Wilkinson, A. V., 328
Wilkinson, J., 277
Willer, B., 356
Willett, J. B., 350
Williams, D. R., 317
Williams, J. E., 386
Williams, S., 279
Williams, T., 189, 305
Williams, V. A., 189, 190
Williams-Russo, P., 329
Willinger, M., 436
Willoughby, T., 223
Wilsnack, S. C., 412
Wilson, A. E., 138
Wilson, B., 50
Wilson, D. K., 335
Wilson, D. S., 266
Wilson, K. S., 158
Wilson, R. S., 49
Wilson, S., 445
Wilson, W. J., 316, 319, 326, 329,
    330, 333, 337
Windle, M., 195, 196
Wingood, G. M., 412

Winslow, J. T., 34, 36
Wismer Fries, A. B., 34, 36
Wissow, L. S., 135
Witherspoon, D. P., 89, 316
Witkowska, E., 305
Witt, P., 435
Wojslawowicz, J., 168
Wojslawowicz Bowker, J., 167
Wolchik, S., 436
Wolfe, C., 80
Wolfe, D. A., 412, 414, 415
Wolff, L. S., 137
Wolitzky-Taylor, K. B., 305
Wood, D., 328
Wood, D. J., 273
Wood, G., 189
Wood, W., 291, 292, 300
Woodard, E., 275, 299
Worthman, C. M., 375, 377
Wozniak, P., 143
Wright, J., 412, 413
Wright, J. C., 215, 245, 279
Wright, K., 140
Wu, D., 391
Wu, Y., 140
Wyatt, T., 273
Wyman, H., 296
Wyman, P. A., 436

Xie, H., 222
Xu, Y., 164, 388

Yang, C., 212
Yap, M. B. H., 53
Yates, M., 87, 279
Yates, T., 408, 411, 434
Yershova, K., 212
Yip, T., 84
Yoder, A. E., 86, 87, 92
Yoshikawa, H., 375, 434

Young, A. M., 195
Young, L., 252
Young, R. D., 78
Young, W. S., 33
Youngblade, L. M., 410
Youniss, J., 87, 279
Yu, L., 388
Yunger, J., 22
Yurkewicz, C., 276

Zaff, J., 279
Zagefka, H., 319
Zagoory-Sharon, O., 33
Zahavi, A., 267
Zahn-Waxler, C., 4, 59, 208, 209,
    211, 222, 248, 268, 271, 430
Zajac, K., 121
Zambarano, R. J., 136, 144
Zarbatany, L., 163, 166, 214,
    218, 276, 303, 307
Zax, M., 349
Zeanah, C. H., 38
Zeff, K. R., 194
Zeljo, A., 212
Zelli, A., 331
Zeman, J., 52, 57
Zerbinos, E., 299
Zhang, Z., 388
Ziegler, T. E., 34
Zigler, E. F., 416, 420
Zimbardo, P. G., 238
Zimmer-Gembeck, M. J., 187,
    188, 189, 408, 410
Zimmerman, H. R., 101, 103
Zimmermann, P., 31, 168
Ziv, E., 318
Ziv, Y., 91
Zoll, D., 407
Zucker, K. J., 90, 412
Zukow, P. G., 384

Subject Index

f following a page number indicates a figure; *t* following a page number indicates a table.

Ability, 80
Abuse. *see* Child maltreatment; Neglect; Physical abuse; Sexual abuse
Academic achievement. *see also* School functioning and adjustment
  child care and, 350
  discrimination and, 335
  peer relationships and, 360–361
  socioeconomic status (SES) and, 323
Acceptance, 360, 361
Accomplishment of natural growth, 333
Adaptation, 427–431, 429*t*–430*t*, 440
ADD–Health Longitudinal Survey, 181–182
Adjustment
  aggression and, 212–213
  emotion regulation and, 57–59
  gender and, 307
  identity and, 89
  peer relationships and, 155–156
  romantic relationships and, 192
  school system and, 361–362
  stages of romantic development and, 187–188
Adolescence. *see also* Late childhood; Romantic relationships
  aggression and, 219–223
  child maltreatment and, 408*t*

culture and, 389–391
discipline and, 139–141
emotion regulation and, 53
gender and, 303–307
identity and, 84
peer relationships and, 165–170
prevention and intervention and, 446–447
prosocial behavior and, 275–278
self-esteem and, 83
stages of romantic development and, 184–188
Adolescent Self-Regulatory Inventory, 54
Adrenocortical activity, 50–51
Adult Attachment Interview (AAI), 108–109, 110–111
Adulthood, 83, 110–111
Affective experience, 164
Affective intuition models, 250–252
Affiliative goals, 299–300, 305–306
Agency, 256–257
Aggression. *see also* Anger
  adolescence and, 219–223
  child maltreatment and, 407, 408*t*, 411
  culture and, 387
  definitions and subtypes of, 208–209
  early childhood and, 209–213
  emotion regulation and, 58–59

future directions in the study of, 224–225
gender and, 209, 295, 300, 301–302, 306
middle childhood and, 213–219
overview, 207–209
parenting and, 137
peer relationships and, 163, 169, 360, 361
prevention and intervention and, 223–224
race, ethnicity, and SES and, 335
romantic relationships and, 193
school system and, 362
serotonin and, 31
sexual harassment and, 304–305, 306–307
Altruism, 266. *see also* Prosocial behavior
Androgyny, 303
Anger. *see also* Aggression
  emotion regulation and, 58–59
  historical views of child development and, 8
  race, ethnicity, and SES and, 335
  serotonin and, 31
Animal studies, 20–23, 31–38, 103
Antecedents hypotheses, 113–114
Antipathies, 165
Antisocial behavior, 137, 360, 408*t*

Anxiety
    aggression and, 219
    attachment and, 117–118
    corumination and, 307
    discrimination and, 335
    gender and, 307
    peer relationships and, 156
Appraisals, 82
Approach–avoidance conflict
    behaviors, 407
Argumentativeness, 193
Assertive goals, 299–300,
    305–306
Assessment
    aggression and, 216
    attachment and, 107–110, 119
    emotion regulation and, 54
    identity and, 84–85
    moral development and, 239
    psychobiological assessments,
        49–51
    socioeconomic status (SES)
        and, 321–325
    temperament and, 48–51
Assets, 429t
Attachment
    child care and, 352–354
    child maltreatment and, 407
    cortisol and, 36–38
    culture and, 381–382
    future directions in the study
        of, 119–121
    intergenerational continuity
        of maltreatment and, 418t
    oxytocin and, 34–35
    serotonin and, 31–33
Attachment Q-Set (AQS),
    107–108, 109
Attachment relationships, 115–
    119. see also Relationships
Attachment Script Assessment
    (ASA), 111
Attachment security, 37
Attachment Story Completion
    Task (ASCT), 110
Attachment style. see also
    Attachment; Insecure
    attachment; Secure
    attachments
    adult attachment and,
        110–111
    child maltreatment and, 407
    individual differences and,
        106–111
    peer relationships and, 168
    self-esteem and, 81
Attachment theory. see also
    Attachment
    developmental psychology
        and, 111–115

ethological and evolutionary
        theories and, 22–23
    future directions in the study
        of, 119–121
    historical overview of,
        102–105
    individual differences and,
        106–111
    moral development and, 249
    as a normative account of
        human development,
        105–106
    overview, 9–10, 12–13, 21,
        101–102
    romantic relationships and,
        183–184, 192
    teacher–child relationships
        and, 358
Attentional difficulties, 156
Attention-deficit/hyperactivity
    disorder (ADHD), 216
Attributional style, 409t
Authoritarian parenting
    style, 131–132. see also
    Parenting
Authoritative parenting style,
    131–132, 139–140, 192.
    see also Parenting
Autonomy support, 130
Avoidance, 117–118, 407

Bandura's theory, 15
Battered child syndrome,
    404. see also Child
    maltreatment
Behavior
    gender and, 295–295, 300,
        304–305
    race, ethnicity, and SES and,
        334–335
Behavioral factors. see also
    Prosocial behavior
    aggression and, 210
    attachment theory and,
        104–105
    identity development and,
        87–88
    self-esteem and, 80
Behavioral genetics, 8–9. see
    also Genetic factors
Behavioral theory, 13–14,
    237
Behaviorism, 6
Belief systems, 334–335,
    377–378
Benefit–cost analyses, 449–450
Best practices, 430t, 440,
    448–449
Biases, 252–253, 334
Big Brothers Big Sisters of
    America (BBBSA),
    443–445

Biological factors
    aggression and, 224–225
    attachment and, 118–119
    brain development and,
        38–39
    future directions in the study
        of, 39–40
    moral development and,
        249
    overview, 29–38
    race and, 318
Black–African American
    identity development,
        336–337
Black–White racial identity,
    336–337
Body image, 303–304, 306–
    307
Bonding, 116–117
Borderline personality disorder,
    222–223
Bossiness, 58–59
Bowlby's theories, 12–13,
    22–23. see also
    Attachment theory
Brain development, 38–39, 50.
    see also Biological factors
Breakups, romantic, 182, 190–
    191. see also Romantic
    relationships
Brofenbrenner's framework,
    378
Bulimia symptoms, 223
Bullying, 163–164, 193. see also
    Aggression

Care moral orientation,
    242–245
Caregiver–child relationship/
    interactions, 348, 353–
    354
Caregivers, 348
Caregiving behavior, 56,
    105–106, 381–382. see
    also Maternal behavior;
    Parenting
Categorical self, 73–74. see also
    Self
Causal risk factor, 429t
Causal theory, 429t, 435–436
Causality, 132–133, 169–170,
    281
Chicago Study, 348
Child abuse. see Abuse; Child
    maltreatment
Child Abuse Potential
    Inventory, 420
Child Abuse Prevention and
    Treatment Act (CAPTA),
    404
Child Behavior Checklist,
    216

Child care
    caregiver–parent partnership
        and, 356
    ecological model and,
        348–350
    future directions in the study
        of, 362–363
    long-term effects of, 356–357
    overview, 347–349, 350–357
Child Care and Family Study,
    348
Child development
    aggression and, 210,
        215–216, 219, 221
    attachment theory and,
        111–115
    emotion regulation and, 62
    gender and, 295–307
    historical views of, 4–9
    overview, 3–4
    prosocial behavior and,
        269–280
    stages of romantic
        development and, 184–188
    temperament and, 45–47
    theoretical views, 9–24
Child maltreatment. see also
        Abuse; Neglect
    attachment and, 407
    history of, 403–406, 405t
    impact of on social
        development, 406–420,
        408t–410t, 413t–415t,
        417t–419t
    incidence rates of, 405t
    intergenerational continuity
        of, 416–420, 417t–419t
    overview, 403, 420–421
    peer relationships and,
        401–411, 408t–410t
    romantic relationships and,
        411–415, 413t–415t
Child-effects method, 131
Child-rearing practices,
    4–5, 129–134. see also
    Parenting
Chores, 384–385
Class, social. see Social class
Classroom environment, 21,
    215–216
Cliques, 166–167. see also Peer
    relationships
Co-construction, 155
Coercive cycles, 137, 140–141,
    210
Cognitive factors
    gender and, 296, 300–301,
        305–306
    identity development and,
        87–88
Cognitive functioning, 335

Cognitive regulation, 59
Cognitive revolution, 9
Cognitive social learning theory,
    6, 14–15
Cognitive-developmental
        theory, 8
    gender and, 292–293
    moral development and, 237,
        240
    overview, 15–18
Collective socialization model,
    330
Collectivist cultures, 280. see
    also Cultural diversity
Communication styles, 296–
    297, 301, 303, 307
Communities That Care (CTC)
    system, 448–449
Community factors, 329–331,
    372–374, 389. see also
    Culture
Compensatory factors, 429t
Competence hypothesis, 115
Competence promotion, 429t,
    436–437
Competition model, 330
Concerted cultivation, 332–333
Concrete operations stage of
    development, 17
Conduct disorder, 156
Conduct Problems Prevention
    Research Group, 224
Conflict, 190–191, 407
Construct validity, 242
Constructivist perspective, 9,
    17–18, 242
Contagion/epidemic model,
    330
Contextual factors, 86–87,
    146–147
Control
    middle childhood and, 138
    parenting and, 137
    prosocial behavior and, 270
Control domain of socialization,
    270, 272–273, 275, 277.
    see also Socialization
Conversation, 163, 166, 375
Cooperation, 163
Coparenting, 144. see also
    Parenting
Corporal punishment. see
    Physical punishment
Cortisol, 35–38
Corumination, 307
Cost, Quality, and Outcomes
    Study, 348
Criminal behavior. see also
    Aggression; Delinquency
Cultural diversity
    discipline and, 143–145
    family structures and, 129

parenting and, 131
    prosocial behavior and, 280
Cultural knowledge, 382–383
Cultural learning environment.
    see also Learning
    ecological and resource
        influences on, 380–381
    overview, 377–378
    play and, 385–386
Cultural models, 391–392. see
    also Culture
Cultural niche, 332–334,
    334–335
Cultural socialization, 333–334.
    see also Socialization
Cultural-comparative database
    and theory, 392–393
Cultural–historical theory, 19
Culture. see also Community
        factors; Cultural diversity
    adolescence and, 389–391
    cultural models and,
        391–392
    heterogeneity and, 391
    importance of, 372–374
    infancy and, 378–383
    middle childhood and,
        383–389
    overview, 376–377, 392–393
    research methods and,
        374–376
Cumulative risk, 429t, 430

Darwinian theory, 5–6, 21–22
Data, 304
Dating activities. see also
        Romantic relationships
    child maltreatment and,
        411–415, 413t–415t
    overview, 181
    stages of romantic
        development and, 184–188
Decision making, 253
Defining Issues Test (DIT), 241
Delinquency. see also
        Aggression
    adolescence and, 221
    parenting and, 137
    peer relationships and, 156
    romantic relationships and,
        195–196
Depression
    aggression and, 212–213,
        219
    corumination and, 307
    discrimination and, 335
    gender and, 303–304, 307
    romantic relationships and,
        194–195
    sexual harassment and, 307
Depressive symptoms, 156,
    169

Developmental factors
 prevention and intervention
  and, 435
 resilience and, 432–434
 self-esteem and, 81–82, 83
Developmental intergroup
 theory, 294
Developmental niche, 377–378,
 378–383
Developmental tasks, 429t
Developmental theory, 429t,
 436f
Developmental-contextual
 theory, 183–188
Differential treatment,
 297–298, 301–302
Discipline. see also Parenting
 aggression and, 213–214
 effectiveness of, 139–143
 future directions in the study
  of, 146–147
 moral development and, 249
 overview, 127–129, 134–145,
  135f, 147
 politics of, 145–146
Discrimination, 328–329, 335
Disequilibrium, 240
Dismissing attachment style,
 111. see also Attachment
 style
Disorganized attachment, 37,
 407
Dispositions, 334–335
Dissemination, 430t, 440–441
Distal outcomes, 435
Divorce. see also Family factors
 family structures and, 128
 romantic relationships and,
  192
 stages of romantic
  development and, 188
DNA information, 9, 269
Domain theory, 245–247,
 269–280
DRD4 receptor, 273
Drive Reduction theory, 103
Duality of self, 74–75
Dual-process theories, 250,
 254–255
Dynamic systems theory, 23–24

Early childhood. see also
 Preschool age children
 aggression and, 208–213
 attachment and, 109–110
 child maltreatment and, 407
 culture and, 383–389
 discipline and, 136–137
 gender and, 295–299
 moral development and,
  245–246, 248–249

peer relationships and,
 154–155, 157–162
prosocial behavior and,
 271–274
self-concept development
 and, 77
self-esteem and, 83
Early Childhood Longitudinal
 Study—Kindergarten
 cohort, 348
Eating disorder symptoms,
 223
Ecocultural theories, 377–378
Ecological model of
 development
 child care and school context
  and, 362–363
 culture and, 380–381
 overview, 348–350
Ecological systems theory, 24
Education level, 323, 326
Effectiveness, 430t, 440
Efficacy, 430t, 439–440
Egalitarianism, 334. see also
 Socialization
Ego, 11
Electroencephalogram (EEG),
 50
Emotion regulation, 44–45,
 51–59, 60–62
Emotion Regulation Checklist
 (ERC), 54
Emotional development,
 155–156
Emotional maltreatment,
 404, 405t. see also Child
 maltreatment
Emotion-Based Prevention
 Program (EBP), 62
Emotions, 247–249, 387–388
Empathy
 gender and, 300
 middle childhood and, 138
 moral development and,
  248–249
 prosocial behavior and, 272
Employment status, 323–324
Environmental factors. see also
 Classroom environment;
 Family factors; Media;
 Parenting; Peer
 relationships; Socialization
 gender and, 296–299,
  301–303, 306–307
 prosocial behavior and,
  269–270
 risk, resilience and prevention
  and, 430–431
Equality
 gender and, 290, 296–297
 peer relationships and,
  155–156

race, ethnicity, and SES and,
 328–329
social class and, 320–321
socioeconomic status (SES)
 and, 320
Erikson's theory, 12, 84
Ethnic Identity Development
 Model, 336
Ethnicity. see also Race
 compared to race, 318–319
 culture and, 376
 effect of on social
  development, 325–337
 family structures and, 129
 future directions in the study
  of, 338
 identity and, 84, 89, 335–337
 overview, 316–325
 parenting research and,
  133–134
 romantic relationships and,
  183
Ethnography, 375
Ethnopsychology, 380–381
Ethological theories, 20–23
Ethology, 21
Event-related potential (ERP)
 studies, 30
Evidence-based programs, 430t,
 440, 441–447, 448–449
Evolutionary analysis, 22
Evolutionary theories, 20–23,
 266–267
Exchange stage of moral
 development, 238. see also
 Moral development
Existential self, 73–74. see also
 Self
Expectations stage of moral
 development, 238. see also
 Moral development
Expertise, moral development
 and, 253
Extended Objective Measure of
 Ego Identity Status, 84–85
Externalizing problems
 aggression and, 216,
  222–223
 child care and, 354–355
 child maltreatment and, 411
 peer relationships and, 156

Face processing, 34–35, 39
Family factors. see also
 Minority families;
 Parenting
 aggression and, 213, 217,
  220–221
 culture and, 390–391
 discipline and, 143–145
 future directions in the study
  of, 146–147

Family factors (*continued*)
    identity development and, 86
    intergenerational continuity
        of maltreatment and,
        416–420, 417*t*–419*t*
    neighborhood characteristics
        and, 330–331
    overview, 127–129, 147
    race, ethnicity, and SES and,
        331–334
    risk, resilience and prevention
        and, 427–428, 432
    school system and, 361–
        362
Family structures. *see also*
        Minority families
    culture and, 389
    discipline and, 143–145
    overview, 128–129
    romantic relationships and,
        192
    stages of romantic
        development and, 188
Family values, 390–391
FAST Track interventions 224,
    437–439
Fathers, 281, 297. *see also*
    Parents
Fearfulness, 38, 249
Fidelity, 430*t*, 440
Fighting, 221. *see also*
    Aggression
5-HIAA, 31–33
5-HTTLPR genotypes, 32–33
Formal operations stage of
    development, 17
Fourth National Incidence
    Study of Child Abuse and
    Neglect, 405–406, 405*t*
Freudian theory, 7, 103. *see also*
    Psychoanalytic theory
Friendships. *see also*
    Peer relationships;
    Relationships
    adolescence and, 165–
        170
    aggression and, 218
    child maltreatment and,
        407–411, 408*t*–410*t*
    early childhood and,
        160–161
    middle childhood and,
        164–165
    romantic relationships and,
        191–194, 197
    school system and, 360–
        361
    social competence and, 44
Functional magnetic resonance
    image (fMRI), 9, 91,
    252

Gender
    adolescence and, 303–307
    aggression and, 209, 211,
        220, 222–223, 225, 387
    child care and, 355–356
    child maltreatment and, 406,
        413*t*–415*t*
    culture and, 386, 387
    discipline and, 143–144
    future directions in the study
        of, 307–308
    identity and, 84, 90
    infancy and early childhood
        and, 295–299
    middle childhood and,
        299–303
    moral development and,
        242–245
    overview, 289–294
    peer relationships and,
        159–160, 166–167, 170
    prosocial behavior and, 276
    romantic relationships and,
        182–183, 187, 197
    self-esteem and, 81
    socially distributed care and,
        384–385
    theoretical views, 291–292
Gender bias, 245, 302
Gender roles, 290. *see also*
    Gender
Gender schema theory, 293
Gendered moral obligations,
    242–245
Generosity, 163
Genetic factors
    aggression and, 210, 213, 217
    attachment and, 118–119,
        120–121
    prosocial behavior and,
        267–269, 273
    self-esteem and, 81
    serotonin and, 32
Genotyping, 9
Geography, 376
Global Initiative to End All
    Corporal Punishment of
    Children, 146
Globalization, 393. *see also*
    Culture
Goal-corrected partnership, 106
Goal-oriented behavior,
    130–131
Good Behavior Game, 224
Goodness of fit, 46, 249
Gossip. *see also* Social
    aggression
    gender and, 307
    peer relationships and, 163,
        221
    sexual harassment and, 305
Group membership, 294

Group participation domain
    of socialization, 270,
    274, 275, 278. *see also*
    Socialization
Guided learning domain of
    socialization, 270, 273,
    278. *see also* Socialization

Health, 319–320
Health promotion, 429*t*,
    436–437
Heart rate measures, 49–50
Helpfulness, 163
Hereditary factors, 81. *see also*
    Genetic factors
Heterogeneity, 391
Heteronomy stage of moral
    development, 238. *see also*
    Moral development
Heuristic intuition models,
    252–253
History, culture and, 376
Hostile attribution bias,
    213–214
Hostility, 193
Human Relations Area Files
    (HRAF), 375–376
Humanistic rationalism, 5

Id, 11
Identity
    overview, 73–74, 84–90, 85*f*
    race, ethnicity, and SES and,
        334–337
Identity, integrated, 256–257
Identity achievement, 84–86,
    85*f*, 88, 89–90
Identity crisis, 84
Identity diffusion
    ethnicity and, 89–90
    future directions in the study
        of, 91–92
    overview, 84–86, 85*f*, 88–89
Identity foreclosure
    ethnicity and, 89–90
    overview, 84–86, 85*f*, 88
Identity moratorium, 84–86,
    85*f*, 88, 89–90
Imprinting process, 21
Impulsivity, 58–59, 295
Income, 322–323, 326
Indicated prevention, 430*t*,
    437–439, 438*f*, 439*f*. *see
    also* Prevention
Indirect forms of aggression,
    163, 209. *see also*
    Aggression; Social
    aggression
Individual differences
    attachment theory and, 105,
        106–111
    gender and, 291

peer relationships and, 160–162
personality development and, 10–11
risk, resilience and prevention and, 431–432
romantic relationships and, 187–188
school system and, 361–362
temperament and, 47
Individual processes, 334–337
Individualist cultures, 280. *see also* Cultural diversity
Infancy
attachment and, 105–106, 106–109
child maltreatment and, 407
culture and, 378–383
discipline and, 134–136, 135*f*
emotion regulation and, 54–56
gender and, 295–299
moral development and, 248–249
peer relationships and, 158
prevention and intervention and, 441–443
prosocial behavior and, 271–274
self-recognition and, 75–76
self-understanding and, 74
Information-processing approach, 293
Inhibition, 38, 387–388
Insecure attachment. *see also* Attachment style
child maltreatment and, 407
cortisol and, 37
overview, 117–118
romantic relationships and, 192, 195
self-esteem and, 81
Institutional racism, 329. *see also* Racism
Instrumental aggression, 208. *see also* Aggression
Integrated identity, 256–257
Intergenerational continuity, 416–420, 417*t*–419*t*
Internal working models
attachment and, 105, 120–121
overview, 12
self-esteem and, 81
Internalizing problems, 156, 219, 223
Intervention. *see also* Prevention
aggression and, 223–224
child maltreatment and, 421

emotion regulation and, 62
evaluating intervention programs, 439–440
examples of, 441–447
risk, resilience and prevention and, 429*t*–430*t*
spectrum of, 437–439, 438*f*, 439*f*
theory and, 435–436, 436*f*
Intimacy
aggression and, 218
child maltreatment and, 409*t*
gender and, 304
romantic relationships and, 189–190
Intuition, 250–254
IQ, 431
"I-self," 73–74. *see also* Self

Justice moral orientation, 242–245

Kohlberg's theories, 17, 237, 238–239

Laboratory Temperament Assessment Battery (LAB-TAB), 48–49, 54
Language development
aggression and, 212
culture and, 376, 382–383
emotion regulation and, 52
gender and, 295, 302
Language socialization, 382–383. *see also* Language development; Socialization
Late childhood. *see also* Adolescence; Middle childhood
aggression and, 219–223
attachment and, 109–110
culture and, 389–391
discipline and, 137–139
emotion regulation and, 53
gender and, 303–307
peer relationships and, 162–165, 165–170
prevention and intervention and, 446–447
prosocial behavior and, 275–278
self-concept development and, 77–78
self-esteem and, 82, 83
Law of effect, 142
Learning, 273, 376–378
Life cycle, 153–154
Limit setting, 139–140
Logic model, 429*t*, 436*f*

Loneliness
aggression and, 223
culture and, 387–388
peer relationships and, 156, 168–169

Macro processes, 327–329
Magnetic resonance imaging (MRI), 91. *see also* Neuroimaging technologies
Maltreatment, child. *see* Child maltreatment
Marcia's theory, 84–86, 85*f*
Marital conflict, 213, 217
Marxist theories, 320
Maternal behavior. *see also* Parenting
attachment theory and, 103–104
cortisol and, 36–37
emotion regulation and, 56
oxytocin and, 33–34
prosocial behavior and, 271–272
self-esteem and, 81–82
serotonin and, 32–33
stress and, 37–38
Media
aggression and, 214–215, 218–219
gender and, 299, 302, 306
Mediator, 429*t*
Medication, 224
Mental health, 319–320
Mentoring programs, 443–445
"Me-self," 73–74. *see also* Self
Methodology, 51
Middle childhood
aggression and, 213–219
attachment and, 109–110
culture and, 383–389
discipline and, 137–139
gender and, 299–303
peer relationships and, 162–165
prevention and intervention and, 443–445
prosocial behavior and, 274–275
self-concept development and, 77–78
self-esteem and, 82, 83
Minnesota Longitudinal Study of Parents and Children, 115
Minnesota Study of Risk and Adaptation, 12–13

Minority families, 325–337. *see also* Ethnicity; Family factors; Family structures; Race; Socioeconomic status (SES)
Mirror-directed social behavior, 75
Mobility, 327–328
Moderators, 435
Modifiable risk factor, 429*t*
Modified Strange Situation Procedure (MSSP), 109
Molecular genetics, 8–9, 118–119, 269. *see also* Genetic factors
Momentary-process approach, 131
Monitoring, 140
Mood, 31
Moral development
  domains, 245–247
  emotions and, 247–249
  future directions in the study of, 257–258
  interplay of science and morality and, 235–237
  intuition and, 250–254
  orientations, 242–245
  overview, 235, 237, 247
  personality and, 254–257
  schemas and, 241–242
  stages of, 238–240
Moral Judgment Interview (MJI), 239
Moral reasoning, 237, 257–258
Moral schemas, 241–242
Morality, 218, 235–237
Mothers, 297, 352–353. *see also* Parents
Motivational factors
  gender and, 296, 300–301, 305–306
  peer relationships and, 360
Multidimensional Model of Racial Identity (MMRI), 336–337
Multidimensional Treatment Foster Care (MTFC), 224
Multilevel selection theory, 266–267
Mutual reciprocity, 270, 281

National Center on Child Abuse and Neglect (NCCAN), 404, 405
National Education Longitudinal Study, 348
National Longitudinal Study of Adolescent Health, 416
National Longitudinal Survey of Youth in Canada, 216

National Youth Survey (NYS), 221
Natural selection, 266
Neglect, 38–39, 404, 405*t*. *see also* Child maltreatment
Neighborhood factors, 329–331
Neo-analytic developmental theories, 24
Neo-Kohlbergian approach, 241–242
Neuroimaging technologies, 9, 31, 91
Neurotransmitters, 30–38
NICHD Early Child Care Research Network (NICHD ECCRN)
  long-term effects of child care, 356–357
  overview, 348–349
  parent–child relationship and, 351–353
  relationships and, 354–355
NICHD Study of Early Child Care
  aggression and, 211–212, 216
  attachment theory and, 114
  bullying and, 163
  overview, 348
  parent–child relationship and, 351–353
  relationships and, 354–355
Nigrescence Model, 336–337
Normativity hypothesis, 112–113, 145
Nurse–Family Partnership (NFP) program, 441–443

Oakland Growth Study, 7–8
Occupational factors, 323–324
Office of Child Abuse and Neglect (OCAN), 405. *see also* National Center on Child Abuse and Neglect (NCCAN)
Ontogeny, 128
Operant conditioning, 6
Oppositional defiant disorder (ODD), 216
Oppression, 328–329
Oregon Social Learning Center (OSLC), 15
Other-oriented emotions, 248–249
Oxytocin, 33–35

Parent management training, 224
Parental monitoring, 140
Parental social cognition, 131

Parent–child relationship. *see also* Relationships
  adolescence and, 139
  biological factors in, 29–38
  child care and, 351–353
  moral development and, 244, 249
  psychoanalytic theory and, 11–12
Parent–infant attachments, 13
Parent–infant interactions, 21, 103–104
Parenting. *see also* Child-rearing practices; Discipline; Family factors
  aggression and, 210, 212, 213–214, 217, 220–221, 224
  attachment development and, 105–106
  child care and, 351–353
  child maltreatment and, 404
  cultural diversity and, 129
  culture and, 373, 378–380, 389
  emotion regulation and, 56
  future directions in the study of, 146–147
  gender and, 296–298, 301–302, 306
  historical views of child development and, 4–5
  intergenerational continuity of maltreatment and, 416–420, 417*t*–419*t*
  moral development and, 244
  overview, 127–129, 129–134, 147
  oxytocin and, 35
  parenting traits, 131
  prosocial behavior and, 271–272, 273, 276, 281
  race, ethnicity, and SES and, 331–334
  romantic relationships and, 183, 191–194
  self-esteem and, 81–82
  study of, 131–132
  styles of, 130, 146–147
Parents
  aggression and, 213, 217
  culture and, 377–378
  identity development and, 86
  parent–teacher relationships and, 359–360
  prosocial behavior and, 281
  romantic relationships and, 191–194
Parent–teacher relationships, 359–360
Passion, 188–189
PATHS curriculum, 224

Peer acceptance
  child maltreatment and,
    408t–410t, 410–411
  school system and, 360, 361
Peer groups, 161, 216. *see also*
    Peer relationships
Peer norms, 302–303
Peer play behavior, 21
Peer rejection
  adjustment and, 156
  aggression and, 212–213,
    215–216, 219
  child maltreatment and,
    408t, 411
  gender and, 300
  social competence and, 44
Peer relationships. *see also*
    Friendships; Relationships;
    Romantic relationships
  adjustment and, 155–156
  adolescence and, 165–170,
    275–276
  aggression and, 212–213,
    214, 215–216, 218, 219,
    222–223
  child care and, 354–355
  child maltreatment and,
    407–411, 408t–410t
  culture and, 387
  early childhood and,
    157–162
  future directions in the study
    of, 171
  gender and, 298–299, 300,
    302–303, 304–305,
    306–307
  identity development and, 86
  moral development and,
    244
  overview, 153–154, 171
  parenting and, 137, 138–139
  prosocial behavior and,
    275–276
  reasons to study, 154–157
  romantic relationships and,
    191–194
  school system and, 360–
    362
  school-age period, 162–165
  social aggression and,
    222–223
  social competence and, 44
  stages of romantic
    development and, 188
Peer status, 161–162. *see also*
    Peer relationships
Permissive parenting style,
    131–132
Personal pronoun use, 75–76
Personal–impersonal dimension,
    251–252

Personality
  culture and, 387–388
  historical views of child
    development and, 7–8
  identity development and,
    87–88
  moral development and,
    254–257
  psychoanalytic theory and,
    10–11
Person/Process/Context/Time
    model, 378
Phenomenological Variant of
    Ecological Systems Theory
    (PVEST), 336, 337, 338
Physical abuse. *see also* Child
    maltreatment
  aggression and, 213–214
  brain development and,
    38–39
  incidence rates of, 405t
  overview, 404
  serotonin and, 32
  spanking as, 145
Physical aggression. *see also*
    Aggression
  adolescence and, 219–221
  early childhood and,
    209–212
  future directions in the study
    of, 225
  gender and, 209, 300
  middle childhood and,
    213–216
  overview, 208
Physical punishment. *see also*
    Discipline; Parenting
  adolescence and, 140–141
  early childhood and,
    136–137
  effectiveness of, 142, 143
  middle childhood and, 138
  overview, 133–134, 135f
  politics of, 145–146
Piaget's theories, 8, 15–18,
    239
Play
  culture and, 385–386
  early childhood and,
    157–162
  gender and, 294, 295, 297,
    300, 301–302, 386
  overview, 21
  peer relationships and,
    157–162
Political factors, 145–146,
    376
Popularity, 222–223, 360
Positron emission tomography
    (PET) scans, 31. *see
    also* Neuroimaging
    technologies

Posttraumatic stress disorder
    (PTSD) symptoms, 415,
    421
Poverty. *see also* Social class;
    Socioeconomic status (SES)
  child care and, 355–356
  intergenerational continuity
    of maltreatment and, 420
  school system and, 349–350
  socioeconomic status (SES)
    and, 322–323
Practices, 130, 377–378
Pregnancy, 36
Preoccupied attachment style,
    111. *see also* Attachment
    style
Preoperational stage of
    development, 16–17
Preparation for bias, 334. *see
    also* Socialization
Preschool age children. *see also*
    Early childhood
  aggression and, 209–213
  attachment and, 109–110
  discipline and, 136–137
  emotion regulation and,
    52–53, 56
  moral development and,
    245–246
  peer relationships and,
    154–155, 157–162
  self-concept development
    and, 77
  self-esteem and, 82
Prevention. *see also* Intervention
  aggression and, 223–224
  child maltreatment and, 421
  developmental processes and,
    434
  examples of, 441–447
  future directions in the study
    of, 447–450
  origins of prevention science,
    434–435
  overview, 427–428, 450
  risk and resilience and,
    429t–430t, 434–447, 436f,
    438f, 439f
Principal component analyses
    (PCAs), 108–109
Prior rights and social
    contract stage of moral
    development, 238–239. *see
    also* Moral development
Program theory, 429t
Promoting Alternative
    THinking Strategies
    (PATHS) program,
    443–445
Promotion of mistrust, 334. *see
    also* Socialization
Promotive factors, 429t

Prosocial behavior. *see also*
Behavioral factors
adolescence and, 275–278
challenges in studying,
263–266
child maltreatment and,
408*t*, 411
cultural differences in,
280
development of, 270–280
evolution of, 266–267
future directions in the study
of, 281
gender and, 300
genetic underpinnings of,
267–269
infancy and early childhood
and, 271–274
middle childhood and,
274–275
moral development and,
248–249
overview, 263, 265–266,
280–281
peer relationships and, 360
socialization and, 269–270
volunteerism, 278–280
Protection domain of
socialization, 270,
271–272, 274, 276. *see
also* Socialization
Protective processes, 433. *see
also* Resilience
Proximal outcomes, 435
Psychoanalytic theory, 7, 10–
13
Psychobiological assessments,
49–51. *see also* Assessment
Psychological control, 141
Psychological functioning and
adjustment, 57–59. *see
also* Adjustment
Psychological maltreatment,
404, 405*t*. *see also* Child
maltreatment
Psychosexual stages, 11
Psychosocial competence,
429*t*
Psychosocial theory, 84
Puberty
culture and, 389–391
gender and, 304
stages of romantic
development and,
185–186, 188
Punishment, 133–134, 154,
213–214. *see also*
Discipline; Parenting;
Physical punishment

Quantitative behavior genetics,
267–269. *see also* Genetic
factors

Race. *see also* Ethnicity
affect of on social
development, 325–337
compared to ethnicity, 318–319
family structures and, 129
future directions in the study
of, 338
identity and, 84, 335–337
overview, 316–325
parenting research and,
133–134
romantic relationships and,
183
Racism, 328–329
Randomized controlled trial
(RCT), 430*t*, 439–440
Reactive aggression, 208, 213–
214. *see also* Aggression
Reactivity, 46–47, 53
Reasoning, 137–138, 253, 383
Reciprocity domain of
socialization, 270, 272,
274, 276–277. *see also*
Socialization
Reconciliation model, 256–257
Regulatory processes, 53. *see
also* Emotion regulation;
Self-regulation
Reinforcement, 277
Rejecting/neglecting parenting
style, 132
Relational aggression, 163. *see
also* Aggression; Social
aggression
Relationships. *see also*
Attachment relationships;
Caregiver–child
relationship/interactions;
Parent–child relationship;
Peer relationships;
Romantic relationships;
Social competence;
Social relationships;
Teacher–child relationship/
interactions
child care and, 354–355
overview, 348
risk, resilience and prevention
and, 432
school system and, 361–362
Relative deprivation model, 330
Religion, 145, 390
Resilience
correlates of, 431–432
developmental processes and,
432–434
future directions in the study
of, 447–450
overview, 427–431,
429*t*–430*t*, 450
prevention and intervention
and, 434–447, 436*t*, 438*f*,
439*f*

Resources, 380–381, 429*t*
Responsibility, 383–384
Responsiveness, 130
Rewards, 154, 273, 321
Risk
developmental processes and,
434
future directions in the study
of, 447–450
overview, 220–221, 427–431,
429*t*–430*t*, 450
prevention and intervention and,
434–447, 436*t*, 438*f*, 439*f*
Risk reduction, 429*t*, 436–437
Role modeling, 296–297, 301
Role-dependent selves, 79
Romantic relationships.
see also Adolescence;
Peer relationships;
Relationships
aggression and, 305
characteristics of, 188–190
child maltreatment and,
411–415, 413*t*–415*t*
conflict and, 190–191
future directions in the study
of, 196–197
gender and, 304, 305
overview, 180–183
parents and friends and,
191–194
prevalence of, 181–183
stages of romantic
development and, 184–188
theoretical views, 183–184
well-being and, 194–196

Same-sex romantic attractions,
183. *see also* Romantic
relationships
Schemas
gender and, 293, 295, 296, 301
moral development and,
241–242
School context, 362–363
School factors, 87
School functioning and
adjustment; *see also*
Adjustment
aggression and, 220–221
discrimination and, 335
emotion regulation and, 57–59
overview, 357–362
peer relationships and, 156,
360–361
socioeconomic status (SES)
and, 323
teacher–child relationships
and, 358–359
School system
discipline and, 145
ecological model and,
348–350

future directions in the study of, 362–363
overview, 347–349, 357–362
parent–teacher relationships and, 359–360
School Transition Environment Program (STEP), 446–447
School-age children, 383–389. see Early childhood; Late childhood; Middle childhood
Science, 235–237
Secure attachments. see also Attachment style
adult attachment and, 110–111
child care and, 353–354
culture and, 381–382
moral development and, 249
overview, 117–118
self-esteem and, 81
Secure–autonomous attachment style, 110–111. see also Attachment style
Segregation, 329. see also Neighborhood factors
Selective prevention, 429t, 437–439, 438f, 439f. see also Prevention
Self
duality of, 74–75
future directions in the study of, 91–92
gender and, 294
overview, 73–74
peer relationships and, 155–156
self-concept development and, 76–79
self-esteem, 79–83
self-recognition and, 75–76
social cognitive theory and, 294
Self as object, 73–74. see also Self
Self as subject, 73–74. see also Self
Self-blame, 409t
Self-concept
development of, 76–79
gender and, 295, 299–300, 303–304
peer relationships and, 155–156
race, ethnicity, and SES and, 334–337
Self-consciousness, 248
Self-control, 295, 300
Self-description, 76–79. see also Self-concept
Self-disclosure, 307
Self-efficacy, 294

Self-esteem
discrimination and, 335
future directions in the study of, 91
gender and, 303–304
overview, 73–74, 79–83
parenting and, 140
peer relationships and, 156, 168–170
romantic relationships and, 194
sexual harassment and, 307
Self-organization, 23
Self-presentation, 303
Self-recognition, 75–76
Self-regulation, 46–47, 57–59, 60–62
Self-talk, 20
Self-understanding, 73–74. see also Self
Sensorimotor stage of development, 16
Separation, 32, 104
Separation Anxiety Test (SAT), 110
Serotonin, 31–33
Sexual abuse. see also Child maltreatment
incidence rates of, 405t
intergenerational continuity of maltreatment and, 417t–419t
overview, 404
romantic relationships and, 412, 413t–415t
Sexual behavior, 192, 194–195
Sexual harassment, 304–305, 306–307
Sexual minority youths, 183. see also Romantic relationships
Shame, child maltreatment and, 409t
Shyness, culture and, 387–388
Sibling caretaking, 384–385
Single parenthood. see also Family factors
discipline and, 143–145
overview, 128–129
romantic relationships and, 192
stages of romantic development and, 188
Skinner's theories, 14, 237. see also Behavioral theory
Social aggression. see also Aggression; Indirect forms of aggression; Relational aggression
adolescence and, 221–223
early childhood and, 212–213
future directions in the study of, 225

gender and, 209
middle childhood and, 216–219
overview, 208
peer relationships and, 163, 221
Social Aggression Prevention Program (SAPP), 224
Social behavior, 265–266. see also Behavioral factors; Prosocial behavior
Social bonds, 34–35
Social class, 316–325, 406
Social cognitive theory, 293–294
Social comparisons, 82
Social competence. see also Relationships
emotion regulation and, 51–59
future directions in the study of, 60–62
overview, 44
temperament and, 45–51
Social construction, 318
Social disorganization theory, 330
Social functioning and adjustment, 57–59. see also Adjustment
Social groups, 84. see also Ethnicity; Gender; Race
Social information-processing theory, 24, 218
Social intelligence, 383
Social interactions, 295
Social intuitionist model, 250–251
Social knowledge, 246–247
Social learning, 131, 154–155
Social networks, 161, 360–362. see also Peer relationships
Social obligation, 384
Social reinforcement, 277
Social relatedness, 360
Social relationships, 35–36, 38–39. see also Relationships
Social role theory, 292
Social skills, 167–168
Social stratification, 320–321, 329–330, 332. see also Social class
Social systems and conscience stage of moral development, 238. see also Moral development
Social trust, 381–382
Social withdrawal, 362, 411
Social-address approach, 131
Socialization
aggression and, 211

Socialization (*continued*)
  culture and, 382–383
  family factors and, 333–334
  gender and, 296
  moral development and, 249
  neighborhood characteristics
    and, 329–331
  parenting and, 130–131
  prosocial behavior and,
    264–265, 269–280
  race, ethnicity, and SES and,
    327
Socially distributed care,
    384–385
Sociocultural perspective, 9,
    18–20
Socioeconomic status (SES)
  affect of on social
    development, 325–337
  child care and, 355–356
  child maltreatment and, 406
  culture and, 379
  future directions in the study
    of, 338
  identity and, 335–337
  intergenerational continuity
    of maltreatment and, 420
  measurements of, 321–325
  overview, 316–325
  risk, resilience and prevention
    and, 430, 432
  school system and, 349–350
Socioemotional selectivity
    theory, 24
Sociohistorical context, 87
Spanking. *see also* Discipline;
    Parenting
  effectiveness of, 142, 143
  overview, 135*f*
  parenting research and,
    133–134
  politics of, 145–146
Sports, 276–277
Stability and lawful change
    hypotheses, 114
Stage theory, 184–188, 238–
    240
Stereotypes
  gender and, 297, 298–299, 301
  peer relationships and,
    298–299
  race, ethnicity, and SES and,
    328–329
Strange Situation
  adult attachment and,
    110–111
  overview, 107–108, 109–110,
    119
Strengthening Family Program
    for 10–14-year-olds (SFP
    10–14) program, 445–446

Stress, 37–38
Stress hormone. *see* Cortisol
Structural equation modeling,
    131, 418*t*
Structural-developmental
    model, 239
Structure, 130
Subjective assessments, 325. *see
    also* Assessment
Substance abuse, 156
Superego, 11
Sustainability, 430*t*, 441
Symbolic interactionism,
    155–156
Systems theory, 23–24

Teacher–child relationship/
    interactions, 348,
    357–359, 359–360
Teachers, 348, 359–360,
    361–362
Teen Outreach Program (TOP),
    446–447
Television
  aggression and, 214–215,
    218–219
  gender and, 299, 302,
    306
Temperament
  aggression and, 210, 213
  attachment and, 117–118
  child care and, 350, 355–
    356
  culture and, 378–383,
    387–388
  development of, 47–48
  emotion regulation and,
    54–57
  future directions in the study
    of, 60–62
  historical views of child
    development and, 7–8
  measurements of, 48–49
  moral development and,
    249
  overview, 45–51
  prosocial behavior and,
    271
  social competence and,
    44–45
Temperament theory, 45–
    47
Theoretical eclecticism, 9–
    10
Theory
  child development and, 9–
    24
  gender and, 291–292
  historical views of child
    development and, 7–8
  overview, 24–25

socioeconomic status (SES)
    and, 320–321
  temperament and, 51
Theory of mind, 137
Toddlers, 134–136, 135*f*, 158.
    see also Early childhood;
    Infancy; Preschool age
    children
Transitions, 192
Transmission gap, 119–120
Trust, 381–382

Universal ethical principles
    stage of moral
    development, 239. *see also*
    Moral development
Universal prevention, 429*t*,
    437–439, 438*f*, 439*f*. *see
    also* Prevention
Universality, 105–106, 112
Universality hypothesis, 112
Unresolved attachment style,
    111. *see also* Attachment
    style

Values, family, 390–391
Verbal aggression, 163, 300. *see
    also* Aggression
Victimization, 163–164
Violence. *see also* Aggression
  adolescence and, 221
  child maltreatment and,
    411–415, 413*t*–415*t*
  dating violence, 411–415,
    413*t*–415*t*
  in the media, 214–215
  race, ethnicity, and SES and,
    335
Volunteerism, 278–280
Vygotsky's theories, 18–20

Warmth, 130
Watson's theories, 13, 127–
    128. *see also* Behavioral
    theory
Wealth, 324–325
Well-being
  parenting and,
    333
  race, ethnicity, and SES and,
    335
  romantic relationships and,
    194–196
  socioeconomic status (SES)
    and, 319–320
Work ethic, 327–328
Working models, 12, 81
Worldviews, 335–337

Zone of proximal development,
    19, 270